# MEDICAL RADIOLOGY

## Diagnostic Imaging

Editors:
A. L. Baert, Leuven
M. Knauth, Göttingen
K. Sartor, Heidelberg

M. F. Reiser · C. R. Becker · K. Nikolaou
G. Glazer (Eds.)

# Multislice CT

## 3rd Revised Edition

With Contributions by

H. Alkadhi · G. Antoch · A. Ba-Ssalamah · A. Baur-Melnyk · C. R. Becker · C. Behrmann
T. A. Bley · D. Böckler · J. Boese · G. Brix · T. Brunner · A. Dirisamer · A. Dörfler
B. Ertl-Wagner · D. Fleischmann · T. Flohr · G. Glazer · A. Graser · J. Griebel
M. Hacker · P. Hallscheidt · C. Hassan · B. Heigl · C. J. Herold · C. P. Heußel
C. Hoeschen · M. H. K. Hoffmann · R.-T. Hoffmann · M. Hoheisel · F. Iafrate · L. Jäger
T. F. Jakobs · T. R. C. Johnson · W. A. Kalender · H.-U. Kauczor
K. Klingenbeck-Regn · C. Kölblinger · M. Körner · S. Kösling · A. Laghi · G. Lauritsch
A. Lembcke · J. Ley-Zaporozhan · U. Linsenmaier · J. Lutz · M. Macari · D. Maintz
O. Meissner · D. Morhard · U. G. Mueller-Lisse · C. Mueller-Mang · M. Nagel
E. A. Nekolla · K. Neumann · K. Nikolaou · M. Owsijewitsch · M. Pfister · C. Plank
G. Pöpperl · D. Regulla · M. F. Reiser · G. Richter · H. Ringl · P. Rogalla
E.-P. Rührnschopf · U. Saueressig · W. Schima · H. Schlattl · B. Scholz · B. Schreiber
H. Seifarth · B. Sommer · W. H. Sommer · M. Spahn · P. Stolzmann · N. Strobel
H. von Tengg-Kobligk · D. Theisen · C. G. Trumm · S. Ulzheimer · T. F. Weber
J.-E. Wildberger · M. Wintermark · B. J. Wintersperger · M. Zankl · C. J. Zech
M. Zellerhoff

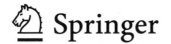 Springer

MAXIMILIAN F. REISER, MD, Professor
CHRISTOPH R. BECKER, MD
KONSTANTIN NIKOLAOU, MD
Institute of Clinical Radiology
Ludwig-Maximilians University
Munich University Hospital
Marchioninistrasse 15
81377 Munich
Germany

GARY GLAZER, MD, Professor
Department of Radiology
Stanford University, School of Medicine
Room P-263
1201 Welch Road
Palo Alto, CA 94304
USA

MEDICAL RADIOLOGY · Diagnostic Imaging and Radiation Oncology
Series Editors:
A.L. Baert · L.W. Brady · H.-P. Heilmann · M. Knauth · M. Molls · C. Nieder · K. Sartor

Continuation of Handbuch der medizinischen Radiologie
Encyclopedia of Medical Radiology

ISBN   978-3-540-33124-7          e-ISBN 978-3-540-33125-4

DOI 10.1007/978-3-540-33125-4

Library of Congress Control Number: 2008926739

© 2009 Springer-Verlag Berlin Heidelberg

*Cover design*: Verlagsservice Teichmann, Mauer, Germany
*Production, reproduction and typesetting*: le-tex publishing services oHG, Leipzig, Germany

Printed on acid-free paper

9 8 7 6 5 4 3 2 1

springer.com

# Foreword

It is a great pleasure to introduce this third, completely revised and updated edition of the successful volume on multislice CT, which was first published in 2002.

It is amazing to observe the continuing rapid technological development in multislice CT and its new clinical applications. This volume again offers a comprehensive overview of all recent new experimental and clinical research in this field, but it also includes new chapters on dynamic volume CT with 320 detector rows and on flat detector CT. Numerous new and excellent illustrations help to push this book into an even higher scientific orbit.

I am again deeply indebted to the editors, M.F. Reiser, C.R. Becker, K. Nikolaou, and G. Glazer, for their high level of dedication and efforts to edit this 3rd volume in such a short time period in order to include all the latest advances in multislice CT. I also congratulate the editors and the contributing authors, all internationally well-known CT experts, on the in-depth coverage of the individual chapters.

This volume is a must for certified radiologists to update their knowledge and a source of basic information on CT for radiologists in training. Referring medical and surgical specialists will find it very useful for the daily clinical management of their patients.

Leuven

ALBERT L. BAERT
Series Editor

# Preface

Multi-detector row technology has become an established CT imaging modality worldwide. Nowadays, clinical applications such as multi-detector row CT angiography, and in particular cardiac CT, assume greater importance in daily routine. Furthermore, the scope of multi-detector row CT applications has expanded and requires different investigation strategies.

To exploit the full potential of multi-detector row CT, a fundamental knowledge of the technique and optimal investigation strategies in terms of patient preparation, contrast medium administration, and image interpretation is mandatory. The new generation of CT scanners, in particular dual-source CT, provides new opportunities and challenges by expanding the clinical applications.

The 5th International Symposium on Multi-Detector Row CT has brought together a variety of CT specialists with individual areas of expertise. This conference had a mission to educate the participants in multi-detector row CT skills rather than simply presenting the recent developments in technology and research. With about 1,000 attendees, this conference was a tremendous success and gained wide attention all over the world.

This volume has not been designed primarily as a reference book on multi-detector row CT. The idea of this book was rather to provide fundamental knowledge combined with an update on the latest CT scanner technology in challenging clinical areas. The book therefore supports the mission of the conference perfectly, with its profound discussion of different applications and investigation strategies.

We are grateful to Prof. Albert Baert for stimulating us to edit again this volume of the "Medical Radiology" series. The publisher, Springer-Verlag, enthusiastically supported the idea and provided us with invaluable assistance. We hope this book will be valuable to all those interested in multi-detector row CT.

| | |
|---|---|
| Munich | Maximilian F. Reiser |
| Munich | Christoph R. Becker |
| Munich | Konstantin Nikolaou |
| Stanford | Gary Glazer |

# Contents

## Neuro / Ear-Nose-Throat

## Cardiovascular Imaging

## Lung

## Oncology

## Intervention

## Trauma Imaging / Acute Care

# Technique

# Multislice CT: Current Technology and Future Developments

Stefan Ulzheimer and Thomas Flohr

## CONTENTS

S. Ulzheimer, PhD
Siemens Medical Solutions U.S.A., Inc., Computed Tomography
Division, 51 Valley Stream Parkway, Malvern, PA, 19355, USA

T. Flohr, PhD
Siemens AG, Healthcare Sector, Business Unit Computed
Tomography, Siemensstr. 1, 91301 Forchheim, Germany

### ABSTRACT

Since its introduction in the early 1970s, computed tomography (CT) has undergone tremendous improvements in terms of technology, performance and clinical applications. Based on the historic evolution of CT and basic CT physics, this chapter describes the status quo of the technology and tries to anticipate future developments. Besides the description of key components of CT systems, a special focus is placed on breakthrough developments, such as multi-slice CT and dedicated scan modes for cardiac imaging.

## 1.1 Introduction

In 1972, the English engineer G.N. Hounsfield built the first commercial medical X-ray computed tomography (CT) scanner for the company EMI Ltd. as a pure head scanner with a conventional X-ray tube and a dual-row detector system moving incrementally around the patient. It was able to acquire 12 slices, each with a 13-mm slice thickness, and reconstruct the images with a matrix of 80×80 pixels (Fig. 1.1a) in approximately 35 min. Even though the performance of CT scanners increased dramatically over time until 1989, there were no principally new developments in conventional CT. By then, the acquisition time for one image decreased from 300 s in 1972 to 1–2 s, thin slices of down to 1 mm became possible, and the in-plane resolution increased from three line pairs per cm (lp/cm) to 10–15 lp/cm with typically 512×512 matrices.

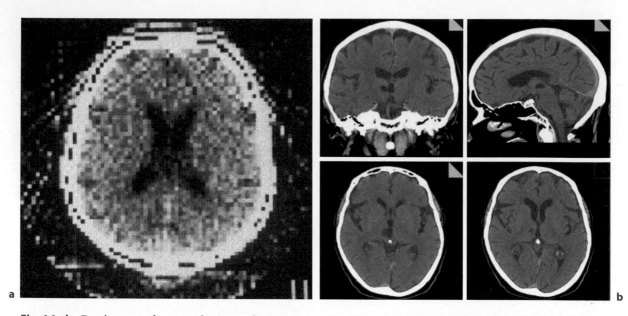

**Fig. 1.1a,b.** Development of computed tomography over time. **a** Cross-sectional image of a brain in the year 1971 and (**b**) the whole brain with sagittal, coronal and cross-sectional slices in the year 2007. (Image courtesy of Mayo Clinic Rochester)

As it was foreseen in the late 1970s that acquisition times of mechanical CT scanners would be far too long for high quality cardiac imaging for the next years or even decades to come, a completely new technical concept for a CT scanner without moving parts for extremely fast data acquisition of 50 ms was suggested and promoted as a cardiovascular CT (CVCT) scanner. Later, these scanners were also called "ultrafast CT" scanners or "electron beam CT" (EBT or EBCT) scanners. High cost and limited image quality combined with low volume coverage prevented the wide propagation of the modality, and the production and distribution of these scanners were discontinued.

Based on the introduction of slip ring technology to get power to and data off the rotating gantry, continuous rotation of the X-ray tube and the detector became possible. The ability of continuous rotation led to the development of spiral CT scanners in the early 1990s (Crawford and King 1990; Kalender et al. 1990), a method proposed already several years before (Mori 1986; Nishimura and Miyazaki 1988). Volume data could be acquired without the danger of mis- or double-registration of anatomical details. Images could be reconstructed at any position along the patient axis (longitudinal axis, z-axis), and overlapping image reconstruction could be used to improve longitudinal resolution. Volume data became the very basis for applications such as CT angiography (CTA) (Rubin et al. 1995), which has revolutionized non-invasive assessment of vascular disease. The ability to acquire vol-

ume data was the prerequisite for the development of three-dimensional image processing techniques such as multi-planar reformations (MPR), maximum intensity projections (MIP), surface shaded displays (SSD) or volume-rendering techniques (VRT), which have become a vital component of medical imaging today.

Main drawbacks of single-slice spiral CT are either insufficient volume coverage within one breath-hold time of the patient or missing spatial resolution in the z-axis due to wide collimation. With single-slice spiral CT, the ideal isotropic resolution, i.e., of equal resolution in all three spatial axes, can only be achieved for very limited scan ranges (Kalender 1995).

Larger volume coverage in shorter scan times and improved longitudinal resolution became feasible after the broad introduction of four-slice CT systems by all major CT manufacturers in 1998 (Klingenbeck-Regn et al. 1999; McCollough and Zink 1999; Hu et al. 2000). The increased performance allowed for the optimization of a variety of clinical protocols. Examination times for standard protocols could be significantly reduced; alternatively, scan ranges could be significantly extended. Furthermore, a given anatomic volume could be scanned within a given scan time with substantially reduced slice width. This way, for many clinical applications the goal of isotropic resolution was within reach with four-slice CT systems. Multi-detector row CT (MDCT) also dramatically expanded into areas previously considered beyond the scope of third-generation CT scanners based on the mechanical rotation of the

X-ray tube and detector, such as cardiac imaging with the addition of the ECG gating capability enabled by gantry rotation times down to 0.5 s (KACHELRIESS et al. 2000; OHNESORGE et al. 2000). Despite all these promising advances, clinical challenges and limitations remained for four-slice CT systems. True isotropic resolution for routine applications had not yet been achieved for many applications requiring extended scan ranges, since wider collimated slices (4×2.5 mm or 4×3.75 mm) had to be chosen to complete the scan within a reasonable timeframe. For ECG-gated coronary CTA, stents or severely calcified arteries constituted a diagnostic dilemma, mainly due to partial volume artifacts as a consequence of insufficient longitudinal resolution (NIEMAN et al. 2001), and reliable imaging of patients with higher heart rates was not possible due to limited temporal resolution.

As a next step, the introduction of an eight-slice CT system in 2000 enabled shorter scan times, but did not yet provide improved longitudinal resolution (thinnest collimation 8×1.25 mm). The latter was achieved with the introduction of 16-slice CT (FLOHR et al. 2002a, 2002b), which made it possible to routinely acquire substantial anatomic volumes with isotropic sub-millimeter spatial resolution. ECG-gated cardiac scanning was enhanced by both improved temporal resolution achieved by gantry rotation time down to 0.375 s and improved spatial resolution (NIEMAN et al. 2002; ROPERS et al. 2003).

The generation of 64-slice CT systems introduced in 2004 is currently the established standard in the high-end segment of the market. Two different scanner concepts were introduced by the different vendors: the "volume concept" was pursued by GE, while Philips and Toshiba aimed at a further increase in volume coverage speed by using 64 detector rows instead of 16 without changing the physical parameters of the scanner compared to the respective 16-slice version. The "resolution concept" pursued by Siemens uses 32 physical detector rows in combination with double $z$-sampling, a refined $z$-sampling technique enabled by a periodic motion of the focal spot in the $z$-direction, to simultaneously acquire 64 overlapping slices with the goal of pitch-independent increase of longitudinal resolution and reduction of spiral artifacts (FLOHR et al. 2004, 2005a). With this scanner generation, CT angiographic examinations with sub-millimeter resolution in the pure arterial phase become feasible even for extended anatomical ranges. The improved temporal resolution due to gantry rotation times down to 0.33 s has the potential to increase clinical robustness of ECG-gated scanning at higher heart rates, thereby significantly reducing the number of patients requiring heart rate

control and facilitating the successful integration of CT coronary angiography into routine clinical algorithms (LESCHKA et al. 2005; RAFF et al. 2005). Today, high-end single-source scanners offer rotation times of down to 0.30 s and can acquire up to 128 slices with an isotropic resolution of down to 0.3 mm (Siemens SOMATOM Definition AS+). In late 2007, two manufacturers, Philips and Toshiba, introduced single-source scanners that can acquire 256 and 320 slices during one rotation, respectively, keeping "Moore's law of multi-slice CT (MSCT)" intact. When looking at the number of slices of multi-slice CT systems versus the year of their market introduction, the number of slices has increased exponentially as a function of time, roughly doubling every 2 years. This is an interesting parallel to Moore's law in the microelectronics sector. It remains to be seen how the recent enhancements in the number of slices translate into clinical benefits of these systems as only clinical performance will be able to justify the additional costs of such large detectors.

Pursuing a different path of technological advancement, in 2005, the first dual-source CT (DSCT) system, i.e., a CT system with two X-ray tubes and two corresponding detectors offset by 90°, was introduced by one vendor (FLOHR et al. 2006). The key benefit of DSCT for cardiac scanning is the improved temporal resolution. A scanner of this type provides temporal resolution of a quarter of the gantry rotation time, independent of the patient's heart rate and without the need for multisegment reconstruction techniques. DSCT scanners also show promising properties for general radiology applications. First, both X-ray tubes can be operated simultaneously in a standard spiral or sequential acquisition mode, in this way providing high power reserves when necessary. Additionally, both X-ray tubes can be operated at different kV settings and/or different pre-filtrations, in this way allowing dual-energy acquisitions. Potential applications of dual-energy CT include tissue characterization, calcium quantification and quantification of the local blood volume in contrast-enhanced scans.

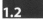

## 1.2
## System Design

The overall performance of a MDCT system depends on several key components. These components include the gantry, X-ray source, a high-powered generator, detector and detector electronics, data transmission systems (slip rings) and the computer system for image reconstruction and manipulation.

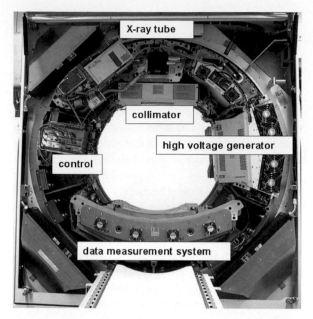

**Fig. 1.2.** Basic system components of a modern third-generation CT system. First-generation systems used a collimated pencil beam and therefore required a translation of the pencil beam and the single detector element before each rotational step to scan the whole object. Second-generation scanner used a small fan beam, but still required translational and rotational patterns of the X-ray source and the small detector array, whereas the fan beam of third-generation scanners the first time covered the whole object and allowed for a pure rotational motion of the tube and the detector around the patient

### 1.2.1
### Gantry

Third-generation CT scanners employ the so-called "rotate/rotate" geometry, in which both the X-ray tube and detector are mounted onto a rotating gantry and rotate around the patient (Fig. 1.2). In a MDCT system, the detector comprises several rows of 700 and more detector elements that cover a scan field of view (SFOV) of usually 50 cm. The X-ray attenuation of the object is measured by the individual detector elements. All measurement values acquired at the same angular position of the measurement system form a "projection" or "view." Typically, 1,000 projections are measured during each 360° rotation. The key requirement for the mechanical design of the gantry is the stability of both focal spot and detector position during rotation, in particular with regard to the rapidly increasing rotational speeds of modern CT systems (from 0.75 s in 1994 to 0.30 s in 2007). Hence, the mechanical support for the X-ray tube, tube collimator and data measurement sys-

tem (DMS) has to be designed so as to withstand the high gravitational forces associated with fast gantry rotation (~17 g for 0.42 s rotation time, ~33 g for 0.33-s rotation time).

### 1.2.2
### X-Ray Tube and Generator

State-of-the-art X-ray tube/generator combinations provide a peak power of 60–100 kW, usually at various, user-selectable voltages, e.g., 80 kV, 100 kV, 120 kV and 140 kV. Different clinical applications require different X-ray spectra and hence different kV settings for optimum image quality and/or the best possible signal-to-noise ratio at the lowest dose. In a conventional tube design, an anode plate of typically 160–220-mm diameter rotates in a vacuum housing (Fig. 1.3). The heat storage capacity of anode plate and tube housing–measured in Mega Heat Units (MHU)–determines the performance level: the bigger the anode plate is, the larger the heat storage capacity, and the more scan-seconds can be delivered until the anode plate reaches its temperature limit. A state-of-the-art X-ray tube has a heat storage capacity of typically 5 to 9 MHU, realized by thick graphite layers attached to the backside of the anode plate. An alternative design is the rotating envelope tube (STRATON, Siemens, Forchheim, Germany, SCHARDT et al. 2004). The anode plate constitutes an outer wall of the rotating tube housing; it is therefore in direct contact with the cooling oil and can be efficiently cooled via thermal conduction (Fig. 1.3). This way, a very high heat dissipation rate of 5 MHU/min is achieved, eliminating the need for heat storage in the anode, which consequently has a heat storage capacity close to zero. Thanks to the fast anode cooling, rotating envelope tubes can perform high power scans in rapid succession. Due to the central rotating cathode, permanent electro-magnetic deflection of the electron beam is needed to position and shape the focal spot on the anode. The electro-magnetic deflection is also used for the double $z$-sampling technology of a 64-slice CT system (FLOHR et al. 2004, 2005a).

### 1.2.3
### MDCT Detector Design and Slice Collimation

Modern CT systems use solid state detectors in general. Each detector element consists of a radiation-sensitive solid-state material (such as cadmium tungstate, gadolinium-oxide or gadolinium oxi-sulfide with suitable dopings), which converts the absorbed X-rays into vis-

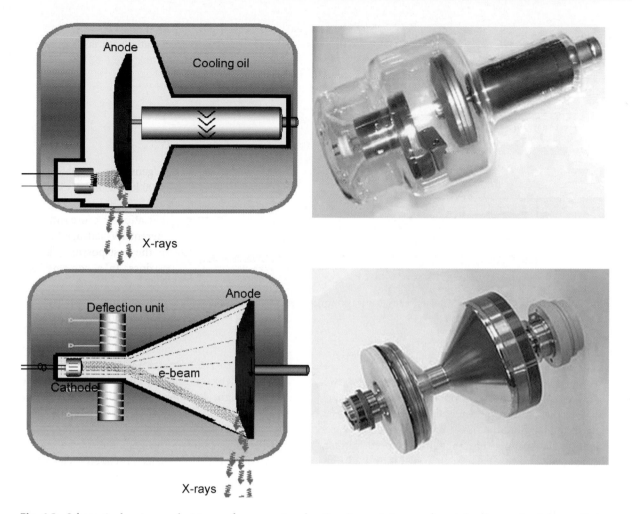

**Fig. 1.3.** Schematic drawings and pictures of a conventional X-ray tube (*top*) and a rotating envelope tube (*bottom*). The electrons emitted by the cathode are represented by *green lines*; the X-rays generated in the anode are depicted as *purple arrows*. In a conventional X-ray tube, the anode plate rotates in a vacuum housing. Heat is mainly dissipated via thermal radia-tion. In a rotating envelope tube, the anode plate constitutes an outer wall of the tube housing and is in direct contact with the cooling oil. Heat is more efficiently dissipated via thermal conduction, and the cooling rate is significantly increased. Rotating envelope tubes have no moving parts and no bearings in the vacuum. (Images not to scale)

ible light. The light is then detected by a Si photodiode. The resulting electrical current is amplified and converted into a digital signal. Key requirements for a suitable detector material are good detection efficiency, i.e., high atomic number, and very short afterglow time to enable the fast gantry rotation speeds that are essential for ECG-gated cardiac imaging.

CT detectors must provide different slice widths to adjust the optimum scan speed, longitudinal resolution and image noise for each application. With a single-slice CT detector, different collimated slice widths are obtained by pre-patient collimation of the X-ray beam. For a very elementary model of a two-slice CT detector consisting of $M=2$ detector rows, different slice widths can be obtained by pre-patient collimation if the detector is separated midway along the $z$-extent of the X-ray beam.

For $M>2$, this simple design principle must be replaced by more flexible concepts requiring more than $M$ detector rows to simultaneously acquire $M$ slices. Different manufacturers of MDCT scanners have introduced different detector designs. In order to be able to select different slice widths, all scanners combine several detector rows electronically to a smaller number of slices according to the selected beam collimation and the desired slice width.

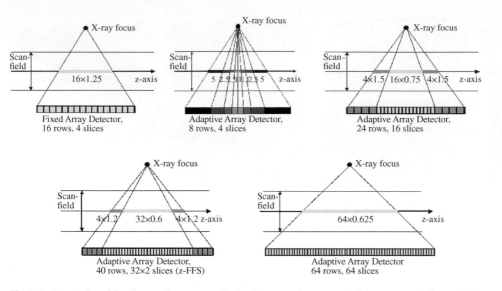

**Fig. 1.4.** Examples of fixed array detectors and adaptive array detectors used in commercially available MDCT systems

For the four-slice CT systems introduced in 1998, two detector types have been commonly used. The fixed array detector consists of detector elements with equal sizes in the longitudinal direction. A representative example for this scanner type, the GE Lightspeed scanner, has 16 detector rows, each of them defining 1.25-mm collimated slice width in the center of rotation (HU et al. 2000; McCOLLOUGH and ZINK 1999). The total coverage in the longitudinal direction is 20 mm at iso-center; due to geometrical magnification, the actual detector is about twice as wide. In order to select different slice widths, several detector rows can be electronically combined to a smaller number of slices. The following slice widths (measured at iso-center) are realized: 4×1.25 mm, 4×2.5 mm, 4×3.75 mm and 4×5 mm (see Fig. 1.4, top left). The same detector design is used for the eight-slice version of this system, providing 8×1.25 and 8×2.5 mm collimated slice width.

A different approach uses an adaptive array detector design, which comprises detector rows with different sizes in the longitudinal direction. Scanners of this type, the Philips MX8000 four-slice scanner and the Siemens SOMATOM Sensation 4 scanner, have eight detector rows (KLINGENBECK-REGN et al. 1999). Their widths in the longitudinal direction range from 1 to 5 mm (at iso-center) and allow for the following collimated slice widths: 2×0.5 mm, 4×1 mm, 4×2.5 mm, 4×5 mm, 2×8 mm and 2×10 mm (see Fig. 1.4, top center).

The 16-slice CT systems have adaptive array detectors in general. A representative example for this scanner type, the Siemens SOMATOM Sensation 16 scanner, uses 24 detector rows (FLOHR et al. 2002a); see Fig. 1.4, top right. By appropriate combination of the signals of the individual detector rows, either 16 slices with 0.75-mm or 1.5-mm collimated slice width can be acquired simultaneously. The GE Lightspeed 16 scanner uses a similar design, which provides 16 slices with either 0.625-mm or 1.25-mm collimated slice width. Yet another design, which is implemented in the Toshiba Aquilion scanner, allows the use of 16 slices with 0.5-mm, 1-mm or 2-mm collimated slice width, with a total coverage of 32 mm at iso-center.

The Siemens SOMATOM Sensation 64 scanner has an adaptive array detector with 40 detector rows (FLOHR et al. 2004). The 32 central rows define 0.6-mm collimated slice width at iso-center; the 4 outer rows on both sides define 1.2-mm collimated slice width (see Fig. 1.4, bottom left). The total coverage in the longitudinal direction is 28.8 mm. Using a periodic motion of the focal spot in the z-direction (z-flying focal spot), 64 overlapping 0.6-mm slices per rotation are acquired. Alternatively, 24 slices with 1.2-mm slice width can be obtained. Toshiba, Philips and GE use fixed array detectors for their 64-slice systems. The Toshiba Aquilion scanner has 64 detector rows with a collimated slice width of 0.5 mm. The total z-coverage at iso-center is 32 mm. Both the GE VCT scanner and the Philips Brilliance 64 have 64 detector rows with a collimated slice width of 0.625 mm, enabling the simultaneous read-out of 64 slices with a total coverage of 40 mm in the longitudinal direction (see Fig. 1.4, bottom right).

## 1.2.4
## Data Rates and Data Transmission

With increasing numbers of detector rows and decreasing gantry rotation times, the data transmission systems of MDCT scanners must be capable of handling significant data rates: a four-slice CT system with 0.5-s rotation time roughly generates $1,000 \times 700 \times 4 \times 2$ bytes = 5.6 MB of data per rotation, corresponding to 11.2 MB/s; a 16-slice CT scanner with the same rotation time generates 45 MB/s, and a 64-slice CT-system can produce up to 180–200 MB/s. This stream of data is a challenge for data transmission off the gantry and for real-time data processing in the subsequent image reconstruction systems. In modern CT systems, contactless transmission technology is generally used for data transfer, which is either laser transmission or electro-magnetic transmission with a coupling between a rotating transmission ring antenna and a stationary receiving antenna. In the image reconstruction, computer images are reconstructed at a rate of up to 40 images/s for a $512 \times 512$ matrix using special array processors.

## 1.2.5
## Dual-Source CT

A recently introduced dual-source CT (DSCT) system is equipped with two X-ray tubes and two corresponding detectors (FLOHR et al. 2006). The two acquisition systems are mounted onto the rotating gantry with an angular offset of 90°. Figure 1.5 illustrates the principle. Using the z-flying focal spot technique (FLOHR et al. 2004, 2005a), each detector acquires 64 overlapping 0.6-mm slices per rotation. The shortest gantry rotation time is 0.33 s. The key benefit of DSCT for cardiac scanning is improved temporal resolution. In a DSCT scanner, the half-scan sinogram in parallel geometry needed for ECG-controlled image reconstruction can be split up into two quarter-scan sinograms that are simultaneously acquired by the two acquisition systems in the same relative phase of the patient`s cardiac cycle and at the same anatomical level due to the 90° angle between both detectors. Details of cardiac reconstruction techniques can be found in Sect. 1.3.3 in this chapter.

With this approach, constant temporal resolution equivalent to a quarter of the gantry rotation time $t_{rot}/4$ is achieved in a centered region of the scan field of view. For $t_{rot} = 0.33$ s, the temporal resolution is $t_{rot}/4 = 83$ ms, independent of the patient's heart rate.

DSCT systems show interesting properties for general radiology applications, too. If both acquisition systems are simultaneously used in a standard spiral or sequential acquisition mode, up to 160 kW X-ray peak power is available. These power reserves are not only beneficial for the examination of morbidly obese patients, whose number is dramatically growing in western societies, but also to maintain adequate X-ray photon flux for standard protocols when high volume coverage speed is necessary. Additionally, both X-ray tubes can be operated at different kV and mA settings, allowing the acquisition of dual-energy data. While dual-energy CT was already evaluated 20 years ago (KALENDER et al. 1986; VETTER et al.1986), technical limitations of the CT scanners at those times prevented the development of routine clinical applications. On the DSCT system, dual-energy data can be acquired nearly simultaneously

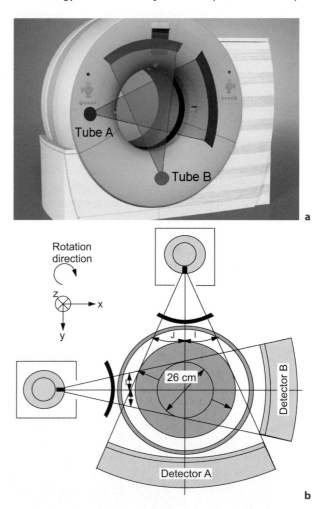

**Fig. 1.5a,b.** Schematic illustration of a dual-source CT (DSCT) system using two tubes and two corresponding detectors offset by 90°. A scanner of this type provides temporal resolution equivalent to a quarter of the gantry rotation time, independent of the patient`s heart rate. In a technical realization, one detector (**a**) covers the entire scan field of view with a diameter of 50 cm, while the other detector (**b**) is restricted to a smaller, central field of view

with sub-second scan times. The ability to overcome data registration problems should provide clinically relevant benefits. The use of dual-energy CT data can in principle add functional information to the morphological information based on X-ray attenuation coefficients that is usually obtained in a CT examination.

Figure 1.6 shows a clinical example to illustrate the clinical performance of DSCT for ECG-gated cardiac scanning.

## 1.3
### Measurement Techniques

The two basic modes of MDCT data acquisition are axial and spiral (helical) scanning.

### 1.3.1
### MDCT Sequential (Axial) Scanning

Using sequential (axial) scanning, the scan volume is covered by subsequent axial scans in a "step-and-shoot" technique. In between the individual axial scans, the table is moved to the next $z$-position. The number of images acquired during an axial scan corresponds to the number of active detector slices. By adding the detector signals of the active slices during image reconstruction, the number of images per scan can be further reduced, and the image slice width can be increased. A scan with 4×1-mm collimation as an example provides either four images with 1-mm section width, two images with 2-mm section width, or one image with 4-mm section

width. The option to realize a wider section by summation of several thin sections is beneficial for examinations that require narrow collimation to avoid partial volume artifacts and low image noise to detect low contrast details, such as examinations of the posterior fossa of the skull or the cervical spine.

With the advent of MDCT, axial "step-and-shoot" scanning has remained in use for only few clinical applications, such as head scanning, high-resolution lung scanning, perfusion CT and interventional applications. A detailed theoretical description to predict the performance of MDCT in step-and-shoot mode has been given (HSIEH 2001).

### 1.3.2
### MDCT Spiral (Helical) Scanning

Spiral/helical scanning is characterized by continuous gantry rotation and continuous data acquisition while the patient table is moving at constant speed; see Fig. 1.7.

### 1.3.2.1
### Pitch

An important parameter to characterize a spiral/helical scan is the pitch $p$. According to IEC specifications (INTERNATIONAL ELECTROTECHNICAL COMMISSION 2002), $p$ is given by:

$p$ = table feed per rotation/total width of the collimated beam

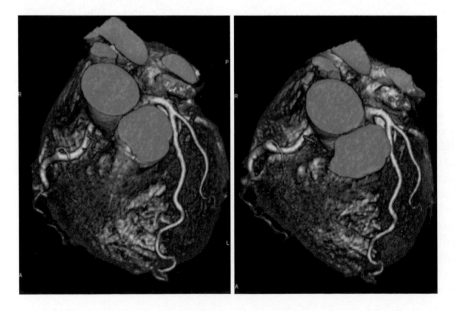

**Fig. 1.6.** Case study illustrating the clinical performance of dual-source CT (DSCT) for ECG-gated cardiac imaging. VRT renderings of a 59-year-old male patient with suspicion of RCA stenosis. The mean heart rate of the patient during the scan was 85 bpm. *Left*: Diastolic reconstruction at 65% of the cardiac cycle. *Right*: End systolic reconstruction at 28% of the cardiac cycle. In both cases the coronary arteries are clearly depicted with few or no motion artifacts

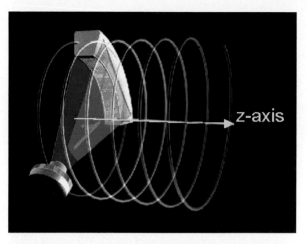

**Fig. 1.7.** Principle of spiral/helical CT scanning: the patient table is continuously translated while multiple rotations of scan data are acquired. The path of X-ray tube and detector relative to the patient is a helix. An interpolation of the acquired measurement data has to be performed in the $z$-direction to estimate a complete CT data set at the desired image position

This definition holds for single-slice CT as well as for MDCT. It shows whether data acquisition occurs with gaps ($p>1$) or with overlap ($p<1$) in the longitudinal direction. With $4\times1$-mm collimation and a table feed of 6 mm/rotation, the pitch is $p = 6/(4\times1) = 6/4 = 1.5$. With $16\times0.75$-mm collimation and a table feed of 18 mm/rotation, the pitch is $p=18/(16\times0.75)=18/12=1.5$, too. For general radiology applications, clinically useful pitch values range from 0.5 to 2. For the special case of ECG-gated cardiac scanning, very low pitch values of 0.2 to 0.4 are applied to ensure gapless volume coverage of the heart during each phase of the cardiac cycle.

### 1.3.2.2
### Collimated and Effective Slice Width

Both single-slice and multi-slice spiral CT require an interpolation of the acquired measurement data in the longitudinal direction to estimate a complete CT data set at the desired plane of reconstruction. As a consequence of this interpolation, the slice profile changes from the trapezoidal, in some cases almost rectangular shape known from axial scanning to a more bell-shaped curve; see Fig. 1.8. The $z$-axis resolution is no longer determined by the collimated beam width $S_{coll}$ alone (as in axial scanning), but by the effective slice width $s$, which is established in the spiral interpolation process. Usu-

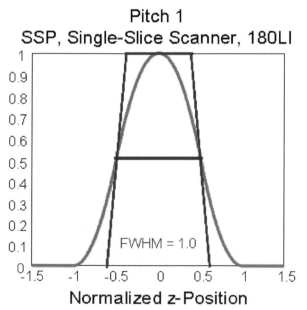

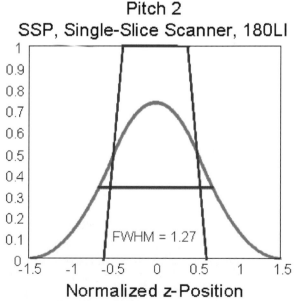

**Fig. 1.8.** Effective slice width in spiral/helical CT: the collimated slice profile, which is a trapezoidal in general, is indicated in *red*. The slice sensitivity profiles (*SSP*) after spiral/helical interpolation are bell-shaped; see the *green curves* for the most commonly used single-slice approach (180-LI) at different pitch values. 180-LI relies on a projection-wise linear interpolation of direct and complementary data. In spiral/helical CT, $z$-axis resolution is no longer determined by the collimated slice width alone, but by the effective slice width, which is defined as the Full Width at Half Maximum (*FWHM*) of the SSP

ally, $S$ is defined as the Full Width at Half Maximum (FWHM) of the Slice Sensitivity Profile (SSP). The wider $S_{coll}$ gets for a given collimated beam width $S_{coll}$, the more the longitudinal resolution degrades. In single-slice CT, $S$ increases with increasing pitch (Fig. 1.9). This is a consequence of the increasing longitudinal distance of the projections used for spiral interpolation. The SSP is not only characterized by its FWHM, but by its entire shape: a SSP that has far-reaching tails degrades longitudinal resolution more than a well-defined, close to rectangular SSP, even if both have the same FWHM and hence the same effective slice width $S$. For a further characterization of spiral SSPs, the Full Width at Tenth Area (FWTA) is often considered in addition.

### 1.3.2.3
### Multi-Slice
### Linear Interpolation and z-Filtering

Multi-slice linear interpolation is characterized by a projection-wise linear interpolation between two rays on either side of the image plane to establish a CT data set at the desired image $z$-position. The interpolation can be performed between the same detector slice at different projection angles (in different rotations) or different detector slices at the same projection angle. In general, scanners relying on this technique provide selected dis-

crete pitch values to the user, such as 0.75 and 1.5 for four-slice scanning (Hu 1999) or 0.5625, 0.9375, 1.375 and 1.75 for 16-slice scanning (Hsieh 2003). The user has to be aware of the pitch-dependent effective slice widths $S$. For low-pitch scanning (at $p = 0.75$ using 4 slices and at $p = 0.5625$ or 0.9375 using 16 slices) $S\sim S_{coll}$ and for a collimated 1.25-mm slice the resulting effective slice width stays at 1.25 mm. The narrow SSP, however, is achieved by conjugate interpolation at the price of increased image noise (Hu et al. 1999; Hsieh 2003). For high-pitch scanning (at $p = 1.5$ using 4 slices and at $p = 1.375$ or 1.75 using 16 slices), $S\sim 1.27S_{coll}$ and a collimated 1.25-mm slice results in an effective 1.5–1.6mm slice. To obtain the same image noise as in an axial scan with the same collimated slice width, 0.73–1.68 times the dose depending on the spiral pitch is required, with the lowest dose at the highest pitch (see Hsieh 2003). Thus, as a "take home point," when selecting the scan protocol for a particular application, scanning at low pitch optimizes image quality and longitudinal resolution at a given collimation, yet at the expense of increased patient dose. To reduce patient dose, either mA settings should be reduced at low pitch or high pitch values should be chosen.

In a $z$-filter multi-slice spiral reconstruction (Taguchi and Aradate 1998; Schaller et al. 2000), the spiral interpolation for each projection angle is no longer restricted to the two rays in closest proximity to the image

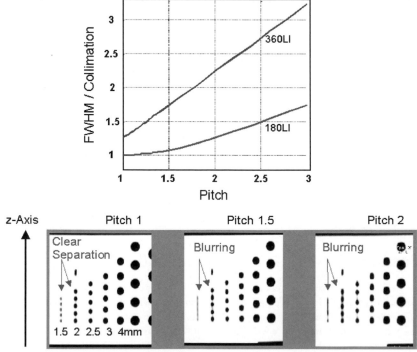

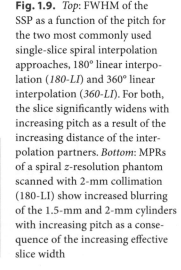

**Fig. 1.9.** *Top*: FWHM of the SSP as a function of the pitch for the two most commonly used single-slice spiral interpolation approaches, 180° linear interpolation (*180-LI*) and 360° linear interpolation (*360-LI*). For both, the slice significantly widens with increasing pitch as a result of the increasing distance of the interpolation partners. *Bottom*: MPRs of a spiral $z$-resolution phantom scanned with 2-mm collimation (180-LI) show increased blurring of the 1.5-mm and 2-mm cylinders with increasing pitch as a consequence of the increasing effective slice width

plane. Instead, all direct and complementary rays within a selectable distance from the image plane contribute to the image. A representative example for a z-filter approach is the Adaptive Axial Interpolation (SCHALLER et al. 2000) implemented in Siemens CT scanners. Another example is the MUSCOT algorithm (TAGUCHI and ARADATE 1998) used by Toshiba. The z-filtering allows the system to trade off z-axis resolution with image noise (which directly correlates with required dose). From the same CT raw data, images with different slice widths can be retrospectively reconstructed. Only slice widths equal to or larger than the sub-beam collimation can be obtained. With the Adaptive Axial Interpolation the effective slice width is kept constant for all pitch values between 0.5 and 1.5 (KLINGENBECK-REGN et al. 1999; SCHALLER et al. 2000; FUCHS et al. 2000). Therefore, longitudinal resolution is independent of the pitch; see Fig. 1.10. As a consequence of the pitch-independent spiral slice width, the image noise for fixed "effective" mAs (that is mAs divided by the pitch p) is nearly independent of the pitch. For 1.25-mm effective slice width reconstructed from 4×1-mm collimation, 0.61–0.69 times the dose is required to maintain the image noise of an axial scan at the same collimation (FUCHS et al. 2000). Radiation dose for fixed effective mAs is independent of the pitch and equals the dose of an axial scan at the same mAs. Thus, as a "take-home point," using higher pitch does not result in dose saving,

which is an important practical consideration with CT systems relying on Adaptive Axial Interpolation and the "effective" mAs concept.

With regard to image quality, narrow collimation is preferable to wide collimation, due to better suppression of partial volume artifacts and a more rectangular SSP, even if the pitch has to be increased for equivalent volume coverage. Similar to single-slice spiral CT, narrow collimation scanning is the key to reduce artifacts and improve image quality. Best suppression of spiral artifacts is achieved by using both narrow collimation relative to the desired slice width and reducing the spiral pitch.

### 1.3.2.4
### 3D Back-Projection and Adaptive Multiple Plane Reconstruction AMPR

For CT scanners with 16 and more slices, modified reconstruction approaches accounting for the cone-beam geometry of the measurement rays have to be considered: the measurement rays in MDCT are tilted by the so-called cone angle with respect to a plane perpendicular to the z-axis. The cone angle is largest for the slices at the outer edges of the detector, and it increases with increasing number of detector rows if their width is kept

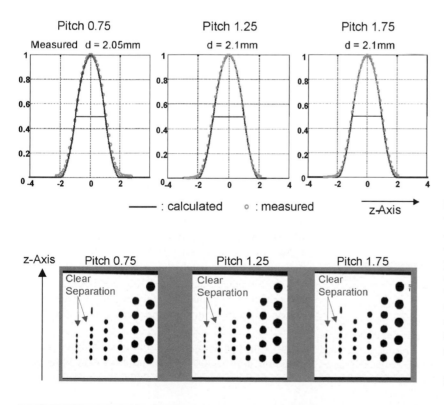

**Fig. 1.10.** Adaptive axial interpolation for a four-slice CT system: SSP of the 2-mm slice (for 4×1-mm collimation) at selected pitch values. The functional form of the SSP, and hence the effective slice width, are independent of the pitch. Consequently, MPRs of a spiral z-resolution phantom scanned with 2-mm slice width show clear separation of the 1.5-mm and 2-mm cylinders for all pitch values

constant. Some manufacturers (Toshiba, Philips) use a 3D filtered back-projection reconstruction (Feldkamp et al. 1984; Wang et al. 1993; Grass et al. 2000; Hein et al. 2003). With this approach, the measurement rays are back-projected into a 3D volume along the lines of measurement, this way accounting for their cone-beam geometry. Other manufacturers use algorithms that split the 3D reconstruction task into a series of conventional 2D reconstructions on tilted intermediate image planes. A representative example is the Adaptive Multiple Plane Reconstruction (AMPR) used by Siemens (Schaller et al. 2001a; Flohr et al. 2003a). Multi-slice spiral scanning using AMPR in combination with the "effective" mAs concept is characterized by the same key properties as Adaptive Axial Interpolation. Thus, all recommendations regarding selection of collimation and pitch that have been discussed there also apply to AMPR.

### 1.3.2.5
### Double z-Sampling

The double z-sampling concept for multi-slice spiral scanning makes use of a periodic motion of the focal spot in the longitudinal direction to improve data sampling along the z-axis (Flohr et al. 2004, 2005a). By continuous electromagnetic deflection of the electron beam in a rotating envelope X-ray tube, the focal spot

is wobbled between two different positions on the anode plate. The amplitude of the periodic z-motion is adjusted in a way that two subsequent readings are shifted by half a collimated slice width in the patient's longitudinal direction (Fig. 1.11). Therefore, the measurement rays of two subsequent readings with collimated slice width $S_{coll}$ interleave in the z-direction, and every two M-slice readings are combined to one 2M-slice projection with a sampling distance of $S_{coll}/2$.

In the SOMATOM Sensation 64 (Siemens, Forchheim, Germany) as an example of a MDCT system relying on double z-sampling, two subsequent 32-slice readings are combined to one 64-slice projection with a sampling distance of 0.3 mm at the iso-center. As a consequence, spatial resolution in the logitudinal direction is increased, and objects <0.4 mm in diameter can be routinely resolved at any pitch; see Fig. 1.12. Another benefit of double z-sampling is the suppression of spiral "windmill" artifacts at any pitch (Fig. 1.13).

### 1.3.3
### ECG-Triggered
### and ECG-Gated Cardio-Vascular CT

### 1.3.3.1
### Principles of ECG Triggering and ECG Gating

For ECG-synchronized examinations of the cardiothoracic anatomy, either ECG-triggered axial scanning or ECG-gated spiral scanning can be used. A technical overview on ECG-controlled CT scanning can be found in Flohr et al. (2003b).

In ECG-triggered axial scanning, the heart volume is covered by subsequent axial scans in a "step-and-shoot" technique. The number of images per scan corresponds to the number of active detector slices. In between the individual axial scans, the table moves to the next z-position. Due to the time necessary for table motion, only every second heart beat can be used for data acquisition, which limits the minimum slice width to 2.5 mm with four-slice or 1.25 mm with eight-slice CT systems if the whole heart volume has to be covered within one breath-hold period. Scan data are acquired with a predefined temporal offset relative to the R-waves of the patient's ECG signal, which can be either relative (given as a certain percentage of the RR-interval time) or absolute (given in ms) and either forward or reverse (Ohnesorge et al. 2000; Flohr and Ohnesorge 2001); see Fig. 1.14.

To improve temporal resolution, modified reconstruction approaches for partial scan data have been proposed (Ohnesorge et al. 2000; Flohr and Ohne-

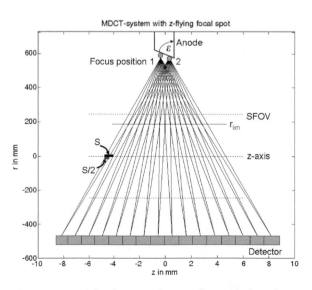

**Fig. 1.11.** Principle of improved z-sampling with the z-flying focal spot technique. Due to a periodic motion of the focal spot in the z-direction, two subsequent M-slice readings are shifted by half a collimated slice width $S_{coll}/2$ at iso-center and can be interleaved to one 2M slice projection

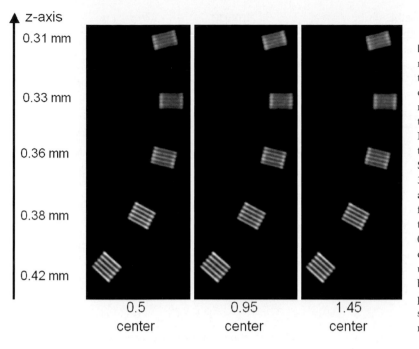

**Fig. 1.12.** Demonstration of z-axis resolution for a MDCT system using the z-flying focal spot technique. MPRs of a z-resolution phantom (high-resolution insert of the CATPHAN, the Phantom Laboratories, Salem, NY, turned by 90°) in the isocenter of the scanner as a function of the pitch. Scan data have been acquired with 32×0.6-mm collimation in a 64-slice acquisition mode using the z-flying focal spot and reconstructed with the narrowest slice width (nominal 0.6 mm) and a sharp body kernel. Independent of the pitch, all bar patterns up to 16 lp/cm can be visualized. The bar patterns with 15 lp/cm are exactly perpendicular to the z-axis, corresponding to 0.33-mm longitudinal resolution

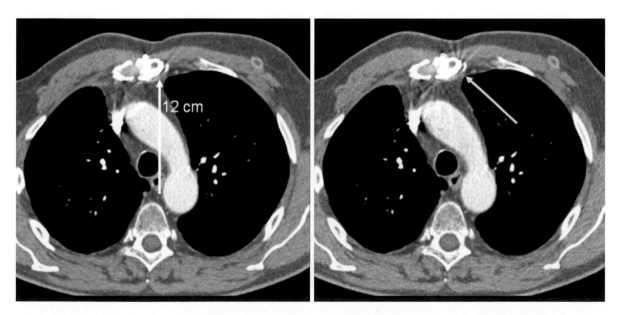

**Fig. 1.13.** Reduction of spiral artifacts with the z-flying focal spot technique. *Left*: Thorax scan with 32×0.6-mm collimation in a 64-slice acquisition mode with z-flying focal spot at pitch 1.5. *Right*: Same scan, using only one focus position of the z-flying focal spot for image reconstruction. This corresponds rea- sonably well to evaluating 32-slice spiral data acquired without z-flying focal spot. Due to the improved longitudinal sampling with z-flying focal spot (*left*), spiral interpolation artifacts (windmill structures at high contrast objects) are suppressed without degradation of z-axis resolution

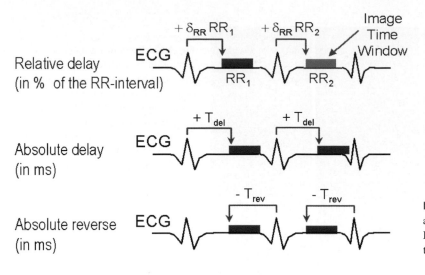

**Fig. 1.14.** Schematic illustration of absolute and relative phase setting for ECG-controlled CT examinations of the cardio-thoracic anatomy

sorge 2001), which provide a temporal resolution up to half the gantry rotation time per image in a sufficiently centered region of interest. The 16-slice and 64-slice CT systems offer gantry rotation times as short as 0.4 s, 0.37 s or even 0.33 s. In this case, temporal resolution can be as good as 200 ms, 185 ms or 165 ms.

With retrospective ECG gating, the heart volume is covered continuously by a spiral scan. The patient's ECG signal is recorded simultaneously to data acqui-

sition to allow for a retrospective selection of the data segments used for image reconstruction. Only scan data acquired in a pre-defined cardiac phase, usually the diastolic phase, are used for image reconstruction (Kachelriess et al. 2000; Ohnesorge et al. 2000; Taguchi et al. 2000; Flohr and Ohnesorge 2001). The data segments contributing to an image start with a user-defined offset relative to the onset of the R-waves, similar to ECG-triggered axial scanning; see Fig. 1.15.

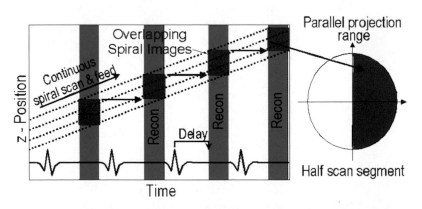

**Fig. 1.15.** Principle of retrospectively ECG-gated spiral scanning with single-segment reconstruction. The patient's ECG signal is indicated as a function of time on the *horizontal axis*, and the position of the detector slices relative to the patient is shown on the *vertical axis* (in this example for a four-slice CT system). The table moves continuously, and continuous spiral scan data of the heart volume are acquired. Only scan data acquired in a pre-defined cardiac phase, usually the diastolic phase, are used for image reconstruction (indicated as *red boxes*). The spiral interpolation is illustrated for some representative projection angles

Image reconstruction generally consists of two parts: multi-detector row spiral interpolation to compensate for the continuous table movement and to obtain scan data at the desired image $z$-position, followed by a partial scan reconstruction of the axial data segments (Fig. 1.15).

### 1.3.3.2
### ECG-Gated Single-Segment and Multi-Segment Reconstruction

In a single-segment reconstruction, consecutive multi-slice spiral data from the same heart period are used to generate the single-slice partial scan data segment for an image; see Fig. 1.15. At low heart rates, a single-segment reconstruction yields the best compromise between sufficient temporal resolution on the one hand and adequate volume coverage with thin slices on the other.

The temporal resolution of an image can be improved up to $t_{rot}/(2N)$ by using scan data of $N$ subsequent heart cycles for image formation in a so-called multi-segment reconstruction (KACHELRIESS et al. 2000; TAGUCHI et al. 2000; CESMELI et al. 2001; FLOHR and OHNESORGE 2001). $t_{rot}$ is the gantry rotation time of the CT scanner. With increased $N$ better temporal resolution is achieved, but at the expense of slower volume coverage: every $z$-position of the heart has to be seen by a detector slice at every time during the $N$ heart cycles. As a consequence, the larger the $N$ and the lower the patient's heart rate are, the more the spiral pitch has to be reduced. With this technique, the patient's heart rate and the gantry rotation time of the scanner have to be properly de-synchronized to allow for improved temporal resolution. Depending on the relationship between the rotation time and the patient heart rate, the temporal resolution is generally not constant, but varies between one half and $1/(2N)$ times the gantry rotation time in a $N$-segment reconstruction. There are "sweet spots," heart rates with optimum temporal resolution and heart rates where temporal resolution cannot be improved beyond half the gantry rotation time. Multi-segment approaches rely on a complete periodicity of the heart motion, and they encounter their limitations for patients with arrhythmia or patients with changing heart rates during examination. They may improve image quality in selected cases, but the reliability of obtaining good quality images with $N$-segment reconstruction goes down with increasing $N$. In general, clinical practice suggests the use of one segment at lower heart rates and $N \geq 2$ segments at higher heart rates (FLOHR and OHNESORGE 2001; FLOHR et al. 2003b). Image reconstruction during different heart phases is feasible by shifting the start points of the data segments used for image reconstruction relative to the R-waves. For a given start position, a stack of images at different $z$-positions covering a small sub-volume of the heart can be reconstructed due to the multi-slice data acquisition (OHNESORGE et al. 2000; FLOHR and OHNESORGE 2001).

Prospective ECG-triggering combined with "step and shoot" acquisition of axial slices has the benefit of smaller patient dose than ECG-gated spiral scanning, since scan data are acquired in the previously selected heart phases only. It does, however, not provide continuous volume coverage with overlapping slices, and mis-registration of anatomical details cannot be avoided. Furthermore, reconstruction of images in different phases of the cardiac cycle for functional evaluation is not possible. Since ECG-triggered axial scanning depends on a reliable prediction of the patient's next RR interval by using the mean of the preceding RR intervals, the method encounters its limitations for patients with severe arrhythmia. To maintain the benefits of ECG-gated spiral CT, but reduce patient dose, ECG-controlled dose modulation has been developed (JAKOBS et al. 2002). During the spiral scan, the output of the X-ray tube is modulated according to the patient's ECG. It is kept at its nominal value during a user-defined phase of the cardiac cycle, in general the mid- to end-diastolic phase. During the rest of the cardiac cycle, the tube output is typically reduced to 20% of its nominal values, although not switched off entirely to allow for image reconstruction throughout the entire cardiac cycle. Depending on the heart rate, dose reduction of 30–50% has been demonstrated in clinical studies (JAKOBS et al. 2002).

The major improvements of 4-slice to 64-slice scanners include improved temporal resolution due to shorter gantry rotation times, better spatial resolution owing to sub-millimeter collimation and considerably reduced examination times (FLOHR and OHNESORGE 2001; FLOHR et al. 2003b); see Fig. 1.16.

### 1.3.4
### Dual-Energy Computed Tomography

One of the limitations of CT is that tissues of different chemical composition but the same X-ray attenuation have the same Hounsfield values. This makes the differentiation and classification of tissue types challenging. Classical examples are the differentiation between calcified plaques and iodinated blood or hyper-dense and contrast-enhanced lesions.

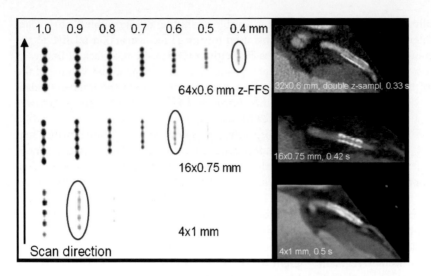

**Fig. 1.16.** Progress in longitudinal resolution for ECG-gated cardiac scanning from 4-slice CT to 64-slice CT. The four-slice CT scanner with 4×1-mm collimation (*bottom*) can resolve 0.9-1.0 mm objects. With 16×0.75-mm collimation, 0.6-mm objects can be delineated (*center*). The 64-slice CT scanner with 64×0.6 mm collimation and double *z*-sampling can routinely resolve 0.4-mm objects (*top*). The corresponding patient examples depict similar clinical situations (a stent in the proximal LAD). With the 64-slice system, an in-stent re-stenosis (*arrow*) can be evaluated. Four-slice case courtesy of Hopital de Coracao, Sao Paulo, Brazil; 16-slice case courtesy of Dr. A. Küttner, Tübingen University, Germany, and 64-slice case courtesy of Dr. C. M. Wong, Hong Kong, China

Besides the issue of differentiation and classification, the ambiguity of CT numbers hampers the reliability of quantitative measurements. Even for the seemingly straightforward quantification of iodine concentration, the accuracy of measured values is limited by the presence of other tissue types. For example, when determining the amount of iodine enhancement of a soft tissue lesion with use of a region of interest in that lesion measurement, the measured mean CT number will reflect not only the enhancement due to iodine, but also the underlying tissue. To overcome this limitation, additional information is required. By looking at attenuation of a material at two different energies, materials such as bone and iodine can be differentiated (Fig. 1.17).

First investigations of dual-energy methods for CT were made already in the 1970s (MACOVSKI et al. 1976; ALVAREZ and MACOVSKI 1976), but never made it into clinical routine, mainly because data for the different tube voltages had to be acquired at two different points in time. In the 1980s, it was possible to acquire dual-en-

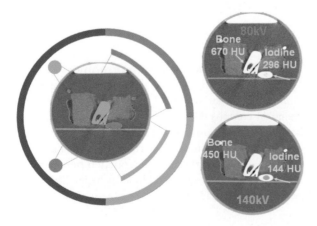

**Fig. 1.17.** Dual-energy principle: Using the two tubes and detectors in the Siemens SOMATOM Definition, the two tubes can be operated at different energies (80 kV and 140 kV) emitting different X-ray spectra. In a phantom with structures with similar attenuation at one energy, such as in this example of a phantom with bone (*green*) and tubes filled with iodine (*orange*), this additional information can be used to charactize and differentiate the two materials due to their different HU values at different energies

ergy data nearly simultaneously using a modified commercial CT system (KALENDER et al. 1987). During the rotation of the tube-detector pair, the tube voltage was switched quickly for each detector reading between the high and low settings so that two sets of raw data (projections) were acquired nearly simultaneously at two different tube voltages. The only application at that time was bone densitometry measurement; however, this application alone did not justify the additional costs, and dual-energy capabilities were not implemented in subsequent CT scanner generations.

With the introduction of dual-source CT, a new approach for dual-energy CT became clinically feasible. The design of this scanner allows adjusting not only the tube voltage, but also the tube current for both tube/detector pairs and allows simultaneous data acquisition. Images from both tube-detector pairs are reconstructed separately, and image-based post processing then is used to extract the dual-energy information.

Besides this approach, other acquisition methods for image-based dual-energy CT using single-source systems have been proposed. Approaches with two subsequent spiral acquisitions or two subsequent sequential scans have been reported. For static anatomical structures without any contrast enhancement dynamics, this acquisition technique appears feasible. However, for most patient scans, this prerequisite is not fulfilled. Motion, pulsation or change in contrast agent concentration between both acquisitions would lead to registration artifacts and false dual-energy information. Closer detail on the technical background and clinical applications of dual-energy CT can be found in Chaps. 5 and 36, respectively.

## 1.4
## Future Developments

The trend towards a larger number of slices will not be driven by the need to increase scan speed in spiral acquisition modes, but rather by new clinical applications that potentially become possible with these detector and system designs. Dynamic volume imaging becomes feasible, opening up a whole spectrum of new applications, such as functional or volume perfusion studies. Recently, both Toshiba and Siemens introduced systems targeting these applications, again pursuing different technological paths to reach the same goal. Toshiba introduced a 320-slice scanner that allows covering whole organs during one rotation. It is based on the prototype scanner with 256×0.5-mm detector elements (MORI et al. 2004, 2006). Siemens introduced a 128-slice scanner with a dynamic spiral shuttle mode that also allows acquiring 4D data of large volumes. Figure 1.18 shows an example of a perfusion scan of the complete brain acquired with that technology.

Prototype systems exist that use CsI-aSi flat-panel detector technology, originally used for conventional catheter angiography, which is limited in low contrast resolution and scan speed. Short gantry rotation times <0.5 s, which are a prerequisite for successful examination of moving organs such as the heart, are beyond the scope of such systems. Spatial resolution is excellent, though, due to the small detector pixel size (GUPTA et al. 2006). In pre-clinical installations, potential clinical applications of flat-panel volume CT systems are currently being evaluated (KNOLLMANN et al. 2003; GUPTA et al. 2003). The application spectrum ranges from ultra-high resolution bone imaging to dynamic CT angiographic studies and functional examinations.

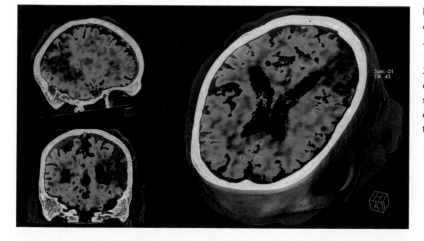

**Fig. 1.18.** Whole brain perfusion study on a Siemens SOMATOM Definition AS+: Using a detector configuration of 128×0.6 mm and a detector coverage of 38.4 mm, whole brain perfusion studies can be carried out by using a special spiral shuttle mode that uses a sinosoidal motion of the patient table to cover the whole brain for a period of 30 s

The combination of area detectors that provide sufficient image quality with fast gantry rotation speeds will be a promising technical concept for medical CT systems. C-arm systems already offering 3D CT capabilities are commercially available and will be discussed in Chap. 3. Compared to dedicated CT systems, which increasingly also offer support for image-guided interventions (Fig. 1.19), these scanners still offer limited image quality, but can be useful for intra-interventional imaging.

Nevertheless, it must be always kept in mind that a potential increase in spatial resolution to the level of flat-panel CT will be associated with increased dose demands, and the clinical benefit has to be carefully considered in the light of the applied patient dose. Therefore, another continued trend is saving patient dose for all kinds of clinical applications. Examples that demonstrate these efforts by the manufacturers are the introduction of dynamic collimators that eliminate the increasing problem of over-radiation in spiral scans, which was increasing with increasing detector width (Fig. 1.20), or the optimization of acquisition modes in cardiac CT, an application especially in the focus of dose discussion in the past years (Fig. 1.21).

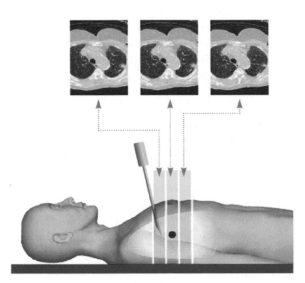

Conventional 2D Intervention

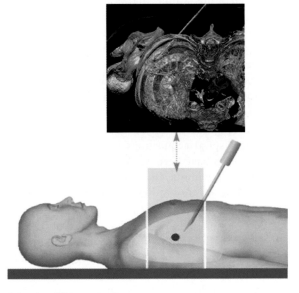

Adaptive 3D Intervention

**Fig. 1.19.** Wider and wider detectors can also be used for interventional applications. Previously interventional CT was a 2D application due to the still limited detector coverage of up to 64 slice detectors (*left*). New visualization methods and scan modes allow real-time 3D interventions with the new generation of 128-slice scanners (*right*)

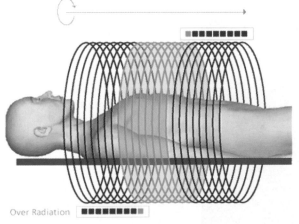

Over Radiation

**Fig. 1.20.** Since the introduction of multislice detectors, it is a known issue that at the start and the end of each spiral scan, a region is irradiated for which no images can be reconstructed (*red*). That portion depends on the width of the detector and becomes more severe the wider the detector becomes and the shorter the scan region is. That problem can be overcome, but introducing a tube side collimator that continuously opens at the start of the scan and closes at the end of the scan. The Siemens SOMATOM Definition AS+ is the first scanner offering that technology, which saves 10–25 % dose depending on the application. Typical dose savings using this technology are 10% for abdominal, 15% for thorax, 20% for head and 25% for cardiac examinations

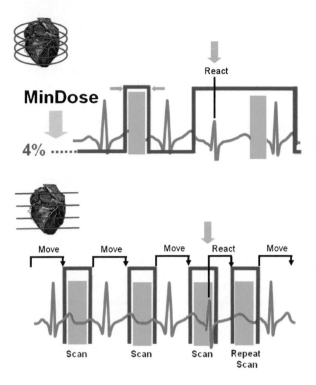

**Fig. 1.21.** Two competing technologies for cardiac examinations are spiral scanning using retrospective gating (*top*) and sequential scanning using prospective ECG triggering (*bottom*). Typically, retrospective gating is more robust and offers superior image quality, while prospective triggering offers additional possibilities to save dose. The recently introduced above approaches are used to make prospective triggering more robust and to save additional dose in retrospective gating. On the Siemens SOMATOM Definition platform, a functionality called "MinDose" is available that reduces the dose in heart phases that are not of interest to 4%. Additionally, it immediately reacts to irregularities in the ECG signal and raises the dose so that retrospective ECG editing becomes possible. A similar functionality was added to prospective triggering modes to make sure data are only acquired in regular heart cycles

## References

Alvarez RE, Macovski A (1976) Energy-selective reconstructions in X-ray computerized tomography. Phys Med Biol 21:733-744

Cesmeli E, Edic M, Iatrou M, Pfoh A (2001) A novel reconstruction algorithm for multiphasic cardiac imaging using multislice CT. Proc SPIE Int Symp Med Imag 4320:645-654

Crawford CR, King KF (1990) Computed tomography scanning with simultaneous patient translation. Med Phys 17:967-982

Feldkamp LA, Davis LC, Kress JW (1984) Practical cone-beam algorithm. J Opt Soc Am A:612-619

Flohr T, Ohnesorge B (2001) Heart rate adaptive optimization of spatial and temporal resolution for ECG-gated multislice spiral CT of the heart. JCAT 25:907-923

Flohr T, Stierstorfer K, Bruder H, Simon J, Schaller S (2002a) New technical developments in multislice CT, part 1: Approaching isotropic resolution with sub-millimeter 16-slice scanning. Röfo Fortschr Geb Rontgenstr Neuen Bildgeb Verfahr 174:839-845

Flohr T, Bruder H, Stierstorfer K, Simon J, Schaller S, Ohnesorge B (2002b) New technical developments in multislice CT, part 2: sub-millimeter 16-slice scanning and increased gantry rotation speed for cardiac imaging. Röfo Fortschr Geb Rontgenstr Neuen Bildgeb Verfahr 174:1022-1027

Flohr T, Stierstorfer K, Bruder H, Simon J, Polacin A, Schaller S (2003a) Image reconstruction and image quality evaluation for a 16-slice CT scanner. Med Phys 30:832-845

Flohr T, Schoepf U J, Kuettner A, Halliburton S, Bruder H, Suess C, Schmidt B, Hofmann L, Yucel E K, Schaller S, Ohnesorge B (2003b) Advances in cardiac imaging with 16-section CT systems. Acad Radiol 10:386-401

Flohr T, Stierstorfer K, Raupach R, Ulzheimer S, Bruder H (2004) Performance evaluation of a 64-slice CT system with z-flying focal spot. Röfo Fortschr Geb Rontgenstr Neuen Bildgeb Verfahr 176:1803-1810

Flohr TG, Stierstorfer K, Ulzheimer S, Bruder H, Primak AN, McCollough CH (2005a) Image reconstruction and image quality evaluation for a 64-slice CT scanner with z-flying focal spot. Med Phys 32:2536-2547

Flohr TG, Schaller S, Stierstorfer K, Bruder H, Ohnesorge BM, Schoepf UJ (2005b) Multi-detector row CT systems and image reconstruction techniques. Radiology 235:756-773

Flohr T, McCollough CH, Bruder H, Petersilka M, Gruber K, Süß C et al. (2006) First performance evaluation of a dual-source CT (DSCT) system. Eur Radiol 16:256-268

Fuchs T, Krause J, Schaller S, Flohr T, Kalender WA (2000) Spiral interpolation algorithms for multislice spiral CT–Part 2: Measurement and evaluation of slice sensitivity profiles and noise at a clinical multislice system. IEEE Trans Med Imag 19:835-847

Grass M, Köhler T, Proksa R (2000) Three-dimensional cone-beam CT reconstruction for circular trajectories. Phys Med Biol 45:329-347

Gupta R, Stierstorfer K, Popescu S, Flohr T, Schaller S, Curtin HD (2003) Temporal bone imaging using a large field-of-view rotating flat-panel CT scanner. Abstract Book of the 89th Scientific Assembly and Annual Meeting of the RSNA 2003, p 375

Gupta R, Grasruck M, Süß C, Bartling SH, Schmidt B, Stierstorfer K, Popescu S, Brady T, Flohr T (2006) Ultra-high resolution flat-panel volume CT: fundamental principles, design architecture, and system characterization. Eur Radiol 16:1191

Hein I, Taguchi K, Silver M D, Kazarna M, Mori I (2003) Feldkamp-based cone-beam reconstruction for gantry-tilted helical multislice CT. Med Phys 30:3233-3242

Hsieh J (2001) Investigation of the slice sensitivity profile for step-and-shoot mode multi-slice computed tomography. Med Phys 28:491-500

Hsieh J (2003) Analytical models for multi-slice helical CT performance parameters. Med Phys 30:169-178

Hu H (1999) Multi-slice helical CT: Scan and reconstruction. Med Phys 26:5-18

Hu H, He HD, Foley WD, Fox SH (2000) Four multidetector-row helical CT: Image quality and volume coverage speed. Radiology 215: 55-62

Jakobs TF, Becker CR, Ohnesorge B, Flohr T, Suess C, Schoepf UJ, Reiser MF (2002) Multislice helical CT of the heart with retrospective ECG gating: reduction of radiation exposure by ECG-controlled tube current modulation. Eur Radiol 12:1081-1086

Kachelriess M, Ulzheimer S, Kalender W (2000) ECG-correlated image reconstruction from subsecond multi-slice spiral CT scans of the heart. Med Phys 27:1881-1902

Kalender WA, Perman WH, Vetter JR, Klotz E (1986) Evaluation of a prototype dual-energy computed tomographic apparatus. I. Phantom studies. Med Phys13:334-339

Kalender WA, Klotz E, Suess C (1987) Vertebral bone mineral analysis: an integrated approach with CT. Radiology 164:419-423.

Kalender W, Seissler W, Klotz E, Vock P (1990) Spiral volumetric CT with single-breath-hold technique, continuous transport and continuous scanner rotation. Radiology 176:181-183

Kalender W (1995) Thin-section three-dimensional spiral CT: is isotropic imaging possible? Radiology 197:578-580

Klingenbeck-Regn K, Schaller S, Flohr T, Ohnesorge B, Kopp AF, Baum U (1999) Subsecond multi-slice computed tomography: basics and applications. EJR 31:110-124

Knollmann F, Pfoh A (2003) Image in cardiovascular medicine. Coronary artery imaging with flat-panel computed tomography. Circulation 107:1209

Leschka S, Alkadhi H, Plass A, Desbiolles L, Grunenfelder J, Marincek B, Wildermuth S (2005) Accuracy of MSCT coronary angiography with 64-slice technology: first experience. Eur Heart J 26:1482-1487

Macovski A, Alvarez RE, Chan JL, Stonestrom JP, Zatz LM (1976) Energy dependent reconstruction in X-ray computerized tomography. Comput Biol Med, 6:325-336

McCollough CH, Zink FE (1999) Performance evaluation of a multi-slice CT System. Med Phys 26:2223-2230

Mori I (1986) Computerized tomographic apparatus utilizing a radiation source. US Patent 4,630,202

Mori S, Endo M, Tsunoo T, Kandatsu S, Tanada S, Aradate H et al. (2004) Physical performance evaluation of a 256-slice CT-scanner for four-dimensional imaging. Med Phys 31:1348-1356

Mori S, Endo M, Obata T, Tsunoo T, Susumu K, Tanada S (2006) Properties of the prototype 256-row (cone beam) CT scanner. Eur Radiol 16:2100-2108

Nieman K, Oudkerk M, Rensing B, van Oijen P, Munne A, van Geuns R, de Feyter P (2001) Coronary angiography with multi-slice computed tomography. Lancet 357:599-603

Nieman K, Cademartiri F, Lemos PA, Raaijmakers R, Pattynama PMT, de Feyter PJ (2002) Reliable noninvasive coronary angiography with fast submillimeter multislice spiral computed tomography. Circulation 106:2051-2054.

Nishimura H, Miyazaki O (1988) CT system for spirally scanning subject on a movable bed synchronized to X-ray tube revolution. US Patent 4,789,929

Ohnesorge B, Flohr T, Becker C, Kopp A, Schoepf U, Baum U, Knez A, Klingenbeck-Regn K, Reiser M (2000) Cardiac imaging by means of electrocardiographically gated multisection spiral CT–Initial experience. Radiology 217:564-571

Raff GL, Gallagher MJ, O'Neill WW, Goldstein JA (2005) Diagnostic accuracy of non-invasive coronary angiography using 64-slice spiral computed tomography. JACC 46:552-557

Ropers D, Baum U, Pohle K, et al. (2003) Detection of coronary artery stenoses with thin-slice multi-detector row spiral computed tomography and multiplanar reconstruction. Circulation 107:664-666

Rubin GD, Dake MD, Semba CP (1995) Current status of three-dimensional spiral CT scanning for imaging the vasculature. Radiol Clin North Am 33:51-70 (Review)

Schaller S, Flohr T, Klingenbeck K, Krause J, Fuchs T, Kalender WA (2000) Spiral interpolation algorithm for multi-slice spiral CT–Part I: Theory. IEEE Trans Med Imag 19:822-834

Schaller S, Stierstorfer K, Bruder H, Kachelrieß M, Flohr T (2001a) Novel approximate approach for high-quality image reconstruction in helical cone beam CT at arbitrary pitch. Proc SPIE Int Symp Med Imag 4322:113-127

Schaller S, Niethammer MU, Chen X, Klotz E, Wildberger JE, Flohr T (2001b) Comparison of signal-to-noise and dose values at different tube voltages for protocol optimization in pediatric CT. Abstract Book of the 87th Scientific Assembly and Annual Meeting of the RSNA 2001, p 366

Schardt P, Deuringer J, Freudenberger J, Hell E, Knuepfer W, Mattern D, Schild M (2004) New X-ray tube performance in computed tomography by introducing the rotating envelope tube technology. Med Phys 31:2699-2706

Taguchi T, Aradate H (1998) Algorithm for image reconstruction in multi-slice helical CT. Med Phys 25:550-561

Taguchi K, Anno H (2000) High temporal resolution for multi-slice helical computed tomography. Med Phys 27:861-872

Vetter JR, Perman WH, Kalender WA, Mazess RB, Holden JE (1986) Evaluation of a prototype dual-energy computed tomographic apparatus. II. Determination of vertebral bone mineral content. Med Phys 13:340-343

Wang G, Lin T, Cheng P (1993) A general cone-beam reconstruction algorithm. IEEE Trans Med Imag 12:486-496

# Dynamic Volume CT with 320-Detector Rows: Technology and Clinical Applications

**2**

Patrik Rogalla

## CONTENTS

### ABSTRACT

Dynamic volume CT is another milestone in the development of CT technology. The use of wide detectors will most probably impact a number of clinical applications and has the potential to significantly reduce radiation exposure. Dynamic scanning of organs and organ regions and post-processing evaluation of the data open up new clinical applications and pose new challenges to programmers and radiologists alike. What remains to be determined is how the display of function and the calculation of organ and tumor perfusion with powerful computers will actually translate into clinical benefits for the patient

## Introduction

After the introduction of spiral CT technology into clinical practice in 1998–1999, the advantages of being able to scan larger areas of anatomy in a single breath hold quickly became apparent (MORI 1986; KALENDER et al. 1990). However, due to the limited detector width available in conventional helical CT scanners, a slice thickness of 5–10 mm had to be used, resulting in multiplanar reconstructed (MPR) images with much poorer resolution compared with axial images. Multidetector configurations consisting of several rows along the patient's longitudinal axis dramatically improved spatial with the additional benefit of shorter scan times (KOPKA et al. 2002; BAUM et al. 2000; PROKOP 2000; BLOBEL et al. 2003). Sixty-four-detector-row CT scanners are now available from all vendors, with detectors varying in width from 3.2 to 4 cm, allowing acquisition of slices ranging from 0.5 to 0.625 mm in thickness,

P. ROGALLA, MD
Institut für Radiologie, Charité–Universitätsmedizin Berlin, Charité Campus Mitte, Charitéplatz 1, 10117 Berlin, Germany

which provides reconstruction with isotropic resolution in all reformatting planes.

As the X-ray cone angle is proportional to the detector size, a further increase in detector width was long thought to be virtually impossible due to the hardware and reconstruction algorithm limitations.

The 320-detector-row CT scanner (dynamic volume CT system) introduced for clinical application in 2007 has a detector width of 16 cm, resulting in a cone angle of 15.2°, and offers new imaging options for a variety of organs.

## 2.2
## Technology

The new dynamic volume CT scanner (Toshiba Aquilion ONE, Ottawara, Japan) comprises a conventional gantry with an aperture of 70 cm and a 70-kW X-ray tube with an opposing solid-state detector. The detector is 16 cm in width along the rotational axis of the gantry and consists of 320 rows of 0.5-mm-thick elements. Each detector row consists of 896 elements, which are read out 900 to 3,600 times per rotation, depending on the gantry revolution time. Revolution times can be varied between 350 ms to 3 s for 360° data acquisition. A maximum of 320 slices or 640 slices with 50% overlap can be acquired with each gantry rotation.

The cone-beam angle of 15.2° is a function of the detector width and the tube focus-to-detector distance as compared with an angle of 3.05° for 64-detector-row CT scanners of the same series (Fig. 2.1). The source data is reconstructed using an exact cone-beam algorithm, which nearly eliminates all artifacts (Fig. 2.2), typically degrading cone-beam CT (ENDO et al. 2006). The geometric configuration of the scan area resulting from the geometry of the X-ray beam when scanning with a stationary table results in images with masked data as seen in the coronal plan (Fig. 2.1c). The missing image data (truncation) could theoretically be reconstructed from the raw data (ANOOP et al. 2007; LENG et al. 2005), but the computation power necessary to do so exceeds the capacity of current generation computers.

Four-scanning modes, which can be freely combined in one examination, are available on the 320-detector-row CT scanner.

### 2.2.1
### Helical Scan Mode

Helical scanning is performed as with conventional 64-detector-row CT. The images generated during one examination are displayed on the monitor in the form of preliminary reconstructions in real time. In a second computational step, the image data is reconstructed as a volume data set with variable slice thick-

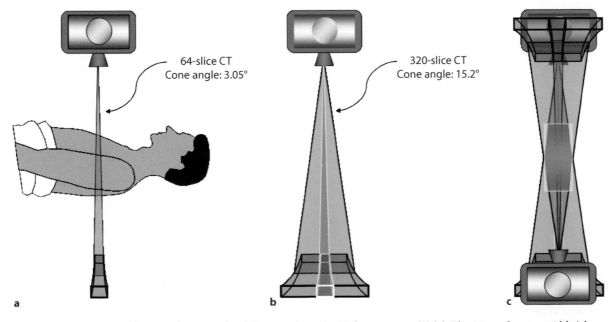

**Fig. 2.1a–c.** Diagram of the typical cone angle of the X-ray beam in 64-detector-row CT (**a**). The 16-cm detector width (along the rotational axis of the gantry) results in a 16° cone angle in dynamic volume CT (**b**) and a rhomboid shape of the image data (**c**)

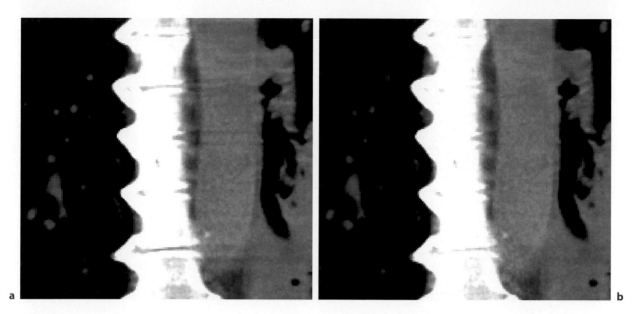

**Fig. 2.2a,b.** Primary reconstruction without correction yields images with cone-beam artifacts seen as horizontal dark lines (**a**). Correction nearly completely eliminates the artifacts (**b**). The correction has no impact on low-contrast resolution

ness (0.5–10 mm). MPRs at any slice thickness can be automatically generated in all three planes and, depending on the protocol used, automatically sent to up to 20 target computers or archives. Once image reconstruction has been completed, all image data is immediately available on a second console for further processing. The scanner can also be operated in a 32-, 16- and 4-detector-row mode, in which case only the respective number of rows is exposed to the X-ray beam.

## 2.2.2
## Wide Volume (Stitching) Scan Mode

In wide volume scan mode, the number of detector rows used is automatically adjusted, depending on the coverage required for the target anatomy.

Wide volume coverage is achieved by sequentially moving the table and stitching together the acquired scans (Fig. 2.3). The table length of 2 m defines the maximum scan length. The time required for shifting the table between scans amounts to 1.4 s. The overlap necessary between two consecutive scans is automatically calculated while planning the examination. The typical scan overlap is 17% and depends on the scan field, which in most cases is determined by the diameter of the patient.

The software automatically generates a single un-interrupted volume data set allowing for three-dimensional postprocessing, identical to a single-scan acquisition. Patient movement during the scan may cause visible stair-step artifacts or contour disruptions at the stitched positions. In helical scanning, the same patient movement should present as a wide spread motion blur.

## 2.2.3
## Dynamic Volume Scan Mode

Dynamic volume scanning provides volumetric imaging over time with a scan range of up to 16 cm, offering functional analysis of entire organs. As there is no table movement during scanning, each individual volume demonstrates just one instance in time.

Dynamic scanning can be performed as a continuous acquisition with uninterrupted radiation exposure or as an intermittent series with variable intervals ranging from 0.5 to 30 s between acquisitions. Additionally, as a low-dose technique is preferable, several rotations can be combined to generate one time-averaged acquisition to reduce noise and improve image quality. The rotation time, tube current, and voltage can be set individually for each acquisition, and it is possible to switch from continuous to intermittent acquisition and vice versa.

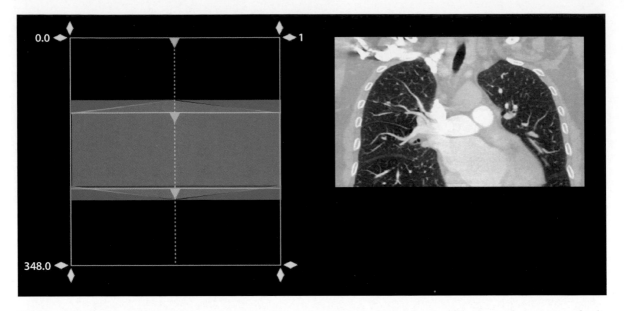

**Fig. 2.3.** Diagram of the wide volume-stitching mode. A large continuous volume is covered by sequential acquisition of individual shots. The thorax is usually covered with three shots, which are joined to form a seamless image

## 2.2.4
## Electrocardiographic-Triggering/-Gating (Prospective, Retrospective) Scan Modes

When an electrocardiogram (ECG) is recorded during scanning, cardiac imaging can be performed with both prospective triggering and retrospective gating, although with volumetric imaging there is no strict separation between both modes. As the start and end of the exposure is controlled by the ECG signal, the scan is always "triggered," and the phase of reconstruction is retrospectively selected from the available acquisition window. If the window is limited to a single rotation at a predefined point in time within the R–R interval (shortest scan time, minimal radiation exposure), then the scan technique is comparable to prospectively triggered 64-detector-row CT, but with complete coverage of the

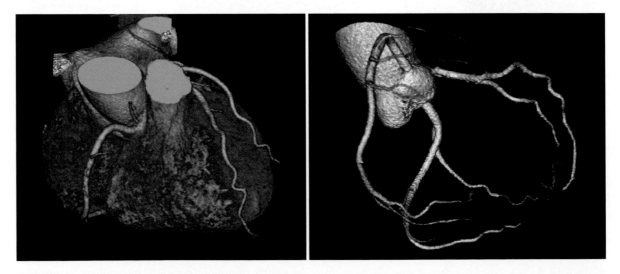

**Fig. 2.4.** Cardiac CT (heart rate of 61 beats per minute). Prospective triggering at 75% of a single R–R interval

heart (Fig. 2.4). A scan window extending over the entire R–R interval enables retrospective reconstruction over all cardiac phases, which in turn allows dynamic display of cardiac motion for calculating ejection fraction and myocardial motility. Tube current modulation can be used to reduce the dose to approximately 20% for the cardiac phases needed for ejection fraction calculation, with the full exposure used only for coronary artery imaging (Fig. 2.5).

The minimum temporal resolution for a prospective single shot scan is 175 ms and is associated with a radiation dose of 2–4 mSv, depending on the parameter settings used. When two serial single shots are combined, the effective temporal resolution is reduced to 87 ms as a result of segmentation during image reconstruction (Fig. 2.6), while the radiation dose is doubled (4–8 mSv). Technically, up to five segments can be combined, resulting in an effective minimum temporal resolution of 35 ms.

The reconstruction filters (kernels) are the same for all four-scan modes, leading to a uniform image appearance when different modes are combined. All image data can be automatically or retrospectively sent to different network nodes (PCs, workstations, archives) in the conventional DICOM format; the new enhanced-CT DICOM format is also available, which is faster and requires less storage capacity.

The low-contrast and high-contrast resolution of the 320-detector-row CT does not differ from the conventional 64-detector-row CT scan from the same manufacturer. Phantom measurements demonstrated a low-contrast resolution of 2 mm at 0.3% Hounsfield unit (HU) difference and a high-contrast resolution of 0.35 mm.

## 2.3
## Clinical Use

Implementation of the complete functionality of 64-detector capabilities in the 320-detector-row system enables use of all whole-body CT protocols and applications developed for 64-detector-row scanners. The wide volume-stitching mode is slightly faster than the helical technique is and likewise, requires no special training since the integrated software automatically joins the individual volumes and adjusts the effective detector width.

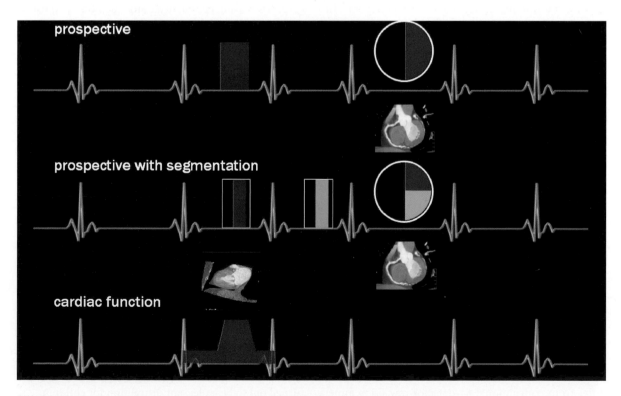

**Fig. 2.5.** Overview of the acquisition options available in the ECG-gated acquisition mode

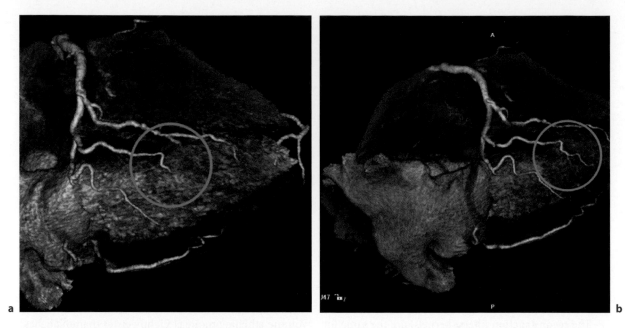

a                                                                    b

**Fig. 2.6.a,b** Three-dimensional reconstruction of a heart acquired with two prospective exposures (two-beat acquisition). **a** Reconstruction from the first beat, **b** from both beats with segmentation. Note the improved detail visualization achieved with segmentation (effective temporal resolution: 87 ms)

Gated imaging without table movement requires a new way of thinking in terms of protocol selection. The smooth transition between prospective triggering and retrospective reconstruction offers the user complete freedom in tailoring the scan to the clinical question. For each patient, the protocol is optimized balancing the required cardiac phases, temporal resolution, and the radiation dose. Patient comfort is also increased due to the very short breath hold times and no distracting table movement.

Patient motion during a CT scan is a common occurrence that is easily identifiable with wide volume scan mode. The resulting geometrical and anatomical differences that may occur between two individual scans are noticeable as abrupt contour shifts. During the infusion of an intravenous contrast agent, there will be visible attenuation differences, e.g., in vessels, due to the time delay between acquisitions. In principle, such differences also occur in helical CT; however, the differences in attenuation are "blurred" over a larger area and are therefore less conspicuous than are the abrupt differences seen at the interface between two images joined in the stitching mode.

The experience available so far suggests that the helical mode on the 320-detector-row scanner does not differ from conventional 64-detector-row CT scanners in terms of contrast medium usage, scan delay, patient preparation, image quality, and radiation exposure. Differences between the helical and wide volume scan modes appear to have no clinical relevance for general applications or CT angiography, except for the above-mentioned differences in the effects of patient movement and heterogeneous vascular opacification.

The dynamic display of motion and perfusion is a new application, which is enabled by the continuous or repeat acquisition of the target volume without table feed. The 16-cm detector width allows coverage of several organs including the pancreas, orthotopically located kidneys, the neck, the brain, and above all, the heart. When devising scan protocols for dynamic imaging, great care must be taken to minimize radiation exposure.

The short examination time with a single volume rotation scan offers important clinical advantages when examining newborns and infants. No sedation was needed in the 21 patients (ranging in age from 3 days to 6.7 years) we have examined so far. Even when the patients were restless, motion artifacts did not degrade the images. Alternatively, ventilation can be interrupted for just 1 s in critically ventilated infants. The display of a short cartoon in the integrated gantry monitor has also turned out to be a pleasant distraction for children.

## 2.4

### Role of Dynamic Volume CT

After the advent of the first helical multi-detector-row CT scanner, manufacturers soon began a race for even more detectors. Following an initial controversy about the most suitable type of detector for 4-detector-row CT—adaptive width (asymmetrical detector) versus detectors with identically sized elements—all manufacturers finally adopted the detector configuration with symmetrically arranged elements of identical size. A confusing factor in the race for the most rows was that doubling of projections using a moving focus of the X-ray source led to an apparent doubling of the number of rows, although the number of slices that could be reconstructed per rotation was that of the actual number of detector rows available. Clinically, this technology offers no real-world benefit in terms of scan speed compared with CT systems with a greater number of detector rows. The 320-detector-row CT scanner represents the current pinnacle in the nominal number of slices that can be scanned per gantry rotation.

The increase in effective detector width is associated with a proportionate increase in the effect of over ranging in the helical scan mode, and therefore, increased proportion of the overall radiation exposure from the first and last half rotation that does not contribute to image reconstruction. This effect is more significant when smaller volumes are imaged, e.g., when examining children, where this effect may account for up to 50% of the overall dose. The only effective means to reduce this excess radiation is the use of an active collimator in front of the X-ray tube, which is commercially available.

Over ranging can be avoided altogether by acquisition of a series of individual images instead of using the helical mode. However, to scan a large volume in roughly the same time as with multi-detector-row helical CT, the detector must be wide enough to cover the target anatomy with a minimum of steps. On the 320-detector-row CT scanner, three to five acquisitions are typically required to scan the chest or abdomen, while the heart can be imaged with a single rotation without table feed.

A substantial increase in patient dose results from helical acquisition in cardiac CT. Regardless of the number of X-ray tubes, the table feed must be sufficiently slow such that projection data of 180° gantry rotation are available for image reconstruction at all points in time and space even in patients with variable heart rate. Though radiation exposure can be markedly reduced

by tube current modulation and use of a smaller safety window for variable heart rates, the principle of overlapping data acquisition in helical scanning and the ensuing higher radiation exposure remain. Use of a detector that is wide enough for whole-heart coverage makes helical scanning superfluous and can reduce radiation exposure by up to 80%. The same reduction in radiation exposure can be achieved by a "step-and-shoot" acquisition with narrower detectors and initial clinical results are already available (HSIEH et al. 2006).

A novel application of the 320-detector-row CT is the ability of dynamically scanning an organ or an organ group over time without table feed. However, the principle of dynamic CT is not new since nearly all CT scanners enable dynamic perfusion imaging of stroke patients. Moreover, the perfusion of many organs (e.g., focal liver lesions) and tissues after radiotherapy has been analyzed by means of dynamic CT. One of the reasons why CT is so popular for perfusion studies is that there is a linear relationship between the concentration of contrast medium in a tissue and the resulting CT attenuation, which enables use of simple perfusion models. The detector widths, those were available before the advent of 320-detector-row CT presented a major obstacle to whole-organ coverage. While the so-called joggle-scan technique (back-and-forth table movement during scanning) provides coverage of the target anatomy over an extended period, the temporal distribution is heterogeneous and precludes uniform temporal display of perfusion.

An important issue in perfusion imaging is to obtain diagnostic information with a reasonable radiation exposure, which increases with the number of scans acquired. Only strict use of low-dose techniques (e.g., 80 kV with a dramatically reduced mA) will restrict radiation exposure to the scope of a conventional diagnostic CT examination.

Dynamic volume CT is another milestone in the development of CT technology. The wider detector will directly impact many clinical applications and has the potential to dramatically reduce radiation exposure. Dynamic scanning of organs and organ regions and postprocessing evaluation of the data open up new clinical applications and pose new challenges to programmers and radiologists alike. What remains to be determined is how the display of function and the calculation of organ and tumor perfusion with powerful computers will actually translate into clinical benefits for the patient.

## References

Anoop KP, Rajgopal K (2007) Estimation of missing data using windowed linear prediction in laterally truncated projections in cone-beam CT. Conf Proc IEEE Eng Med Biol Soc 2007:2903–2906

Baum U, Greess H, Lell M, Nomayr A, Lenz M (2000) Imaging of head and neck tumors—methods: CT, spiral-CT, multi-detector-row-spiral-CT. Eur J Radiol 33:153–160

Blobel J, Baartman H, Rogalla P, Mews J, Lembcke A (2003) Spatial and temporal resolution with 16-slice computed tomography for cardiac imaging. Rofo 175:1264–1271

Endo M, Mori S, Tsunoo T, Miyazaki H (2006) Magnitude and effects of x-ray scatter in a 256-slice CT scanner. Med Phys 33:3359–3368

Hsieh J, Londt J, Vass M, Li J, Tang X, Okerlund D (2006) Step-and-shoot data acquisition and reconstruction for cardiac x-ray computed tomography. Med Phys 33:4236–4248

Kalender WA, Seissler W, Klotz E, Vock P (1990) Spiral volumetric CT with single-breath-hold technique, continuous transport, and continuous scanner rotation. Radiology 176:181–183

Kopka L, Rogalla P, Hamm B (2002) Multi-detector-row CT of the abdomen—current indications and future trends. Rofo 174:273–282

Leng S, Zhuang T, Nett BE, Chen GH (2005) Exact fan-beam image reconstruction algorithm for truncated projection data acquired from an asymmetric half-size detector. Phys Med Biol 50:1805–1820

Mori I (1986) Computerized tomographic apparatus utilizing a radiation source. US Patent 4,630,202, 16 September 1986

Prokop M (2000) Multi-detector-row CT angiography. Eur J Radiol 36:86–96

# Imaging with Flat-Detector C-Arm Systems

## 3

Norbert Strobel, Oliver Meissner, Jan Boese, Thomas Brunner, Benno Heigl,
Martin Hoheisel, Günter Lauritsch, Markus Nagel, Marcus Pfister,
Ernst-Peter Rührnschopf, Bernhard Scholz, Bernd Schreiber,
Martin Spahn, Michael Zellerhoff and Klaus Klingenbeck-Regn

## CONTENTS

## ABSTRACT

Three-dimensional (3D) C-arm computed tomography is a new and innovative imaging technique. It uses two-dimensional (2D) X-ray projections acquired with a flat-panel detector C-arm angiography system to generate CT-like images. To this end, the C-arm system performs a sweep around the patient, acquiring up to several hundred 2D views. They serve as input for 3D cone-beam reconstruction. Resulting voxel data sets can be visualized either as cross-sectional images or as 3D data sets using different volume rendering techniques. Initially targeted at 3D high-contrast neurovascular applications, 3D C-arm imaging has been continuously improved over the years and is now capable of providing CT-like soft-tissue image quality. In combination with 2D fluoroscopic or radiographic imaging, information provided by 3D C-arm imaging can be valuable for therapy planning, guidance, and outcome assessment all in the interventional suite.

M. Nagel, PhD
CAS innovations, Heusteg 47, 91056 Erlangen, Germany

N. Strobel, PhD, O. Meissner, MD,
J. Boese, PhD, T. Brunner, PhD, B. Heigl, PhD,
M. Hoheisel, PhD, G. Lauritsch, PhD,
M. Pfister, PhD, E.-P. Rührnschopf,
B. Scholz, PhD, B. Schreiber, PhD,
M. Spahn, PhD, M. Zellerhoff, PhD,
and K. Klingenbeck-Regn, PhD
Siemens AG, Healthcare Sector, MED AX, Siemensstrasse 1,
91301 Forchheim, Germany

## 3.1
### Introduction

Three-dimensional (3D) C-arm computed tomography is a new and innovative imaging technique. Also referred to as C-arm CT, it uses two-dimensional (2D) X-ray projection data acquired with flat-panel detector C-arm angiography systems to generate CT-like images (SAINT-FELIX et al. 1994; KOPPE et al. 1995; FAHRIG et al. 1997; BANI-HASHEMI et al. 1998; JAFFRAY and SIEWERDSEN 2000; GROH et al. 2002; ZELLERHOFF et al. 2005; RITTER et al. 2007; KALENDER and KYRIAKU 2007). To obtain 2D radiographic projection data, the C-arm performs a sweep around the patient, e.g., over 200°. Up to several hundred images are acquired depending on the acquisition protocol selected. Reconstruction of three-dimensional voxel data sets from 2D raw projection data is performed using a 3D cone-beam reconstruction algorithm. Resulting voxel data sets can be visualized either as cross-sectional images or as 3D data sets using different volume rendering techniques.

Initially targeted at neuroendovascular imaging of contrast-enhanced vascular structures, 3D C-arm imaging has been continuously improved over the years. It is now capable of providing CT-like soft-tissue image quality directly in the interventional radiology suite. Beyond their use for trans-arterial catheter procedures, these 3D data sets are also valuable for guidance and optimization of percutaneous treatments such as liver tumor ablations. In combination with 2D fluoroscopic or radiographic imaging, information provided by 3D C-arm imaging can be very valuable for therapy planning, guidance, and outcome assessment-in particular for complicated interventions (MISSLER et al. 2000; ANXIONNAT et al. 2001; HERAN 2006; MEYER et al. 2007; WALLACE et al. 2007).

C-arm CT requires state-of-the-art C-arm systems equipped with flat-panel detector (FD) devices. It is commercially available from various vendors, e.g., marketed as *syngo* DynaCT (Siemens AG, Healthcare Sector, Forchheim, Germany), XperCT (Philips Healthcare, Andover, MA), or Innova CT (GE Healthcare, Chalfont St. Giles, UK).

The goal of this book chapter is to provide an overview of how 3D C-arm imaging works and for what it can be used. To this end, we focus on important C-arm system components first. Then we explain how X-ray input images are acquired and take a look at the resulting patient dose. In the next step, we cover three-dimensional image reconstruction and the correction methods needed to obtain low-contrast 3D results with CT-like image quality. After we explained how C-arm CT images are generated, we analyze them in terms of spatial resolution and contrast resolution. In the remainder of this chapter, we look at clinical imaging results and C-arm CT applications including instrument guidance.

## 3.2
### Technology of C-Arm CT Systems

### 3.2.1
### C-Arm System Components

#### 3.2.1.1
#### X-Ray Beam Generation and Exposure Control

The X-ray tube, X-ray generator, and X-ray control system are crucial components of any C-arm imaging system. They determine tube voltage, tube current, and irradiation time, respectively. These exposure parameters are essential for X-ray imaging, since contrast-detail perceptibility and dose depend on them.

Better contrast visibility, in particular of iodine, is the main reason why angiographic C-arm systems usually operate at lower tube voltages than CT scanners. Since decreasing tube voltage can lead to an increase in image noise, the question arises if better low contrast visibility at lower tube voltages can compensate for higher noise or not. Recent studies not only support this hypothesis, but they also indicate that there is great potential for dose reduction by scanning with lower tube voltages (MCCOLLOUGH 2005; NAKAYAMA et al. 2005).

The requirement to obtain high 2D image quality for fluoroscopic and radiographic imaging led to C-arm systems equipped with automatic exposure control (AEC). The use of AEC turns out to be extremely beneficial for C-arm CT imaging as well. In fact, it is very similar to attenuation-based tube current modulation used in CT. Tube current modulation can either improve image quality through noise reduction at a given dose, or it can reduce radiation exposure without impairing image quality (GIES et al. 1999; KALENDER et al. 1999).

#### 3.2.1.2
#### Flat-Panel Detector Technology

Until the 1990s, C-arm systems for real-time angiographic imaging used to rely on X-ray image intensifiers (XRIIs). Although optimized over decades, this technology has a number of inherent disadvantages that limit its utility for low-contrast C-arm CT imaging. For example, the convex input screen of XRIIs results in a non-homogeneous image quality across the output image. In addition, scatter processes of light and electrons within the image intensifier limit the coarse contrast resolution. This effect is also known as veiling glare (ROWLANDS and YORKSTON 2000). Yet another critical point with large image intensifier formats is patient access as well as the flexibility during angulation due to the large size of XRIIs.

Flat detectors, on the other hand, either avoid or at least reduce some of the major disadvantages of image intensifiers (GRANFORS et al. 2001; BRUIJNS et al. 2002; BUSSE et al. 2002; CHOQUETTE et al. 2001; COLBETH et al. 2001). The most important technical advantages of flat detectors are:

- Homogeneous image quality across the entire image area resulting in distortion-free images and position-independent spatial resolution.
- High 'low-contrast resolution,' i.e., good 2D soft-tissue imaging performance.
- High detective quantum efficiency (DQE) across all dose levels, in particular for CsI/aSi-based flat detectors.
- High dynamic range at all dose levels from fluoroscopy to digital subtraction angiography (DSA) facilitated by A/D converters with 14 bits.
- Tightly enclosed square or rectangular active imaging areas offering improved patient access.

The most widely used flat detector (FD) design is based on a two-level, indirect conversion process of X-rays to light (GRANFORS et al. 2001; ANTONUK et al. 1997; SPAHN et al. 2000; YAMAZAKI et al. 2004; DUCOURANT et al. 2003). In the first step, the X-ray quantum is absorbed by a fluorescence scintillator screen, e.g., a cesium iodide (CsI) substrate, converting it into visible light. In the second step, this light is received by a photodiode array, e.g., based on amorphous silicon (a-Si), and converted into electrical charge.

Besides good intrinsic X-ray absorption properties of the material itself, scintillator thickness is an important design parameter for X-ray detectors. A larger scintillator thickness improves the energy absorption efficiency and therefore the X-ray sensitivity of the detector. Unfortunately, it also reduces the spatial resolution due to optical diffusion blur. Thus, an optimum has to be found between X-ray sensitivity and spatial resolution. This is where CsI's columnar, needle-like microscopic crystalline structure provides a particular advantage. By limiting lateral optical light spread, CsI enables high spatial resolution at a larger phosphor thickness and, hence, increased X-ray sensitivity. As a result, CsI

is the scintillator material of choice for high-resolution X-ray applications at low dose levels. A typical value of the effective CsI scintillator thickness for FDs used in today's C-arm systems is around 500 μm.

A schematic view of an indirect converting flat detector based on CsI is presented in Fig. 3.1. An individual pixel is shown in detail, comprising a large photodiode and a small thin-film transistor (TFT). Pixel readout is initiated when the TFT is switched on. This causes the charge to flow to dedicated low-noise readout electronics, where it is amplified and subsequently converted into a digital signal.

Flat detector technology is subject to further development and continuous improvement. Miniaturized electronics will allow for even thinner and lighter detectors required for mobile or portable applications. Higher bit depths of 16 bits or even 18 bits will improve C-arm CT image quality, allowing it to further approach the low-contrast resolution of multi-slice computed tomography (MSCT).

### 3.2.1.3
### C-Arm Gantries

An angiography device for 3D C-arm imaging comprises a stand and a C-arm to which the detector, X-ray tube, and collimator are attached. The C-arm keeps the X-ray tube, collimator, and flat-panel detector exactly aligned under varying view angles. Thanks to an open design maximizing the number of degrees of freedom

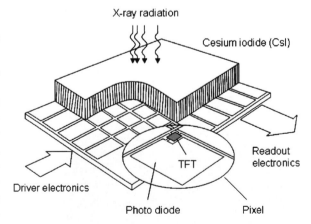

**Fig. 3.1.** Schematic view of an indirect converting flat detector based on CsI and an amorphous silicon active readout matrix, including driver and readout electronics. An individual pixel is shown in detail. It comprises a large photodiode and a small thin-film transistor (*TFT*)

for movements while minimizing the required space for the gantry itself, C-arm systems achieve high positioning flexibility and provide excellent patient access. As a result, C-arm systems are in use for interventional radiology, neuroradiology, cardiology, as well as for surgical applications.

In some cases, such as ceiling-mounted C-arm systems, the whole gantry can be rotated and translated to increase patient coverage and access. This traditional gantry design, shown in Fig. 3.2a, involves a mechanically fixed center of rotation commonly referred to as the isocenter. To further increase positioning flexibility, a new type of multi-axis C-arm system has recently been introduced (Artis **zeego**, Siemens AG, Healthcare Sector, Forchheim, Germany). Illustrated in Fig. 3.2b, this system involves a robotic stand moving a light-weight C-arm. Since the multi-axis stand facilitates greater flexibility, more accurate, faster movements, and better patient coverage, such systems are especially well suited for minimally invasive procedures and surgery.

### 3.2.2
### C-Arm CT Image Acquisition and Dose

Although C-arm CT data acquisition is increasingly automated for ease of use, the following steps are usually involved. First, the patient needs to be optimally positioned such that the region of interest is visible in all X-ray views acquired during a spin around the patient. With the patient properly placed, the C-arm is initially driven into a position, which will be the scan end position. Then a safety run is performed during which the C-arm is slowly moved into the actual C-arm CT start position. This safety run is required to rule out collision during the actual scan. After the C-arm has reached its start position, a short fluoroscopic X-ray pulse is applied to initialize the automatic exposure control. At this point, the system is ready to begin a 3D run during which the C-arm rotates from the start position into its end position. Raw data acquisition is performed by activating a dead-man switch. The rotational scan is stopped at once if the switch is released to prevent accidental X-ray exposure. On state-of-the-art C-arm CT systems, such as the Artis **zee** family (Siemens AG, Healthcare Sector, Forchheim, Germany), raw data acquisition and 3D reconstruction can be faster than 1 min depending on the scan protocol chosen.

Since C-arm CT is usually performed in an interventional setting, intra-arterial access is typically available. As a consequence, selective intra-arterial contrast injections can be used to enhance vessels as well as corresponding tissue regions during C-arm CT data acquisition.

X-ray input projections for C-arm CT can either be taken subtracted or native. Subtracted data acquisition involves a mask run without and a fill run after injection of contrast agent. Native data acquisition, on the other

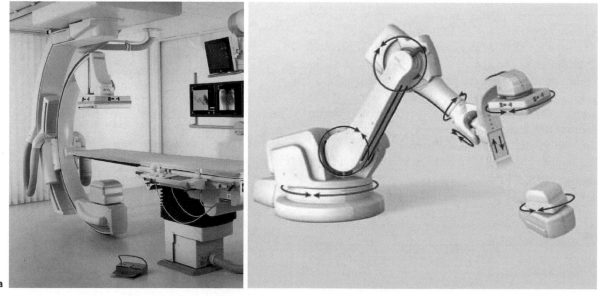

a                                                                                                                                          b

**Fig. 3.2a,b.** C-arm gantries: An Artis **zee** ceiling-mounted C-arm (**a**) is shown on the *left*, while the Artis **zeego** (**b**) is depicted on the *right* (both Siemens AG, Healthcare Sector, Forchheim, Germany). The C-arm keeps the detector (positioned on *top*) exactly aligned with collimator and X-ray source (bottom-mounted). Detector and collimator rotate in synchronization as shown in (**b**). The X-ray source is built into the C-arm below the collimator

hand, involves only one set of input projections-often taken without (but conceivably also with) contrast.

C-arm CT systems with automatic exposure control (AEC) adjust X-ray exposure parameters such that the detector entrance dose remains constant. Detector entrance dose is the X-ray dose measured behind the antiscatter grid. System dose is the detector entrance dose evaluated at a reference detector zoom format. System dose is an important set-up parameter for C-arm CT imaging protocols on Artis **zee** systems (Siemens AG, Healthcare Sector, Forchheim, Germany). Due to internal adjustments, the detector entrance dose for C-arm CT is about half the system dose.

One way to monitor and report dose is to rely on an index such as the CT dose index (CTDI). A recent study investigating weighted CTDI ($CTDI_w$) and image quality for C-arm CT of the head demonstrated that the weighted CT dose index was within accepted limits (FAHRIG et al. 2006). Besides CTDI, the dose to the patient may also be quantified in terms of effective dose. For this purpose, anthropomorphic phantoms with embedded thermoluminescence detectors (TLDs) are used (BALTER et al. 2005). These phantoms have realistic body sizes and absorption values. Once the TLDs have been placed at selected positions inside a phantom, e.g., an Alderson phantom (Alderson Research Laboratories Inc., Long Island City, NY), it can be scanned using a particular C-arm CT examination protocol. The dose applied to single organs is derived by weighted summation of the individual TLD dose recordings. Effective dose is quantified in mSv instead of mGy. The worldwide average background dose for a human being is about 2.4 mSv per year (UNSCEAR 2000).

Although technical constraints and clinical requirements make it a non-trivial task to establish a practical set of clinical C-arm CT scan protocols, application-specific techniques can be established. This requires a careful choice of imaging parameters such as system dose, scan time, and pixel binning at the detector. Pixel binning means that the outputs of neighboring detector pixels are combined into one reading. For example, 2 × 2 binning implies that a total of four neighboring detector pixels that are adjacent in the horizontal and vertical direction, respectively, are taken together. Pixel binning determines spatial resolution, because it controls effective pixel size. The detector frame rate depends on pixel binning as well, because the amount of data is proportional to the number of pixels.

For C-arm CT data acquisition using an Artis **zee** system (Siemens AG, Healthcare Sector, Forchheim, Germany), the FD is mostly operated either in a 2 × 2 binning mode or in a 4 × 4 binning mode. For 2 × 2 binning, usually used for 3D C-arm imaging in the head,

we get a detector frame rate of 30 frames per second ($fs^{-1}$). In case of 4 × 4 binning, the frame rate increases to 60 $fs^{-1}$. The 4 × 4 binning mode is a clinically accepted setting for soft-tissue imaging in the abdomen, because it facilitates acquisition of a higher number of X-ray views in a shorter scan time.

Two sets of C-arm CT scan parameters and effective dose are presented below for Artis **zee** systems (Siemens AG, Healthcare Sector, Forchheim, Germany). They include mean effective dose values for the head and liver regions determined using a normal-size, male Alderson phantom with embedded TLDs. Since effective dose depends on phantom positioning and size, however, measurement outcomes may vary. This is why great care was taken to position the phantom identically for all experiments to obtain comparable results.

In Table 3.1, we summarize common high-contrast C-arm CT scan protocols and the resulting effective doses. These scan protocols are often used for subtracted runs involving injection of contrast agent to image vascular malformations such as aneurysms, arteriovenous malformations (AVMs), and stenoses. Tumor feeders can be visualized this way as well. Subtracted data acquisition is indicated in Table 3.1 by using a plus sign for the number of frames acquired. For 3D C-arm imaging where motion can be an issue, e.g., in the body, non-subtracted runs are usually the method of choice. Interventional imaging applications in the body that can benefit from C-arm CT include abdominal aortic aneurysms (AAAs), transjugular intrahepatic portosystemic shunts (TIPSs), non-vascular therapies, e.g., biliary duct treatments and tumors. The effective body dose stated in Table 3.1 was determined inside the liver region of an Alderson phantom using TLDs.

Table 3.2 lists two often-used scan parameter sets together with the resulting effective dose for low-contrast C-arm CT imaging in the head (therapy control, complication management) and in the body, e.g., for liver tumor treatment. Effective dose in the body was measured inside the liver region of an Alderson phantom using TLDs. A comprehensive list of C-arm CT scan protocols, including proper 3D reconstruction parameter settings for Artis **zee** systems (Siemens AG, Healthcare Sector, Forchheim, Germany), can be found in an application protocol book for these systems (MOORE and ROHM 2006).

Various adult effective doses for CT scans have been reported in the literature. For example, BECKER et al. (1998) obtained an effective dose of 6 mSv for a spiral scan of the abdomen. In a comprehensive review, McCOLLOUGH and SCHUELER (2000) provide an effective dose between 1.9 mSv and 2.6 mSv for a (male) CT head scan and 7.3 mSv to 7.8 mSv for a (male) CT abdo-

**Table 3.1.** Common high-contrast C-arm CT scan protocols for Artis **zee** C-arm systems (Siemens AG, Healthcare Sector, Forchheim, Germany) and the resulting effective doses

| Clinical application | System dose (µGy/view) | Scan time (s) | Binning | No. frames | C-arm CT dose (mSv) |
|---|---|---|---|---|---|
| Head: vascular malformations, e.g., aneurysms, AVMs, stenoses, and tumor feeders | 0.36 | 5 | 2 × 2 | 133 + 133 | 0.3 |
| Body: AAA,TIPS, non-vascular therapies (e.g., biliary duct), and tumor feeders | 0.36 | 5 | 2 × 2 | 133 | 1.5 |

**Table 3.2.** Common low-contrast C-arm CT scan protocols for Artis **zee** C-arm systems (Siemens AG, Healthcare Sector, Forchheim, Germany) and the resulting effective doses

| Clinical application | System dose (µGy/view) | Scan time (s) | Binning | No. frames | C-arm CT dose (mSv) |
|---|---|---|---|---|---|
| Head: therapy control, complication management | 1.20 | 20 | 2 × 2 | 496 | 2 |
| Body: liver tumor treatment | 0.36 | 8 | 4 × 4 | 397 | 5 |

men scan, respectively. Comparing these values to the entries in Table 3.1 and Table 3.2, we see that high-contrast C-arm CT scan protocols result in a significantly lower dose to a patient, while the effective dose for a low-contrast C-arm CT examination appears similar to what is applied in regular CT scans.

### 3.2.3
### C-Arm CT and Image Quality

### 3.2.3.1
### Cone-Beam
### Reconstruction Algorithm

If C-arm systems can rotate around a patient along a sufficiently large angular scan range, then it is possible to use the acquired X-ray projections for tomographic image reconstruction. Usually a minimum angular scan range of 180° plus the so-called fan-angle is required (KAK and SLANEY 1999). For typical C-arm CT devices, this results in an angular scan range requirement of at least 200°.

In 1984, FELDKAMP et al. (1984) suggested a 3D reconstruction algorithm that has become the de-facto standard for 3D C-arm imaging. Originally designed

for a 360° scan along a perfectly circular trajectory, some modifications are, however, required before it can successfully process X-ray projections acquired along a C-arm CT scan trajectory. For example, a data weighting scheme is needed to compensate for the fact that during a partial circle scan some data are taken once, while other measurements are observed twice (PARKER 1982). In addition, a method may be needed with which to account for a C-arm system's irregular yet reproducible scan trajectory (ROUGEE et al. 1993; NAVAB et al. 1996; NAVAB et al. 1998; WIESENT et al. 2000).

Although predominately used for stationary objects, C-arm CT can also be applied to quasi-stationary 3D reconstruction problems, such as imaging the moving heart. To this end, the C-arm system performs multiple runs around the patient while the ECG signal is monitored. A continuous injection of contrast media is necessary to enhance the heart throughout data acquisition. The raw data obtained over the multiple runs can be resorted for a particular phase of the cardiac cycle using retrospective ECG gating. Since resorting of the acquired 2D X-ray views yields a valid input data set associated with the heart 'frozen' at a selected cardiac cycle, a standard C-arm CT reconstruction algorithm can be applied (LAURITSCH et al. 2006; PRUEMMER et al. 2007).

Sophisticated correction techniques are needed to obtain C-arm CT results with good low-contrast visibility. They are explained below. We start with overexposure correction, then turn to scatter correction, and next look into beam-hardening correction. After that, we briefly visit truncation correction and finish up with ring correction.

## 3.2.3.2
## Overexposure Correction

While the dynamic range provided by 14-bit A/D converters of state-of-the-art flat-panel detectors is usually sufficient for conventional 2D fluoroscopic or radiographic imaging, it may not be high enough to rule out overexposure in all projections acquired during a C-arm CT scan. In this case, an object is X-rayed from many orientations. As a result, strong direct radiation may hit certain detector regions in some views and overexpose them.

Three-dimensional reconstruction from overexposed projections may result in incorrect density values and also produce a capping artifact. This means that gray values of a homogeneous object get increasingly smaller the further they are away from the object center. Since a capping artifact can impair the display of low-contrast objects, an overexposure correction is needed. It is applied to saturated image areas only. By correcting for overexposure, one may be able to obtain results without any apparent capping artifact.

## 3.2.3.3
## Scatter Correction

Once overexposed image areas have been processed, scatter correction can be performed. Scattered X-ray quanta are photons that were deflected from their straight (primary) direction. They are detected at positions away from where a straight primary ray would hit the detector. As a result, the primary intensity distribution for tomographic reconstruction is impaired by a secondary distribution due to scattered radiation.

With single-row detectors of third generation CT scanners, scatter is almost negligible, because the irradiated patient volume is reduced to a small slice by collimation near the X-ray source. However, when working with flat-panel detectors, the collimator at the X-ray source is usually opened much more widely, and a considerable amount of scattered radiation may be produced. It can reach a multiple of the primary intensity in case of abdominal X-ray projections and up

to the order of magnitude of the primary intensity in head images (AICHINGER et al. 2004; SIEWERDSEN and JAFFRAY 2001).

The impact of scatter on image quality is determined by the scatter-to-primary intensity ratio (SPR) at every detector pixel. Effective SPR reduction of up to about a factor of five can be obtained with anti-scatter grids (KYRIAKOU and KALENDER 2007). Unfortunately, even with an anti-scatter grid, scatter can still degrade image quality after tomographic reconstruction. Typical image quality problems caused by scatter are:

- Smooth gray value deviations within homogenous regions (cupping).
- Streaks, bars, or shadows in soft tissue regions, especially in the vicinity and between high contrast objects such as bones.
- Reduction of contrast differences in soft tissue regions.
- Increase of noise.

The appearance of cupping and shadowing artifacts due to scatter can be very similar to those created by beam hardening (RUEHRNSCHOPF and KALENDER 1981). Contrary to beam hardening, however, a decrease in differential contrast and an increase in noise are typical consequences of scatter.

Efficient scatter suppression and additional correction procedures are essential for C-arm CT to achieve CT-like image quality. A variety of scatter correction approaches exist. They comprise measurement techniques, software models, and hybrid approaches (NING et al. 2002; SIEWERDSEN et al. 2006; ZHU et al. 2008). Since measurement techniques require additional hardware, software approaches are often preferable. Fast and efficient algorithms are available that operate directly on the projection images acquired (ZELLERHOFF et al. 2005; RINKEL et al. 2007). Iterative approaches appear promising to obtain further improvements beyond state-of-the art scatter correction methods (KYRIAKOU et al. 2006).

The impact of scatter correction can be appreciated by looking at Fig. 3.3. As part of an overview illustrating the effect of C-arm CT correction methods provided by *syngo* DynaCT (Siemens AG, Healthcare Sector, Forchheim, Germany), we show an abdominal cross-section reconstructed without applying scatter correction in Fig. 3.3a. This data set suffers from a considerable cupping artifact. A reference result obtained after applying all correction steps is displayed in Fig. 3.3d. A comparison between Fig. 3.3a and Fig. 3.3d demonstrates that the cupping artifact due to scatter could be removed.

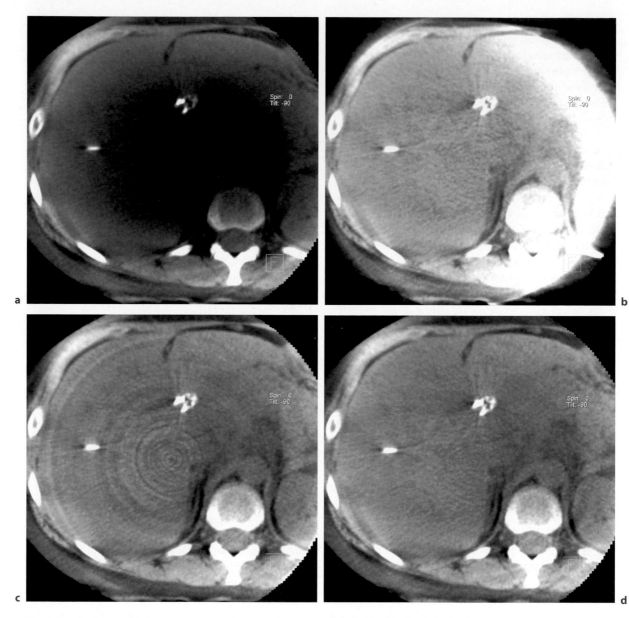

**Fig. 3.3a–d.** C-arm CT data sets computed using *syngo* DynaCT based on 2D X-ray projections acquired on an AXIOM Artis dTA system (both Siemens AG, Healthcare Sector, Forchheim, Germany) with correction techniques turned off/on. An axial abdominal slice without scatter correction is shown in (**a**). The same image reconstructed without truncation correction is depicted in (**b**). Another result obtained without ring correction can be found in (**c**), and a reference section involving all correction steps is demonstrated in (**d**) (images courtesy of Dr. Loose and Dr. Adamus, Department of Radiology, Klinikum Nuremberg Nord, Germany)

### 3.2.3.4
### Beam Hardening Correction

After dealing with overexposure and scatter removal, 2D projections can be corrected for beam hardening. X-ray tubes emit photons with different energies. Low-energy photons are absorbed and attenuated more strongly by matter than higher energy photons. As a consequence, the mean energy of an X-ray beam's poly-energetic spectrum gets increasingly higher (harder) the further X-rays penetrate into an attenuating object. This physical effect is commonly referred to as beam hardening (Barrett and Swindell 1981; Hsieh 2003).

Because of beam hardening, the linear relationship between attenuation value and object thickness no longer applies. As a result, attenuation values towards the center of a large object may be underestimated, causing a cupping artifact. This means that density values for a homogeneous object get increasingly larger away from the center. In case of inhomogeneous objects, composed of tissue and bone, beam-hardening artifacts may also show up as streak artifacts between highly attenuating components, e.g., between bony structures surrounded by soft tissue.

The reduction of the two types of beam hardening artifacts requires two different correction approaches. The cupping artifact can be compensated by restoring a linear relationship between attenuation value and path length through an assumed water-equivalent object. This correction step, applied before carrying out any 3D reconstruction, is usually called 'water correction.' On the other hand, to reduce streak artifacts, one can make the assumption that the attenuating object is composed of water-equivalent tissue and bones and then design an algorithm to correct for beam hardening caused by the two different materials (JOSEPH and SPITAL 1978).

## 3.2.3.5
### Truncation Correction

Unlike in MSCT systems, where detectors are usually wide enough to always capture a patient's full X-ray profile irrespective of view direction, FDs of today's C-arm systems may not be large enough to accomplish this in any case. As a result, it is possible that X-ray projections are truncated in some or even all views. Truncated projections can be problematic for tomographic reconstruction algorithms, because they may generate bright circular artifacts and result in incorrectly reconstructed density values as shown in Fig. 3.3b.

Truncation artifacts and density errors can be reduced by applying row-wise extrapolation techniques (OHNESORGE et al. 2000; STARMAN et al. 2005; SOURBELLE et al. 2005; ZELLERHOFF et al. 2005; HSIEH et al. 2004). Since row-wise extrapolation only depends on neighboring data in a horizontal direction, this approach is adaptive, and it can be very effective, as shown in Fig. 3.3d.

New multi-axis C-arm gantry designs, such as the Artis **zeego** (Siemens AG, Healthcare Sector, Forchheim, Germany) shown in Fig. 3.2b, can be operated in a large-volume scan mode. This approach almost doubles the object size that can be reconstructed without truncation artifacts, because two C-arm runs are performed with the detector positioned such that it captures one half of an X-ray projection in one run while recording the remaining half in the other.

## 3.2.3.6
### Ring Artifact Correction

Ring artifacts are caused by detector gain inhomogeneities or defective detector pixels. Fortunately, elaborate detector calibration and built-in FD defect correction can usually correct detector pixel problems to a large extent, thus preventing most serious ring artifacts right at the detector.

Nevertheless, with the steadily improving image quality of C-arm CT, even the slightest 3D image imperfections start to show up. This is why a ring correction algorithm is needed. Implemented as a post-processing algorithm, it first generates a ring image using sophisticated image processing techniques. This ring image is then subtracted from the initial reconstruction result to obtain a cleaned-up image as depicted in Fig. 3.3c and Fig. 3.3d (FLOHR 2000; ZELLERHOFF et al. 2005).

## 3.2.3.7
### Image Quality

Thanks to a detector optimized for high-resolution 2D fluoroscopic and radiographic imaging, the spatial resolution provided by C-arm CT can be very high. For example, a common FD for large-plate C-arm systems, such as the 30 cm × 40 cm Pixium 4700 flat-panel detector (Trixell, Moirans, France), offers a native pixel pitch of 154 μm in a 1,920 × 2,480 matrix. Although this leads to an excellent spatial resolution, taking full advantage of it reduces the FD frame rate in overview mode to 7.5 fs$^{-1}$. Such a low frame rate limits its clinical use to certain high-contrast applications unless special read-out techniques are applied. Higher frame rates are possible by applying 2 × 2 binning or 4 × 4 binning of detector pixels. Since pixel binning combines neighboring detector elements, the effective pixel width and height increases to 308 μm (2 × 2 binning) or to 616 μm (4 × 4 binning), respectively.

To arrive at a first estimate of how detector pixel width is related to spatial resolution, let us start with an example based on a detector pixel pitch of 308 μm. This is the pixel width of the Pixium 4700 FD when operated in 2 × 2 binning mode. Taking into account a cone-beam magnification factor between isocenter and detector of 1.5, we arrive at an effective pixel size at isocenter of 205 μm. This suggests that a spatial (in-plane) resolution of up to 2.4 LP/mm should be achievable after tomographic reconstruction (1/0.410 mm), if imaging conditions were ideal. Unfortunately, additional factors such as finite focal spot size, gantry motion, and 3D reconstruction kernel may lower spatial resolution. For example, the spatial resolution after tomographic reconstruction for an Artis **zee** system using *syngo* DynaCT (both Siemens AG, Healthcare Sector, Forchheim, Germany) is not 2.4 LP/mm as estimated above, but rather 2.0 LP/mm as depicted in Fig. 3.4. The smallest high contrast object that can be resolved at 2.0 LP/mm has a size of about 250 µm or 0.25 mm. At native detector resolution (154 µm pixel pitch), the spatial resolution encountered in phantom measurements reaches almost 4.0 LP/mm. This means that details may be resolved that are as small as 0.13 mm. If 4 × 4 binning is applied, then the spatial resolution seen in bar-pattern experiments is about 1.0 LP/mm, i.e., the system can be expected to resolve objects with a size of around 0.50 mm. This value is only slightly less than results obtained with current multi-slice CT devices. In fact, the 4 × 4 binning mode is a clinically well accepted acquisition technique for low-contrast C-arm CT imaging, e.g., in the abdomen, because the increased detector frame rate enables the acquisition of a higher number of views in a shorter time frame. The higher number of views results in improved low-contrast detectability, while the shorter scan time reduces the chance of artifacts due to patient motion, breathing, or peristalsis.

Contrast resolution characterizes a C-arm CT system's capacity to resolve soft tissue differences. For good low-contrast imaging results, it is advantageous to acquire a high number of views, because this reduces streak artifacts. To further reduce noise in applications such as head scans, an additional option may be to increase system dose.

With a properly selected image acquisition protocol, state-of-the-art C-arm CT systems such as *syngo* DynaCT (Siemens AG, Healthcare Sector, Forchheim, Germany) can at least resolve 5-mm (10-mm) diameter objects with a contrast difference of 10 HU (5 HU) (FAHRIG et al. 2006). Even better results are sometimes possible as demonstrated in Fig. 3.5. From a clinical point of view, the low-contrast imaging performance of today's C-arm systems not only can be expected to differentiate between fat and muscle tissue, but C-arm CT can also resolve smaller contrast differences and possibly even visualize bleeds.

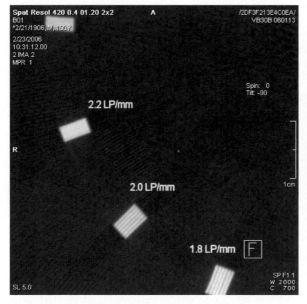

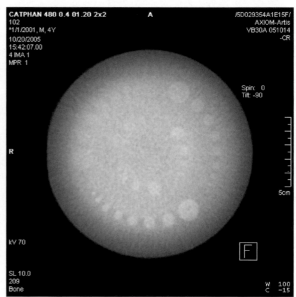

**Fig. 3.4.** Spatial resolution experiment involving an axial slice through a spatial resolution phantom. The 3D spatial resolution from 2D X-ray projections acquired with a Trixell Pixium 4700 detector is about 2.0 LP/mm, if 2 × 2-pixel binning is applied. Projection data were acquired on an Artis **zee** C-arm system, and reconstruction was performed with *syngo* DynaCT (both Siemens AG, Healthcare Sector, Forchheim, Germany)

**Fig. 3.5.** C-arm CT reconstruction of the CTP515 CATPHAN image quality segment (Phantom Laboratory, Salem, NY) using *syngo* DynaCT (Siemens AG, Healthcare Sector, Forchheim, Germany). A 10-mm-thick MPR slice is shown. It comprises low-contrast-equivalent insets with a density difference of 10 HU (5 o'clock to 8 o'clock), 5 HU (1 o'clock to 4 o'clock), and 3 HU (9 o'clock to 12 o'clock). The diameters of the individual insets are 15, 9, 8, 7, 6, 5, 4, 3, and 2 mm, respectively. The 3D data set was reconstructed from 538 raw input projections acquired on an Artis **zee** system at 70 kV tube voltage (Siemens AG, Healthcare Sector, Forchheim, Germany). The associated weighted CT dose index ($CTDI_w$) was 50 mGy

## Applications

### 3.3.1
### Interventional Imaging Using C-Arm CT

#### 3.3.1.1
#### Neurovascular Imaging

Two-dimensional digital subtraction angiography (DSA) is still considered a gold-standard imaging technique for diagnostic and therapeutic imaging of intracranial vessels. One of DSA's advantages is its superb spatial resolution. Today, however, many clinicians often rely on 3D C-arm imaging as well-at least for complex cases. In fact, several studies comparing 2D DSA to 3D C-arm imaging concluded that 3D images can offer more detailed anatomical information for the therapy of intracranial aneurysms than 2D DSA (Hoff et al. 1994; Tu et al. 1996; Missler et al. 2000; Sugahara et al. 2002; Hochmuth et al. 2002). In addition to providing more information about the aneurysm neck, the available 3D geometry can also be used to find optimal C-arm working views (Anxionnat et al. 2001; Mitschke and Navab

2000). This is illustrated in Fig. 3.6 for a lobulated intracranial aneurysm. Once a proper view orientation has been found by interactively inspecting a rendered volume, the C-arm can be automatically positioned at the selected view angle for 2D imaging. On *syngo* X-workplace systems (Siemens AG, Healthcare Sector, Forchheim, Germany), a little blue icon is used to denote C-arm positions that can be reached safely. A red icon indicates that the C-arm cannot be aligned with a certain volume-rendered view due to collision control or mechanical constraints.

When using 3D C-arm imaging for the visualization of stents, physicians again found that access to 3D information during the intervention facilitated better clinical outcomes (VAN DEN BERG et al. 2002; BENNDORF et al. 2005, 2006; RICHTER et al. 2007a). BENNDORF et al., for example, valued the clear visualization of both the stent struts and their adaptation to arterial walls and aneurismal lumen.

Another important C-arm CT application in the brain is tumor imaging. For example, intra-arterially contrast-enhanced 3D C-arm imaging can reveal both vascularity and blood supply of a meningioma of the olfactory groove, as illustrated in Fig. 3.7a–c. An axial slice is displayed in Fig. 3.7a, a sagittal cross-section is

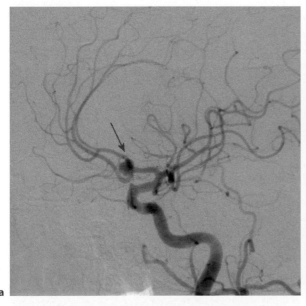
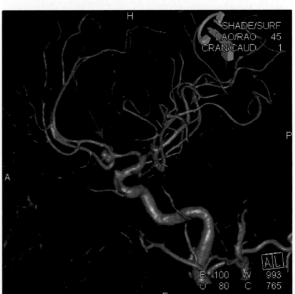

a    b

**Fig. 3.6a,b.** View-aligned DSA and C-arm CT data sets. C-arm systems can be brought into proper 2D working views by rendering a 3D data set interactively under various orientations, choosing the most suitable view, and initiating an automatic C-arm move. This is displayed for a DSA sequence (**a**) and a volume rerendered 3D vessel tree (**b**) depicting a lobulated intracranial aneurysm (*red arrow*). Images were acquired on an AXIOM Artis dBA system and reconstructed on a *syngo* X-workplace running *syngo* DynaCT (all Siemens AG, Healthcare Sector, Forchheim, Germany). DSA sequence and 3D vessel tree are both seen under LAO/RAO = 45° and CRAN/CAUD = 1° (images courtesy of Prof. Knauth, Department of Neuroradiology, University Göttingen, Germany)

shown in Fig. 3.7b, and a coronal cut through the lesion can be found in Fig. 3.7c, respectively. A volume rendered display is presented in Fig. 3.7d. This information can be useful to determine the best treatment option. The C-arm CT images were obtained with *syngo* DynaCT running on a *syngo* X-workplace (both Siemens AG, Healthcare Sector, Forchheim, Germany). X-ray projections were acquired on an AXIOM Artis dBA angiography system (Siemens AG, Healthcare Sector, Forchheim, Germany).

### 3.3.1.2
### Abdominal Imaging

Besides endovascular treatments in the brain, C-arm CT is also well suited to support abdominal applications. In fact, C-arm CT has already received considerable attention for minimally invasive liver tumor treatments. Innovative therapeutic approaches, such as local chemotherapy, chemoembolization, or selective internal radiation therapy (SIRT), may all benefit,

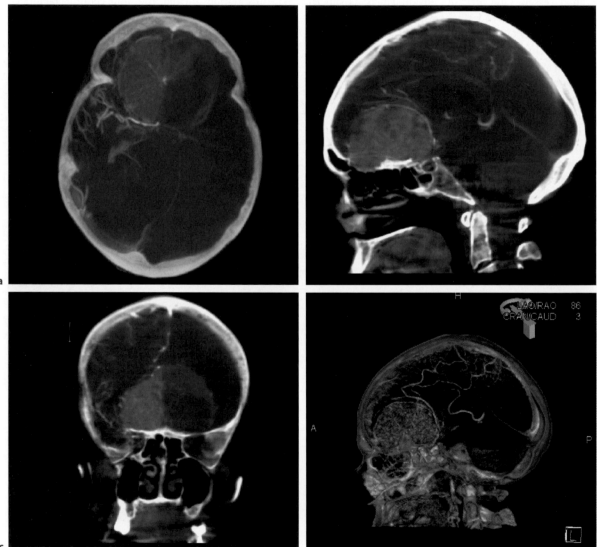

**Fig. 3.7a–d.** C-arm CT images showing a meningioma of the olfactory groove: axial (**a**), sagittal (**b**), coronal cross-section (**c**), and volume rendered display (**d**). The C-arm CT results were obtained with *syngo* DynaCT running on a *syngo* X-workplace (both Siemens AG, Healthcare Sector, Forchheim, Germany). X-ray projections were acquired on an AXIOM Artis dBA angiography system (images courtesy of Prof. Doerfler, Department of Neuroradiology, University Erlangen-Nuremberg, Germany)

because C-arm CT can be used to image both feeder vessels and soft tissue. For example, MEYER et al. recently presented five cases involving abdominal transarterial chemoembolization in which C-arm CT had a considerable impact on the course of the treatment (MEYER et al. 2007). Based on their experience, MEYER et al. (2007) concluded that C-arm CT has the potential to expedite any interventional procedure that requires three-dimensional information and navigation. Similarly, WALLACE et al. (2007) found that C-arm CT

provided additional imaging information beyond DSA in approximately 60% of all cases. In about 19% of all procedures, procedure management changed. When VIRMANI et al. (2007) investigated the usefulness of C-arm CT for transcatheter arterial chemoembolization (TACE) of unresectable liver tumors, they observed that 3D C-arm imaging led to different catheter positions in 39% of all cases, while improving the diagnostic confidence in 78% of all patients.

Another procedure that can benefit from 2D and 3D X-ray imaging is uterine fibroid embolization. In addition to 2D fluoroscopic imaging for catheter guidance, C-arm CT can confirm blood supply to fibroids in 3D as well. This is illustrated in Fig. 3.8. Data sets were generated on an Artis **zeego** system (Siemens AG, Healthcare Sector, Forchheim, Germany). Figure 3.8a was obtained with the catheter in the left uterine artery revealing blood supply to two fibroids. Figure 3.8a also demonstrates single-run C-arm CT volume coverage. Figure 3.8b, on the other hand, was acquired using Artis **zeego**'s large-volume scan mode involving two scans with the detector positioned such that it captures one half of an X-ray projection in one run and the remaining half in the other. For this data set, the catheter was placed in the right uterine artery to confirm if it also supplies blood to the fibroids or not. The Artis **zeego**'s large-volume C-arm CT imaging mode increases the width of the field-of-view from 25 cm, displayed in Fig. 3.8a, to 47 cm, illustrated in Fig. 3.8b. Figure 3.8b demonstrates that large-volume *syngo* DynaCT (Siemens AG, Healthcare Sector, Forchheim, Germany) provides superior organ coverage.

Additional clinical applications in the body that can benefit from C-arm CT are drainages and punctures. When performing percutaneous biliary drainage procedures, FROEHLICH et al. (2000), for example, found that C-arm CT resulted in decreased procedure and fluoroscopy times. C-arm CT can also be beneficial for complicated transjugular intrahepatic portosystemic shunt cases (SZE et al. 2006). BINKERT et al. (2006) described another successful application for C-arm devices providing both 2D and 3D imaging. They used the 3D cross-sectional information for needle placement and 2D fluoroscopy to perform embolization of translumbar type II endoleaks.

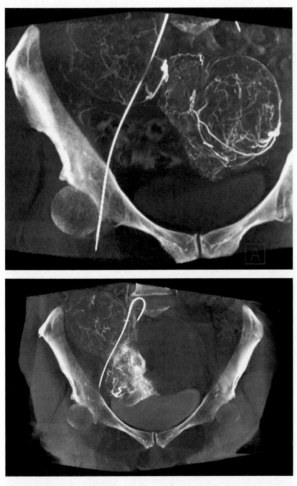

a

b

**Fig. 3.8a,b.** Uterine fibroid embolization. A maximum-intensity-projection (MIP) image of a C-arm CT data set obtained with the catheter in the left uterine artery is shown in (**a**). Another MIP image with the catheter in the right uterine artery is displayed in (**b**). Results were obtained with an Artis **zeego** multi-axis C-arm system (Siemens AG, Healthcare Sector, Forchheim, Germany) using the regular C-arm CT data acquisition mode (**a**) and the large-volume mode (**b**) (images courtesy of Dr. Waggershauser, Department of Clinical Radiology, University of Munich, Germany)

### 3.3.1.3
### Cardiac Imaging

Cardiac imaging for electrophysiology treatments is another promising field for C-arm CT imaging. It can provide accurate morphological information in the interventional suite immediately before, during, and after an ablation procedure, whereas preoperative CT images may be limited in accuracy due to changes in anatomical heart structures over time.

First clinical results obtained with *syngo* DynaCT Cardiac (Siemens AG, Healthcare Sector, Forchheim, Germany) are shown in Fig. 3.9a–d. Three multiplanar reformatted images are displayed with a slice thickness of 2.1 mm. They illustrate important anatomical structures, such as the four heart chambers (Fig. 3.9a) and the left ventricle together with the ascending aorta and the aortic valve (Fig. 3.9b). In this case, even a coronary artery could be successfully imaged, as shown in Fig. 3.9c. A volume rendered posterior view of the contrast-enhanced heart is displayed in Fig. 3.9d. There, the esophagus was enhanced using barium (see yellow arrow) to obtain information about its position relative to the left atrium.

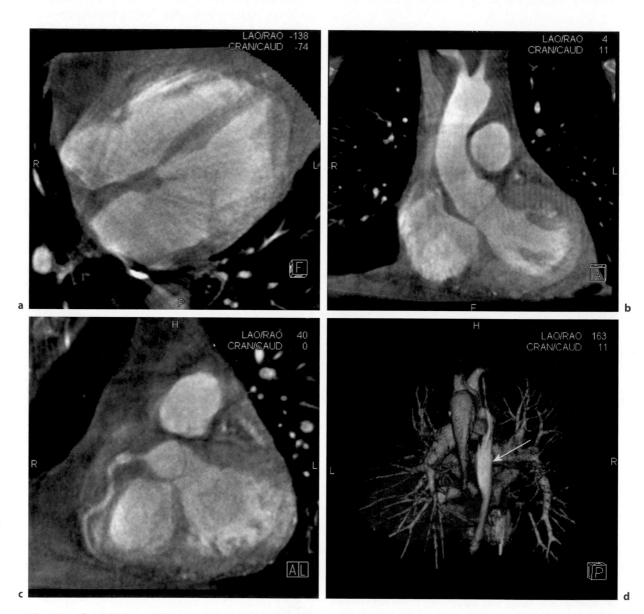

**Fig. 3.9a–d.** Multiplanar reformatted images (*MPRs*) reconstructed using an ECG-based multi-segment C-arm CT technique such as *syngo* DynaCT Cardiac (Siemens AG, Healthcare Sector, Forchheim, Germany). Images are rendered with a slice thickness of 2.1 mm. A four-chamber view is shown in the upper left (**a**). The left ventricle, ascending aorta, and aortic valve can be found in the *upper right* (**b**). In the *lower left*, the proximal right coronary artery is depicted (**c**). A volume rendered posterior 3D view of the contrast-enhanced heart is displayed in the *lower right* (**d**). The *yellow arrow* points to the barium-enhanced esophagus (images courtesy of Prof. Brachmann and Dr. Nölker, Klinikum Coburg, Germany)

### 3.3.2
### Guidance of Interventional Procedures Using C-Arm CT

In the past, image guidance in the interventional suite has been limited to 2D X-ray fluoroscopic imaging. With the emergence of C-arm CT, however, it is now possible to generate 3D data sets and perform real-time 2D imaging in the same room without having to relocate the patient.

### 3.3.2.1
### Enhanced X-Ray Navigation

Two-dimensional fluoroscopic images, which are usually acquired to guide interventional procedures at very low X-ray dose, offer excellent spatial and temporal resolution. Unfortunately, fluoroscopic images lack both contrast resolution and 3D information. This may cause difficulties when localizing devices with respect to treatment regions. Three-dimensional C-arm CT data sets, on the other hand, can provide both low-contrast resolution and a 3D spatial orientation, but not in real-time. By integrating 2D fluoroscopic imaging with 3D C-arm CT, the strengths of both methods can be combined. The result is an auto-registered (hybrid) system integrating 2D and 3D X-ray imaging.

Since 2D and 3D imaging modalities are mechanically coregistered, 3D C-arm CT data sets can be used for (augmented) real-time visualization of 2D fluoroscopic projections (RICHTER et al. 2007b). This is illustrated in Fig. 3.10. Figure 3.10a depicts a 3D vascular segment (in red) overlaid onto a coiled aneurysm. Fig. 3.10b shows a volume-rendered roadmap with vessels (in light orange) to facilitate guidewire navigation. Since a volume-rendered roadmap can be recomputed in real-time, changes in C-arm viewing angles, source-detector-distance, zoom, and table movements can all be taken into account without any need to acquire another 2D roadmap. From a clinical point of view, volume-rendered roadmapping can reduce the amount of contrast medium administered to a patient and lessen X-ray dose. It can also save some procedure time (SOEDERMAN et al. 2005).

Live 2D fluoroscopy augmented with anatomical overlays derived from C-arm CT data sets can be further enhanced by including an additional treatment plan for instrument guidance. Such a plan can be generated by annotating a C-arm CT data set, e.g., by adding points and drawing lines. This treatment plan can then be superimposed on 2D X-ray projections either together with an anatomical overlay or even without it. Similar to anatomical overlays, the 2D appearance of a treatment plan set up in 3D is also updated whenever the C-arm view orientation changes. This way, an appropriate

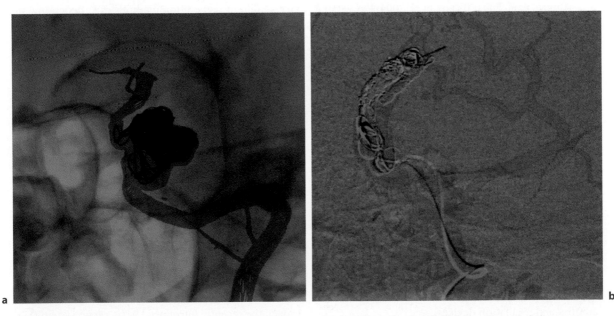

**Fig. 3.10a,b.** Enhanced X-ray navigation: Scene (**a**) depicts a 3D vascular segment (in *red*) overlaid onto a coiled aneurysm. Scene (**b**) shows a volume-rerendered roadmap with vessels (in *orange*). Both results were generated with *syngo* iPilot (Siemens AG, Healthcare Sector, Forchheim, Germany) (images courtesy of Prof. Mawad, Baylor College of Medicine, Department of Radiology, Houston, TX)

overlay view of both anatomy and treatment plan can be obtained under each C-arm projection angle.

An interesting clinical application that can benefit from the use of graphical treatment plans is percutaneous needle guidance. The advantage of using a C-arm system for percutaneous needle procedures is superior access to bigger patients and better support for complex, double-oblique needle trajectories. To set up a treatment plan, the physician specifies a target point and a needle trajectory in 3D first. To this end, a C-arm CT data set may be used. In the next step, the C-arm is moved into a bull's eye view (down-the-barrel view) that aligns X-ray view orientation and needle path. This view orientation is used to insert the needle. After the needle has been placed, the C-arm is driven back and forth between two suitably chosen progression views to monitor needle advancement. If needed, C-arm CT data sets can be generated throughout the procedure to confirm the needle position in 3D. If a thin slice is sufficient, narrow collimation may be preferable as it reduces patient dose. Needle guidance for C-arm systems is commercially available as iGuide (Siemens AG, Healthcare Sector, Forchheim, Germany) or XperGuide (Philips Healthcare, Andover, MA).

One challenge for X-ray guidance involving C-arm CT volume data is that the relation between the 3D data sets and the 2D projection images needs to be maintained at all times. This requires stabilizing or tracking the patient. However, if misalignment does occur, then 2D-3D registration algorithms are available to correct for it (Byrne et al. 2004; Baert et al. 2004; Pruemmer et al. 2006).

### 3.3.2.2
### Electromagnetic Navigation / Tracking (EMT)

Electromagnetic (EM) tracking (EMT) systems receive an increasing amount of attention in interventional radiology. These tracking systems use a transmitter located in the vicinity of the patient. It houses several coils generating a complex EM field that extends to some 50 cm in front of the device. If a small coil (position sensor) is brought into the EM field, the voltage induced can be used to calculate sensor position and orientation. With modern systems, a position accuracy of around 1 mm can be achieved. Positions sensors are usually located in the tip of interventional instruments, e.g., needles used for biopsy, drainage, vertebroplasty, or radiofrequency ablation devices.

The workflow of an electromagnetically navigated intervention is as follows. First, the patient is placed on the table of the C-arm CT system possibly immobilized

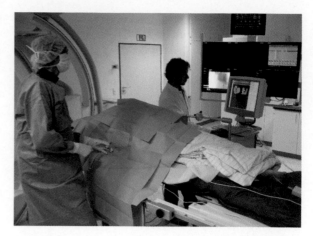

**Fig. 3.11.** Typical setup of an electromagnetic (*EM*) navigation system. The transmitter, held by the flexible arm shown in the *center* of the image, is placed underneath sterile covers. Since the needle has an integrated localization sensor, the tracking system can show its position inside a registered C-arm CT data set. The 3D data was generated with an AXIOM Artis dBA C-arm system (Siemens AG, Healthcare Sector, Forchheim, Germany), while EM navigation was performed with a CAPPA IRAD EMT navigation system (CAS innovations, Erlangen, Germany) (image courtesy of Prof. Wacker, Charité, Berlin, Germany)

using a vacuum mattress. In the next step, a C-arm CT data set is generated. Afterwards, the C-arm CT data set is registered to the coordinate system of the tracking device. Different registration methods exist depending on the EM tracking system used (Nagel et al. 2007). After registration, the EM tracking system can display real-time instrument movement within a C-arm CT data set using a graphical instrument representation as shown in Fig. 3.11. It is also possible to mark target and skin entry point in the 3D data set and, based on this information, use EMT to navigate the needle to the desired position. Initial clinical results obtained for percutaneous procedures have demonstrated that EM navigation based on C-arm CT data sets can be safe and effective (Nagel et al. 2008).

### 3.4
### Future Perspectives of C-Arm CT

The technical progress in C-arm CT is going to continue. In fact, the recently introduced Artis **zeego** system (Siemens AG, Healthcare Sector, Forchheim, Germany) already provides a glimpse into the future of advanced C-arm devices. Based on a new multi-axis platform combined with a light-weight C-arm, these systems are not only going to offer better patient access, but they will also support faster, more flexible image acquisition trajectories for increased 3D coverage. Latest C-arm gantry designs together with further optimized X-ray generation components, more advanced flat detectors, and increasingly sophisticated 3D reconstruction algorithms will improve C-arm CT image quality beyond what is currently available. Since navigation techniques and instruments are continuously upgraded as well, it seems safe to predict that future C-arm systems are going to be integrated medical devices seamlessly combining high-quality C-arm CT with 2D live imaging and device navigation for therapy planning, guidance, and outcome assessment all in the interventional suite.

## Acknowledgements

We would like to thank Angelika Hench and Sabine Wich for their help with the clinical image data sets.

## References

Aichinger H, Dierker J, Joite-Barfuß S, et al. (2004) Radiation exposure and image quality in X-ray diagnostic radiology-Physical principles and clinical applications. Springer, Heidelberg Berlin New York

Antonuk LE, El-Mohri Y, Siewerdsen JH, et al. (1997) Empirical investigation of the signal performance of a high-resolution, indirect detection, active matrix flat-panel imager (AMFPI) for fluoroscopic and radiographic operation. Med Phys 24 :51–70

Anxionnat R, Bracard S, Ducrocq X, et al. (2001) Intracranial aneurysms: Clinical value of 3D digital subtraction angiography in the therapeutic decision and endovascular treatment. Radiology 218:799–808

Baert SAM, Penney GP, van Walsum T, et al. (2004) Precalibration versus 2D-3D registration for 3D guide wire display in endovascular interventions. In: Medical Image Computing and Computer-Assisted Intervention–MICCAI, pp 577–584

Balter S, Banckwitz R, Joite-Barfuß S, et al. (2005) Protocol for evaluating CT reconstructions acquired on an angiographic C-arm. Biomedizinische Technik 50 (Suppl 1, part 1):475–476

Bani-Hashemi A, Navab N, Nadar M, et al. (1998) Interventional 3D-angiography: calibration, reconstruction and visualization system. In: Navab N (ed) Fourth IEEE Workshop on Applications of Computer Vision, 1998. WACV '98. Proceedings, pp. 246–247

Barrett HH, Swindell W (1981) Radiological Imaging. Academic Press, New York

Becker CR, Schätzl M, Feist H, et al. (1998) Radiation dose for investigation of the chest and abdomen. Comparison of sequential, spiral and electron beam computed tomography. Radiologe 38:726–729

Benndorf G, Strother CM, Claus B, et al. (2005) Angiographic CT in cerebrovascular stenting. Am J Neuroradiol 26:1813–1818

Benndorf G, Klucznik RP, Strother CM (2006) Angiographic computed tomography for imaging of underdeployed intracranial stent. Circulation 114 :499–500

Binkert CA, Alencar H, Singh J, et al. (2006) Translumbar type II endoleak repair using angiographic CT. J Vasc Intervent Radiol 17:1349–1353

Bruijns TJC, Bastiaens RJM, Hoornaert B, et al. (2002) Image quality of a large-area dynamic flat detector: comparison with a state-of-the-art II/TV system. In: Medical Imaging 2002: Physics of Medical Imaging. San Diego, pp 332–343

Busse F, Ruetten W, Sandkamp B, et al. (2002) Design and performance of a high-quality cardiac flat detector. In: Medical Imaging 2002: Physics of Medical Imaging. San Diego, CA, pp 819–827

Byrne JV, Colominas C, Hipwell J, et al. (2004) Assessment of a technique for 2D-3D registration of cerebral intra-arterial angiography. Br J Radiol 77:123–128

Choquette M, Demers Y, Shukri Z, et al. (2001) Performance of a real-time selenium-based X-ray detector for fluoroscopy. In: Medical Imaging 2001: Physics of Medical Imaging. San Diego, CA, pp 501–508

Colbeth RE, Boyce SJ, Fong R, et al. (2001) 40×30 cm flat-panel imager for angiography, R&F, and cone-beam CT applications. In: Medical Imaging 2001: Physics of Medical Imaging. San Diego, CA, pp 94–102

Ducourant T, Couder D, Wirth T, et al. (2003) Image quality of digital radiography using flat detector technology. In: Medical Imaging 2003: Physics of Medical Imaging. San Diego, CA, pp 203–214

Fahrig R, Fox AJ, Lownie S, et al. (1997) Use of a C-arm system to generate true three-dimensional computed rotational angiograms: preliminary in vitro and in vivo results. Am J Neuroradiol 18:1507–1514

Fahrig R, Dixon R, Payne T, et al. (2006) Dose and image quality for a cone-beam C-arm CT system. Med Phys 33:4541–4550

Feldkamp L, Davis L, Kress J (1984) Practical cone-beam algorithm. J Opt Soc Am A 1:612–619

Flohr T (2000) Method for post-processing of a tomogram and computed tomography apparatus operating in accordance with the method. US Patent 6047039, Siemens AG, Germany

Froelich JJ, Wagner H-J, Ishaque N, et al. (2000) Comparison of C-arm CT fluoroscopy and conventional fluoroscopy for percutaneous biliary drainage procedures. J Vasc Intervent Radiol 11:477–482

Gies M, Kalender WA, Wolf H, et al. (1999) Dose reduction in CT by anatomically adapted tube current modulation. I. Simulation studies. Med Phys 26:2235–2247

Granfors PR, Albagli D, Tkaczyk JE, et al. (2001) Performance of a flat-panel cardiac detector. In: Medical Imaging 2001: Physics of Medical Imaging. San Diego, CA, pp 77–86

Groh BA, Siewerdsen JH, Drake DG, et al. (2002) A performance comparison of flat-panel imager-based MV and kV cone-beam CT. Med Phy 29:967–975

Heran NS, Song JK, Namba K, et al. (2006) The Utility of DynaCT in neuroendovascular procedures. A J Neuroradiol 27:330–332

Hochmuth A, Spetzger U, Schumacher M (2002) Comparison of three-dimensional rotational angiography with digital subtraction angiography in the assessment of ruptured cerebral aneurysms. Am J Neuroradiol 23:1199–1205

Hoff DJ, Wallace MC, terBrugge KG, et al. (1994) Rotational angiography assessment of cerebral aneurysms. Am J Neuroradiol 15:1945–1948

Hsieh J (2003) Computed Tomography. SPIE Press, Bellingham, WA

Hsieh J, Chao E, Thibault J, et al. (2004) A novel reconstruction algorithm to extend the CT scan field-of-view. Med Phys 31:2385–2391

Jaffray DA, Siewerdsen JH (2000) Cone-beam computed tomography with a flat-panel imager: Initial performance characterization. Med Phys 27:1311–1323

Joseph PM, Spital RD (1978) A method for correcting bone-induced artifacts in computed tomography scanners. J Comp Ass Tomography 2:100–108

Kalender W, Wolf H, Suess C (1999) Dose reduction in CT by anatomically adapted tube current modulation. II. Phantom measurements. Med Phys 26:2248–2253

Kalender W, Kyriakou Y (2007) Flat-detector computed tomography (FD-CT). Eur Radiol 17:2767–2779

Kak AC, Slaney M (1988) Principles of Computerized Tomographic Imaging. IEEE, New York

Koppe R, Klotz E, de Beek JO, et al. (1995) Three-dimensional vessel reconstruction based on rotational angiography. In: Lemke HU, Inamura K, Jaffe CC, et al. (eds) Proc Int Symp Computer Assisted Radiology. Springer, Berlin Heidelberg New York, pp 101–107

Kyriakou Y, Riedel T, Kalender W (2006) Combining deterministic and Monte Carlo calculations for fast estimation of scatter intensities in CT. Phys Med Biol 51:4567–4586

Kyriakou Y, Kalender W (2007) Efficiency of antiscatter grids for flat-detector CT. Phys Med Biol 52:6275–6293

Lauritsch G, Boese J, Wigstrom L, et al. (2006) Towards cardiac C-arm computed tomography. IEEE Transact Med Imaging 25:922–934

McCollough CH, Schueler BA (2000) Calculation of effective dose. Med Phys 27:828–837

McCollough CH (2005) Automatic exposure control in CT: Are we done yet? Radiology 237:755–756

Meyer B, Frericks B, Albrecht T, et al. (2007) Contrast-enhanced abdominal angiographic CT for intra-abdominal tumor embolization: A new tool for vessel and soft tissue visualization. Cardiovasc Intervent Radiol 30:743–749

Missler U, Hundt C, Wiesmann M, et al. (2000) Three-dimensional reconstructed rotational digital subtraction angiography in planning treatment of intracranial aneurysms. Eur Radiol 10:564–568

Mitschke MM, Navab N (2000) Recovering projection geometry: How a cheap camera can outperform an expensive stereo system. CVPR 2000:1193–1200

Moore T, Rohm E (2006) Application protocol book for Artis **zee** 3D applications. Siemens AG

Nagel M, Hoheisel M, Petzold R, et al. (2007) Needle and catheter navigation using electromagnetic tracking for computer-assisted C-arm CT interventions. In: Medical Imaging 2007: Visualization and Image-Guided Procedures. San Diego, CA, pp 65090J

Nagel M, Hoheisel M, Bill U, et al. (2008) Electromagnetic tracking system for minimal invasive interventions using a C-arm system with CT option: First clinical results. In: Medical Imaging 2008: Visualization and Image-Guided Procedures. San Diego, CA, pp 69180G

Nakayama Y, Awai K, Funama Y et al. (2005) Abdominal CT with low tube voltage: Preliminary observations about radiation dose, contrast enhancement, image quality, and noise. Radiology 237:945–951

Navab N, Bani-Hashemi AR, Mitschke MM, et al. (1996) Dynamic geometrical calibration for 3D cerebral angiography. In: Medical Imaging 1996: Physics of Medical Imaging. Newport Beach, CA, pp 361–370

Navab N, Bani-Hashemi A, Nadar M, et al. (1998) Three-dimensional reconstruction from projection matrices in a C-arm based 3D-angiography system. In: Medical image computing and computer-assisted intervention—MICCAI'98, pp 119–129

Ning R, Tang X, Conover DL (2002) X-ray scatter suppression algorithm for cone-beam volume CT. In: Medical Imaging 2002: Physics of Medical Imaging. San Diego, CA, pp 774–781

Ohnesorge B, Flohr T, Schwarz K, et al. (2000) Efficient correction for CT image artifacts caused by objects extending outside the scan field of view. Med Phys 27:39–46

Parker D (1982) Optimal short scan convolution for fanbeam CT. Med Phys 9:254–257

Pruemmer M, Hornegger J, Pfister M, et al. (2006) Multimodal 2D-3D non-rigid registration. In: Medical Imaging 2006: Image Processing. San Diego, CA, pp 61440–61412

Pruemmer M, Fahrig R, Wigstrom L, et al. (2007) Cardiac C-arm CT: 4D non-model based heart motion estimation and its application. In: Medical Imaging 2007: Physics of Medical Imaging. San Diego, CA, pp 651015–651012

Richter G, Engelhorn T, Struffert T, et al. (2007a) Flat panel detector angiographic CT for stent-assisted coil embolization of broad-based cerebral aneurysms. Am J Neuroradiol 28:1902–1908

Richter G, Pfister M, Struffert T, et al. (2007b) Visualization of self-expandable stents using 2D-3D coregistration of angiographic computed tomography data to facilitate stent assisted coil embolization of broad based intracranial aneurysms: in vitro feasibility study. In: 42. Jahrestagung der Deutschen Gesellschaft für Neuroradiologie, Frankfurt am Main

Rinkel J, Gerfault L, Esteve F, et al. (2007) A new method for X-ray scatter correction: First assessment on a cone-beam CT experimental setup. Phys Med Biol 52:4633–4652

Ritter D, Orman J, Schmidgunst C, et al. (2007) Three-dimensional soft tissue imaging with a mobile C-arm. Comput Med Imaging Graphics 31:91–102

Rowlands JA, Yorkston J (2000) Flat panel detectors for digital radiography. In: Metter RLV, Beutel J, Kundel HL (eds) Handbook of Medical Imaging. SPIE Press, Bellingham, WA, pp 223–328

Rougee A, Picard CL, Trousset YL, et al. (1993) Geometrical calibration for 3D X-ray imaging. In: Medical Imaging 1993: Image Capture, Formatting, and Display. Newport Beach, CA, pp 161–169

Rührnschopf E-P, Kalender W (1981) Artifacts caused by non-linear partial volume and spectral hardening effects in computerized tomography. Electromedica 2:96–105

Saint-Felix D, Trousset Y, Picard C, et al. (1994) In vivo evaluation of a new system for 3D computerized angiography. Phys Med Biol 39:583–595

Siewerdsen JH, Jaffray DA (2001) Cone-beam computed tomography with a flat-panel imager: Magnitude and effects of X-ray scatter. Med Phys 28:220–231

Siewerdsen JH, Daly MJ, Bakhtiar B, et al. (2006) A simple, direct method for X-ray scatter estimation and correction in digital radiography and cone-beam CT. Med Phys 33:187–197

Soederman M, Babic D, Homan R, et al. (2005) Three-dimensional roadmap in neuroangiography: Technique and clinical interest. Neuroradiology 47:735–740

Sourbelle K, Kachelriess M, Kalender W (2005) Reconstruction from truncated projections in CT using adaptive detruncation. Eur Radiol 15:1008–1014

Spahn M, Strotzer M, Voelk M, et al. (2000) Digital radiography with a large-area, amorphous-silicon, flat-panel X-ray detector system. Invest Radiol 35:260–266

Starman J, Pelc N, Strobel N, et al. (2005) Estimating $0^{th}$ and $1^{st}$ moments in C-arm CT data for extrapolating truncated projections. In: Medical Imaging 2005: Image Processing. San Diego, CA, pp 378–387

Sugahara T, Korogi Y, Nakashima K, et al. (2002) Comparison of 2D and 3D digital subtraction angiography in evaluation of intracranial aneurysms. Am J Neuroradiol 23:1545–1552

Sze DY, Strobel N, Fahrig R, et al. (2006) Transjugular intrahepatic portosystemic shunt creation in a polycystic liver facilitated by hybrid cross-sectional/angiographic imaging. J Vasc Intervent Radiol 17:711–715

Tu RK, Cohen WA, Maravilla KR, et al. (1996) Digital subtraction rotational angiography for aneurysms of the intracranial anterior circulation: injection method and optimization. Am J Neuroradiol 17:1127–1136

United Nations Scientific Committee on the Effects of Atomic Radiation (UNSCEAR) (2000) Sources and effects of ionizing radiation, vol II: Effects. In: Report to the General Assembly, with scientific annexes. United Nations, Geneva New York

van den Berg JC, Overtoom TTC, de Valois JC, et al. (2002) Using three-dimensional rotational angiography for sizing of covered stents. Am J Roentgenol 178:149–152

Virmani S, Ryu RK, Sato KT, et al. (2007) Effect of C-arm angiographic CT on transcatheter arterial chemoembolization of liver tumors. J Vasc Intervent Radiol 18:1305–1309

Wallace MJ, Murthy R, Kamat PP, et al. (2007) Impact of C-arm CT on hepatic arterial interventions for hepatic malignancies. J Vasc Intervent Radiol 18:1500–1507

Wiesent K, Barth K, Navab N, et al. (2000) Enhanced 3-D-reconstruction algorithm for C-arm systems suitable for interventional procedures. IEEE Transact Med Imaging 19:391–403

Yamazaki T, Tamura T, Nokita M, et al. (2004) Performance of a novel 43-cm × 43-cm flat-panel detector with CsI:Tl scintillator. In: Medical Imaging 2004: Physics of Medical Imaging. San Diego, CA, pp 379–385

Zellerhoff M, Scholz B, Rührnschopf EP, et al. (2005) Low contrast 3D reconstruction from C-arm data. In: Medical imaging 2005: Physics of medical imaging. SPIE, San Diego, CA, pp 646–655

Zhu L, Bennett NR, Fahrig R (2006) Scatter correction method for X-ray CT using primary modulation: Theory and preliminary results. IEEE Transact Med Imaging 25:1573–1587

# Radiation Exposure and Protection in Multislice CT

## 4

Christoph Hoeschen, Dieter Regulla, Maria Zankl,
Helmut Schlattl and Gunnar Brix

## CONTENTS

C. Hoeschen, PhD
Helmholtz Zentrum München, German Research Center
for Environmental Health, Institute of Radiation Protection,
Ingolstädter Landstr. 1, 85764 Neuherberg, Germany

D. Regulla, PhD
Helmholtz Zentrum München, German Research Center
for Environmental Health, Institute of Radiation Protection,
Ingolstädter Landstr. 1, 85764 Neuherberg, Germany

M. Zankl, PhD
Helmholtz Zentrum München, German Research Center
for Environmental Health, Institute of Radiation Protection,
Ingolstädter Landstr. 1, 85764 Neuherberg, Germany

H. Schlattl, PhD
Helmholtz Zentrum München, German Research Center
for Environmental Health, Institute of Radiation Protection,
Ingolstädter Landstr. 1, 85764 Neuherberg, Germany

G. Brix, PhD
Federal Office for Radiation Protection, Department of
Radiation Protection and Health, Ingolstädter Landstr. 1,
85764 Neuherberg, Germany

## ABSTRACT

Technical progress in computed tomography (CT) has substantially increased the clinical efficacy of CT procedures and offered promising new applications in diagnostic imaging. On the other hand, data from various national surveys have confirmed, as a general pattern, the growing impact of CT as a major source of patient and population exposure. From a radiation-hygienic point of view, it is thus necessary to optimize the medical benefit of CT examinations to patients, while strictly controlling and reducing their risk from the radiation exposure. It is the purpose of this chapter to summarize relevant dosimetric concepts for dose assessment in CT, to give an overview on the specific factors determining radiation exposure to patients in MSCT, and to provide suggestions for the optimization of MSCT protocols to balance patient exposure against image quality.

## 4.1
## Introduction–General Remarks on Radiation Exposure Related to Medical Diagnosis

Projection radiography and even more tomographic imaging technologies such as CT are of great importance for the diagnosis of diseases as well as for therapy planning and monitoring. Digital X-ray imaging technologies and the possibilities of fast and large volume data acquisition in multi-slice CT (MSCT) have changed the clinical praxis to a large extent. On the other hand, the technical progress results in a rise of the radiation exposure to patients, although the dose per investigation has been reduced in the last decades. In most health-care level-I countries, medical radiation exposure is now by far the greatest single component of radiation exposure to the population, summing up to as much as the overall radiation exposure coming from natural sources on average.

According to recent studies (RADIOLOGICAL SOCIETY OF NORTH AMERICA 2004; REGULLA and EDER 2005; UNSCEAR 2000), the mean effective dose per person and year in these countries is ranging between 0.4 and 4 mSv, mainly due to exposures from CT, angiographic and interventional investigations. In the USA, for instance, the value of the annual mean exposure *per caput* from medical X-ray examinations has recently been reported to have increased from the long-term value (1980-2000) of 0.5 mSv effective dose to now 3.2 mSv (METTLER 2007).

This trend is obviously ongoing. It corresponds to the development and spreading of new powerful MSCT systems that allow new types of investigations due to their fast acquisition modes. In Germany, for example, the frequency of CT examinations has increased from about four percent of all X-ray examinations in 1997 to about six percent in 2003 (e.g., BRIX et al. 2005; BUNDESAMT FÜR STRAHLENSCHUTZ 2006; REGULLA et al. 2003). As a consequence, CT is currently causing more than 50% of the annual mean effective dose administered to individual members of the public due to medical X-ray procedures.

The effective doses of a single patient from CT examinations can vary between about a few millisieverts up to more than 100 mSv. Effective doses below 100 mSv are classified as low-dose applications (BEIR VII; COMMITTEE TO ASSESS HEALTH RISKS FROM EXPOSURE TO LOW LEVELS OF IONIZING RADIATION; NUCLEAR AND RADIATION STUDIES BOARD 2006). On the other hand, it is worth noticing that effective doses in the range of 5 to 50 mSv are comparable, with the lowest range of exposures for persons among the atomic bomb survivors. In this dose range, stochastic radiation risks are of relevance. In accordance with recent recommendations of international bodies such as the ICRP (International Commission on Radiological Protection; ICRP 2007a), it is assumed that the risk is proportional to the radiation dose (linear non-threshold hypothesis). Despite the broad discussions concerning the harm of low radiation doses to humans (BRECKOW 2006; BRENNER and SACHS 2006; TRABALKA and KOCHER 2007; WAMBERSIE et al. 2005), this hypothesis provides a conservative approach for risk assessment.

## General Radiation Protection Principles and Their Applicability to Medical X-Ray Diagnosis

Radiation protection is governed by three fundamental principles that are designed to establish a level of protection based on what is deemed acceptable (ICRP 2007a). These principles are: justification, optimization of protection, and application of dose limits. In the following, the meaningfulness of these principles in medical X-ray diagnosis–in particular, MSCT–is discussed:

Justification: "Any decision that alters the radiation exposure situation should do more good than harm" (ICRP 2007a). This means that the potential benefits of a CT examination must be balanced against the individual detriment that may be caused by radiation exposure. There must be sufficient net benefit for the individual patient, considering the efficacy, benefits and risks of available alternative imaging techniques that involve no exposure to ionizing radiation or result in lower patient doses.

Optimization of protection: "The likelihood of incurring exposures, the number of people exposed, and the magnitude of their individual doses should all be kept as low as reasonably achievable, taking into account economic and societal factors" (ICRP 2007a). This means that examinations have to be optimized in order to define an acceptable balance between patient exposure and necessary diagnostic image quality.

Application of Dose Limits–Diagnostic Reference Levels: "The total dose to any individual from regulated sources in planned exposure situations other than medical exposure of patients should not exceed the appropriate limits" (ICRP 2007a): this means that a clearly justified medical examination employing ionizing radiation is not limited by a specific dose value. The explicit exemption of medical exposure from the principle of dose limitation is owed both to the assumption that medical exposures are generally for the benefit of the patient and the perception that medical diagnostic procedures may lead to comparatively high doses to individual patients, e.g., when interventional procedures are considered. However, it is also recognized that the magnitude of patient exposures varies considerably among different radiological departments due to both equipment and skill of the personnel. Therefore, the ICRP recommends in its publication on 'Radiological Protection and Safety in Medicine' (ICRP 1996) the use of Diagnostic Reference Levels (DRLs) for patient examinations as a measure of adequacy of protection. The DRLs apply to an easily measurable operational dose quantity and are intended for use as a simple test for identifying situations where the levels of patient dose are unusually high. If patient doses related to a specific procedure are consistently exceeding the corresponding DRL, there should be a local review of the procedures and equipment. Measures aimed at the reduction of dose levels should be taken, if necessary. The COUNCIL OF THE EUROPEAN UNION (1997) has adopted this concept in the Council Directive 97/43/EURATOM. By this means, the member states of the EU are obliged to adopt the DRLs into national legislation and regulations concerning radiation protection in medical diagnostics (for Germany: Bundesamt für Strahlenschutz 2003).

## 4.3
## How to Quantify Radiation Exposure to Patients Related to CT Examinations

### 4.3.1
### Fundamental Dose Quantities

The most comprehensive way to quantify the exposure of a patient undergoing a specific investigation is to determine a dose for each organ. The absorbed dose averaged over an organ is called the organ dose. However, the complexity inherent to a large number of dose values makes it difficult to compare patient doses from different investigations or even different equipment. For such a comparison, it is desirable to have one single value–the effective dose, $E$.

This dosimetric quantity is defined by a weighted sum of organ (or tissue) equivalent doses[1] as

$$E = \sum_T w_T H_T \qquad (1)$$

where $w_T$ is the tissue-weighting factor for tissue $T$, $H_T$ the equivalent dose of tissue $T$, and $\sum w_T = 1$ (ICRP 1991). The sum is performed over all organs and tissues of the human body considered to be sensitive to the induction of stochastic radiation effects. The $w_T$ values are chosen to represent the contributions of individual organs and tissues to overall radiation detriment from

stochastic effects. The organs and tissues for which tissue weighting factors are specified are given in Table 4.1. As indicated, these factors have recently been changed for some organs. All effective dose values given in this chapter are computed with the weighting factors specified in 1991 (ICRP 1991).

Although introduced for radiological protection of workers and the general public, the "effective dose can be of value for comparing doses from different diagnostic procedures and for comparing the use of similar technologies and procedures in different hospitals and countries as well as the use of different technologies for the same medical examination. However, for planning the exposure of patients and risk-benefit assessments, the equivalent dose or the absorbed dose to irradiated tissues is the relevant quantity" (ICRP 2007a). Potential applications of this quantity in patient dosimetry should therefore be confined to the above considerations, and the limitations of this quantity concerning personalized dosimetry have to be kept in mind.

### 4.3.2
### Determination of Organ and Tissue Doses

In general, organ doses cannot be measured directly; they have to be calculated by radiation transport simulations, mostly using Monte Carlo techniques and computational models of the human body. The results of these calculations are so-called organ dose conversion coefficients, i.e., mean organ doses normalized to a measurable dose quantity, such as the *CTDI* (see below).

In the past, dose estimates have been based upon schematic representations of the human body where the shape of the body and its internal organs are described by relatively simple geometric bodies such as spheres, ellipsoids, elliptical cylinders and parts and combinations thereof (CRISTY and ECKERMAN 1987; SNYDER et al. 1978). Using these "mathematical" models, various radiation protection organizations around the world have simulated X-ray examinations to determine organ dose conversion coefficients (DREXLER et al. 1990; HART et al. 1994a, b; ROSENSTEIN 1976, 1992; STERN et al. 1995; WALL 2004). During the last 2 decades, voxel models were introduced that are derived mostly from (whole-body) medical image data of real persons. Examples of voxel models are shown in Fig. 4.1. Typically, they represent realistic models of the human anatomy and offer a clear improvement compared to the mathematical models whose organs are described by relatively simple geometrical bodies. As a consequence, the dose coefficients estimated for voxel models deviate system-

---

1 The equivalent dose, $H$, is the absorbed dose, $D$, multiplied with a radiation weighting factor. For photons and electrons of all energies, the radiation weighting factor is equal to unity, and absorbed doses and equivalent doses are numerically identical.

**Table 4.1.** Tissue-weighting factors, $w_T$, given by the ICRP in 1991 (ICRP 1991) and 2007 (ICRP 2007a) reflecting the relative susceptibility of various tissues and organs to ionizing radiation

| Tissue or organ | $w_T$ |
|---|---|
| **ICRP 1991** | |
| Gonads | 0.20 |
| Bone marrow, lungs, colon, stomach | 0.12 |
| Liver, thyroid, esophagus, breast, bladder | 0.05 |
| Bone surface, skin | 0.01 |
| Remainder tissues[a] | 0.05 |
| **ICRP 2007** | |
| Bone marrow (red), colon, lung, stomach, breast, remainder tissues[b] | 0.12 |
| Gonads | 0.08 |
| Bladder, esophagus, liver, thyroid, | 0.04 |
| Bone surface, brain, salivary glands, skin | 0.01 |

The remainder tissues consist of a group of additional organs and tissues with a lower sensitivity for radiation-induced effects for which the average dose must be used:

[a] Small intestine, brain, spleen, muscle tissue, adrenals, kidneys, pancreas, thymus and uterus, extrathoracic region

[b] Adrenals, extrathoracic region, gall bladder, heart, kidneys, lymphatic nodes, muscle, oral mucosa, pancreas, prostate, small intestine, spleen, thymus, uterus/cervix

atically from those calculated for mathematical models (Zankl et al. 2002, Schlattl et al. 2007, Winslow et al. 2004).

### 4.3.3
### Measurable Dose Quantities in CT

The dosimetric quantities typically used in CT are the "CT dose index" (*CTDI*) and the "dose length product" (*DLP*). The *CTDI* is defined for an axial CT scan (one rotation of the X-ray tube) by dividing the integral of the absorbed dose along the *z* axis by the nominal beam width. As shown in Fig. 4.2, this value is equivalent to the dose within the nominal width of the slice assuming that the absorbed dose has a rectangular profile with a constant dose inside the nominal width and zero dose outside.

The *CTDI* is measured either free in air (*CTDI*$_{air}$) or in a specified phantom made of PMMA. Different phantom sizes are used to reflect differences in body anatomy. This is mainly realized by different phantom diameters (16-cm diameter for head investigations, 32-cm diameter for body investigations). In practice, *CTDI* measurements are usually performed with a pencil ionization chamber with an active length of 100 mm, which is positioned at the center (*CTDI*$_{100,c}$) and at the periphery (*CTDI*$_{100,p}$) of either a standard head or body CT dosimetry phantom. On the assumption that the dose decreases linearly with the radial position from the surface to the center of the phantom, the average dose is given by the "weighted *CTDI*" (*CTDI*$_w$) that is a weighted linear combination of the central and peripheral *CTDI* values:

$$CTDI_w = \frac{1}{3}CTDI_{100,c} + \frac{2}{3}CTDI_{100,p}. \qquad (2)$$

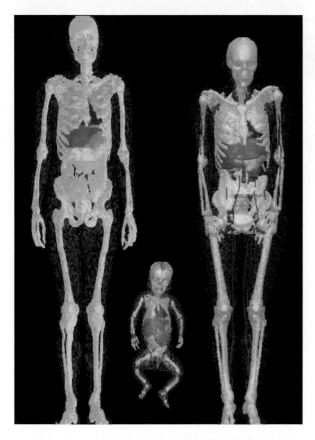

**Fig. 4.1.** Three voxel phantoms of a man (*left*), baby (*middle*), and woman (*right*) developed by the Helmholtz Zentrum München, German Research Center for Environmental Health (Fill et al. 2004; Petoussi-Henss et al. 2002; Zankl et al. 2002)

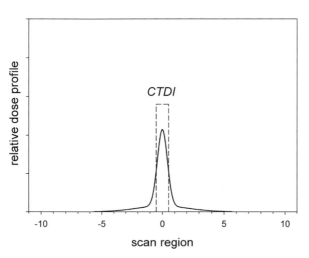

**Fig. 4.2.** Schematic presentation of the meaning of the normalized *CTDI*

The *CTDI* is directly proportional to the electrical current-time product (i.e., charge, $Q_{el}$, in mAs) chosen for the scan; when the *CTDI* is divided by the $Q_{el}$ value, it is called "normalized *CTDI*" (n*CTDI*). $CTDI_w$ values have to be measured for all combinations of tube potentials (*U* in kV) and slice collimations that can be realized at the specific type of scanner, but only for a fixed $Q_{el}$ value. It should be noted that the $CTDI_w$ is a system specific parameter from which neither a value for a patient dose nor the dose requirements of a system can be deduced directly, without additional knowledge of specific scan parameters, such as collimation and number of rotations.

According to the revised IEC standard 60601-2-44, the dose quantity displayed at the operator's console of a CT system is the "volume *CTDI*."

$$CTDI_{Vol} = \frac{CTDI_w}{p}, \qquad (3)$$

where *p* is the pitch, i.e., the ratio of table feed per gantry rotation and the total beam collimation *h*. The $CTDI_{vol}$ is the principal dose descriptor in CT, reflecting not only the combined effect of the scan parameters $Q_{el}$, *U*, *p*, and *h* on the local dose level, but also of scanner specific factors, such as beam filtration, beam-shaping filter, geometry, and overbeaming (see below). The volume *CTDI* ($CTDI_{vol}$) describes the average local dose for the patient within the volume of investigation given in mGy.

A better representation of the overall energy delivered by a given scan protocol is the dose-length product (*DLP*) that is the volume *CTDI* multiplied with the total scan length, $L_{tot}$:

$$DLP = CTDI_{Vol} \cdot L_{tot} \qquad (4)$$

According to the "European Guidelines on Quality Criteria for CT" (European Commission 1999), DRLs for CT examinations are given in terms of $CTDI_w$ or $CTDI_{vol}$ and *DLP*. DRLs valid in Germany for some of the most frequent CT examinations are listed in Table 4.2.

### 4.3.4
### Determination of the Effective Dose from Device and Scan Parameters

A simple, but coarse estimation of effective dose can be derived from the *DLP* using representative conversion coefficients provided by the ICRP (ICRP 2007b):

$$E = k \cdot DLP, \qquad (5)$$

**Table 4.2.** Diagnostic Reference Levels for some CT investigations of adults, valid in Germany since 2003

| CT investigation | $CTDI_w$ [mGy] | $CTDI_{Vol}$ [mGy] | $DLP$ [mGy × cm] |
|---|---|---|---|
| Brain | 60 | 60 | 1,050 |
| Face and sinuses | 35 | 28 | 360 |
| Thoracic scan | 22 | 17 | 650 |
| Abdominal scan | 24 | 19 | 1,500 |
| Pelvis | 28 | 23 | 750 |
| Upper abdomen | 25 | 20 | 770 |
| Lumbar spine | 47 | 44 | 280 |

where $k$ are conversion coefficients (in $mSv \cdot mGy^{-1} \cdot cm^{-1}$), depending on the scanned body region and patient size (respectively age). Some values of $k$ for adult patients are presented in Table 4.3.

Alternatively, and based on the above quantities, one can calculate all relevant parameters for dose estimates from the scan parameters and some system-specific components. The basic principle is summarized in Table 4.4. In the first column the needed or calculated parameters are described; the corresponding symbols are given in column 2, while in column 3 the appropriate units are specified. (To achieve meaningful results, it is indispensable to express the quantities in their correct units. If required, suitable conversions from other units

have to be made prior to applying respective values in the following calculation scheme.)

There are various software tools commercially available that can be used to estimate organ and effective dose values for a variety of CT protocols and scanners from measured $CTDI_A$ values (BRIX et al. 2004; STAMM et al., VAMP). The user should make sure, however, to employ software versions that cover the special aspects of MSCT discussed in the following. Table 4.5 summarizes representative dose values determined in a nationwide survey in Germany for the most common tyes of CT examinations (BRIX et al. 2003).

### 4.3.5
### Special Aspects of MSCT

The larger acquisition volumes per rotation in multislice compared to single-slice CT results in considerably shorter scan times. The resulting improvement in scanner performance has not only increased the clinical efficacy of CT procedures, but also offered promising new applications in diagnostic imaging due to a reduction of motion artifacts compared to single-slice CT. On the other hand, the radiologist may be tempted to scan a larger body region than necessary or to apply imaging protocols resulting in the best attainable image quality to every patient. However, larger scan ranges and, usually, higher image quality are connected with higher patient doses. For instance, a lower pitch corresponds typically to a higher image quality, but also to a higher dose to the patient. On the other hand, and in view of the requested optimization of protection, the radiologist is obliged to apply the lowest dose resulting in an

**Table 4.3.** Normalized effective dose per dose-length product (*DLP*) for adults (standard physique) for various body regions (ICRP 2007b)

| Body region | $k$ ($mSv \cdot mGy^{-1} \cdot cm^{-1}$) |
|---|---|
| Head and neck | 0.0031 |
| Head | 0.0021 |
| Neck | 0.0059 |
| Chest | 0.014 |
| Abdomen and pelvis | 0.015 |
| Trunk | 0.015 |

**Table 4.4.** Calculation scheme for determining patient doses from device-specific and measurable quantities (example values mostly from STAMM et al.)

| Quantity | Symbol | Unit | Example |
|---|---|---|---|
| Current | $I$ | mA | 120 |
| × Time | $t$ | s | 1.5 |
| = Charge | $Q$ | mAs | 180 |
| × Normalized $CTDI$ in air | $_nCTDI_A$ | mGy/mAs | 0.2 |
| × Correction for beam quality [a] | $k_V$ | 1 | $(140/120)^2$ |
| = Dose at axis free in air | $CTDI_A$ | mGy | 49 |
| × Collimation (# rows × thickness of rows) | $h$ | cm | 2.1 |
| × Number of rotations | $N$ | 1 | 10 |
| = Dose length product (free in air) | $DLP_A$ | mGy cm | 1,029 |
| × Conversion factor [b] | $fav$ | mSv/(mGy cm) | 0.01 |
| × System correction factor [c] | $kCT$ | 1 | 0.8 |
| × Correction for beam quality [d] | $kV,2$ | 1 | $(140/120)^{1/2}$ |
| = Effective dose | $E$ | mSv | 8.9 |

[a] $k_V$ is the square of the ratio of the tube voltage at which the examination is performed to the tube voltage where the $CTDI$ measurements have been performed

[b] Effective dose conversion coefficient for the examined body region (e.g., STAMM et al.)

[c] Device-specific parameter

[d] $k_{V,2}$ is the square root of the ratio of the tube voltage at which the examination is performed to the tube voltage where the conversion coefficients $f_{av}$ have been calculated

image quality (determined by slice thickness, slice resolution, pitch, noise and contrast) with which a reliable diagnosis is possible. In the following, different aspects that have to be considered in MSCT imaging are discussed.

*Resolution:* In order to keep the statistical noise level constant, considerably higher doses are required for higher resolution. For instance, halving the slice thickness requires a four times higher radiation dose for the patient to keep the noise level constant. On the other hand, the so-called partial volume effect, which leads to a reduced contrast for details smaller than the slice thickness, is reduced with decreasing slice thicknesses. That means, if small details are considered, an increase of the slice resolution by a factor of two would not require a four times higher radiation dose to keep the contrast-to-noise ratio constant. Unfortunately, this is not true for larger objects; therefore, in most cases the required dose for the whole scan volume is indeed larger with smaller slice thicknesses. (In principle, the same relations hold for both dimensions of the in-plane resolution. However, higher in-plane resolution is not a consequence of MSCT technology, but of contemporary faster reconstruction computers and higher-resolution detectors.)

*Overscanning:* Using a spiral scan technique, an additional half turn at both ends of the scan volume of interest is required to acquire sufficient data for the image reconstruction. However, only a fraction of this additional data can be used for the reconstruction. As a consequence, the body region exposed to ionizing radiation is larger than the imaged body region. Since the number of detector rows and the scanned volume per rotation is larger in MSCT than in single-slice CT, the amount of the additional radiation exposure is higher in MSCT (VEIT et al. 2005). Figure 4.3 illustrates how the effective

**Table 4.5.** Typical dose values from MSCT examinations, as determined in a nationwide survey performed in Germany in 2002 (BRIX et al. 2003)

| Examinations | Dose values per scan | | |
|---|---|---|---|
| Type | $CTDI_{vol}$ (mGy) | DLP (mGy cm) | E (mSv) |
| Brain | 60.6 | 813 | 2.2 |
| Face and sinuses | 26.7 | 272 | 0.8 |
| Face and neck | 14.4 | 288 | 1.9 |
| Chest | 10.9 | 339 | 5.5 |
| Abdomen and pelvis | 12.6 | 529 | 9.7 |
| Pelvis | 14.8 | 349 | 6.3 |
| Liver/kidney | 12.8 | 292 | 5.5 |
| Whole trunk | 12.8 | 836 | 14.5 |
| Aorta, thoracic | 12.6 | 361 | 6.1 |
| Aorta, abdominal | 12.8 | 484 | 9.0 |
| Pulmonary vessels | 12.8 | 300 | 5.2 |
| Pelvis, skeleton | 19.4 | 438 | 8.2 |
| Cervical spine | 27.0 | 275 | 2.9 |
| Lumbar spine | 32.4 | 441 | 8.1 |
| Extremities | 14.4 | 169 | -- |
| Coronary CTA | 43.1 | 564 | 10.2 |
| Calcium scoring | 12.4 | 171 | 3.1 |
| Virtual colonoscopy | 11.4 | 440 | 8.0 |

reconstructed volume is reduced for a four-slice compared to a single-slice system when the same body region is exposed in both systems. In practice, this means that for the same reconstructed body region, the irradiated body region increases with the detector width. Overscanning is, of course, only relevant for system operation in a spiral mode. If the system is used in a single table position or in a step-by-step (axial) mode, overscanning is avoided. Another possibility for reducing the additional patient dose is currently becoming available: Adaptive collimation at the beginning and the end of a spiral scan reduces the–clearly unwanted–exposure that does not serve for the image reconstruction.

*Overbeaming:* This effect is caused by the finite size of the focal spot, which–together with the collimator blades–leads to a penumbra outside the edges of the collimation. The penumbra size depends on the size of the focal spot and the collimator-to-focus distance only and thus has a constant value. While this additional radiation can be detected in single-slice systems, this is not possible in MSCT. Thus, the resulting overbeaming causes an increase of radiation dose compared to single-slice scanners. Obviously, the relative contribution of overbeaming becomes smaller with an increasing number of detector rows (BRIX et al. 2003).

*Detector geometry:* A small proportion of the radiation entering the patient is not used for diagnostic imaging, since it impinges at the borders between the single detector elements and is hence not detected. In the new detector generation, these areas are considerably smaller, and thus the proportion of the additional dose to the patient is reduced.

*Scatter radiation:* The amount of scatter radiation is increasing with total collimation. Scatter radiation causes an additional signal in the detectors, which is superimposing the signal from the attenuated primary

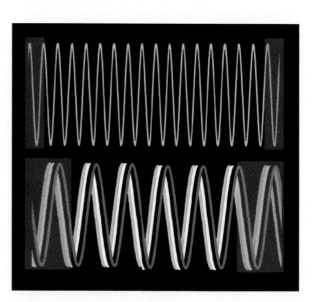

**Fig. 4.3.** Schematic representation of the overscanning effect, for single-slice (*upper part*) and multislice CT (*lower part*). The amount of volume that is exposed additionally (*green shaded part*) is larger in MSCT, since the axial extension of one helical movement of the source is larger in MSCT due to the increased height of the detector array. It is obvious that scanning of small body sections with MSCT in spiral mode is not appropriate

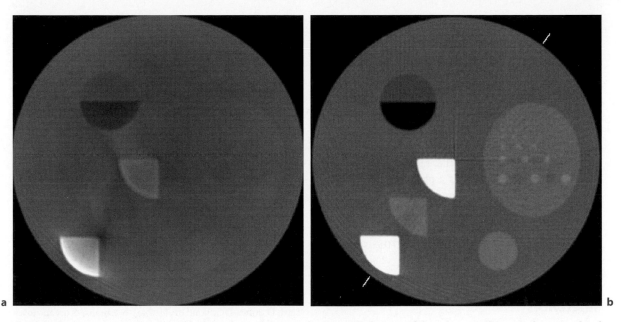

a

b

**Fig. 4.4a,b.** Reconstructed image of a physical test object in a fictitious CT device with large beam collimation from simulated data (**a**) including scatter, (**b**) excluding scatter (i.e., attenuated primary radiation only)

radiation (that contains the structural information) and thus reduces the contrast. Besides, the scatter signal itself is noisy, which further increases the noise of the image. The effect of the scatter is more dominant with larger collimation such as in the actual scanners with 64, 128, 256 or 320 detector rows. It also plays a crucial role in systems with two sources (dual-source CT), where scatter radiation is not only recorded by the detector opposite of the source, but also the second detector. To demonstrate how scatter radiation is deteriorating image quality in large collimation systems, various simulations have been performed to quantify the scatter signal.

A simulation of the amount of scatter radiation in two different CT geometries showed that the scatter radiation fraction remains below about 30% in an MSCT system (32 slices) with a collimation of 40 mm; in a circular flat-panel CT with collimation 400 mm (simulating the "worst case" in MSCT), this fraction amounts to almost 80%. In other words, for the flat-panel CT, the magnitude of the undesirable scatter radiation signal is about four times higher than that of the primary signal, whereas for the MSCT, it is about a factor of two lower than the primary signal (SCHLATTL et al. 2006).

Figure 4.4 demonstrates the effect of scatter radiation for image reconstruction for a physical test object in a large collimation CT system. The strongly reduced contrast due to large amounts of scatter is obvious (SCHLATTL and HOESCHEN 2008)

## 4.4
## Conclusions

MSCT is a technology under steady development. It offers great possibilities, but contributes also largely to radiation exposure of the population. Therefore, it is very important that radiologists use this imaging technology with appropriate caution and for the patients' benefit. This includes questions like:

- Is a radiological investigation necessary (i.e., justified)?
- Are there other types of investigations–involving less or no radiation–possible?
- Is the radiation susceptibility of a specific patient higher than average (e.g., pediatric patients)?
- Which values of in-plane resolution and slice thickness are required for a reliable diagnosis?
- Which pitch value is appropriate to achieve the optimal relation between radiation exposure and diagnostic output?
- Which level of image noise is acceptable?
- What is the scan range required to image the body region to be examined?
- Is the relation of the body region to be examined and the range exposed due to overscanning reasonable?
- In summary: Is the examination justified (in view of a net benefit to the patient) and is the radiation protection optimized?

Certainly, novel developments are to be expected in the fields of medical physics, medical technology, and engineering that will reduce the dose per investigation, such as adaptive collimation, step-by-step data acquisition with large collimation, scatter reduction, structure-saving noise reduction, and more effective reconstruction algorithms. However, even if the dose per examination could be reduced substantially due to these technical developments, this progress will never ease the radiologist's responsibility for a specific radiological investigation. Obviously, this requires a profound education as well as continuous further professional training. Additionally, aid towards the justified use of MSCT is offered by suitable guidance documents [e.g., EUROPEAN COMMISSION 2001; STRAHLENSCHUTZKOMMISSION (SSK) 2006].

# References

Breckow J (2006) Linear-no-threshold is a radiation-protection standard rather than a mechanistic effect model. Radiat Environ Biophys 44:257-260

Brenner DJ, Sachs RK (2006) Estimating radiation-induced cancer risks at very low doses: rationale for using a linear no-threshold approach. Radiat Environ Biophys 44:253-256

Brix G, Nekolla EA, Griebel J (2005) Strahlenexposition von Patienten durch diagnostische und interventionelle Röntgenanwendungen: Fakten, Bewertung und Trends. Der Radiologe 45:340-349

Brix G, Nagel HD, Stamm G et al. (2003) Radiation exposure in multi-slice versus single-slice spiral CT: results of a nationwide survey. Eur Radiol 13:1979-1991

Brix G, Lechel U, Veit R et al. (2004) Assessment of a theoretical formalism for dose estimation in CT: an anthropomorphic phantom study. Eur Radiol 14:1275-1284

Bundesamt für Strahlenschutz (2003) Bekanntmachung der diagnostischen Referenzwerte für radiologische und nuklearmedizinische Untersuchungen. Bundesanzeiger 143:17503

Bundesamt für Strahlenschutz (2006) Umweltradioaktivität und Strahlenbelastung im Jahr 2005. Bundesministerium für Umwelt, Naturschutz und Reaktorsicherheit, Berlin

Committee to Assess Health Risks from Exposure to Low Levels of Ionizing Radiation; Nuclear and Radiation Studies Board DoEaLS, National Research Council of the National Academies (2006) Health risks from exposure to low levels of ionizing radiation: BEIR VII Phase 2. The National Academies Press, Washington, DC

Council of the European Union (1997) Council directive 97/43/Euratom of 30 June 1997 on health protection against the dangers of ionizing radiation in relation to medical exposure, and repealing directive

Cristy M, Eckerman KF (1987) Specific absorbed fractions of energy at various ages from internal photon sources, part I: Methods. ORNL Report TM-8381/V1. Oak Ridge National Laboratory, Oak Ridge, TN

Drexler G, Panzer W, Widenmann L et al. (1990) The calculation of dose from external photon exposures using reference human phantoms and Monte Carlo methods, part III: Organ doses in X-ray diagnosis. GSF-Report 11/90. GSF-National Research Center for Environment and Health, Neuherberg, Germany

European Commission (1999) European Guidelines on quality criteria for computed tomography. Report EUR 16262 EN. European Commission, Brussels

European Commission (2001) Referral guidelines for imaging. Radiation Protection Series 118. European Commission, Luxembourg

Fill U, Zankl M, Petoussi-Henss N et al. (2004) Adult female voxel models of different stature and photon conversion coefficients for radiation protection. Health Phys 86:253-272

Hart D, Jones DG, Wall BF (1994a) Normalised organ doses for medical x-ray examinations calculated using Monte Carlo techniques. NRPB Report SR262. National Radiological Protection Board, Chilton, Didcot, UK

Hart D, Jones DG, Wall BF (1994b) Estimation of effective dose in diagnostic radiology from entrance surface dose and dose-area product measurements. NRPB Report 262. National Radiological Protection Board, Chilton, Didcot, UK

ICRP (1991) 1990 Recommendations of the International Commission on Radiological Protection. ICRP Publication 60. Pergamon Press, Oxford, UK

ICRP (1996) Radiological protection and safety in medicine. ICRP Publication 73. Pergamon Press, Oxford, UK

ICRP (2007a) The 2007 recommendations of the International Commission on Radiological Protection. ICRP Publication 103 International Commission on Radiological Protection

ICRP (2007b) Managing patient dose in multi-detector computed tomography (MDCT). ICRP Publication 102. Elsevier Ltd, Amsterdam

Mettler FAJ (2007) Magnitude of radiation uses and doses in the United States: NCRP Scientific Committee 6-2 analysis of medical exposures.

Petoussi-Henss N, Zankl M, Fill U et al. (2002) The GSF family of voxel phantoms. Phys Med Biol 47:89-106

Radiological Society of North America (2004) Radiation exposure in X-ray examinations

Regulla D, Eder H (2005) Patient exposure in medical X-ray imaging in Europe. Radiat Prot Dosim 114:11-25

Regulla D, Griebel J, Noßke D et al. (2003) Erfassung und Bewertung der Patientenexposition in der diagnostischen Radiologie und Nuklearmedizin. Zeitschrift für Medizinische Physik 13:127-135

Rosenstein M (1976) Organ doses in diagnostic radiology. HEW Publication (FDA) 76-8030. Bureau of Radiological Health, Rockville, MD

Rosenstein M, Suleiman OH, Burkhart RL et al. (1992) Handbook of selected tissue doses for the upper gastrointestinal fluoroscopic examination. HHS Publication FDA 92-8282. US Department of Health and Human Service, Center for Devices and Radiological Health, Rockville, MD

Schlattl H, Hoeschen C (2008) The built-in capacity of CT D'OR's static ring for scatter correction. In: Hsieh J, Samei E (eds) Medical imaging. SPIE, San Diego, CA

Schlattl H, Tischenko O, Hoeschen C (2006) Modeling realistic raw data for image reconstruction–Quantifying scattering noise in different CT geometries. In: Flynn MJ, Hsieh J (eds) Medical imaging 2006: Physics of medical imaging. Bellingham, WA. SPIE, San Diego, CA, pp 1656-1662

Schlattl H, Zankl M, Hausleiter J et al. (2007) Local organ dose conversion coefficients for angiographic examinations of coronary arteries. Phys Med Biol 52:4393-4408

Snyder WS, Ford MR, Warner GG (1978) Estimates of specific absorbed fractions for monoenergetic photon sources uniformly distributed in various organs of a heterogeneous phantom. MIRD pamphlet 5, revised. Society of Nuclear Medicine, New York, NY

Stamm G, Nagel H-D, Galanski M CT- Expo. http://www99.mh-hannover.de/kliniken/radiologie/str_04.html

Stern SH, Rosenstein M, Renaud L et al. (1995) Handbook of selected tissue doses for fluoroscopic and cineangiographic examination of the coronary arteries (in SI units). HHS Publication FDA 95-8289. US Department of Health and Human Services, Food and Drug Administration, Center for Devices and Radiological Health, Rockville, MD

Strahlenschutzkommission (SSK) (2006) Orientierungshilfe für radiologische und nuklearmedizinische Untersuchungen, Strahlenschutzkommission (SSK) des Bundesministeriums für Umwelt NuR (ed) H. Hoffmann. GmbH–Fachverlag, Berlin

Trabalka JR, Kocher DC (2007) Energy dependence of dose and dose-rate effectiveness factor for low-LET radiations: Potential importance to estimation of cancer risks and relationship to biological effectiveness. Health Phys 93:17-27

UNSCEAR (2000) Sources and effects of ionizing radiation. United Nations Scientific Committee on the Effects of Atomic Radiation, New York

VAMP ImPactDose. http://www.vamp-gmbh.de/software/impactdose.php

Veit R, Lechel U, Truckenbrodt R et al. (2005) Does the consideration of 'overranging' in the calculation of effective doses for CT examinations improve the correlation of calculated with measured doses? Biomed Tech (Berl) 50:1328-1329

Wall BF (2004) Radiation protection dosimetry for diagnostic radiology patients. Radiat Prot Dosim 109:409-419

Wambersie A, Zoetelief J, Menzel HG et al. (2005) The ICRU (International Commission on Radiation Units and Measurements): its contribution to dosimetry in diagnostic and interventional radiology. Radiat Prot Dosim 117:7-12

Winslow M, Huda W, Xu XG et al. (2004) Use of the VIP-Man model to calculate energy imparted and effective dose for X-ray examinations. Health Phys 86:174-182

Zankl M, Fill U, Petoussi-Henss N et al. (2002) Organ dose conversion coefficients for external photon irradiation of male and female voxel models. Phys Med Biol 47:2367-2385

# Dual-Energy CT–Technical Background

Thorsten R. C. Johnson

CONTENTS

## ABSTRACT

With the development of Dual Source CT, simultaneously acquired Dual Energy CT has become feasible in a clinical setting. Running both x-ray tubes at different potentials, different x-ray spectra can be obtained. Thus, elements with a strongly energy dependent absorption such as iodine or xenon gas can be differentiated from other materials. A three material decomposition algorithm is applied to map the distribution of such a substance in a CT image.

This approach can be used to extract further clinically relevant information from CT scans acquired at normal dose levels. For example, it is possible to identify iodine in liver or kidney tissue and to display the contrast enhancement either by color-coding it in the CT image or by subtracting it to obtain virtual unenhanced images. This also works in lung tissue for the evaluation of pulmonary perfusion. Also, bones can be eliminated from angiography datasets by the spectral properties of calcium so that the evaluation of vessels becomes easier and faster in a maximum intensity projection. Applications without contrast material include the differentiation of kidney stones and the depiction of tendons and ligaments.

## 5.1
## Introduction

T. R. C. Johnson, MD
Department of Clinical Radiology, Ludwig-Maximilians-University of Munich, Munich University Hospitals, Marchioninistrasse 15, 81377 Munich, Germany

First attempts to use spectral information in computed tomography date back to the late 1970s (Avrin et al. 1978; Chiro et al. 1979; Genant and Boyd 1977; Millner et al. 1979). At that time, two separate scans were acquired, and either projection data or reconstructed data were post-processed. However, the lacking stability of the CT density values, the long scan times, the limited spatial resolution and the difficulty of post-processing were the main reasons why the method never achieved broad clinical acceptance (KELCZ et al. 1979). With the necessity to acquire both scans separately, the use of contrast material and its differentiation by dual-energy or spectral analysis were impossible. Other approaches with double-layer or 'sandwich' detectors that aim to differentiate energies of photons from one X-ray source have not been more successful. This changed fundamentally with the advent of dual-source CT (FLOHR et al. 2006; JOHNSON et al. 2007). Of course, the technology was primarily developed to increase the temporal resolution for cardiac imaging to achieve reliable diagnostic coronary angiographies even in fast or irregularly beating hearts. Quite a few clinical studies have meanwhile proven the success of this technology in this respect (JOHNSON et al. 2006, 2007, 2007; ACHENBACH et al. 2006; SCHEFFEL et al. 2006; LEBER et al. 2007). But obviously, this dual-source CT also offers the opportunity to operate both X-ray tubes at different potentials to obtain different X-ray spectra and to use spectral information for diagnostic purposes. Although this idea is quite obvious, the integration is not quite as simple.

## 5.2
## Technical Background

One primary requirement is that the difference between the X-ray spectra is large enough to obtain differences in attenuation and that the amount and energy of the applied quanta are still acceptable for diagnostic purposes. Figure 5.1 shows the X-ray spectra that are obtained from the Straton tubes of the Siemens Somatom Definition when they are operated at 140 and 80 kV. The higher energy spectrum is dominated by the characteristic lines of the tungsten anode, while the lower energy spectrum mainly consists of Bremsstrahlung. The mean photon energies are 71 and 53 keV, respectively. Therefore, these lowest and highest potentials are always used for dual-energy acquisitions to obtain the largest possible difference between the spectra. On the other hand, a tube voltage lower than 80 kV would not be useful because too much of the quanta would be absorbed by the human body, and values higher than 140 kV would result in so little soft tissue contrast that it likely could not contribute to a further tissue differentiation. As evident in the diagram (Fig. 5.1), the area under the curve for equivalent tube currents differs by a factor of about 4.5, and the tube current needs to be adapted to obtain a similar output of quanta from both tubes. Also, tube current modulation (McCOLLOUGH et al. 2006) is especially desirable for dual-energy scanning to obtain sufficient quanta from the 80 kV tube for dense body regions, such as the pelvis or the shoulders in lateral projection, and the modulation has to regulate both tubes analogously to avoid variations in the relation between tube currents. Not only the photon output, but also the data acquisition and processing of raw data have to be optimized for this purpose. Apart from the photo effect, which causes desirable differences in attenuation at different spectra, attenuation is mainly a result of Compton scatter. The problem is that a significant part of the photons is scattered at an angle of about 90°, which means that they hit the other detector of the dual-source CT scanner, i.e., a large part of the quanta from the 140 kV tube contaminate the data of the detector that are supposed to correspond to the 80-kV tube. Therefore, a precise correction of cross scatter is required in order to obtain valid dual-energy information. Also, the kernels that are used for filtered back-projection in CT usually blur or accentuate edges or contours in the image. However, as this effect would be different at different spectra, this would be deleterious for spectral information. Specific dual-energy reconstruction kernels vary in sharpness, but do not alter object edges.

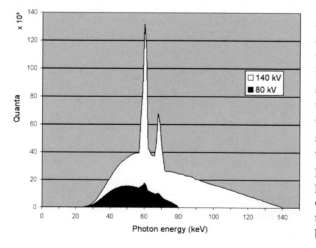

**Fig. 5.1.** Spectra of the Straton tube at 140 and 80 kV potential. The peaks represent the characteristic lines of the tungsten anode and the continuous spectrum is a result of Bremsstrahlung. The mean photon energies are 53 and 71 keV, respectively

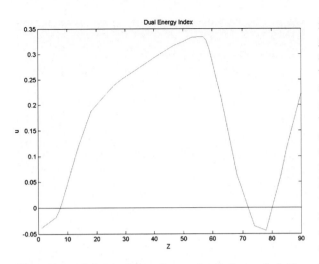

**Fig. 5.2.** Dual-Energy Index of atoms in relation to their element number ($z$). The relation is unique, but only reversible up to a value of 55

i.e., hydrogen (1), oxygen (8), carbon (6) and nitrogen (7), have low element numbers and hence do not show a sufficient photo effect and spectral behavior that would allow a differentiation. The low element numbers and the lacking photo effect explain why their similar spectral behavior is so similar (MICHAEL 1992). Bone with its high content in calcium (20) and fat, which only consists of hydrogen and carbon, represent tissues that differ from others significantly, but their differentiation from other body tissues clearly does not pose a problem in CT, although there have been approaches to use this for the quantification of obesity or for the identification of calcifications in pulmonary nodules (CANN et al. 1982; SVENDSEN et al. 1993). Therefore, the most clinically useful application of dual-energy CT can be expected for the differentiation of iodine (KRUGER et al. 1977; RIEDERER and MISTRETTA 1977; NAKAYAMA et al. 2005), which is generally used in CT as a contrast agent anyway and whose distribution can be masked by the underlying tissue.

## 5.3 Post Processing

The post processing of the acquired projection data primarily requires a normal image reconstruction by filtered back-projection. The fact that the acquired projection data have an offset of ninety degrees at equal $z$-axis positions means that a primary post-processing of projection data is impossible because there are no equivalent projections. A conceivable, but very laborious workaround would be a mathematical back and forward projection of the data from one detector. Another mechanical alternative would be to move the one tube by a quarter of the total collimated width in $z$-direction for dual-energy acquisitions, which would set the foci of the tubes onto an equal spiral path and result in equivalent projections. The post-processing based on reconstructed images is the feasible approach that was primarily implemented in the system. This implies a little disadvantage, which is that a correction of beam hardening or streak artifacts from very dense objects, such as metallic implants, is not as easily possible. On the other hand, there are multiple advantages to this approach: The post-processing is a lot faster, the data can be archived as DICOM files in a normal PACS system, the image data can be read by normal workstations and viewing software, the raw projection data do not need to be stored, and a post-processing can be performed repeatedly with variable settings.

On the other hand, the object that is to be analyzed with dual-energy techniques has to have properties that allow a diagnostically useful differentiation. In order to quantify the spectral behavior of different materials, a Dual-Energy Index can be calculated independently from the mere CT density as the relation of attenuations of the same voxel divided by its mean attenuation at the different tube potentials (Eq. 5.1):

$$u \approx \frac{\mu_{80} - \mu_{140}}{\mu_{80} + \mu_{140}} \qquad (1)$$

As Hounsfield units should be related linearly with attenuation, the calculation can be performed based on CT density values measured for the respective substance. However, as the definition of Hounsfield units implies that an attenuation of 0 is reflected by a value of -1,000 for air, the formula for the Dual-Energy Index resolves to (Eq. 5.2):

$$u \approx \frac{x_{80} - x_{140}}{x_{80} + x_{140} + 2000} \qquad (2)$$

Compton scatter, which makes the largest contribution to attenuation at diagnostically relevant photon energies, is related to the electron density and not to the element number of the atoms under investigation (McCULLOUGH 1975). However, the photo effect, which also causes significant attenuation in many atoms, is related to their element number. As evident in Fig. 5.2, high values apply for $z$-values of 53 (iodine) or 54 (xenon). The elements that make up the human,

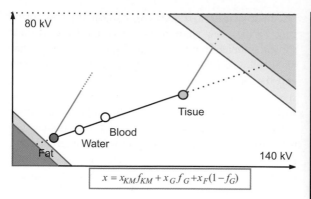

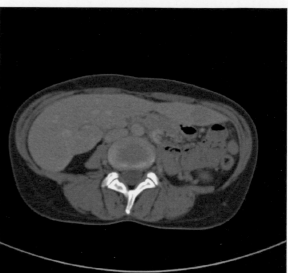

$$x = x_{KM}f_{KM} + x_G f_G + x_F(1-f_G)$$

**Fig. 5.3.** Diagram of the three-material decomposition showing the relation of CT densities of a voxel at 140 and 80 kVp for different body tissues. The *blue lines* indicate beam hardening by additional iodine content in a voxel

**Fig. 5.4. a** An 140-kVp image; **b** 80-kVp image acquired simultaneously. **c** Map of the iodine content semi-quantified by three-material decomposition of fat, soft tissue and iodine. Note that the system only works in soft tissue organs. **d** Virtual unenhanced image obtained by subtraction of the iodine map from the average image. **e** Average image with color-coded superimposition of the iodine distribution

Initial trials have shown that a mere adjustment of the window level of the images reconstructed from both tubes is not sufficient to interactively display the diagnostically relevant spectral information. The post-processing that has been perceived to work most effectively is three-material decomposition. Figure 5.3 shows a diagram of CT density values of the same voxel at 80 and 140 kVp. For most atoms and body tissues, the attenuation will show a linear behavior, i.e., the CT density values will remain close to the bisecting line. However, with beam hardening caused by substances with high $z$-values such as iodine, the density will increase at 80 kVp over the 140 kVp value, and the voxels come off the bisecting line. With this information, voxels that remain on the line can be interpreted as a mixture of two materials, for example, fat and soft tissue in the liver. If a voxel has an offset from the line, this can be attributed to a content of iodine, i.e., uptake of contrast material. The displacement from the line is largely linearly related to the iodine content, which thus can be semi-quantified. This information can be used to color code the iodine distribution in a CT image. Figure 5.4 shows an example of an abdominal scan. Parts a and b show the acquired 140 and 80 kVp images; c shows a map of the iodine distribution. Of course, the beam hardening caused by the calcium in the bone is misinterpreted as iodine because it is not defined in the system of fat, soft

tissue and iodine. Part d show the result of a subtraction of c from the average of a and b, i.e., the iodine-related density has been removed, and the result is a virtually unenhanced image. This approach may be applied to discard unenhanced scans. Apart from the reduced radiation exposure, the advantage is that a misregistration due to different breathing positions is impossible. Part e shows the color-coded iodine distribution superimposed on the normal average image.

## 5.4
## Clinical Applications

Due to the high dual-energy index of iodine, the mapping of the iodine distribution offers a high signal-to-noise ratio without the necessity to invest more doses compared to a routine protocol for the respective body region. There are multiple possible applications of this technique, among them the mapping of lung perfusion, the assessment of iodine distribution in the liver parenchyma or in unclear masses. Figure 5.5a shows the color-coded perfusion of the lungs. The segmental defect corresponds to an occlusive segmental pulmonary embolus in this patient. In part b, small peripheral perfusion defects indicate recurrent subsegmental thromboembolism,

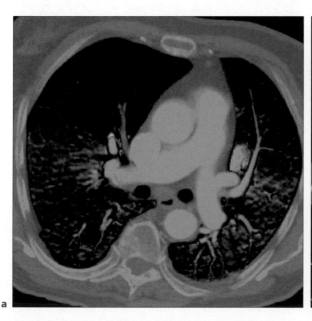

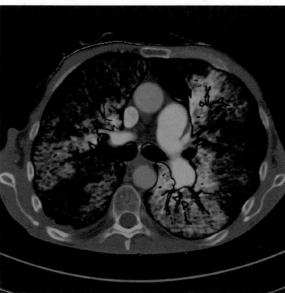

a                                                                                                                                      b

**Fig. 5.5. a** Color-coded lung perfusion as a result of three-material decomposition of air, soft tissue and iodine. Note the perfusion defect caused by the embolus in the segmental vessel. **b** In another patient with chronic recurrent pulmonary embolism, a patchy perfusion with multiple small subpleural defects can be shown, although no emboli are evident in the corresponding vessels

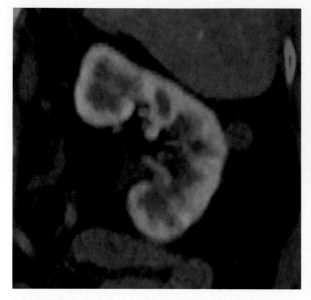

**Fig. 5.6.** The color coding of the iodine distribution confirms that the exophytic cortical mass represents a hemorrhagic cyst and not perfused tissue

which can be diagnosed as the cause of pulmonary hypertension for this patient. Figure 5.6 shows a kidney lesion with a high density of 70-80 HU. The iodine map shows that this lesion does not contain iodine and can thus be attributed to a hemorrhagic cyst. Similar to iodine, xenon gas can be differentiated and can be used to map lung ventilation, which has also been shown in initial trials (WINKLER et al. 1977; HOFFMAN and CHON 2005).

An attractive application of dual-energy differentiation is the separation of bones and iodine in angiography datasets so that a display of a maximum intensity projection makes a fast and easy assessment of large datasets feasible. Although iodine has a high dual-energy index, the calcium in the bone behaves somewhat similarly so that the difference between both is limited. However, additional factors can be taken into account to differentiate bones and vessels to reduce mis-assigned voxels. In the algorithm that has been implemented for this purpose, an averaging over several voxels is used to more reliably identify the course of vessels, and the three-dimensional area over which the algorithm averages is not uniformly round, but prefers areas in which there are other voxels with an iodine-like spectral behavior. Additionally, mixed voxels of fat and bone, which can have a similar spectral behavior, are identified by their inhomogeneous, broad configuration. With these refinements, a quite reliable bone removal is feasible, as evident in Fig. 5.7, showing a carotid angiography in part a and an angiography of the run-off vessels in part b.

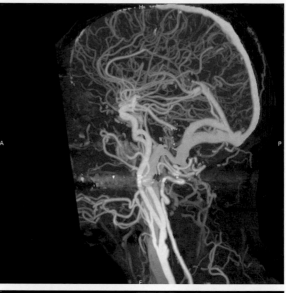

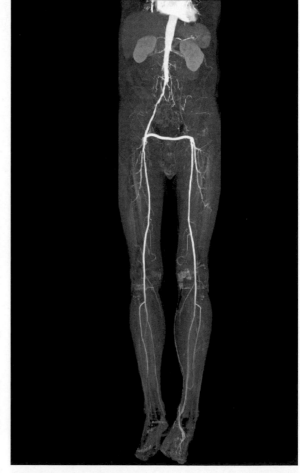

**Fig. 5.7. a** With the automatic dual-energy bone removal, an angiography of the cerebral vessels can be evaluated easily on maximum intensity projections. **b** Similarly, a runoff angiography can be primarily assessed on one maximum intensity projection

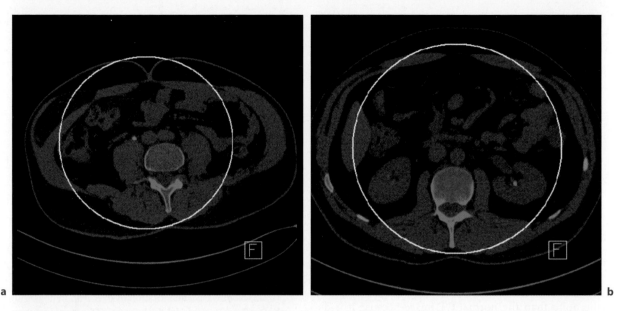

a         b

**Fig. 5.8. a** The calculus in the right ureter is color coded in *red*, indicating that it consists of uric acid. **b** A caliceal stone of another patient is shown in *blue* to indicate that it is calcified

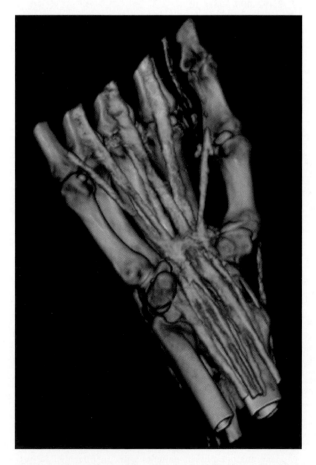

**Fig. 5.9.** The tendons of the wrist can be differentiated by dual-energy CT and displayed without other surrounding soft tissue

Apart from the applications that exploit the spectral properties of iodine, there are a few other algorithms. One can differentiate different types of kidney stones by their spectral properties. While uric acid has a low dual-energy index, other calculi have a stronger beam-hardening effect. Thus, these calculi can be differentiated in spite of their similar CT density. Figure 5.8 shows an in-vivo example of a uric acid calculus in the ureter encoded red in part a and a calcified stone in the lower caliceal group encoded blue in part b. The identification of uric acid is even possible in gout tophi (JOHNSON et al. 2007). Another application is based on the observation that collagen-containing tissues do have dual-energy properties. The exact physical correlate is, to the best of my knowledge, not clear. A possible explanation is the dense packing of the unique hydroxy-proline and hydroxy-lysine amino acids in the side chains of the collagen molecule. By their spectral properties, collagen-containing structures can be differentiated and depicted without surrounding soft tissue. As shown in Fig. 5.9, this works well for most tendons. However, ligaments are frequently too thin to display them in their full continuity. Thus, the clinical value of this application remains to be further investigated. Among other potential applications is the differentiation of iron or copper in the liver parenchyma to quantify the overload of the respective metal in hemochromatosis or Wilson's disease (CHAPMAN et al. 1980; GOLDBERG et al. 1982; OELCKERS and GRAEFF 1996). However, it has been shown that the quantification of iron only works reliably with a normal fat content in the liver, i.e., in the absence of steatosis (WANG et al. 2003; MENDLER et al. 1998), which can usually not be assumed in patients with this disease. Still, the method should be useful to differentiate local fatty infiltration from other hypodense liver masses (RAPTOPOULOS et al. 1991).

## 5.5
## Radiation Exposure

Regarding radiation exposure, dual-energy CT does not require a higher patient dose than a routine CT scan of the same body region. It is possible to tailor the tube current so that the dose from both tubes matches that of a routine single source CT protocol (JOHNSON et al. 2007). The dual-energy information is affected more by the noise than the normal CT image because it is derived from the individual images acquired at 140 and 80 kVp at half dose. Therefore, the noise could of course be reduced, and the results of most applications could be improved significantly if a higher dose was applied, but this seems hard to justify as long as the additional spectral information represents additional, not primarily requested diagnostic information.

## 5.6
## Summary

In summary, dual-energy CT offers the possibility to exploit spectral information for diagnostic purposes in routine clinical examinations. The mapping of iodine distribution in the lung, liver or kidneys and the bone removal from angiography datasets can be regarded as very promising applications. The differentiation of kidney stones represents another clinically useful implementation.

## References

Achenbach S, Ropers D, Kuettner A, Flohr T, Ohnesorge B, Bruder H, Theessen H, Karakaya M, Daniel WG, Bautz W, Kalender WA, Anders K (2006) Contrast-enhanced coronary artery visualization by dual-source computed tomography–initial experience. Eur J Radiol 57:331–335

Avrin DE, Macovski A, Zatz LE (1978) Clinical application of Compton and photo-electric reconstruction in computed tomography: preliminary results. Invest Radiol 13:217–222

Cann CE, Gamsu G, Birnberg FA, Webb WR (1982) Quantification of calcium in solitary pulmonary nodules using single- and dual-energy CT. Radiology 145:493–496

Chapman RW, Williams G, Bydder G, Dick R, Sherlock S, Kreel L (1980) Computed tomography for determining liver iron content in primary haemochromatosis. Br Med J 280:440–442

Chiro GD, Brooks RA, Kessler RM, Johnston GS, Jones AE, Herdt JR, Sheridan WT (1979) Tissue signatures with dual-energy computed tomography. Radiology 131:521–523

Flohr TG, McCollough CH, Bruder H, Petersilka M, Gruber K, Suss C, Grasruck M, Stierstorfer K, Krauss B, Raupach R, Primak AN, Kuttner A, Achenbach S, Becker C, Kopp A, Ohnesorge BM (2006) First performance evaluation of a dual-source CT (DSCT) system. Eur Radiol 16:256–268

Genant HK, Boyd D (1977) Quantitative bone mineral analysis using dual energy computed tomography. Invest Radiol 12:545–551

Goldberg HI, Cann CE, Moss AA, Ohto M, Brito A, Federle M (1982) Noninvasive quantitation of liver iron in dogs with hemochromatosis using dual-energy CT scanning. Invest Radiol 17:375–380

Hoffman EA, Chon D (2005) Computed tomography studies of lung ventilation and perfusion. Proc Am Thorac Soc 2:492–498, 506

Johnson TR, Weckbach S, Kellner H, Reiser MF, Becker CR (2007) Clinical image: Dual-energy computed tomographic molecular imaging of gout. Arthritis Rheum 56:2809 Johnson TR, Krauss B, Sedlmair M, Grasruck M, Bruder H, Morhard D, Fink C, Weckbach S, Lenhard M, Schmidt B, Flohr T, Reiser MF, Becker CR (2007) Material differentiation by dual energy CT: initial experience. Eur Radiol 17:1510–1517

Johnson TR, Nikolaou K, Wintersperger BJ, Leber AW, von Ziegler F, Rist C, Buhmann S, Knez A, Reiser MF, Becker CR (2006) Dual-source CT cardiac imaging: initial experience. Eur Radiol 16:1409–1415

Johnson TR, Nikolaou K, Fink C, Becker A, Knez A, Rist C, Reiser MF, Becker CR (2007) [Dual-source CT in chest pain diagnosis]. Radiologe 47:301–309

Johnson TR, Clevert DA, Busch S, Schweyer M, Nikolaou K, Reiser MF, Becker CR (2007) Evaluation of left atrial myxoma by dual-source CT. Cardiovasc Intervent Radiol 30:1085–1086 Millner MR, McDavid WD, Waggener RG, Dennis MJ, Payne WH, Sank VJ (1979) Extraction of information from CT scans at different energies. Med Phys 6:70–71

Kelcz F, Joseph PM, Hilal SK (1979) Noise considerations in dual energy CT scanning. Med Phys 6:418–425

Kruger RA, Riederer SJ, Mistretta CA (1977) Relative properties of tomography, K-edge imaging, and K-edge tomography. Med Phys 4:244–249

Leber AW, Johnson T, Becker A, von Ziegler F, Tittus J, Nikolaou K, Reiser M, Steinbeck G, Becker CR, Knez A (2007) Diagnostic accuracy of dual-source multi-slice CT-coronary angiography in patients with an intermediate pretest likelihood for coronary artery disease. Eur Heart J 28:2354–2360

McCollough CH, Bruesewitz MR, Kofler JM Jr (2006) CT dose reduction and dose management tools: overview of available options. Radiographics 26:503–512

McCullough EC (1975) Photon attenuation in computed tomography. Med Phys 2:307–320

Mendler MH, Bouillet P, Le Sidaner A, Lavoine E, Labrousse F, Sautereau D, Pillegand B (1998) Dual-energy CT in the diagnosis and quantification of fatty liver: Limited clinical value in comparison to ultrasound scan and single-energy CT, with special reference to iron overload. J Hepatol 28:785–794

Michael GJ (1992) Tissue analysis using dual energy CT. Australas Phys Eng Sci Med 15:75–87

Nakayama Y, Awai K, Funama Y, Hatemura M, Imuta M, Nakaura T, Ryu D, Morishita S, Sultana S, Sato N, Yamashita Y (2005) Abdominal CT with low tube voltage: preliminary observations about radiation dose, contrast enhancement, image quality, and noise. Radiology 237:945–951

Oelckers S, Graeff W (1996) In situ measurement of iron overload in liver tissue by dual-energy methods. Phys Med Biol 41:1149–1165

Raptopoulos V, Karellas A, Bernstein J, Reale FR, Constantinou C, Zawacki JK (1991) Value of dual-energy CT in differentiating focal fatty infiltration of the liver from low-density masses. AJR Am J Roentgenol 157:721–725

Riederer SJ, Mistretta CA (1977) Selective iodine imaging using K-edge energies in computerized X-ray tomography. Med Phys 4:474–481

Scheffel H, Alkadhi H, Plass A, Vachenauer R, Desbiolles L, Gaemperli O, Schepis T, Frauenfelder T, Schertler T, Husmann L, Grunenfelder J, Genoni M, Kaufmann PA, Marincek B, Leschka S (2006) Accuracy of dual-source CT coronary angiography: first experience in a high pre-test probability population without heart rate control. Eur Radiol (Epub 2006 Sep 19)

Svendsen OL, Hassager C, Bergmann I, Christiansen C (1993) Measurement of abdominal and intra-abdominal fat in postmenopausal women by dual energy X-ray absorptiometry and anthropometry: comparison with computerized tomography. Int J Obes Relat Metab Disord 17:45–51

Wang B, Gao Z, Zou Q, Li L (2003) Quantitative diagnosis of fatty liver with dual-energy CT. An experimental study in rabbits. Acta Radiol 44:92–97

Winkler SS, Holden JE, Sackett JF, Flemming DC, Alexander SC (1977) Xenon and krypton as radiographic inhalation contrast media with computerized tomography: preliminary note. Invest Radiol 12:19–20

# Radiation Dose in Multislice Cardiac CT

## 6

Ulrich Saueressig and Thorsten A. Bley

## CONTENTS

### ABSTRACT

The development of computed tomography of the heart is still making rapid progress regarding the applied radiation dose. The peak of dose exposure has been reached with 10 to 15 mSv in 64-slice CTCA with a standard protocol (120 kV, 800 $mAs_{eff}$, 0.2 pitch). New inventions like dual-source CT decrease the dose to 8 mSv. Initial data from prospectively gated CT scans promise even less dose exposure in the range of 3 mSv. However, basic underlying facts of dose optimization in cardiac CT remain of great importance. The effective dose in women is generally higher than in men, because radiation sensitive breast tissue is inevitably within the scan range. ECG-controlled tube current modulation (ECTCM) significantly lowers the effective dose. Efficacy of ECTCM up to the introduction of dual-source CT benefits from lowering the heart rate with ß-blockers. Exact planning of a cardiac examination can help to shorten scan length and directly save radiation. A milestone in argumentative discussion will be reached if the effective dose of a cardiac scan consistently lies below 5 mSv, the alleged dose of a diagnostic catheter angiography of the coronary arteries.

U. Saueressig, MD
Abteilung Röntgendiagnostik, Radiologische Universitätsklinik
Freiburg, Hugstetter Str. 55, 79106 Freiburg, Germany

T. A. Bley, MD
Abteilung Röntgendiagnostik, Radiologische Universitätsklinik
Freiburg, Hugstetter Str. 55, 79106 Freiburg, Germany

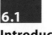

## 6.1
## Introduction

Examinations of the heart and the coronary arteries with multislice CT (computed tomography coronary angiography, CTCA) require high standards of temporal and spatial resolution for optimal diagnostic imaging. Comparatively high exposure of ionizing radiation is due to a low pitch value, which depends on the demand for fast gantry rotation speeds (Primak et al. 2006). Unlike in other multislice examinations, data of overlapping slices cannot be used to improve image quality. Typically, estimated dose values given in the literature range from 8–20 mSv for 16- and 64-slice CT (Einstein et al. 2007). In Table 6.1, a selection of effective dose values is presented.

The increased reliability of cardiac CT has led to new indications, such as assessment of coronary artery bypass grafts or chest pain protocols, increasing the number of examinations (Pache et al. 2006; d'Agostino et al. 2006; Johnson et al. 2007). From

early on, dose reduction mechanisms have been used to reduce radiation, most importantly the adaptation of tube current according to the patient's cardiac cycle. With new generation CT scanners, much focus was placed on the radiation-saving aspects of cardiac examinations.

All mentioned radiation dose estimates in this article refer to the coronary angiography part of the examination of the heart. However, in many cases a calcium scoring scan precedes CTCA. The scan can be executed with prospective gating; the dose ranges between 0.5 and 1.8 mSv (Flohr et al. 2003; Trabold et al. 2003; Poll et al. 2002). Of note, in case of severe coronary

**Table 6.1.** Selection of effective dose values taken from the literature

| Author, year | Without ECTCM [mSv] | With ECTCM [mSv] | Dose estimation method | Comments |
|---|---|---|---|---|
| 16-slice CT | | | | |
| Trabold 2003 | 8.1 (m) 10.9 (f) | 4.3 (m) 5.6 (f) | Alderson-Rando-Phantom | 60 bpm scan length 10 cm 400 mAs Table feed: 5.7 mm/2.8 mm |
| Hohl 2006 | 8.2–12.1 | | ImpactDose | 80 bpm scan length 12 cm 100–120 kV 550–600 mAs |
| Hausleiter 2006 | 10.6 ± 1.2 | 6.4 ± 0.9 (120kV) 5.0 ± 0.3 (100kV) | Conversion factor | 60 bpm Scan length 12.5 cm 100–120 kV |
| Coles 2006 | 13.5–14.5 | | ImpactDose | 60 bpm Scan length 15 cm 500–550 mAs |
| Flohr 2003 | 6.8–7.1 (m) 10.1–10.5 (f) | | WinDose 2.0 a | Scan length 10 cm 500–555 mAs |
| 64-slice CT | | | | |
| Raff 2005 | 13 (m) 18 (f) | | Not stated | |
| Hausleiter 2006 | 14.8 ± 1.8 | 9.4 ± 1.0 (120kV) 5.4 ± 1.1 (100kV) | Conversion factor | 60 bpm Scan length 12.5 cm 100–120 kV |
| DS-CT | | | | |
| Stolzmann 2007 | | 8.8 ± 0.7 7.8 ± 1.1 MinDose | Conversion factor | 70 ± 17 bpm Scan length 12.4 cm 2 × 350 mAs MinDose = minimal mAs 4% of maximum |

ECTCM = ECG tube current modulation; m = male; f = female

calcifications, which may hamper image quality in such a way that a diagnostic evaluation becomes impossible, the angiography scan can be omitted, and the unnecessary radiation can be avoided.

## 6.2
## Dose Estimation: Nomenclature and Methods

### 6.2.1
### Terms for Expressing Radiation Dose

The terms most commonly employed for expressing radiation dose exposure in daily practice are computed tomography dose index in a predefined volume (CTDI$_{vol}$) denoting dose in Gray (Gy), dose-length-product (DLP), which is computed by multiplying CTDI with scan length, and effective dose, which is measured in Sievert (Sv). The former two parameters are commonly displayed on the scanner console. The CTDI$_{vol}$ value is useful for comparing different scanning protocols. The effective dose is the sum of the dose of the exposed organs, weighted by radiation sensitivity. This is not routinely done for every scan, but is the only way to compare the dose of different modalities. Effective dose in computed tomography is always an estimated value and cannot be assigned to an individual patient. The underlying principles stem from phantom measurements and mathematical simulation models (Monte Carlo simulation). Details regarding these underlying concepts have been reported elsewhere (EINSTEIN et al. 2007; MORIN et al. 2003; GERBER et al. 2005).

### 6.2.2
### Estimating Effective Dose

Effective dose of a particular examination is typically estimated by one of the following three different methods. In many cases, a region-specific conversion factor is multiplied with the DLP to obtain a dose value. For cardiac examinations, a conversion factor of 0.017 has been suggested by the European Guidelines on Quality Criteria for Computed Tomography (MENZEL et al. 2000). This leads to a gender-averaged effective dose value. Secondly, a computer program based on Monte Carlo simulations, such as CT-EXPO or ImpactDose, can be employed (VAMP GmbH, Erlangen, Germany) (STAMM and NAGEL 2002). Thirdly, the dose can be physically measured with the help of a phantom (TRABOLD et al. 2003; McCOLLOUGH et al. 2007).

## 6.3
## Strategies for Reducing Dose Exposition in Cardiac CT

### 6.3.1
### Scan Coverage

One of the easiest ways to reduce radiation dose is correct planning of the examination. In 64-slice cardiac CT, for example, 1 cm of scan length equals between 0.5 to 1 mSv of effective dose for the patient. A typical scan should start at the tracheal bifurcation and end beneath the heart. Anatomical information from the calcium scoring scan prior to the CTCA examination can be used to increase the exactitude of the scan (Fig. 6.1). Scan lengths in cardiac CT may range from 8–14 cm, but can ascend to more than 20 cm in patients with coronary bypass grafts.

### 6.3.2
### ECG-Controlled Tube Current Modulation

Modulation of tube current according to the patient's cardiac cycle (ECTCM) is a standard method of reducing radiation in cardiac CT. JAKOBS et al. (2002) described this method in detail. Since the heart moves least during diastole, in most cases it is sufficient to collect information at the end of the heart cycle, typically in an interval of 40 to 80% relative to the R-wave. Technical refinements have rendered faster alternations between high and low tube current possible, as well as significantly lower minimal tube current during systole (McCOLLOUGH et al. 2007). With this technique, the radiation dose can be reduced by 30 to 50%. The effect is lesser in higher heart rates because of shortened systole (POLL et al. 2002) (Fig. 6.2).

### 6.3.3
### Low-Dose Protocol and Adaptation to Patient Morphology

The use of low-dose protocol for cardiac CT has been described in the literature with a variety of approaches (HAUSLEITER et al. 2006; PAUL and ABADA 2007; d'AGOSTINO et al. 2006; JUNG et al. 2003; ABADA et al. 2006). As tube current directly increases the effective dose, it should be set as low as image quality allows. Lowering voltage can also decrease dose, approximately to the voltage squared. When lowered values for tube current and voltage are used, the patient morphology

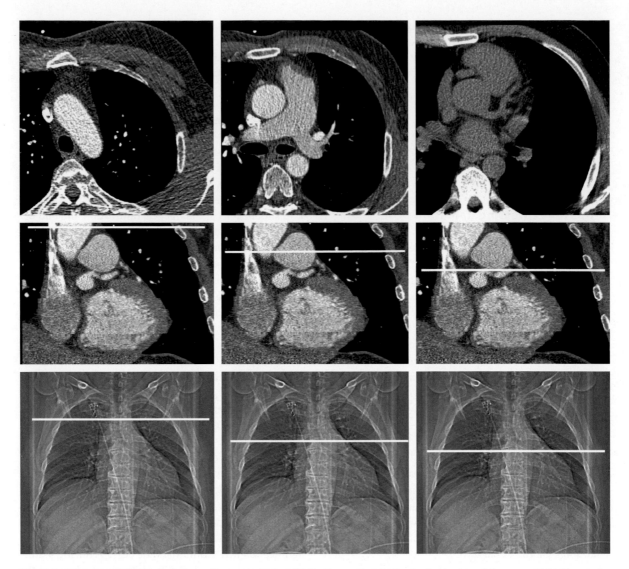

**Fig. 6.1.** Planning of CTCA. *Left*: Start of scan too high. *Middle*: Correct height for the beginning of the scan. *Right*: Shows visibility of coronary arteries in calcium scan

should be taken into consideration. This can either be done with a weight or body mass index approach (JUNG et al. 2003; ABADA et al. 2006), or by measuring image noise (PAUL and ABADA 2007).

### 6.3.4
### Non-Spiral Scanning and Prospective Gating

A new method to acquire cardiac images with reduced radiation has been proposed by HSIEH et al. (2006). In-

stead of helical scanning, a prospective gated step-and-shoot ("SAS") approach is used, combined with a new reconstruction algorithm. This is made more practical by wider detectors, culminating in the 320-row scanner with 16-cm detector width (AquillionOne, Toshiba, Japan). Initial experience demonstrates that dose values lower than 3 mSv seem possible at low heart rates (HUSMANN et al. 2008). With prospective gating, the radiation dose is applied during diastole only, while a sequential scanning mode avoids unnecessary radiation due to overranging.

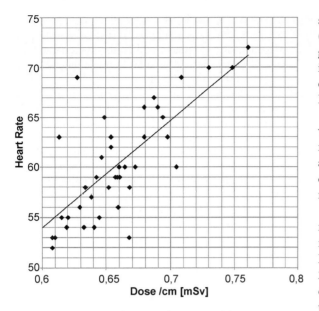

**Fig. 6.2.** Correlation between dose/cm and heart rate in 41 patients with ECTCM (Siemens Somatom 64)

### 6.3.5
### Adaptive Pitch

In most CTCA examinations, a low pitch of around 0.2 is used to ensure gapless coverage of the entire heart in the phases of the cardiac cycle (PRIMAK et al. 2006). Doubling the pitch of an examination reduces the radiation dose by half. For the dual-source CT scanner, the use of adaptive pitch was first described by McCOLLOUGH et al. (2007). Since the higher temporal resolution of up to 83 ms allows the usage of a single segment reconstruction even in patients with higher heart rates, the pitch can be increased up to 0.5. This may result in a significant dose reduction of up to 50% compared to 64-slice CT.

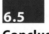

### Implications of Dose Exposition in Cardiac CT

The implications of performing cardiac CT and the corresponding radiation dose exposure are a complex issue with many health policy aspects. Some authors have tried to shed light in those topics. COLES et al. (2006) performed a comparison between 16-slice CTCA and conventional angiography in 91 directly comparable patients. The dose applied in CTCA of 14.7 ± 2.2 mSv was

significantly higher than in conventional angiography (CA) (5.6 ± 3.6 mSv). He states, "A coronary CT angiogram with an effective dose of 14.7 mSv has a risk of inducing a fatal cancer of 1 in 1,400. Conventional coronary angiography (5.6 mSv) has a risk of 1 in 3,600…" ECTCM was not used, and the scan length was 15 cm.

ZANZONICO et al. (2006) compare CTCA and conventional angiography by first evaluating the lifetime risk of death by cancer based on Coles' data and then adding risk of death of interventional angiography as calculated by NOTO et al. (1991). The final values for mortality are 0.07% of CTCA versus 0.13% of CA.

EINSTEIN et al. (2007) estimate a lifetime attributable risk of cancer incidence (LAR) based on the BEIR VII report (COMMITTEE TO ASSESS HEALTH RISKS FROM EXPOSURE TO LOW LEVELS OF IONIZING RADIATION 2006) for 64-slice CTCA with Monte Carlo simulations of male and female patients. According to these estimations, the LAR of a 20-year old woman equals 1 in 143, while an 80-year-old man only suffers a LAR of 1 in 3,261. The estimated LAR of a 60-year-old woman and man were 1 in 466 and 1 in 1,241, respectively, which resembles that of more typical patients for CTCA. The use of ECTCM reduced this LAR to 1 in 715 and 1 in 1,911, respectively.

The methodology leading to the presented risk estimates has serious limitations. Firstly, the risk models are based on extrapolated data of the consequences of radiation exposure, and secondly, the applied Monte Carlo methods use standardized geometrical phantoms not corresponding to different types of patient morphology. However, as Einstein states, "…this study provides a simplified approach, albeit one that we believe is the best available from current data."

### Conclusion

The development of computed tomography of the heart is still making rapid progress regarding the applied radiation dose. The peak of dose exposure has been reached with 10 to 15 mSv in 64-slice CTCA with a standard protocol (120 kV, 800 mAs$_{eff}$, 0.2 pitch). New inventions such as dual-source CT decrease the dose to 8 mSv. Initial data from prospectively gated CT scans promise even less dose exposure. However, basic underlying facts of dose optimization in cardiac CT remain of great importance. The effective dose in women is generally higher than in men, because radiation-sensitive breast tissue is inevitably within the scan range. ECG-controlled tube current modulation significantly lowers the effective dose. The efficacy of ECTCM up to the introduction of dual-source CT benefits from lowering the heart rate with ß-blockers. Exact planning of a cardiac examination can help to shorten scan length and directly save radiation.

Existing studies on low-dose protocols reveal interesting possibilities to reduce radiation exposure. The more widespread use of those protocols could be promoted when included in scanner software combined with automatic noise measurements or mandatory entering of patient weight and height.

While computation of an individual's radiation in computed tomography is not possible, the implications and possible biological and epidemiological effects of exposure to ionizing radiation will remain a point of heated discussion and complex statistical analysis. A milestone in argumentative discussion will be reached if the effective dose of a cardiac scan consistently lies below 5 mSv, the alleged dose of a diagnostic catheter angiography of the coronary arteries.

## References

Abada HT, Larchez C, Daoud B, Sigal-Cinqualbre A, Paul JF (2006) MDCT of the coronary arteries: feasibility of low-dose CT with ECG-pulsed tube current modulation to reduce radiation dose. AJR Am J Roentgenol 186 (6 Suppl 2):S387–390

Coles DR, Smail MA, Negus IS, Wilde P, Oberhoff M, Karsch KR, Baumbach A (2006) Comparison of radiation doses from multislice computed tomography coronary angiography and conventional diagnostic angiography. J Am Coll Cardiol 47:1840–1845

Committee to Assess Health Risks from Exposure to Low Levels of Ionizing Radiation; Nuclear and Radiation Studies Board, Division on Earth and Life Studies, National Research Council of the National Academies (2006) *Health Risks From Exposure to Low Levels of Ionizing Radiation: BEIR VII Phase 2*. The National Academies Press, Washington, DC

Einstein AJ, Henzlova MJ, Rajagopalan S (2007) Estimating risk of cancer associated with radiation exposure from 64-slice computed tomography coronary angiography. JAMA 18;298:317–323

Einstein AJ, Moser KW, Thompson RC, Cerqueira MD, Henzlova MJ (2007) Radiation dose to patients from cardiac diagnostic imaging. Circulation 116:1290–1305

d'Agostino AG, Remy-Jardin M, Khalil C, Delannoy-Deken V, Flohr T, Duhamel A, Remy J (2006) Low-dose ECG-gated 64-slices helical CT angiography of the chest: evaluation of image quality in 105 patients. Eur Radiol 16:2137–2146

Flohr T, Kuttner A, Bruder H, Stierstorfer K, Halliburton SS, Schaller S, Ohnesorge BM (2003) Performance evaluation of a multi-slice CT system with 16-slice detector and increased gantry rotation speed for isotropic submillimeter imaging of the heart. Herz 28:7–19

Flohr TG, Schoepf UJ, Kuettner A, Halliburton S, Bruder H, Suess C, Schmidt B, Hofmann L, Yucel EK, Schaller S, Ohnesorge BM (2003) Advances in cardiac imaging with 16-section CT systems. Acad Radiol 10:386–401

Gerber TC, Kuzo RS, Morin RL (2005) Techniques and parameters for estimating radiation exposure and dose in cardiac computed tomography. Int J Cardiovasc Imaging 21:165–176

Hausleiter J, Meyer T, Hadamitzky M, Huber E, Zankl M, Martinoff S, Kastrati A, Schomig A (2006) Radiation dose estimates from cardiac multislice computed tomography in daily practice: impact of different scanning protocols on effective dose estimates. Circulation 14;113:1305–1310

Hohl C, Mühlenbruch G, Wildberger JE, Leidecker C, Süss C, Schmidt T, Günther RW, Mahnken AH (2006) Estimation of radiation exposure in low-dose multislice computed tomography of the heart and comparison with a calculation program. Eur Radiol 16:1841–1846. Epub 2006 Feb 3

Hsieh J, Londt J, Vass M, Li J, Tang X, Okerlund D (2006) Step-and-shoot data acquisition and reconstruction for cardiac x-ray computed tomography. Med Phys 33:4236–4248

Husmann L, Valenta I, Weber K, Adda O, Veit-Haibach P, Gaemperli O, Kaufmann PA (2008) Cardiac fusion imaging with low-dose computed tomography using prospective electrocardiogram gating. Clin Nucl Med 33(7):490–1

Jakobs TF, Becker CR, Ohnesorge B, Flohr T, Suess C, Schoepf UJ, Reiser MF (2002) Multislice helical CT of the heart with retrospective ECG gating: reduction of radiation exposure by ECG-controlled tube current modulation. Eur Radiol 12:1081–1086

Johnson TR, Nikolaou K, Fink C, Becker A, Knez A, Rist C, Reiser MF, Becker CR (2007) [Dual-source CT in chest pain diagnosis (German).] Radiologe 47:301–309

Jung B, Mahnken AH, Stargardt A, Simon J, Flohr TG, Schaller S, Koos R, Gunther RW, Wildberger JE (2003) Individually weight-adapted examination protocol in retrospectively ECG-gated MSCT of the heart. Eur Radiol 13:2560–2566

McCollough CH, Primak AN, Saba O, Bruder H, Stierstorfer K, Raupach R, Suess C, Schmidt B, Ohnesorge BM, Flohr TG (2007) Dose performance of a 64-channel dual-source CT scanner. Radiology 243:775–784

Menzel HG, Schibilla H, Teunen D (eds) European guidelines on quality criteria for computed tomography. Luxembourg: European Commission; 2000. Publication no. EUR 16262 EN

Morin RL, Gerber TC, McCollough CH (2003) Radiation dose in computed tomography of the heart. Circulation 107:917–922

Noto TJ Jr, Johnson LW, Krone R, Weaver WF, Clark DA, Kramer JR, Jr., Vetrovec GW (1991) Cardiac catheterization 1990: a report of the Registry of the Society for Cardiac Angiography and Interventions (SCA&I). Cathet Cardiovasc Diagn 24:75–83

Pache G, Saueressig U, Frydrychowicz A, Foell D, Ghanem N, Kotter E, Geibel-Zehender A, Bode C, Langer M, Bley T (2006) Initial experience with 64-slice cardiac CT: noninvasive visualization of coronary artery bypass grafts. Eur Heart J 27:976–980

Paul JF, Abada HT (2007) Strategies for reduction of radiation dose in cardiac multislice CT. Eur Radiol 17:2028–2037

Poll LW, Cohnen M, Brachten S, Ewen K, Modder U (2002) Dose reduction in multi-slice CT of the heart by use of ECG-controlled tube current modulation ("ECG pulsing"): phantom measurements. Rofo 174:1500–1505

Primak AN, McCollough CH, Bruesewitz MR, Zhang J, Fletcher JG (2006) Relationship between noise, dose, and pitch in cardiac multi-detector row CT. Radiographics 26:1785–1794

Raff GL, Gallagher MJ, O'Neill WW, Goldstein JA (2005) Diagnostic accuracy of noninvasive coronary angiography using 64-slice spiral computed tomography. J Am Coll Cardiol 46:552–557

Stamm G, Nagel HD (2002) CT-expo—a novel program for dose evaluation in CT (German). Rofo 174:1570–1576

Tatsugami F, von Schulthess GK, Kaufmann PA (2008) Feasibility of low-dose coronary CT angiography: first experience with prospective ECG-gating. Eur Heart J 29:191–197

Stolzmann P, Scheffel H, Schertler T, Frauenfelder T, Leschka S, Husmann L, Flohr TG, Marincek B, Kaufmann PA, Alkadhi H (2007) Radiation dose estimates in dual-source computed tomography coronary angiography. Eur Radiol (Epub Oct 2007)

Trabold T, Buchgeister M, Kuttner A, Heuschmid M, Kopp AF, Schroder S, Claussen CD (2003) Estimation of radiation exposure in 16-detector row computed tomography of the heart with retrospective ECG-gating. Rofo 175:1051–1055

Zanzonico P, Rothenberg LN, Strauss HW. Radiation exposure of computed tomography and direct intracoronary angiography: risk has its reward. J Am Coll Cardiol 2;47:1846–1849

# Radiation Risks Associated with CT Screening Procedures

## 7

Elke A. Nekolla, Jürgen Griebel and Gunnar Brix

## CONTENTS

### ABSTRACT

In screening procedures, a test is offered to asymptomatic persons in order to detect either risk factors for developing a disease or the disease itself at an early stage where an efficient treatment may improve outcome and prognosis. However, if radiological imaging procedures are used as screening tools, some risk due to the exposure to ionizing radiation is inhered. Although radiation risks at low exposure levels have a hypothetical character, this issue has to be thoroughly evaluated since asymptomatic persons are involved. This can be done by estimating the lifetime attributable risks, LAR, based on radiation risk models recently published by the BEIR VII committee. To exemplify the impact of radiation risk due to CT screening, the LAR for four specified CT screening scenarios (calcium scoring, virtual colonoscopy, lung cancer, and whole body screening) were calculated indicating considerable radiation risks that should not be neglected from a radiation protection perspective. On the other hand, there are, to date, no valid data from randomized controlled trials demonstrating a benefit, i.e. a significant reduction in cancer mortality due to CT screening. Scientific evidence is, therefore, at present, insufficient to recommend organized CT screening programmes.

E. A. Nekolla, PhD
Federal Office for Radiation Protection, Germany, Department "Radiation Protection and Health", Ingolstaedter Landstrasse 1, 85764 Oberschleißheim, Germany

J. Griebel, MD
Federal Office for Radiation Protection, Germany, Department "Radiation Protection and Health", Ingolstaedter Landstrasse 1, 85764 Oberschleißheim, Germany

G. Brix, PhD
Federal Office for Radiation Protection, Germany, Department "Radiation Protection and Health", Ingolstaedter Landstrasse 1, 85764 Oberschleißheim, Germany

## 7.1
### Introduction

Medical X-ray exposures have been by far the largest man-made source of population exposure to ionizing radiation in industrialized countries for many years. Recent developments in medical imaging, particularly with respect to computed tomography (CT), have led to rapid increases in the number of relatively high-dose X-ray examinations performed, with significant consequences for individual patient doses and for the collective dose to the population as a whole. It is therefore important for the radiation protection and healthcare authorities in each country to make regular assessments of the magnitude and distribution of this large and increasing source of population exposure. In Germany, the Federal Office for Radiation Protection (BfS) has been collecting and evaluating data for medical radiation exposure of the general population for many years. The predominant objectives of the population dose assessment are to observe trends in the annual collective dose and the annual average per caput dose from medical X-rays with time, and to determine the contributions of different imaging modalities and types of examination to the total collective dose from all medical X-rays. The most recent German survey reveals a steady increase in the annual collective effective dose per caput between 1996 and 2004 (see Fig. 7.1). From Fig. 7.2, which relates to the survey in 2004, it can be concluded that this increase is mainly caused by CT, which contributes more than 50% to the collective effective dose.

Radiological imaging techniques always pose some radiation risk of adverse health effects to patients or – in the case of screening and preventive diagnosis – asymptomatic persons. Therefore, benefit risk considerations are of major concern. In this context, two applications of CT can be distinguished. The first one refers to CT being performed in a patient within the scope of medical diagnosis or treatment, i.e., within healthcare. The second one refers to CT screening procedures performed in asymptomatic persons.

In case of CT being performed within the scope of healthcare, multi-slice CT provides fascinating new capabilities for diagnosis and therapy management of

patients. Like all medical exposures, CT has to be justified on an individual basis by offsetting the radiation risk for the patient with the usually very substantial benefit from improved diagnosis by CT leading to more effective treatment. Furthermore, from a public health perspective, it has to be taken into account that medical radiation exposures do not affect the entire population. Instead, only a small fraction of the population receives a medical exposure in any year, in particular elderly and severely ill persons. For a significant fraction of these patients, the life expectancy – and thus their risk to develop a clinically manifest radiation-induced cancer – is shorter than that of the general population. Therefore, for the healthcare scenario, the justification process is usually based on sound arguments. In the following, special emphasis will, thus, be placed on the benefit and the radiation risk associated with CT screening procedures.

## 7.2
## Screening for Diseases

In the past, health strategies focused on individual patients presenting to a medical doctor with recognized symptoms. Screening fundamentally deviates from this clinical model of care, because apparently healthy individuals are offered a test. An effective screening detects either risk factors for developing a disease or the dis-

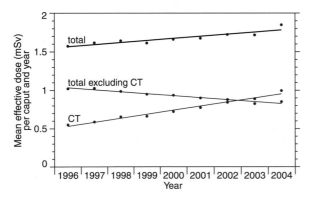

**Fig. 7.1.** Annual per caput effective dose (mSv) due to X-ray procedures in Germany for 1996 to 2004

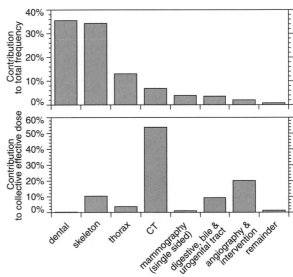

**Fig. 7.2.** Relative frequencies (*upper* panel) of various X-ray examination categories and their relative contribution to the collective effective dose (*lower* panel) in Germany in 2004

ease itself at an early stage where treatment can improve clinical outcome. The aim is to identify those individuals who are more likely to be helped than harmed by further diagnostic tests or treatment (BRITISH MEDICAL ASSOCIATION 2005). Organized screening programs systematically invite all members of a certain population to take a screening test. For example, several breast screening programs in Europe were established where all women in a given population, for instance, between 50 and 69 years of age, routinely receive invitations to have an X-ray mammography. These programs are evidence based and meet stringent quality requirements (IARC 2002).

It is important to distinguish from these organized screening programs more informal arrangements where clinical guidance and/or patient choice results in an ad hoc screening ("opportunistic screening" or "individual screening"). The most prominent example is whole-body CT screening, which is promoted – especially in the USA (FENTON and DEYO 2003) – by private providers in the last years. Up to now, opportunistic CT screening may not play a dominant role in medical exposures. However, this could change dramatically within the next years, if CT screening is extensively advertised by providers and – as a consequence – is widely accepted by the public. This kind of advertisement must be critically questioned as long as there is a lack of evidence supporting the screening procedures on offer, because opportunistic screening potentially puts individuals at risk. This is especially the case as the service is unlikely to be properly quality assured or coordinated. Furthermore, in an opportunistic screening, individuals are unlikely to receive sufficient information to enable them to make an informed decision as to whether or not to undertake the screening test.

Even for well-established screening programs, the ratio between benefits and undesired adverse health effects can be unfavorable. Due to the typically low prevalence of serious diseases in an asymptomatic population, the vast majority of individuals undergoing screening is not affected by the disease. These individuals do not derive a direct health effect, but can be harmed.

The adverse effects most relevant to any screening are false-positive results and overdiagnosis. False positives potentially may cause psychological impairment and/or physical harm because they lead to unnecessary interventions, such as biopsy. The term overdiagnosis refers to lesions detected by a screening procedure that never would have led to a clinically meaningful disease (e.g., invasive cancer) and death (MEISSNER et al. 2004).

The ultimate objective of screening for a specific disease is to reduce mortality from that disease in the target population (MEISSNER et al. 2004). Even if a screening program is able to identify many persons with the disease in a pre-clinical state, it will have little public health impact if early diagnosis and treatment do not affect mortality of these cases. At the early phase of follow-up of a screening study or program, surrogate parameters, such as stage distribution at diagnosis and survival (case fatality), are commonly used to evaluate the success of screening. However, although absence of a change in these parameters may mean that a screening is not effective, a positive change does not provide an adequate measure of evaluation due to length bias, lead-time bias, and overdiagnosis bias (DOS SANTOS SILVA 1999). *Length bias* refers to the phenomenon that the distribution of cases detected by screening (i.e., in an asymptomatic population) is not necessarily identical to the distribution of cases in a symptomatic population, because in a screening population a larger part of the cases might be those that are slow growing, i.e., those with a long pre-clinical phase potentially having a more favorable prognosis resulting in favorable survival compared to those cases detected by clinical symptoms (DOS SANTOS SILVA 1999). The *lead-time* is the time by which diagnosis is extended due to screening, i.e., the interval between the time when the disease can be first diagnosed by screening and the time when it is usually diagnosed in patients presenting with symptoms. Even in case the early detection of the disease does not translate into longer life, the time interval between diagnosis and death, and thus survival, will nevertheless automatically be enhanced by screening (= *lead-time bias*). Therefore, survival is not the appropriate quantity to demonstrate a screening benefit except if a reliable estimate of the lead-time exists and can be accounted for (DOS SANTOS SILVA 1999).

Large randomized controlled trials (RCT) with long follow-up are considered to be the gold standard to demonstrate a significant mortality reduction due to screening.

Predominantly the following CT screening procedures are discussed at present:

1. Lung CT for early detection of lung cancer, in particular in smokers and asbestos workers (I-ELCAP INVESTIGATORS 2006, BLACK et al. 2006, BACH et al. 2007);

2. Virtual CT colonoscopy for early detection of intestinal polyps (which might be pre-cancerous lesions) and colorectal cancer (MULHALL et al. 2005);

3. CT quantification of coronary artery calcification (which is considered as sensitive marker of arteriosclerosis) (WAUGH et al. 2006);

4. Whole-body CT, particularly for early detection of cancer (ILLES et al. 2003).

### 7.2.1
### Lung Cancer Screening

In 2002, lung cancer was the second most common cancer in men, the third most common cancer in women, and the most common cause of cancer-related death in men in Western and Northern Europe (FERLAY et al. 2004). The major risk factor for lung cancer is cigarette smoking. In Europe, smoking tobacco is responsible for about 90% or 60% of lung cancer cases in men or women (SIMONATO et al. 2001). Lung cancer has one of the lowest survival outcomes of any cancer because the majority of cases are diagnosed at a late stage. In Germany, for example, the relative 5-year lung cancer survival rate (i.e., adjusted for the normal life expectancy of the general population) is around 12% for men and about 14% for women. To improve the survival rates, early detection of lung cancer is thus considered to be very important.

Lung cancer is the only site where RCTs are performed to find out whether a benefit of CT screening exists. There are two RCTs, the National Lung Screening Trial (NLST) sponsored by the National Cancer Institute of the United States (CHURCH 2003) and the NELSON trial from the Netherlands/Belgium (VAN IERSEL et al. 2007). The NLST is comparing spiral CT and standard chest X-ray for detecting lung cancer. The study opened for enrollment in September 2002 and closed in February 2004. By February 2004, nearly 50,000 current or former smokers had joined NLST at more than 30 study sites across the USA. However, results are not expected before 2010. The NELSON trial started in August 2003 and intends to show whether screening for lung cancer by multi-slice low-dose CT in current or former smokers (about 20,000 participants) will lead to a 25% decrease in lung cancer mortality. Results are not expected before 2015.

Besides these RCTs, there are several feasibility studies (mainly on risk patients like smokers/ex-smokers) from the USA, Japan, and Europe on lung cancer CT screening. Most of them reported on shifts towards less advanced stages and improved survival rates.

A recently published report of the International Early Lung Cancer Action Program (I-ELCAP 2006) contributes substantial data concerning the clinical effectiveness of CT lung cancer screening. The I-ELCAP involved about 32,000 asymptomatic persons who were at increased risk for lung cancer (mostly current or former smokers). It was concluded by the authors that annual spiral CT screening has the potential to detect lung cancer that is curable: among participants

in the study who received a diagnosis of lung cancer based on spiral CT screening and a resulting biopsy, 85 percent had stage I lung cancer. The statistically estimated 10-year survival among these patients was 88%. However, as mentioned above, this cannot be taken as proof that CT screening for lung cancer decreases mortality.

Other reports also demonstrate limitations of lung cancer screening by CT (BACH et al. 2007; DIEDERICH et al. 2004). BACH et al. (2007) concluded from an analysis of asymptomatic current and former smokers screened for lung cancer that screening may increase the rate of lung cancer diagnosis and treatment (i.e., overdiagnosis), but may not significantly reduce lung cancer mortality.

### 7.2.2
### Colorectal Cancer Screening

Colorectal cancer is the third most common cancer, and the third and second leading cause of cancer death in Northern and Western Europe (FERLAY 2004). In case of colorectal cancer, the rationale of early detection is that the disease itself can be prevented by the detection and removal of benign, neoplastic adenomatous polyps (adenomas), from which more than 95% of cancers arise (BOND 2000). Besides, early diagnosis of colorectal cancer increases survival rates considerably. It has been demonstrated that fecal occult blood (FOB) screening can significantly reduce mortality and morbidity from colorectal cancer (SCHOLEFIELD et al. 2002), although FOB testing often fails due to false-negative or false-positive results. Alternatively, examination with use of optical colonoscopy is recommended by many organizations. In Germany, for example, FOB testing from age 45 and two colonoscopies at ages 55 and 65 are part of the national program for early diagnosis of cancer. Another tool for colorectal cancer screening is double contrast barium enema.

Yet, there is low public acceptability of screening for colorectal cancer by colonoscopy, and a higher rate of patient compliance can be expected with CT colonoscopy (GLUECKER et al. 2003), although the patient must undergo a colonic preparation, as with double-contrast barium enema or colonoscopy. Besides, if polyps or tumors are diagnosed by CT, conventional colonoscopy is required to verify the diagnosis, to obtain a biopsy sample, and to remove them.

There is no published evidence from RCTs examining the effectiveness of CT colonoscopy. Yet, CT colonoscopy has been evaluated by several comparisons with conventional colonoscopy and compares favorably in terms of detecting clinically relevant lesions, i.e., polyps at least 8 mm in diameter (PICKHARDT et al. 2003). The detection of polyps of less than 5 mm in diameter on virtual colonoscopy and subsequent matching on optical colonoscopy are both unreliable. However, there appears to be a majority opinion that colonic polyps of less than 5 mm in diameter should be regarded as clinically insignificant (PICKHARDT et al. 2003). PICKHARDT et al. (2003) evaluated that, in case of virtual colonoscopy, 8 mm might be a reasonable threshold for an intervention by optical colonoscopy. Patients with lesions of about 5 to 7 mm could receive short-term follow-up by virtual colonoscopy (in intervals of 2 to 3 years). All other patients could undergo routine follow-up (in intervals of 5 to 10 years).

## 7.2.3
## Calcium Scoring

Quantification of coronary artery calcification (CAC) can identify patients with an increased risk of coronary artery disease (GREENLAND et al. 2004), which ranks among the leading causes of death in Western countries. In symptomatic patients, calcium scoring can be used to confirm a suspected diagnosis in order to decide on the appropriate treatment and on secondary prevention. On the contrary, in asymptomatic persons, the long-term risk of coronary artery disease shall be assessed. This might be helpful especially for those persons at intermediate risk where clinical decision making is most uncertain (GREENLAND et al. 2004). Several studies assessed the association between CAC scores on CT and cardiac events in asymptomatic people. However, it remains unclear whether CT screening for CAC would provide sufficient extra information over risk factor scoring (e.g., via Framingham risk scores) for it to be worthwhile (WAUGH et al. 2006).

## 7.2.4
## Whole-Body Screening

To date, there is no scientific evidence demonstrating that whole-body CT of asymptomatic persons provides more benefit than harm. Whole-body CT screening is controversially discussed (BEINFELD et al. 2005). There are few firm data on which to base the potential benefit of whole-body CT. A retrospective study evaluated the frequency and spectrum of findings reported with whole-body CT (FURTADO et al. 2005). On average,

2.8 suspect findings per patient were detected, most of them benign, and in 37% of cases additional tests were necessary for further clarification.

## 7.3
## Health Effects Induced by Ionizing Radiation

Exposure to ionizing radiation may lead to early or late health effects, which may be either stochastic or non-stochastic. A non-stochastic effect is an effect where the severity increases with increasing dose (e.g., damage of the skin: erythema at low doses, severe tissue damage at high doses). A stochastic effect, on the other hand, is an effect where the severity is independent of dose, but the probability of inducing the effect does increase with increasing dose. Examples for stochastic effects are cancer or hereditary disorders. In the following, only cancer induction is considered.

Cancers caused by ionizing radiation occur several years after the exposure has taken place. They do not differ in their clinical appearance from cancers that are caused by other factors. A radiation-induced cancer cannot be recognized as such, and it is only by means of epidemiological studies that increases in the spontaneous cancer incidence rates of irradiated groups can be detected. Ionizing radiation is the carcinogen that has been most intensely studied.

Increased cancer rates have been demonstrated in humans through various radio-epidemiological studies at moderate or high doses, i.e., organ or whole-body doses exceeding 50 to 100 mSv, delivered acutely or over a prolonged period.

The so-called *Life Span Study* (LSS) of the survivors of the atomic bombings in Hiroshima and Nagasaki is the most important of these studies (PRESTON et al. 2007). The follow-up of the atomic bomb survivors has provided detailed knowledge of the relationships between radiation risk and a variety of factors, such as absorbed dose, age at exposure, age at diagnosis, and other parameters. The LSS provides data with good radio-epidemiologic evidence due to the large size of the study population (about 86,600 individuals with individual dose estimates), the broad age- and dose-distribution, the long follow-up period (about half a century), and an internal control group (individuals exposed only at a minute level or not at all) (BEIR VII 2006). The LSS is, therefore, generally used for predicting radiation-induced risks for the general population.

However, radiation risk estimates are not merely based on the follow-up of the atomic bomb survivors.

They are also largely supported by a multitude of smaller studies, mostly on groups of persons exposed for medical reasons, both in diagnostics and therapy (BEIR VII 2006).

There is considerable controversy regarding the risk of low levels of radiation, typical for diagnostic radiation exposures, since radiation risks evaluated at low dose levels are not based on experimental and epidemiological evidence. Given this lack of evidence, estimates on risk, derived from high doses, have been extrapolated down to low dose levels by various scientific bodies, including the International Commission on Radiological Protection (ICRP), the United Nations Scientific Committee on the Effects of Atomic Radiation (UNSCEAR), and the BEIR (Biological Effects on Ionizing Radiation) committee. Estimates on risk per unit of dose have been derived using the so-called linear, non-threshold (LNT) hypothesis, which is based on the assumptions that

1. any radiation dose – no matter how small – may cause an increase in risk and
2. the probability of this increase is proportional to the dose absorbed in the tissue.

Although the risks evaluated at low dose levels are hypothetical, a majority of scientists recognize the assumption of linearity as a pragmatic guideline adopted in the absence of scientific certainty. It is for this reason that current radiation protection standards as well as risk assessments are generally based on the LNT hypothesis.

For extrapolating results from high dose-rate exposures to low dose-rate situations, the so-called dose and dose-rate effectiveness factor, DDREF, can be applied. ICRP estimated the DDREF to be 2, i.e., for low doses and dose protraction, risk estimates are to be reduced by a factor of 2 (ICRP 1991). UNSCEAR and the BEIR VII committee suggested a DDREF of 1.5 (UNSCEAR 2000, BEIR VII 2006). In the risk estimates presented below, no DDREF adjustment was made.

### 7.3.1
### Assessment of Radiation Risks

The risk estimates proposed by ICRP (1991) and UN-SCEAR (2000) – for use in radiation protection – provide simple and robust estimates for the lifetime excess risk to die from radiation-induced cancer. But they facilitate only an overall, not an organ-specific estimate and are aimed at age- and gender-averaged groups of persons, such as the working population or the whole population of a country.

An assessment of radiation risks induced by screening procedures such as X-ray mammography or CT has to take into account that these procedures typically are aimed at members of a certain population, such as – for example – women between 50 and 69 years in breast

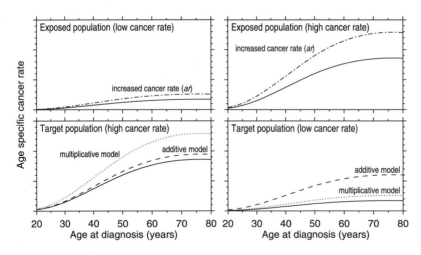

**Fig. 7.3.** Transfer of risk in a population with low to a population with high cancer rates (*left panel*) and transfer of risk in a population with high to a population with low cancer rates (*right panel*). The *broken lines* in the *upper panels* are the increased cancer rates representing a relative excess of 50%. The transfer of the excess relative rate of 0.5 ("multiplicative model") to a population with diverging cancer rates (*solid lines below*) results in the *dotted lines* in the *lower panels*. A transfer of the excess absolute rate ("additive model"), i.e., the difference between the *solid* and the *broken lines* in the *upper panels*, results in the *dashed lines* in *lower panels*

cancer screening. Furthermore, the radiation-induced risk to be diseased with cancer, i.e., the incidence, is of major concern, not only the radiation-induced risk to die from cancer, i.e., the mortality, because incidence data are of better diagnostic quality, and they provide larger numbers of cases for several cancer sites. Finally, screening procedures using ionizing radiation typically expose only parts of the body and, thus, organ-related absorbed doses and risk estimates are necessary for a reliable risk assessment.

Analyses of radio-epidemiological data, e.g., the A-bomb survivors' data, can be based on the assumption of an excess *relative* risk (*ERR*) model or an excess *absolute* risk (*EAR*) model. The *ERR* model assumes that the excess risk is proportional to the baseline (or spontaneous) risk, the cancer risk for a person to be diseased with a specific cancer in the absence of radiation. The *EAR* model expresses the risk as difference in the total risk and the baseline risk. The choice whether the *ERR* or the *EAR* model is taken to estimate radiation risks can be a crucial point due to the fact that risk estimates based on an *ERR* or an *EAR* model can vary considerably when individual tumor sites are considered. This issue is also called "transport (or transfer) of risks from the exposed population to the target population" (e.g., from a Japanese to a European population) and corresponds to the question whether the *ERR* or the *EAR* is taken to be the same in the exposed population and in the reference population (see below). Section 3.3 elaborates on the issue of radiation risk transfer, and Fig. 7.3 gives an illustration.

## 7.3.2
### Radiation Risk Models by BEIR VII

The BEIR VII report, published in 2006, is the seventh in a series of titles from the National Research Council of the United States that addresses the effects of exposure to low levels of exposure to ionizing radiation. The report offers a full review of the available biological, biophysical, and epidemiological literature since the last BEIR report on the subject (BEIR V, 1990). In addition to cancer mortality, the BEIR VII committee developed risk estimates for cancer incidence.

The models by the BEIR VII committee have primarily been developed from A-bomb survivors' data, namely data on cancer mortality with follow-up period 1950 to 2000, and from data on cancer incidence with follow-up period 1958 to 1998. The BEIR VII committee used both *ERR* (Eq. 7.1) and *EAR* (Eq. 7.2) models to calculate the absolute rate, *ar*:

$$ar(e, a, D, s) = r_0(a,s) \cdot (1+err(e, a, D, s)), \qquad (7.1)$$

$$ar(e, a, D, s) = r_0(a,s) + ear(e, a, D, s). \qquad (7.2)$$

The absolute rate, *ar*, denotes the total risk of a person of gender *s*, after an exposure to organ dose, *D*, at the age *e*, to be clinically diseased with cancer at the age *a* or, more specifically, in the interval [*a*, *a*+1). $r_0(a,s)$ is the baseline rate for a person of gender *s* to be diseased with a specific cancer at age *a*. The excess absolute rate, *ear*, is the absolute cancer rate, *ar*, in an exposed population minus the baseline rate, i.e., the rate in an unexposed population. The excess relative rate, *err*, is the ratio of the cancer rate in the exposed population and the baseline rate minus 1. In other words, *err* = 1 means that the additional (radiation-related) cancer rate equals the baseline cancer rate.

Site-specific BEIR VII models for those exposed at age 30 years or later are dependent on organ dose, *D*, and attained age, *a*. The *err* decreases and the *ear* increases with increasing attained age, *a*. For those exposed before the age of 30, the BEIR VII models include an additional term dependent on age at exposure, *e* (*err* and *ear* decreasing with increasing age at exposure).

For breast and thyroid cancer as well as for leukemia, different models were chosen by BEIR VII. The breast cancer model is based on a pooled analysis of data from eight breast cancer incidence studies by PRESTON et al. (2002). The thyroid cancer model is based on a pooled analysis of data from seven thyroid cancer incidence studies by RON et al. (1995). For leukemia, the BEIR VII model includes a time, *t* (= *a*−*e*), since exposure dependence (decreasing with increasing *t*) and a linear-quadratic function of dose.

In the BEIR VII report, risk models for the following individual cancer sites are presented: stomach, colon, liver, lung, female breast, prostate, uterus, ovary, bladder, other solid cancer, thyroid, and red bone marrow (leukemia). Other cancer sites can be accounted for by applying the BEIR VII risk model for "other solid cancer" and adjusting it by means of the baseline rates of the cancer of concern.

It is important to notice that in previous analyses of the A-bomb data, the *ERR* for lung cancer diverged from the usual pattern of decreasing with increasing age at exposure, instead increasing with age (THOMPSON et al. 1994). As was demonstrated by PIERCE et al. in 2003, this effect was an artifact caused by the influence of smoking on lung cancer risk. After adjusting for smoking, there was evidence of a decline of the *ERR* with increasing age comparable to other cancer sites.

### 7.3.3
### Transfer of Risk
### between Populations
### with Different Cancer Rates

For many cancer sites, the baseline risks are different between Japanese and Western populations. On the one hand, e.g., breast and bladder cancer rates are considerably lower in Japan compared to Western populations. On the other hand, e.g., stomach and liver cancer rates are much higher in Japan (FERLAY et al. 2004). Likewise, considerable differences in site-specific relative and absolute risk estimates were demonstrated in several radio-epidemiological studies, and it is therefore essential whether the excess relative risk or the excess absolute risk is taken to estimate radiation risks. The BEIR VII committee decided to apply a mixed approach, i.e., to calculate weighted geometric averages with a weight of 0.7 for the relative risk estimate and a weight of 0.3 for the absolute risk estimate for sites other than breast, thyroid, and lung. The larger weight for the relative risk estimate is based on the somewhat greater support for a relative risk transport. Moreover, relative risk estimates are commonly more robust. For lung cancer, the BEIR VII weighting procedure is inverted, i.e., the additive risk estimate is attached greater weight (0.7) because of evidence that the additive model is valid in case of interaction of radiation and smoking in the LSS of atomic bomb survivors (PIERCE et al. 2003). For breast and thyroid cancer, the BEIR VII models are based on pooled analyses of both Japanese as well as Western populations. For thyroid cancer, merely a relative risk model was derived by RON et al. (1995). For breast cancer, the BEIR VII committee prefers the absolute risk model predicting considerably lower absolute risk estimates

compared to the multiplicative model for exposure ages above 25 years. To be precautious, in the risk estimates presented below a mixed approach was applied on radiation risk for breast cancer, i.e., for the absolute risk estimate a weight of 0.7 and for the relative risk estimate a weight of 0.3 were utilized (analogous to the BEIR VII weighting procedure in case of lung cancer).

### 7.3.4
### Calculating Lifetime Excess Risks

Lifetime excess risks, also referred to as lifetime attributable risks (KELLERER et al. 2001, BEIR VII 2006), *LAR*, are calculated by means of site-specific risk models, site-specific baseline rates on cancer incidence (or cancer mortality), and life-table data to account for competing risks:

$$LAR = \sum_{site} \left( \sum_{e} \left( \int_{e+L}^{a_{max}} ear(e, a, D, s) \cdot S(a)/S(e) \mathrm{d}a \right) \right)$$

(7.3)

where $L$ is the minimum latency period and $a_{max}$ is the maximum attained age (assumed to be 100). The minimum latency period denotes the time interval following radiation exposure during which an excess of tumors is not expected to be observed. It is understood as the minimum period for a tumor to develop to a detectable size after an irradiation. Usually, a minimum latency period of 5 or 10 years for solid cancer and of 2 years for leukemia is applied. The survival function, i.e., the probability at birth to reach at least age a is denoted by $S(a)$. The ratio $S(a)/S(e)$ is the conditional probability of a person alive at age $e$ to reach at least age $a$.

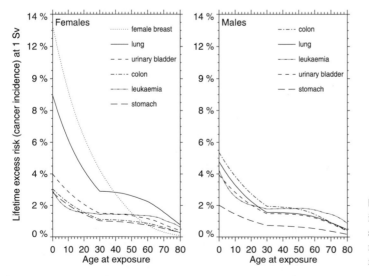

**Fig. 7.4.** Lifetime excess risk at 1 Sv organ dose in dependence on age at exposure for those cancer sites attributing most to the total excess lifetime risk according to BEIR VII risk models and German life tables and German cancer incidence rates

Applying the BEIR VII risk models and German disease and life table data (Statistisches Bundesamt 2006, DeStatis 2004, GEKID and RKI 2006), Fig. 7.4 gives *LAR* estimates for cancer incidence for organ doses of 1 Sv for those cancer sites contributing most to the total *LAR* in dependence on age at exposure. To derive risk estimates for organ doses, *D*, other than 1 Sv, the *LAR* has to be multiplied by *D* for solid cancer and by the factor $(0.53 \cdot D + 0.47 \cdot D^2)$ for leukemia.

### 7.3.5
### How to Assess
### Radiation Risks from CT Screening

Risk analyses for CT screening have been presented by Brenner and colleagues for lung cancer CT, virtual colonoscopy, and whole-body CT screening (Brenner 2004, Brenner and Georgsson 2005, Brenner and Elliston 2004, Brenner and Hall 2007). For lung CT and virtual colonoscopy, they are based on risk estimates derived from cancer incidence data of the Japanese atomic bomb survivors with follow-up period 1958 to 1987 (Thompson et al. 1994); for whole-body CT screening they are based on risk estimates for cancer mortality given by the Biological Effects of Ionizing Radiation (BEIR) V committee in 1990. Brenner et al. used representative scanning protocols to estimate organ doses and gave radiation risk estimates for a US population. The main results presented by Brenner are given in Table 7.1.

In a present study performed by our group, a risk assessment was conducted for the CT screening procedures mentioned above applying the most recent risk models presented by the BEIR VII committee in 2006 and utilizing disease and life table data for a German population (Statistisches Bundesamt 2006, DeStatis 2004, GEKID and RKI 2006). The BEIR VII risk models were applied to estimate age-, gender-, and organ-specific lifetime excess risks, *LAR*, for stomach,

colon, liver, lung, female breast, prostate, uterus, ovary, bladder, thyroid, esophagus, kidney, and other solid cancer as well as for leukemia.

Four screening procedures were accounted for:
1. Annual lung cancer screening from age 50 to 69 years (i.e., 20 CT examinations) in a smoking population (i.e., lung cancer baseline rates for smokers were assumed). Scan parameters: scan length 34 cm; current time product: 35 mAs; pitch1.8; collimation 4 * 1 mm; 120 kV; $CTDI_{vol}$: 3.8 mGy.
2. Three virtual colonoscopies (paired CT scans: supine and prone position) at intervals of 10 years from age 50 to 70 years. Scan parameters: scan length 45 cm; current time product: 40 mAs; pitch 1.35; collimation 4 * 2.5 mm; 120 kV; $CTDI_{vol}$: 7.1 mGy.
3. Calcium scoring at intervals of 4 years from age 50 to 66 years (i.e., five CT examinations). Scan parameters: scan length 12 cm; current time product: 37 mAs; pitch 0.37; collimation 4 * 2.5 mm; 120 kV; $CTDI_{vol}$: 9 mGy.
4. Whole-body CT screening every 2 years from age 50 to 68 years (i.e., 10 CT examinations). Scan parameters: scan length 77 cm; current time product: 200 mAs; pitch 1.75; collimation 4 * 2.5 mm; 120 kV; $CTDI_{vol}$: 10.3.

Effective and organ doses were calculated for certain CT protocols with the program CT-Expo (version 1.5.1, Stamm and Nagel 2002).

In Table 7.2 the estimated cumulative effective doses are given for the above-mentioned screening procedures. In Table 7.3, the *LAR* estimates for cancer incidence are given in dependence on organ doses for those sites contributing most to the total *LAR*. For the CT screening procedures mentioned above, increased risks in particular of cancer of the lung, female breast, colon, and stomach, as well as of leukemia, are of concern. This is especially valid for whole-body CT, where all of these organs are being exposed to organ doses of about 10 mSv and more.

**Table 7.1.** Estimates of lifetime excess cancer risks for CT screening procedures given by Brenner

| Lung CT (Brenner 2004) | | Virtual colonoscopy (Brenner and Georgsson 2005) | | Whole body CT (Brenner and Elliston 2004) |
|---|---|---|---|---|
| Lifetime excess lung cancer risk for smokers undergoing annual screening from age 50 to 75 | | Lifetime excess total cancer risk from single paired CT at age 50 | | Lifetime excess total cancer mortality risk from annual screening from age 50 to 74 |
| Female | Male | Female | Male | Averaged over both sexes |
| 0.85% | 0.23% | 0.13% | 0.15% | 1.5% |

**Table 7.2.** Cumulative effective doses due to four CT screening scenarios

| | Age of participants (years) | Screening interval (years) | Number of rounds | Cumulative effective dose [a, b] (mSv) | |
|---|---|---|---|---|---|
| | | | | Male | Female |
| Lung cancer screening | 50–69 | 1 | 20 | 34 | 38 |
| Virtual colonoscopy | 50–70 | 10 | 3 | 15 | 20 |
| Calcium scoring | 50–66 | 4 | 5 | 10 | 13 |
| Whole-body screening | 50–68 | 2 | 10 | 114 | 144 |

[a]Tissue-weighting factor for breast tissue for women 0.1, for men 0

[b]Dose values related to the protocols described in the text

**Table 7.3.** Cumulative organ doses due to four CT screening scenarios (see Table 7.2 and text) and corresponding estimates of lifetime attributable risk (*LAR*) to incur cancer/leukemia for those sites contributing most to total *LAR*

| Sites | Cumulative organ doses [a] (mSv) | | *LAR* (incidence) (%) | |
|---|---|---|---|---|
| | Male | Female | Male | Female |
| **Lung cancer screening** | | | | |
| Female breast | – | 114 | – | 0.09 |
| Lung | 114 | 100 | 0.19 | 0.46 |
| **Virtual colonoscopy** | | | | |
| Colon | 27 | 28 | 0.03 | 0.02 |
| Urinary bladder | 28 | 29 | 0.03 | 0.03 |
| Stomach | 30 | 31 | 0.01 | 0.02 |
| **Calcium scoring** | | | | |
| Female breast | – | 69 | – | 0.06 |
| Lung | 48 | 47 | 0.06 | 0.10 |
| **Whole-body screening** | | | | |
| Female breast | – | 173 | – | 0.14 |
| Lung | 169 | 170 | 0.20 | 0.37 |
| Colon | 128 | 135 | 0.17 | 0.11 |
| Stomach | 153 | 157 | 0.08 | 0.11 |
| Urinary bladder | 134 | 141 | 0.15 | 0.16 |
| Red bone marrow | 101 | 107 | 0.07 | 0.06 |

[a]Dose values related to the protocols described in the text

**Table 7.4.** Estimates of total lifetime attributable risk to incur cancer (*LAR*) due to four CT screening scenarios (see Table 7.2 and text) and estimated lifetime baseline risk (from age 50) from dying from the disease of concern (i.e., *a*: lung cancer in a smoking population; *b*: colorectal cancer; *c*: acute myocardial infarction; *d*: all cancers)

| | *LAR* (incidence) (%) | | Remaining lifetime baseline risk (%) for dying from the disease(s) of concern | |
| --- | --- | --- | --- | --- |
| | Male | Female | Male | Female |
| a: Lung cancer screening | 0.23 | 0.59 | 25 | 38 |
| b: Virtual colonoscopy | 0.12 | 0.12 | 3.1 | 3.4 |
| c: Calcium scoring | 0.07 | 0.18 | 11 | 8.3 |
| d: Whole-body screening | 0.80 | 1.08 | 26 | 20 |

Finally, Table 7.4 gives the *total LAR* estimates for cancer incidence. In addition, estimates of the lifetime baseline risks of dying from the disease of concern are provided for comparison.

- In case of lung cancer CT screening, radiation-associated lung cancer contributes most to the *total LAR*. The *LAR* is more than 2.5 times as high for women as for men because on the one hand, the excess lung cancer risk is higher for women. On the other hand, about 15% of the *LAR* arises from the increased breast cancer risk, the accumulated organ dose due to 20 low-dose CT examinations being about three times as high compared to the accumulated organ dose due to a mammography screening (assuming ten examinations in 2-year intervals).

- Although only three paired CT examinations were assumed for screening by virtual CT colonoscopy, organ doses are relatively high for the intestinal sites. Consequently, the estimated *LAR* is high compared to the lifetime baseline risk of colorectal cancer.

- CT calcium scoring inheres relatively high organ doses for breast and lung. Due to the higher radiation-related risk of lung cancer in women and the excess breast cancer risk, the *LAR* for women is 2.5 times higher than for men. However, for men, radiation-related risks due to CT calcium scoring are lower compared to the radiation risks associated with CT screening for cancer.

- Whole-body screening in 2-year intervals between ages 50 and 68 years results in a *LAR* to be diseased with cancer of about 0.8%/1% for men/women, while the baseline lifetime risk for dying from cancer for a 50-year-old male/female person is about 26%/20% in Germany (factor of about 1/30 or 1/20). In contrast, according to the modified BEIR VII

model for breast cancer, the radiation risk associated with breast cancer screening by X-ray mammography for women receiving ten mammographies in 2-year intervals from age 50 years is estimated to be 0.03% while the fatal baseline lifetime breast cancer risk for a 50-year-old German woman is 3.4% (factor of about 1/100).

## 7.4
### Concluding Remarks

The radiation risk due to CT screening procedures can be estimated by means of established methods of risk assessment. The evaluation indicates considerable radiation risks that should not be neglected from a radiation protection perspective. In addition, there are – in contrast to screening X-ray mammography – no valid data from RCTs indicating a benefit, i.e., a significant reduction in cancer mortality due to CT screening. Considering the findings concerning risk and benefit, it can be concluded that scientific evidence is, at present, insufficient to recommend organized screening programs for any of the CT procedures mentioned above.

## References

Bach PB, Jett JR, Pastorino U, Tockman MS, Swensen SJ, Begg CB (2007) Computed tomography screening and lung cancer outcomes. JAMA 297:953–961

Beinfeld MT, Wittenberg E, Gazelle GS (2005) Cost-effectiveness of whole-body CT screening. Radiology 234:415–422

BEIR V: Advisory Committee on the Biological Effects of Ionizing Radiations, National Research Council (1990) Health effects of exposure to low levels of ionizing radiation: BEIR V. National Academy Press, Washington DC

BEIR VII: Committee to Assess Health Risks from Exposure to Low Levels of Ionizing Radiation, National Research Council (2006) Health risks from exposure to low levels of ionizing radiation: BEIR VII Phase 2. The National Academies Press, Washington, DC

Black C, Bagust A, Boland A, Walker S, McLeod C, De Verteuil R, Ayres J, Bain L, Thomas S, Godden D, Waugh N (2006) The clinical effectiveness and cost-effectiveness of computed tomography screening for lung cancer: systematic reviews. Health Technol Assess 10:iii–iv, ix–x, 1–90

Brenner DJ (2004) Radiation risks potentially associated with low-dose CT screening of adult smokers for lung cancer. Radiology 231:440–445

Brenner DJ, Elliston CD (2004) Estimated radiation risks potentially associated with full-body CT screening. Radiology 232:735–738

Brenner DJ, Georgsson MA (2005) Mass screening with CT colonography: should the radiation exposure be of concern? Gastroenterology 129:328–337

Brenner DJ, Hall EJ (2007) Computed tomography – an increasing source of radiation exposure. N Engl J Med 357:2277–2284

British Medical Association (2005) Population screening and genetic testing – A briefing on current programs and technologies. British Medical Association. UK National Screening Committee at www.nsc.nhs.uk

Church TR; National Lung Screening Trial Executive Committee (2003) Chest radiography as the comparison for spiral CT in the National Lung Screening Trial. Acad Radiol 10:713–715

DeStatis (2004) Gesundheitswesen, Todesursachen in Deutschland [Causes of Death in Germany] Fachserie 12 / Reihe 4. Ed: Statistisches Bundesamt [Federal Office for Statistics], Wiesbaden

Diederich S, Thomas M, Semik M, Lenzen H, Roos N, Weber A, Heindel W, Wormanns D (2004) Screening for early lung cancer with low-dose spiral computed tomography: results of annual follow-up examinations in asymptomatic smokers. Eur Radiol 14:691–702

Dos Santos Silva I (1999) Cancer epidemiology: principles and methods. International Agency for Research on Cancer, Lyon, pp 365–379

Fenton JJ, Deyo RA (2003) Patient self-referral for radiologic screening tests: clinical and ethical concerns. J Am Board Fam Pract 16:494–501

Ferlay J, Bray F, Pisani P, Parkin DM (2004) GLOBOCAN 2002. Cancer incidence, mortality and prevalence worldwide. IARC Cancer Base no. 5, version 2.0, IARC Press, Lyon

Furtado CD, Aguirre DA, Sirlin CB, Dang D, Stamato SK, Lee P, Sani F, Brown MA, Levin DL, Casola G (2005) Whole-body CT screening: spectrum of findings and recommendations in 1,192 patients. Radiology 237:385–394

GEKID and RKI (Association of Population-Based Cancer Registries in Germany and Robert-Koch Institute) (2006) Cancer in Germany. Incidence and trends, 5th revised, updated edn, Saarbrücken

Gluecker TM, Johnson CD, Harmsen WS, Offord KP, Harris AM, Wilson LA, Ahlquist DA (2003) Colorectal cancer screening with CT colonography, colonoscopy, and double-contrast barium enema examination: prospective assessment of patient perceptions and preferences. Radiology 227:378–384

Greenland P, LaBree L, Azen SP, Doherty TM, Detrano RC (2004) Coronary artery calcium score combined with Framingham score for risk prediction in asymptomatic individuals. JAMA 291:210–215

IARC: International Agency for Research on Cancer (2002) Handbooks of cancer prevention Vol. 7 Breast Cancer Screening. International Agency for Research on Cancer IARC Press, Lyon

ICRP: International Commission on Radiological Protection (1991) 1990 Recommendations of the ICRP. ICRP Publication 60. Annals of the ICRP 21/1–3. Pergamon Press, New York

I-ELCAP: The International Early Lung Cancer Action Program Investigators (2006) Survival of patients with stage I lung cancer detected on CT screening. N Engl J Med 355:1763–1771

Illes J, Fan E, Koenig BA, Raffin TA, Kann D, Atlas SW (2003) Self-referred whole-body CT imaging: current implications for health care consumers. Radiology 228:346–351

Kellerer AM, Nekolla EA, Walsh L (2001) On the conversion of solid cancer excess relative risk into lifetime attributable risk. Radiat Environ Biophys 40:249–257

Meissner HI, Smith RA, Rimer BK, Wilson KM, Rakowski W, Vernon SW, Briss PA (2004) Promoting cancer screening: Learning from experience. Cancer 101 (Suppl):1107–1117

Mulhall BP, Veerappan GR, Jackson JL (2005) Meta-analysis: computed tomographic colonography. Ann Intern Med 142:635–650

Pickhardt PJ, Choi JR, Hwang I, Butler JA, Puckett ML, Hildebrandt HA, Wong RK, Nugent PA, Mysliwiec PA, Schindler WR (2003) Computed tomographic virtual colonoscopy to screen for colorectal neoplasia in asymptomatic adults. N Engl J Med. 349:2191–2200

Pierce DA, Sharp GB, Mabuchi K (2003) Joint effects of radiation and smoking on lung cancer risk among Atomic bomb survivors. Radiat Res 159:511–520

Preston DL, Mattsson A, Holmberg E, Shore R, Hildreth NG, Boice JD Jr (2002) Radiation effects on breast cancer risk: a pooled analysis of eight cohorts. Radiat Res 158:220–235. Erratum in: Radiat Res 158:666

Preston DL, Ron E, Tokuoka S, Funamoto S, Nishi N, Soda M, Mabuchi K, Kodama K (2007) Solid cancer incidence in atomic bomb survivors: 1958–1998. Radiat Res 168:1–64

Ron E, Lubin JH, Shore RE, Mabuchi K, Modan B, Pottern LM, Schneider AB, Tucker MA, Boice JD Jr (1995) Thyroid cancer after exposure to external radiation: a pooled analysis of seven studies. Radiat Res 141:259–277

Scholefield JH, Moss S, Sufi F, Mangham CM, Hardcastle JD (2002) Effect of faecal occult blood screening on mortality from colorectal cancer: results from a randomised controlled trial. Gut 50:840–844

Simonato L, Agudo A, Ahrens W, Benhamou E, Benhamou S, Boffetta P, Brennan P, Darby SC, Forastiere F, Fortes C, Gaborieau V, Gerken M, Gonzales CA, Jöckel KH, Kreuzer M, Merletti F, Nyberg F, Pershagen G, Pohlabeln H, Rösch F, Whitley E, Wichmann HE, Zambon P (2001) Lung cancer and cigarette smoking in Europe: an update of risk estimates and an assessment of inter-country heterogeneity. Int J Cancer 91:876–87

Stamm G, Nagel HD (2002) CT-Expo – ein neuartiges Programm zur Dosisevaluation in der CT [CT-Expo – a novel program for dose evaluation in CT]. Rofo 174:1570–1576

Statistisches Bundesamt [Federal Office for Statistics] (ed) (2006) Statistisches Jahrbuch 2006 für die Bundesrepublik Deutschland [Statistical Yearbook 2006 for the Federal Republic of Germany]. Metzler-Poeschel, Stuttgart

Thompson DE, Mabuchi K, Ron E, Soda M, Tokunaga M, Ochikubo S, Sugimoto S, Ikeda T, Terasaki M, Izumi S, Preston DL (1994) Cancer incidence in atomic bomb survivors. Part II: Solid tumors, 1958–1987. Radiat Res 137(2 Suppl):S17–S67

UNSCEAR: United Nations Scientific Committee on the Effects of Atomic Radiation (2000) UNSCEAR 2000 Report to the General Assembly, with scientific annexes. Volume I: Sources; Volume II: Effects. United Nations, New York

van Iersel CA, de Koning HJ, Draisma G, Mali WP, Scholten ET, Nackaerts K, Prokop M, Habbema JD, Oudkerk M, van Klaveren RJ (2007) Risk-based selection from the general population in a screening trial: selection criteria, recruitment and power for the Dutch–Belgian randomised lung cancer multi-slice CT screening trial (NELSON). Int J Cancer 120:868–874

Waugh N, Black C, Walker S, McIntyre L, Cummins E, Hillis G (2006) The effectiveness and cost-effectiveness of computed tomography screening for coronary artery disease: systematic review. Health Technol Assess 10: 1–60

# Contrast Agent Application and Protocols

**8**

Martin H. K. Hoffmann

## CONTENTS

## ABSTRACT

Many patient-related and injection-related factors can affect the magnitude and timing of intravenous contrast agent attenuation. MDCT, with its dramatically shorter image acquisition times, permits images with a much better utilization of the peak contrast attenuation. High iodine concentrations of contrast media and newer scanner generations are mutually conditional. The very high iodine flux rates required by cutting-edge angiographic applications can be met by low concentration iodine agents only at very high flow rates resulting in high volumes administered. Sporadic failure, though, is unpreventable at the current stage of development. This is simply due to the fact that the patient's cardiac output is not known prior to scan initiation in most cases. MDCT is a powerful and continuously evolving technology for noninvasive imaging. CA administration is an integral part of this evolution and needs to be continuously adopted and optimized to take full advantage of this technology. A basic understanding of physiologic and pharmacokinetic principles, as well as an understanding of the effects of injection parameters on vascular and parenchymal enhancement, allows the development of optimized contrast agent delivery protocols for current and future MDCT. Scan timing will only then succeed to acquire images at peak enhancement in the tissue of interest.

M. H. K. HOFFMANN, MD
Klinik für Diagnostische und Interventionelle Radiologie, Unikliniken Ulm, Steinhoevelstr. 9, 89075 Ulm Germany

## 8.1
### Basic Rationale

MDCT technology continues to evolve rapidly. At the current stage of development, improvements concentrate on gantry rotational speed (up to 270 ms for a single rotation) and detector width (up to 16 cm with a collimation of 320 × 0.5 mm). This allows for a rapid acquisition of large volumes along the patient's z-axis. Subsequently, contrast agent application is an increasingly demanding task that has to synchronize the timely coincidence of peak enhancement of the tissue at interest and the scan acquisition. For parenchymal imaging such as liver tissue, a wide peak plateau ensues with enough room for securing adequate contrast enhancement. Vascular imaging, on the other hand, has changed tremendously. The peak of contrast attenuation has shortened substantially in order to utilize the contrast agent (CA) efficiently. This is coupled with and enabled by a rapid acquisition of today's scanner generations in less than 10 s. From the aforementioned it is easily deductible that the timing of a scan in relation to the contrast peak is crucial. It demands both semi-automated scanner protocols and individual protocol adaptation.

## 8.2 Factors Affecting Contrast Attenuation

The factors affecting contrast agent attenuation of the tissue of interest can be separated into three general categories: patient related, injection of contrast and CT parameters. The former two factors directly determine and affect the contrast attenuation process itself. The latter, i.e., CT parameters, though only indirectly affecting contrast attenuation, are critical in permitting optimal timing of the acquisition to visualize the peak enhancement of the tissue of interest.

### 8.2.1 Patient-Related Factors

The two relevant patient-derived factors that affect contrast enhancement are body weight and cardiac output (or cardiovascular circulation time). All other patient-related effects on contrast attenuation are negligible.

### Body Weight

Body weight (BW) affects the magnitude of both vascular and parenchymal contrast enhancement (KORMANO et al. 1983; HEIKEN et al. 1995). The contrast agent (CA) administered to the larger blood volume of a heavy patient is more diluted than that administered to a slim patient. Patient weight and the magnitude of

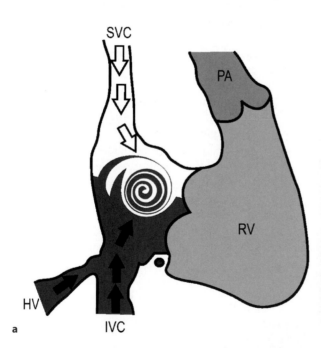

a                                                                          b

**Fig. 8.1a,b.** Mixing of non-contrasted and densely CA containing blood in the right heart. After intravenous administration into an antecubital line the contrast arrives in the right heart via the superior vena cava (*SVC, white arrows* in **a**). In the right atrium, dilution (*swirl*) with non-contrasted blood from the inferior vena cava and hepatic veins (*IVC* and *HV*, *dark arrows* in **a**) is dependent on the flow ratio of SVC:IVC. The contrast distribution in the right atrium is inhomogenous not allowing diagnostic evaluation at early first pass (**b**). The resultant contrast distribution in the right ventricle (*RV*) is homogenous and allows discerning trabeculae in the apex and a floating thrombus (*T* in **b**). *PA*: pulmonary artery

contrast attenuation are inversely related in a linear fashion. However, the timing of enhancement is largely unaffected, due to a concomitant increase of blood volume and cardiac output for an increase in body weight (KIRCHNER et al. 2000).

Hence, for daily clinical application, overall iodine dose should be increased with increasing body weight of the individual patient. This can be effectively achieved by multiplying the body weight with a constant amount of contrast per kg of BW [e.g., 1.2 ml CA (370 mgI/ml) × BW]. The linear increase of CA volume predominantly applies to all parenchymal imaging with a more limited effect on vascular attenuation.

### Cardiac Output

Global cardiac function (measured as cardiac output or cardiovascular circulation time) critically affects the timing of contrast attenuation (BAE et al. 1998b). Decreased cardiac function results in a delay of peak vascular and parenchymal attenuation.

But this is only one parameter affected by cardiac function. The other one critically affected for all vascular or early enhancing scan applications is magnitude of CA enhancement. CA is typically injected via an antecubital vein and therefore arrives at the right heart via the superior vena cava (SVC). For patients with good to high cardiac output, the densely contrasted blood volume is mixed with 1.5-2 times the volume of non-contrasted blood drained from the inferior vena cava (IVC) (Fig. 8.1). For a patient with non-compromised cardiac function at rest, the volume relation of blood drained from IVC and SVC is 1.3:1 or higher (CHENG et al. 2004). For patients with compromised cardiac function, this ratio may drop below 1. It is therefore readily apparent that a patient with a low cardiac output situation will mix the densely contrasted blood volume drained from the SVC with a substantially lower amount of unsaturated blood from the IVC. Subsequently, the magnitude of enhancement in the pulmonary, and systemic vasculature will be higher.

The impact of this theoretical concept on daily clinical routine applies almost exclusively to early phase imaging; this includes angiography, perfusion and early enhancing parenchymal applications. Global cardiac function parameters are usually unknown at CT scan initiation. The test bolus has shown some potential to predict contrast attenuation in situations of variable cardiac output, but the individualization of the scan delay according to automatic bolus tracking is the much more practical approach applied today. The parameters to be adjusted for the individual patient to correct for variable cardiac functions are contrast flow rate and bolus length. Adjustments should be carried out as outlined in Table 8.1.

### Central Venous Return

Central venous blood flow is subject to intrathoracic pressure changes due to respiration (GOSSELIN et al. 2004). In the setting of CM-enhanced CT, this may be particularly harmful if a patient performs an ambitious Valsalva maneuver during breath holding. During a Valsalva maneuver, the intrathoracic pressure increases, which causes a temporary interruption of venous return from the superior vena cava and a temporary increase of (un-opacified) venous blood flow from the inferior vena cava. The effect of this flow alteration is a temporary decrease of vascular opacification. In some cases (especially with fast scan times), this may cause non-diagnostic opacification of the entire pulmonary arterial tree.

Hence, a rehearsal of breath-holding commands should be conducted. The patient should be instructed not to bear down during breath holding. The mouth should be kept open. This may ensue in minor breath holding artifacts, but these may be much more tolerable than the loss of diagnostic quality associated with non-opacified vessels.

### 8.2.2
### Contrast Injection Parameters

Contrast Injection parameters that determine attenuation within the tissue of interest are duration of injection and iodine administration rate or iodine flux. The

**Table 8.1.** Effects of cardiac output on contrast attenuation and homogeneity

| Cardiac output | Attenuation | Flow rate | Homogeneity | Bolus length |
|---|---|---|---|---|
| ↓ | ↑ | ↓ | ↓ | ↑ |
| ↑ | ↓ | ↑ | ↑ | ↓ |

programming of power injectors on the other hand requires volume and rate to be affixed prior to scan initialization. Volume can be easily calculated by multiplying CA flow with duration of injection for that purpose. Another factor that has emerged with the advent of double-barrel injectors is the use of a saline flush for a more efficient utilization of a compact iodine bolus.

### Duration and Flow Rate

The duration of iodine injection critically affects both magnitude and timing of contrast attenuation (AWAI et al. 2004) (Fig. 8.2). Increased injection duration at a fixed flow rate leads to a greater deposition of iodine. This is particularly important for parenchymal imaging with the magnitude of enhancement increased by the amount of iodine administered (MEGIBOW et al. 2001). Peak parenchymal enhancement occurs much later than arterial vascular attenuation. Hence, for dedicated parenchymal protocols, the time frame allowed for contrast agent administration is long and ideally suited for a bolus with a long duration at a reasonable flow rate.

Arterial enhancement depends on iodine administration rate (or iodine flux) and can be controlled by the injection flow rate (ml/s) and/or the iodine concentration of the contrast medium (mgI/ml) (FLEISCHMANN et al. 2000) (Fig. 8.3). Most of the angiography protocols used on 64-detector-row scanners today utilize very high flow rates in order to yield a compact bolus with steep flanks and a high peak.

### Iodine Concentration

The availability of contrast agents with high iodine concentrations (above 350 mgI/ml) has recently attracted a great deal of interest (BECKER et al. 2003; ROOS et al. 2004; SUZUKI et al. 2004). For injections performed with a fixed duration and flow, a contrast agent with a high iodine concentration will deliver a larger total iodine load more rapidly. The resulting magnitude of peak contrast enhancement is increased. The temporal window at a given level of enhancement is wider. Conversely, time-to-peak enhancement is unaffected because duration and rate of injection remain constant.

On the other hand, contrast agents with a higher concentration deliver a constant total iodine mass at a given flow rate in a shorter duration of time. For daily clinical routine, a contrast agent with high iodine concentrations is an alternative approach to using an increased injection rate in order to increase iodine delivery rate. The rapid improvement of current MDCT generations allows an ever increasing scan speed. This consequently allows utilizing shorter and higher contrast peaks, especially for angiographic applications. In other words, higher iodine concentrations are an ideal match for increasing scan speeds. Many of the rapid

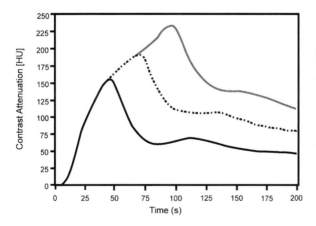

**Fig. 8.2.** Effect of duration of injection on contrast accumulation and peak. Aortic and subsequently parenchymal peak attenuation accumulates with increasing duration or volume of injection. The peak occurs later requiring a modification of scan delays. *Solid line* 75 ml, *dashed line* 125 ml and *dotted line* 175 ml of CA volume. Modified according to BAE and HEIKEN (2000)

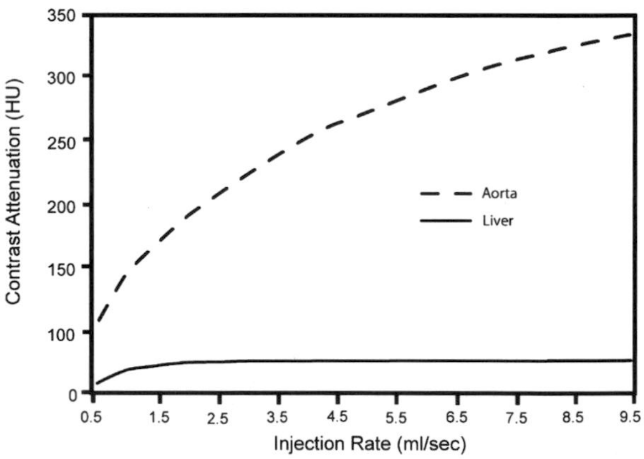

**Fig. 8.3.** Vascular versus parenchymal contrast. Effect of CA injection rate on the magnitude of peak contrast enhancement. For vascular attenuation the increasing injection rate results in substantially higher intraluminal enhancement. For parenchymal imaging the increase of injection rate beyond 2 ml/s does not affect peak enhancement. Modified according to BAE and HEIKEN (2000)

angiographic acquisitions amenable on newest scanner generations can only be utilized relying on the highest iodine concentrations (370-400 mgI/ml) available today. This holds true not only for applications dedicated to the aorta and arterial circulation, but also for pulmonary angiography (SCHOELLNAST et al. 2005).

### Saline Flush

Current double-barrel power injectors are equipped with two syringes. One is filled with non-diluted CA, the other with normal saline. The saline syringe is activated and injects after the contrast bolus has been administered completely. This flushes the arm veins after CA injection and slightly prolongs and increases arterial enhancement (SCHOELLNAST et al. 2004a, 2004b). Pericaval streak artifacts are prevented by this technique for cardio-thoracic applications. The importance of saline flushing increases for smaller amounts of CA applied at higher absolute iodine concentrations. Some injectors allow mixing saline and CA utilizing simultaneous injection from both syringes. This is useful to opacify the right ventricular cavity and pulmonary vasculature for dedicated clinical applications (KÜTTNER et al. 2007).

### Bolus Geometry

Intravenous contrast will travel to the right heart, lung and left heart before reaching the arterial system; this is the "first pass." When the contrast medium is distributed in the intravascular and interstitial space and reenters the right heart, recirculation occurs (FLEISCHMANN 2003b). Both the first pass and recirculation account for the shape, or bolus geometry, of the enhancement curve. In ideal bolus geometry, there is an immediate increase in arterial enhancement at the start of the CT acquisition and uniform enhancement during the data acquisition. With a uniphasic injection (injection at a constant rate), the enhancement increases to a peak and then declines (FLEISCHMANN 2003b). Because CTA will typically be performed during both the upslope and downslope of the curve, enhancement is not uniform throughout the acquisition. Biphasic injection techniques (fast injection followed by slow injection) and exponentially decelerating injection techniques that can increase uniformity of contrast attenuation have been described (BAE et al. 2000, 2004). However, with short scan times, uniformity of contrast attenuation may be less important for a well-defined application, e.g., for

coronary angiography (CADEMARTIRI et al. 2004a). Clinical applications that intend to cover a wider range of vascular territories, though, may well ask for more uniformity with a long plateau phase (VRACHLIOTIS et al. 2007).

### 8.2.3
### CT Parameters

The patient- and injection-related parameters shape the arrival time and distribution of the contrast agent within the organ, tissue or vessel of interest. In order to succeed with an ideally contrasted CT scan that efficiently utilizes the amount of contrast agent administered and that addresses all individualization necessary to account for patient-related factors, the last thing to do correctly is to start the scan at the right time. For scanners with one to four detectors, the determination of scan start times was fairly easy. The scan and subsequently the breath-hold duration was so long that the scan had to be started early. The scan start time was equal to the contrast arrival time determined in a simple test bolus procedure. With the advent of 16 and more detectors in a CT scanner, scans became ever shorter and shorter, allowing for utilization of the maximum height of the contrast bolus peak. These technical developments rendered scan timing much more complicated and demanding.

### Scan Timing

In order to determine scan delays correctly, three factors have to be considered: (1) contrast agent injection duration, (2) contrast arrival time (Carr) and (3) scan duration.

In patients with normal cardiac output, peak arterial contrast is achieved shortly after termination of contrast agent injection (BAE et al. 1998c, 2003). A short, high-flow bolus will therefore result in an early Carr; thus, a short scan delay should be selected for CTA. Conversely, a low flow, long duration bolus will result in delayed peak attenuation, and the scan start has to be delayed. Timing for such a bolus is more critical, and the first choice for CTA is therefore a compact, high-flow bolus.

In addition to injection duration, variable cardiac output parameters of individual patients will have to be addressed. In principle, the two methods to assess the contrast arrival are test bolus techniques and so-called bolus tracking. Both approaches measure Carr and therefore adapt for varying cardiac output. The bolus tracking method is the most efficient, according to our experience. However, the test bolus has the advantage of testing the venous access line with a small volume of contrast before applying the full volume and flow needed for the scan itself. Both techniques utilize a region of interest (ROI) that is placed in a vessel proximal to the organ of interest, e.g., the right ventricle or pulmonary trunk for pulmonary CTA.

Traditionally, for slow CTA studies (single-row and four-detector-row scanners), the scan start was chosen to equal a patient's contrast arrival time (Carr). The scan time of these scanners was not fast enough to allow capturing of the peak of contrast enhancement, but rather to position acquisition around the peak (Fig. 8.4). Logically, this fact resulted in somewhat inhomogeneous contrast distributions in the acquired axial stack.

Faster helical acquisitions available on newer scanner generations (16–64-row detectors and beyond) allow to better utilize the bolus peak (Fig. 8.4). The scan duration fits better to the bolus peak time, and, consequently, both the average magnitude and homogeneity of contrast attenuation within the axial stack improve. But these benefits for CTA will not yield without an additional "diagnostic" delay (ΔT in Fig. 8.4) introduced to better position scan speed in proximity to peak enhancement (BAE 2003; FLEISCHMANN 2003a). It has been proven both empirically (CADEMARTIRI et al. 2004b) and theoretically (BAE 2005) that an accurate ΔT may significantly improve CT image quality. Determination of the additional delay, which is related

to scan speed and injection duration, is critical for fast MDCT. ΔT can be calculated using complex models either assuming normal cardiac function (so called "variable" approach) or they can be more or less empirically determined (BAE et al. 1998a). A so-called "circulation adjusted" approach allows to calculate the "diagnostic" delay with a combined approaches of measuring Carr with bolus tracking (BAE and HEIKEN 2000). As a rule of thumb, the additional "diagnostic" delay or post-threshold delay for bolus tracking should be sufficiently long enough to apply breath-hold commands for the patient. The additional delay has to be longer for faster scanners (e.g., for a 64-detector-row scanner, it is in the range of 6–7 s and should be longer for both faster gantry rotation and larger detectors).

## 8.3
## Sample Protocols

### 8.3.1
### CT Angiography

MDCT has rapidly evolved for pulmonary artery (PA) angiography (SCHOELLNAST et al. 2006; LEE et al. 2007a, 2007b). Today, though never officially acclaimed as the standard of reference, it is the first-line modality in daily clinical life for the detection of pulmonary embolism (CLEMENS and LEEPER 2007). Pulmonary opacification occurs first after mixing of contrast-containing blood in the SVC and non-opacified blood from the IVC in the right heart. In other words, the contrast arrival time (Carr typically in the range of 15 s) is short. The ROI for pulmonary imaging should therefore be placed either in the right ventricle or the pulmonary trunk, and the diagnostic delay time (ΔT) should be short, but long enough to instruct the patient for a convenient inspirational breath hold (JELTSCH et al. 2008). It has already been outlined in the section on central venous return how the impact of flow redistribution between the SVC and IVC can deleteriously affect diagnostic opacification of the pulmonary tree. A sample protocol for a 64-detector-row configuration is given in Table 8.2.

Other vessels further downstream of the vascular territories that are ideally suited for CT imaging are the aorta, the coronary arteries and all other major side-branches of the arterial tree. Aortic imaging utilizing CT is superior to conventional angiography and has therefore replaced most of the arterial catheter-based applications used in the past. This is in part due to the

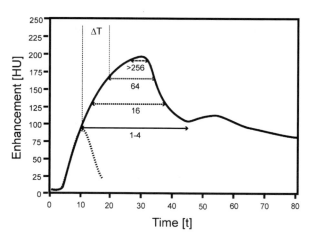

**Fig. 8.4.** Simulated aortic contrast attenuation curve with different scan delays (*ΔT*) designated for multiple scanner generations. ΔT has to be lengthened with shorter scan durations provided by a CT scanner with increasing detector width and rotational speed. A faster scanner may utilize peak contrast enhancement more efficiently than a slower one

**Table 8.2.** Sample protocols for vascular imaging with 64 detector rows

| Parameter | PAD | Coronaries | Aorta | PA | Triple rule-out |
|---|---|---|---|---|---|
| Table speed | ≤30 mm/s | 20 mm/s | 90 | 90 | 20 |
| Scan time | 40 s | 6.5 s | 8 s | 4.4 s | 17.5 s |
| Sample scanner settings | 64 × 0.625 mm, pitch 0.375, gantry rotation time 0.4 s | 64 × 0.625 mm, pitch 0.2, gantry rotation time 0.4 s | 64 × 0.625 mm, pitch 0.9, gantry rotation time 0.4 s | 64 × 0.625 mm, pitch 0.9, gantry rotation time 0.4 s | 64 × 0.625 mm, pitch 0.2, gantry rotation time 0.4 s |
| Scanning delay | Tao + 4 | Tao + 7 | Tao + 6 | Tpa + 4 | Tao + 5 |
| Injection flow rates | First: 5–6 ml/s (1.8 g iodine/sec) for 5 s Second: 3–4 ml/s (0.92 g iodine/s) for remaining scanning time-10 s | Single phase: 6 ml/s (2.4 g iodine/s) for 17 s followed by saline chaser 50 ml at the same flow rate | Single phase: 4.5 ml/s (1.8 g iodine/s) for 20 s and 40 ml saline chaser at the same flow rate | Single phase: 4.5 ml/s (1.8 g iodine/s) for 20 s and 40 ml saline chaser at the same flow rate | First: 5 ml/s (1.8 g iodine/s) for 18 s Second: 2.5 ml/s (1 g iodine/s) for 10 s followed by saline 3 ml/s (50 ml) |

*Tao*: Bolus tracking in the descending aorta, *Tpa*: bolus tracking in the pulmonary trunk

large diameter of the vessel of interest and therefore a reduced propensity for calcium- and metal-induced artifacts. The contrast attenuation within the vessel lumen should be high in order to guarantee adequate opacification in contrast to surrounding structures. One prerequisite to achieve this is a high iodine flux, which may directly be controlled by both flow rate and iodine concentration. The scan delay is best achieved with an ROI placed in the descending aorta at the level of the bronchial bifurcation. The diagnostic delay time ($\Delta T$) should equal peak enhancement of a test bolus for one to four detector rows. A very short $\Delta T$ applies for scanners with 16 detector rows and consecutively longer $\Delta$Ts apply for 32–320 detector rows (Fig. 8.4).

Arterial enhancement continuously increases over time with longer injection durations due to the cumulative effects of bolus broadening and recirculation. Thus, increasing the injection duration also improves vascular opacification. In order to utilize this mechanism in situations with inappropriate vascular access or other reasons restricting injection flow rates, the scan delay has to be adjusted accordingly. $\Delta T$ should be substantially longer to catch the later occurring and higher bolus peak (Fig. 8.4). Provided that a suitable vascular access allows rapid flow rates the injection duration should be timed according to the equation: 15 s + (scan duration/2). This applies to injections with a saline chaser

of 30-40 ml administered at the same flow rate as the preceding contrast agent. For injections without a saline chaser, the above equation should be lengthened by another 5 s.

The strength of an individual's attenuation response to intravenously injected contrast dye is controlled by cardiac output and blood volume, both correlate with body weight. An individual contrast application protocol should therefore be adapted to patient body weight. Whereas the iodine flux rates of Table 8.2 apply for the average 75-80-kg patient, lower flux rates apply for slim patients and higher flux rates for heavier ones. Weight-adapted protocols are less important for vascular attenuation than for parenchymal contrast imaging, but should nevertheless be used in order not to overdose slim patients.

Peripheral arterial disease (PAD) is another potential application for CT angiography. The contrast-related issues for this application center around a highly variable bolus transit time across the territory of interest. The velocity of a contrast bolus to travel from the aorta to the popliteal arteries varies from 29 to 177 mm/s in patients with PAD (FLEISCHMANN and RUBIN 2005). This large variability is unpredictable and does not necessarily correspond to the severity of obstructive disease. In other words, surfing on the bolus peak to guarantee good to excellent magnitude of contrast attenuation at any given z-axis position for such a scan carries the risk of outrunning the bolus. Scanners with 16 and more detector rows are capable of outpacing the bolus along the lower peripheral extremity.

### 8.3.2
### Triple Rule-Out

Patients who present to the emergency department (ED) with chest pain constitute a common and important diagnostic challenge (HAIDARY et al. 2007; WHITE and KUO 2007). In a recent center for disease control and prevention survey, chest pain accounted for the second leading cause of ED presentation. Newer generations of multi-detector CT scanners allow conducting ECG-gated scans of the full chest. This has fueled interest for a comprehensive chest pain evaluation protocol (so-called "triple rule-out" covering pulmonary embolism, coronary disease and aortic dissection evaluation). The demands in terms of contrast opacification of such a protocol are centered on a long homogenous bolus with a reasonably high magnitude. Aortic, coronary and pulmonary tree opacification has to be achieved. That means the bolus peak should be in the aortic root with long tails of the bolus stretching out into the pulmonary and aortic vasculature. The contrast attenuation along the tails should ideally be plateau-like with flat up and down slopes. The most efficient way to achieve this is a biphasic bolus with a rapid initial and slower flow secondary phase as outlined in the paragraph on bolus geometry above. A sample protocol adapted to 64-detector-row platforms has been recently published (HAIDARY et al. 2007). A modification of this protocol is shown in Table 8.2. Modifications account for a higher iodine concentration of a larger detector [4 cm (Table 8.2) compared to 2 cm (protocol of HAIDARY et al.)] and a slower rotational speed [0.4 s (Table 8.2) compared to 0.33 s (protocol of HAIDARY et al.)].

### 8.3.3
### Hepatic Multi-Phasic Imaging

Hepatic multi-phasic imaging is typically conducted at three discrete phases, namely, early arterial phase, late arterial/portal vein inflow phase and hepatic parenchymal phase. The early arterial phase of enhancement is useful primarily for the acquisition of a pure arterial dataset for CTA and has only limited value for liver evaluations per se. The late arterial or portal inflow phase is preferred for the detection of hypervascular primary or metastatic liver lesions (AWAI et al. 2002). The early phase is acquired with a diagnostic delay ($\Delta T$) equivalent to arterial aortic scanning of 6 s. The late arterial phase is best centered at $\Delta T = 20$ s (LAGHI 2007). During this phase, the hypervascular hepatic lesions enhance maximally, while the hepatic parenchyma remain relatively unenhanced, correlating to the relatively small contribution of the hepatic artery to the total blood supply of the organ.

The hepatic parenchymal phase, the period of peak hepatic enhancement, is the phase used for routine abdominal CT imaging. Most hepatic lesions, including most metastases, are hypovascular and are therefore best depicted against the maximally enhanced hepatic parenchyma during this phase. The typical delay for this phase is dependent on indication. A fixed delay preceded by a rather slow (typically 2.5–3 ml/s) injection would suffice for single-phase parenchymal imaging. For a bolus tracking approach that interleaves multiple-phase imaging with an early enhancing arterial and a later parenchymal phase, the typical delay post threshold of the bolus tracker would be in the range of 55–65 s. This delay is dependent on the duration of CA injection.

For some dedicated indications it may be useful to acquire an even later phase of parenchymal imaging (>3 min). This phase has shown potential to discern hepatocellular carcinoma (hypoattenuating) and cholangiocarcinoma (delayed contrast enhancement).

Overall, the most important parameter affecting total peak contrast enhancement for liver and parenchymal imaging is the total iodine mass administered. The administration of iodine is governed by the parameters: total CA volume and iodine concentration. The subsequently most important patient-related parameter that affects the magnitude of parenchymal attenuation is patient weight. For parenchymal imaging per se, it is much more important to adjust the total amount of deposited iodine to the patient weight than for any vascular application. A multicenter study found that 30 HU was the lowest acceptable diagnostic threshold to allow hepatic evaluation. The same study also found that no additional diagnostic benefit was obtained by increasing hepatic enhancement beyond 50 HU. Hence, the recommended iodine dose of 0.5 gI should be injected per kg of a patient's body weight to yield the most efficient diagnostic peak enhancement of 50 HU. Hepatic parenchymal enhancement is much less dependent on flow rate than vascular enhancement (Fig. 8.3), but if combined in multiple-phase imaging, rapid injection rates apply for the early phase. For a single phase application aimed at parenchymal imaging, only an injection rate of ≈3 ml/s is totally sufficient (Fig. 8.3).

### 8.3.4
### Major Trauma Scanning

A major trauma situation necessitating rapid evaluation for life-threatening injuries is so far one of the few accepted indications for full body radiation exposure (Anderson et al. 2006; Hessmann et al. 2006). Multiple-phase acquisitions for vascular and parenchymal imaging require repeated helical acquisitions. In order to minimize the dose exposure, we have adopted an approach to achieve both homogenous contrast distributions in the parenchymal abdominal organs and high-density arterial opacification with a reversed bi-phasic CA application. Based upon a regular 16 detector scanner and a contrast agent with 400 mgI/ml available in the trauma unit, the following flow rates apply: a pre-bolus for parenchymal saturation is injected at a rate of 2 ml/s for a duration of 35 s; after that a compact bolus for vascular enhancement is injected at a rate of 3.5 ml/s for 15 s. This is followed by a saline chaser (40 ml) at the same rate. The bolus tracking procedure is started with a 10-s delay after initiation of the compact vascular bolus phase. The ROI is placed in the descending aorta at the level of the tracheal bifurcation. The diagnostic delay is set at 5 s. A single helical acquisition is acquired with a subsequent bone, lung and soft filter reconstruction. The soft tissue reconstruction allows both assessment of abdominal parenchymal organs for lacerations and diagnostic evaluation of the arterial vascular structures. Head and brain perfusion scans are added to the protocol based upon lesion pattern and trauma presentation.

### 8.3.5
### Perfusion Studies

CT-based perfusion imaging per se has not yet gained a wide-spread clinical acceptance; this is in part due to the technological development just starting to provide CT scanners that cover whole organs in a single rotation. Probably the most promising clinical application of CT would be cerebral perfusion scanning. Perfusion CT relies on the extraction of perfusion parameters from time-attenuation curves derived from the rapid transit of a contrast bolus through the brain. Various algorithms can be used for calculating perfusion values based on nondiffusible indicators, such as iodine contrast, all of which require administration of a compact bolus (Axel 1980). For this reason, the duration of injection should be very short, which subsequently limits the injected volume of contrast. High iodine content seems to substantially improve the diagnostic image quality. A typical brain perfusion protocol injects very rapidly >5 ml/s (≈2 gI/s) for 10 s followed by a saline chaser (Konig et al. 2007).

### 8.4
### Summary

Many patient-related and injection-related factors can affect the magnitude and timing of intravenous contrast agent attenuation. A cross-linked network interrelates all of these factors, but they may be grossly separated into two categories: (1) factors that predominantly affect the magnitude of contrast attenuation (body size, contrast volume, iodine concentration and saline flush) and (2) factors that predominantly affect the temporal pattern of contrast attenuation (cardiac output, contrast injection duration and contrast injection rate).

MDCT, with its dramatically shorter image acquisition times, permits images with a much better utilization of peak contrast attenuation. High iodine concentrations of contrast media and newer scanner generations are mutually conditional. The very high iodine flux rates required by cutting edge angiographic applications can be met by low concentration iodine agents only at very high flow rates resulting in high volumes administered. This is not compatible with compromised cardiac output and may easily result in substantial amounts of contrast retrogradely injected via the right atrium into abdominal venous capacity vessels (Fig. 8.5). Disobeying the basic rules of contrast agent application for MDCT may therefore result in a great deal of non-usable contrast agent being administered. Sporadic failure, though, is unpreventable at the current stage of development. This is simply due to the fact that the patient's cardiac output is not known prior to scan initiation in most cases.

MDCT is a powerful and continuously evolving technology for noninvasive imaging. CA administration is an integral part of this evolution and needs to be continuously adopted and optimized to take full advantage of this technology. A basic understanding of physiologic and pharmacokinetic principles, as well as an understanding of the effects of injection parameters on vascular and parenchymal enhancement, allows the development of optimized contrast agent delivery protocols for current and future MDCT. Scan timing will only then succeed to acquire images at peak enhancement in the tissue of interest.

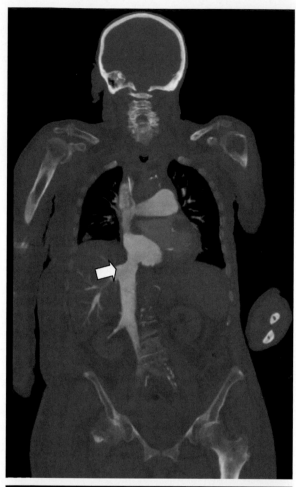

a

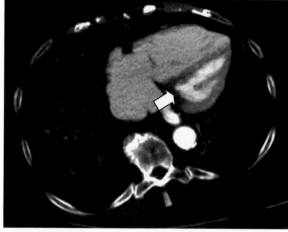

b

**Fig. 8.5a,b.** Sample case with reduced cardiac output due to myocardial infarction. The flow rate of contrast injection for pulmonary angiography was too high resulting in a vast amount of contrast agent injected retrogradely into IVC and branches via the right atrium (**a**). The patient was suffering from compromised cardiac function (or output) induced by an acute myocardial infarction (hypodense area in **b**) in the territory of the right coronary artery

# References

Anderson SW, Lucey BC, Varghese JC, Soto JA (2006) Sixty-four multi-detector row computed tomography in multi-trauma patient imaging: early experience. Curr Probl Diagn Radiol 35:188–198

Awai K, Hiraishi K, Hori S (2004) Effect of contrast material injection duration and rate on aortic peak time and peak enhancement at dynamic CT involving injection protocol with dose tailored to patient weight. Radiology 230:142–150

Awai K, Takada K, Onishi H, Hori S (2002) Aortic and hepatic enhancement and tumor-to-liver contrast: analysis of the effect of different concentrations of contrast material at multi-detector row helical CT. Radiology 224:757–763

Axel L (1980) Cerebral blood flow determination by rapid-sequence computed tomography: theoretical analysis. Radiology 137:679–686

Bae KT (2003) Peak contrast enhancement in CT and MR angiography: when does it occur and why? Pharmacokinetic study in a porcine model. Radiology 227:809–816

Bae KT (2005) Test-bolus versus bolus-tracking techniques for CT angiographic timing. Radiology 236:369–370; author reply 370

Bae KT, Heiken JP (2000) Computer modeling approach to contrast medium administration and scan timing for multidetector CT. In: Marincek B, Ros PR, Reiser M, Baker ME (eds) Multidetector CT: A practical guide. Springer, Berlin Heidelberg New York, pp 28–36

Bae KT, Heiken JP, Brink JA (1998a) Aortic and hepatic contrast medium enhancement at CT. Part I. Prediction with a computer model. Radiology 207:647–655

Bae KT, Heiken JP, Brink JA (1998b) Aortic and hepatic contrast medium enhancement at CT. Part II. Effect of reduced cardiac output in a porcine model. Radiology 207:657–662

Bae KT, Heiken JP, Brink JA (1998c) Aortic and hepatic peak enhancement at CT: effect of contrast medium injection rate-pharmacokinetic analysis and experimental porcine model. Radiology 206:455–464

Bae KT, Tran HQ, Heiken JP (2000) Multiphasic injection method for uniform prolonged vascular enhancement at CT angiography: Pharmacokinetic analysis and experimental porcine model. Radiology 216:872–880

Bae KT, Tran HQ, Heiken JP (2004) Uniform vascular contrast enhancement and reduced contrast medium volume achieved by using exponentially decelerated contrast material injection method. Radiology 231:732–736

Becker CR, Hong C, Knez A, Leber A, Bruening R, Schoepf UJ, Reiser MF (2003) Optimal contrast application for cardiac four-detector-row computed tomography. Invest Radiol 38:690–694

Cademartiri F, Luccichenti G, Marano R, Gualerzi M, Brambilla L, Coruzzi P (2004a) Comparison of monophasic vs biphasic administration of contrast material in non-invasive coronary angiography using a 16-row multidetector computed tomography. Radiol Med (Torino) 107:489–496

Cademartiri F, Nieman K, van der Lugt A, Raaijmakers RH, Mollet N, Pattynama PM, de Feyter PJ, Krestin GP (2004b) Intravenous contrast material administration at 16-detector row helical CT coronary angiography: test bolus versus bolus-tracking technique. Radiology 233:817–823

Cheng CP, Herfkens RJ, Lightner AL, Taylor CA, Feinstein JA (2004) Blood flow conditions in the proximal pulmonary arteries and vena cavae: healthy children during upright cycling exercise. Am J Physiol Heart Circ Physiol 287:H921–926

Clemens S, Leeper KV Jr (2007) Newer modalities for detection of pulmonary emboli. Am J Med 120:S2–12

Fleischmann D (2003a) Use of high-concentration contrast media in multiple-detector-row CT: principles and rationale. Eur Radiol 13 (Suppl 5):M14–20

Fleischmann D (2003b) Use of high concentration contrast media: principles and rationale-vascular district. Eur J Radiol 45 (Suppl 1):S88–93

Fleischmann D, Rubin GD (2005) Quantification of intravenously administered contrast medium transit through the peripheral arteries: implications for CT angiography. Radiology 236:1076–1082

Fleischmann D, Rubin GD, Bankier AA, Hittmair K (2000) Improved uniformity of aortic enhancement with customized contrast medium injection protocols at CT angiography. Radiology 214:363–371

Gosselin MV, Rassner UA, Thieszen SL, Phillips J, Oki A (2004) Contrast dynamics during CT pulmonary angiogram: analysis of an inspiration associated artifact. J Thorac Imaging 19:1–7

Haidary A, Bis K, Vrachiolitis T, Kosuri R, Balasubramaniam M (2007) Enhancement performance of a 64-slice triple rule-out protocol vs 16-slice and 10-slice multidetector CT-angiography protocols for evaluation of aortic and pulmonary vasculature. J Comput Assist Tomogr 31:917–923

Heiken JP, Brink JA, McClennan BL, Sagel SS, Crowe TM, Gaines MV (1995) Dynamic incremental CT: effect of volume and concentration of contrast material and patient weight on hepatic enhancement. Radiology 195:353–357

Hessmann MH, Hofmann A, Kreitner KF, Lott C, Rommens RM (2006) The benefit of multidetector CT in the emergency room management of polytraumatized patients. Acta Chir Belg 106:500–507

Jeltsch M, Klein S, Juchems MS, Hoffmann MHK, Aschoff AJ (2008) Objective evaluation of vessel attenuation in multidetector-row computed tomographic pulmonary angiography using high-density contrast material for the detection of pulmonary embolism. J Comput Assist Tomogr: in press

Kirchner J, Kickuth R, Laufer U, Noack M, Liermann D (2000) Optimized enhancement in helical CT: experiences with a real-time bolus tracking system in 628 patients. Clin Radiol 55:368–373

Konig M, Bultmann E, Bode-Schnurbus L, Koenen D, Mielke E, Heuser L (2007) Image quality in CT perfusion imaging of the brain. The role of iodine concentration. Eur Radiol 17:39–47

Kormano M, Partanen K, Soimakallio S, Kivimaki T (1983) Dynamic contrast enhancement of the upper abdomen: effect of contrast medium and body weight. Invest Radiol 18:364–367

Küttner A, Zunker C, Wüst W, Voit H, Wechsel M, Achenbach S, Anders K, Bautz W (2007) Optimiertes Kontrastmittel-Injektionsprotokoll für die kardiale Bildgebung unter Verwendung einer neuen Dual-Injection Technik. In: Mödder (ed) Deutscher Röntgenkongress. Thieme, Berlin

Laghi A (2007) Multidetector CT (64 slices) of the liver: examination techniques. Eur Radiol 17:675–683

Lee CH, Goo JM, Bae KT, Lee HJ, Kim KG, Chun EJ, Park CM, Im JG (2007a) CTA contrast enhancement of the aorta and pulmonary artery: the effect of saline chase injected at two different rates in a canine experimental model. Invest Radiol 42:486–490

Lee CH, Goo JM, Lee HJ, Kim KG, Im J-G, Bae KT (2007b) Determination of optimal timing window for pulmonary artery MDCT angiography. Am J Roentgenol 188:313–317

Megibow AJ, Jacob G, Heiken JP, Paulson EK, Hopper KD, Sica G, Saini S, Birnbaum BA, Redvanley R, Fishman EK (2001) Quantitative and qualitative evaluation of volume of low osmolality contrast medium needed for routine helical abdominal CT. AJR Am J Roentgenol 176:583–589

Roos JE, Desbiolles LM, Weishaupt D, Wildermuth S, Hilfiker PR, Marincek B, Boehm T (2004) Multi-detector row CT: effect of iodine dose reduction on hepatic and vascular enhancement. Rofo 176:556–563

Schoellnast H, Deutschmann HA, Berghold A, Fritz GA, Schaffler GJ, Tillich M (2006) MDCT angiography of the pulmonary arteries: Influence of body weight, body mass index, and scan length on arterial enhancement at different iodine flow rates. Am. J. Roentgenol. 187:1074–1078

Schoellnast H, Deutschmann HA, Fritz GA, Stessel U, Schaffler GJ, Tillich M (2005) MDCT angiography of the pulmonary arteries: influence of iodine flow concentration on vessel attenuation and visualization. AJR Am J Roentgenol 184:1935–1939

Schoellnast H, Tillich M, Deutschmann HA, Stessel U, Deutschmann MJ, Schaffler GJ, Schoellnast R, Uggowitzer MM (2004a) Improvement of parenchymal and vascular enhancement using saline flush and power injection for multiple-detector-row abdominal CT. Eur Radiol 14:659–664

Schoellnast H, Tillich M, Deutschmann MJ, Deutschmann HA, Schaffler GJ, Portugaller HR (2004b) Aortoiliac enhancement during computed tomography angiography with reduced contrast material dose and saline solution flush: influence on magnitude and uniformity of the contrast column. Invest Radiol 39:20–26

Suzuki H, Oshima H, Shiraki N, Ikeya C, Shibamoto Y (2004) Comparison of two contrast materials with different iodine concentrations in enhancing the density of the the aorta, portal vein and liver at multi-detector row CT: a randomized study. Eur Radiol 14:2099–2104

Vrachliotis TG, Bis KG, Haidary A, Kosuri R, Balasubramaniam M, Gallagher M, Raff G, Ross M, O'Neil B, O'Neill W
(2007) Atypical chest pain: coronary, aortic, and pulmonary vasculature enhancement at biphasic single-injection
64-section CT angiography. Radiology 243:368-376

White CS, Kuo D (2007) Chest pain in the emergency department: Role of multidetector CT. Radiology 245:672–681

# Neuro / Ear-Nose-Throat

# Cerebral Perfusion CT:
# Technique and Clinical Applications

Max Wintermark

## CONTENTS

## ABSTRACT

Perfusion computed tomography (PCT) is an imaging technique that allows rapid, noninvasive, quantitative evaluation of cerebral perfusion by generating maps of cerebral blood flow (CBF), cerebral blood volume (CBV), and mean transit time (MTT). The concepts behind this imaging technique were developed in the 1980s, but its widespread clinical use was allowed by the recent introduction of rapid, large-coverage multidetector-row CT scanners. Key clinical applications for PCT include the diagnosis of cerebral ischemia and infarction, and evaluation of vasospasm after subarachnoid hemorrhage. PCT measurements of cerebrovascular reserve after acetazolamide challenges in patients with intracranial vascular stenoses permit evaluation of candidacy for bypass surgery and endovascular treatment. PCT has also been used to assess cerebral perfusion after head trauma and microvascular permeability in the setting of intracranial neoplasm. Some controversy exists regarding this technique, including questions regarding correct selection of an input vessel, the accuracy of quantitative results, and the reproducibility of results. This article provides an overview of PCT, including details of technique, major clinical applications, and limitations.

M. Wintermark, MD
Department of Radiology, Neuroradiology Section, University of California, 505 Parnassus Avenue, Box 0628, San Francisco, 94143-0628, CA, USA

## Introduction

Multiple imaging techniques have been used to evaluate cerebral perfusion, including positron emission tomography (PET), single photon emission computed tomography (SPECT), xenon computed tomography (CT), and magnetic resonance (MR) perfusion; these modalities, however, are hampered by limited availability, cost, and/or patient tolerance (WINTERMARK et al. 2005b). Perfusion CT (PCT) was introduced as a timely and simple means to evaluate cerebral perfusion. PCT can be performed rapidly with any modern spiral CT scanner and standard power injector. The PCT maps can be generated quickly and easily at a workstation equipped with the appropriate software. Multidetector-row CT scanners are desirable as they allow an increased anatomical coverage. At our institution, PCT is routinely used in acute stroke patients to confirm a suspected diagnosis of stroke and to distinguish between infarct and penumbra or tissue at risk, the target of reperfusion therapies (WINTERMARK et al. 2005a, 2007b; TAN et al. 2007). It has been extended into the evaluation of patients with possible vasospasm after subarachnoid hemorrhage (SAH) (WINTERMARK et al. 2006c) and for the evaluation of cerebrovascular reserve with acetazolamide challenge in patients with carotid artery stenosis who are potential candidates for bypass surgery or endovascular treatment (SMITH et al. 2008). PCT can also be applied to assess cerebral perfusion after head trauma (WINTERMARK et al. 2004a, 2004b, 2006a) and to measure the permeability surface product area (PS) in patients with intracranial neoplasms (ROBERTS et al. 2002a, 2002b; CIANFONI et al. 2006).

## Technique

### 9.2.1
### PCT Data Acquisition Technique

PCT scans at our institution are obtained using a 64-slice CT scanner. After an unenhanced CT of the whole brain, and before a CT angiogram (CTA) of the carotid and vertebral arteries and a post-contrast CT of the brain, 16 5-mm-thick sections are selected to include the level of the basal ganglia and centrum semiovale, where all three supratentorial vascular territories can be evaluated. The CT gantry is tilted both for the unenhanced CT and the PCT so that the selected slices are imaged parallel to the hard palate.

Forty millileters of a nonionic contrast agent (300 mg of iodine per ml) is injected and flushed by 25 ml of saline chase, at a rate of 5 ml/s, using a standard power injector. Contrast administration via an 18–20 gauge line in a right antecubital vein is preferred, as it minimizes pooling of contrast, lowers the risk of extravasation, and minimizes streak artifact at the thoracic inlet during the CTA portion of the exam. All these pitfalls are frequently observed in case of a left antecubital vein injection, because of a compression of the left innominate vein between the sternum and the dolichoid ascending aorta often seen in elderly patients.

At 7 s after initiation of the injection, PCT scanning is initiated with the following technique: 80 kVp, 100 mA. One image per second is acquired in a cine mode for 37 s, followed by one image every 3 s for another 33 s. Total duration of the acquisition is 70 s.

We typically increase the anatomical coverage in our PC protocol by injecting two successive boluses and acquiring two successive PCT series. This is however not feasible in all patients due to renal function. Alternative approaches to increase the anatomic coverage of PCT include the "toggle-table" technique, in which the scanner moves between two different brain levels, obtaining data from each in turn. This method permits imaging of a larger portion of the brain with a single bolus, but sacrifices some temporal resolution due to increased time between sequential images of a single slice (ROBERTS et al. 2001).

When an acute stroke patient is imaged within the therapeutic window, we usually do not wait for the results of creatinine testing, except in case of known history of renal failure or prior serum creatinine measurement that exceeded 1.5 mg/dl, known renal disease, solitary kidney (e.g., prior nephrectomy, congenital absence), diabetes mellitus (insulin-dependent ≥2 years or non-insulin dependent ≥3 years), collagen vascular disease (e.g., lupus), or paraproteinemia syndromes (e.g., myeloma). This approach has been demonstrated as safe in more than 1,000 patients, with only a very low rate of temporary renal failure (0.19%) and no case of permanent renal failure (JOSEPHSON et al. 2005).

If low kVp (80 kVp) and mAs (100 mAs) are used for PCT acquisition (WINTERMARK et al. 2000), the overall effective dose required for PCT (2.0–3.0 mSv) is only slightly higher than that required for routine head CT (1.5–2.5 mSv). This dose equivalent is less than the dose equivalent obtained with PET or SPECT, and is comparable to that of a single-level xenon CT examination (EASTWOOD et al. 2003).

## 9.2.2
## PCT Data Processing Technique

The theoretical basis for PCT imaging is the central volume principle, which relates cerebral blood flow (CBF), cerebral blood volume (CBV), and mean transit time (MTT) as follows: CBF = CBV/MTT. Perfusion data are obtained by monitoring the first pass of an iodinated contrast agent bolus through the cerebral vasculature. The linear relationship between contrast agent concentration and attenuation can be used to calculate the amount of contrast agent in a given region from the degree of transient increase in attenuation. Time versus contrast-concentration curves are created for an arterial and a venous region of interest, as well as for each pixel of the scan. The MTT map derives from deconvolution of arterial and tissue enhancement curves. CBV is calculated as the area under the curve in a parenchymal pixel divided by the area under the curve in the venous pixel. The central volume equation can then be solved for CBF (WINTERMARK et al. 2001a).

Deconvolution softwares allow much lower injection rates—5 ml/s as reported above—compared to other softwares that use different approaches, such as the maximal slope model (WINTERMARK et al. 2001a). These lower injection rates are more practical and tolerable for patients. They do not impair accuracy, since the deconvolution analysis controls for bolus dispersion by comparing the arterial input time-attenuation curve with that of the tissue (WINTERMARK et al. 2001a).

PCT data are analyzed at an imaging workstation. Post-image-collection processing involves semi-automated definition of an input artery and a "vein." In acute stroke patients, selection of different arterial inputs has been demonstrated to have no significant effect on PCT results for an individual patient (WINTERMARK et al. 2007a). As a result, we routinely use the anterior cerebral artery as the arterial input function to provide standardization and facilitate intersubject comparison. In patients with chronic cerebral vascular disease, the situation is different, and we select for each vascular territory its own, specific arterial input function.

The reference "vein" actually needs to be the pixel with the largest area under its contrast-enhancement curve. As such, it must be selected at the center of the largest vascular structure perpendicular to the PCT slices. These requirements are usually met by pixels at the center of the superior sagittal sinus. However, in some instances, other venous structures, or even the supraclinoid internal carotid arteries, can be appropriate "veins" for PCT processing purposes.

## 9.3
## Clinical Indications

### 9.3.1
### Acute Stroke

PCT provides a rapid and simple means to evaluate cerebral perfusion in patients presenting with acute stroke symptoms, most of whom already undergo unenhanced head CT to rule out intracranial hemorrhage. Indeed, findings of acute cerebral ischemia, however, can be subtle or absent on unenhanced CT. In addition, the advent of thrombolytic therapy for acute nonhemorrhagic stroke has intensified the need for a rapid, readily available technique to help identify and quantify the presence and extent of the ischemic penumbra, or tissue at risk. The latter tissue may be salvageable with the administration of thrombolytic agents, while irreversibly damaged infarct will not benefit from reperfusion and may be at increased risk of hemorrhage after thrombolytic therapy. Direct assessment of an individual patient's ischemic penumbra ("penumbra is brain") may allow more personalized, appropriate selection of candidates for intervention than generalized time criteria ("time is brain"), since individuals may have different timelines for evolution of penumbra into infarct.

PCT provides a timely and easy means of identifying ischemic penumbra, permitting rapid triage of patients who may benefit from reperfusion. Distinction between infarct and penumbra from PCT data is based on the concept of cerebral vascular autoregulation. Within the infarct core, autoregulation is lost, and both MTT and CBV are low; within the penumbra, autoregulation is preserved, MTT is again increased, but CBV is preserved or even increased (Fig. 9.1) (WINTERMARK et al. 2002a, 2002b).

In our routine assessment of PCT maps in patients suspected of stroke, we first evaluate the MTT maps, which are the most sensitive, particularly with regard to detection of early stages of minor ischemia. When a MTT abnormality is diagnosed, we use the CBF maps to confirm that CBF is decreased and that we are dealing with an ischemic stroke (MTT can be prolonged in transient ischemic attacks, but then CBF is preserved). Finally, we look at the CBV values within the area with abnormal MTT and CBF to elucidate the underlying pathophysiology (CBV decreased in the infarct core; CBV preserved or increased within the penumbra) (WINTERMARK et al. 2002a, 2002b, 2006b).

PCT provides equivalent results to diffusion/perfusion MRI in terms of characterizing the infarct and

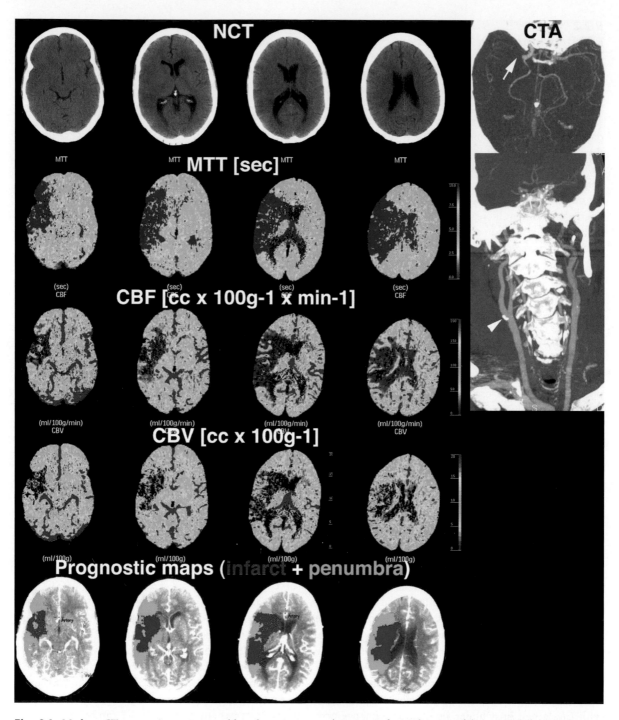

**Fig. 9.1.** Modern CT survey in a 57-year-old male patient admitted to our emergency room with a left hemisyndrome, including an unenhanced CT (*first row*), a perfusion CT (*PCT*) (*rows 2 through 5*) and a CT angiogram (*CTA*) (*right column*). The unenhanced CT ruled out a cerebral hemorrhage. From the PCT raw data, three parametric maps were extracted, relating to mean transit time (*MTT, second row*), cerebral blood flow (*CBF, third row*), and cerebral blood volume (*CBV, fourth row*), respectively. Application of the concept of cerebral vascular autoregulation led to a prognostic map (*fifth row*), describing the infarct in red and the penumbra in green, the latter being the target of acute reperfusion therapies. CTA identified an occlusion at the right M1–M2 junction (*arrow*) as the origin of the hemodynamic disturbance demonstrated by PCT. CTA also revealed a calcified atheromatous plaque at the right carotid bifurcation (*arrowhead*)

penumbra (Wintermark et al. 2002a, 2002b, 2006b) and also in terms of selection of patients for acute reperfusion therapies (Wintermark et al. 2007b). PCT requires a shorter scan time and is usually more widely available in the emergency setting compared to MRI. As such, it represents a very appealing imaging technique to assess acute stroke patients (Wintermark and Bogousslavsky 2003; Kaste 2004). However, there are some specific situations (lacunar infarcts, posterior fossa strokes, young patients) in which MRI is warranted instead of PCT.

### 9.3.2
### Cerebrovascular Reserve

In patients with known chronic cerebral ischemia related to underlying carotid artery stenotic lesions, CBF is usually preserved, at least initially, because of the cerebrovascular reserve. The cerebrovascular reserve represents the vasodilatation ability of cerebral arteries to compensate for a CBF tending to decrease and maintain this CBF at a normal level. In patients with chronic cerebral vascular disorders, it is necessary to quantify the residual cerebrovascular reserve and to distinguish tissue that has used only a limited fraction of its vasodilatation ability and still has cerebrovascular reserve available as a buffer from tissue that has exhausted its vasodilatation ability and cerebrovascular reserve. The latter is at risk of ischemia, which can be triggered by any hemodynamic stress, and requires intervention to increased CBF, usually through carotid stenosis surgery or endovascular treatment, or extracranial-intracranial artery bypass (Nariai et al. 1995).

Hemodynamic stress can be mimicked by using a tolerance test such as acetazolamide administration in conjunction with quantitative measurement of CBF. Although the exact mechanism of action is uncertain, acetazolamide causes vasodilatation of normal cerebral arteries and an increase in CBF in the corresponding territory. Patients with impaired cerebrovascular reserve, however, are already maximally vasodilated due to the response of cerebral autoregulatory mechanisms, and thus cannot respond further to acetazolamide. CBF does not increase, but remains stable or even decreases, because of a steal phenomenon by the "healthy" arteries (Nariai et al. 1995). Acetazolamide is generally well tolerated, with the most common side effects being circumoral numbness, paresthesias, and headache. One case of acetazolamide-associated reversible ischemia has been reported (Komiyama et al. 1997).

Xenon CT (Yonas et al. 1998), PET (Nariai et al. 1995), SPECT (Hirano et al. 1994), transcranial Doppler sonography, and perfusion MR imaging (Detre et al. 1999) have all been used to evaluate cerebrovascular reserve with the acetazolamide test. Recently, PCT has been used to perform acetazolamide challenges (Eastwood et al. 2002; Smith et al. 2008). Implementation of acetazolomide challenges is always the same, independently of the technique used to assess brain perfusion. Patients undergo a first brain perfusion imaging study. Subsequently, 1 g of acetazolamide is administered intravenously, followed 20 min later by another PCT brain perfusion imaging study.

The quantitative results potentially available with PCT may provide an advantage over qualitative techniques such as SPECT and perfusion MR imaging. The ability to measure CBV and MTT may also be an added advantage of PCT. Indeed, a recent study demonstrated that the degree of impairment in cerebrovascular reserve, as assessed by clinical history, correlated most closely with the change in MTT in response to acetazolamide (Smith et al. 2008). This study also showed that increased baseline MTT values may be a static, quantitative indicator of compromised cerebrovascular reserve in at-risk territories (Smith et al. 2008).

### 9.3.3
### Vasospasm

Vasospasm is a frequent complication after aneurysmal subarachnoid hemorrhage (SAH), causing significant morbidity during the early post-SAH clinical course. Angiographic evidence of vasospasm is present in 60%–80% of patients with SAH, with approximately 32% of patients becoming symptomatic. Among patients with aneurysmal SAH who reach neurosurgical referral centers, it is estimated that 7% will be severely disabled, and another 7% will die as a result of vasospasm (Mayberg et al. 1994; Awad et al. 1987). Measurement of CBF can be useful in initial identification of those patients at risk for cerebral ischemia, as well as in guiding therapeutic decisions and monitoring response to therapy (Yonas et al. 1989).

Various methods have been employed to measure cerebral perfusion, including PET, SPECT (Lewis et al. 1992), xenon CT (Yonas et al. 1989), and transcranial Doppler sonography (Clyde et al. 1996). Of these modalities, sonography has been the most widely used, but has many limitations, as it is operator dependent, cannot quantify CBF at the tissue level, and, alone, may not be specific enough to guide therapy.

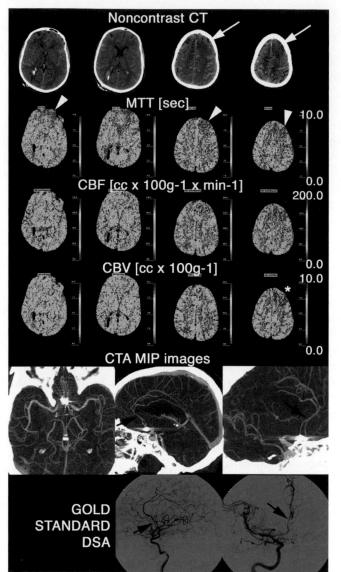

**Fig. 9.2.** Patient transferred at day 8 to our neurovascular intensive care unit (ICU) from an outside institution after coiling of a ruptured anterior communicating artery aneurysm. Unenhanced brain CT obtained at the admission of the patient in our neurovascular ICU demonstrated extensive residual subarachnoid hemorrhage and suspicious loss of gray-white matter contrast in the left superior frontal gyrus (*white arrows*). The tip of a right ventricular drain catheter is also visible. On PCT, significantly abnormal brain perfusion in the distribution of the anterior and inferior branches of the left (and also, to a lesser extent, right) anterior cerebral arteries (ACA) (*arrowheads*) and of the right posterior middle cerebral artery (MCA) branches is seen primarily on MTT maps. The CBF was also slightly decreased in the same territories, whereas CBV was mainly preserved [it is lowered only in the left superior frontal gyrus (*star*)]. CTA confirmed the suspicion of moderate vasospasm of both A2 and A3 segments of the ACA (*arrows*), ultimately verified by gold standard digital subtraction angiography (DSA). No abnormality of the right posterior MCA branches was identified. Of note, the artifacts created by the coils on the CTA images obscure the A1 segments bilaterally and interfere with their evaluation. Endovascular therapy (IA verapamil) was performed in the ACA territories during the DSA

At our institution, PCT is used in combination with CTA to monitor cerebral perfusion in SAH patients with a positive Doppler study (Fig. 9.2). MTT maps are reviewed for arterial territories with prolonged MTT values. Such a territory is considered at risk for vasospasm, and the artery supplying this territory is then evaluated by CTA for vasospasm. If CTA of the corresponding artery is abnormal, the diagnosis of vasospasm is made. Finally, the arterial territories with MTT and CTA suggestion of vasospasm are carefully assessed for a decrease in cortical CBF values. If present, the latter prompts a conventional angiogram for possible endovascular treatment. This approach, which is as sensitive as and more specific than performing Doppler alone, allows obviating unnecessary invasive angiograms in selected lower risk patients (WINTERMARK et al. 2006c).

### 9.3.4
### Head Trauma

PCT has been used in severe head trauma patients, as it affords insight into regional brain perfusion alterations due to head trauma, with the major advantage of being able to detect regional heterogeneity (Fig. 9.3). Its results show specific patterns, linked to cerebral edema and intracranial hypertension. PCT allows distinguish-

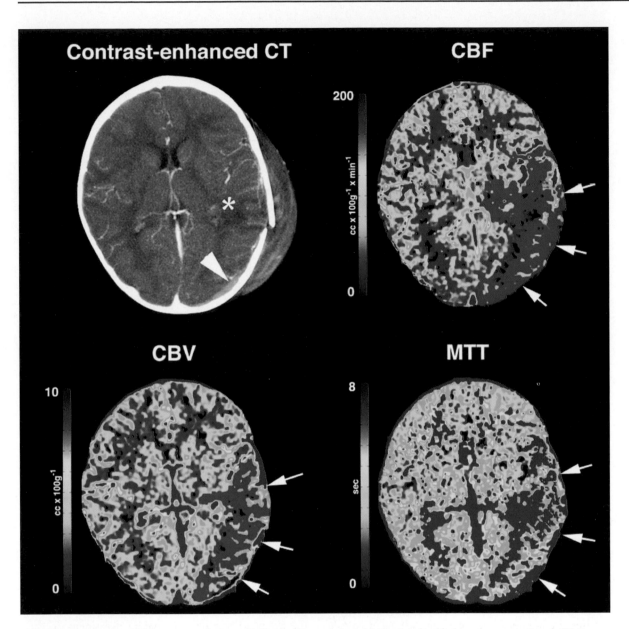

**Fig. 9.3.** Patient who fell from a 6-m height, admitted with a Glasgow Coma Scale score of 9. Neurological examination in the emergency room revealed an asymmetry of tone and deep tendon reflex involving both right upper and lower limbs. Admission contrast-enhanced cerebral CT demonstrated a displaced left parietal skull fracture, associated with a large cephalhematoma. A small left parieto-occipital epidural hematoma (*white arrowhead*) and a small contusion area (*white star*) could also be identified on the conventional CT images. PCT demonstrated a much wider area of brain perfusion compromise (*white arrows*), with involvement of the whole left temporal and parietal lobes, the latter showing increased mean transit time (*MTT*) and decreased cerebral blood flow (CBF) and volume (*CBV*). Thus, PCT afforded a better understanding of the neurological examination findings on admission than conventional CT

ing between patients with preserved autoregulation (or pseudoautoregulation) and those with impaired autoregulation. It may help monitor cytotoxic and vasogenic edema, and guide their treatment (WINTERMARK et al. 2004a, 2006a).

PCT is more sensitive than conventional unenhanced CT in the detection of cerebral contusions, with a sensitivity reaching 87.5% versus 39.6% (WINTERMARK et al. 2004b). PCT can detect altered brain perfusion as a result of compression by an epidural/subdural hematoma (WINTERMARK et al. 2004b). Finally, PCT offers prognostic information with respect to the functional outcome, and this as early as on admission. Normal brain perfusion or hyperemia is observed in case of favorable outcome, and oligemia in case of unfavorable outcome (WINTERMARK et al. 2004b). Head trauma patients with altered brain PCT results might be considered for more aggressive and early treatment to prevent intracranial hypertension, whereas patients with preserved brain perfusion might benefit from less invasive treatment (WINTERMARK et al. 2004a, 2004b, 2006a).

### 9.3.5
### Tumors

Tumors are inherently associated with increased angiogenic activity and neovascularization that results in increased blood volume and hyperpermeability related to the immature vessels (CENIC et al. 2000). Results of previous studies have indicated that microvascular permeability increases with increasing biologic aggressiveness of tumors, while a reduction in permeability in response to antiangiogenic therapy correlates with decreased tumor growth. Results of initial studies in which measurements of CBV and permeability surface product area (PS), a measure of microvascular permeability, were obtained from PCT show PS to be predictive of pathologic grade and to correlate with tumor mitotic activity (CENIC et al. 2000). Elevated PS values are evident only in the tumor and not in the surrounding tissues (ROBERTS et al. 2002a, 2002b). Finally, PCT may help in distinguishing primary glial neoplasms from extraaxial tumors and metastases (Fig. 9.4) (CIANFONI et al. 2006). PCT may prove to be advantageous over MR imaging in the assessment of tumor angiogenesis, given the linear relationship between contrast agent concentration and attenuation changes, the lack of sensitivity to flow, the high spatial resolution, and the absence of susceptibility artifacts. However, the exposure to ionizing radiation, the potential for adverse reaction to the contrast agent, and the limited anatomic coverage are limitations of CT, compared with MR, for evaluation of the microvasculature (ROBERTS et al. 2002b, 2002a).

There are also reports describing the use of PCT to evaluate squamous cell carcinomas of the head and neck. Initial results revealed elevated PS, CBF, and CBV and a lower MTT in the primary tumor site, compared with those values in normal structures (GANDHI et al. 2003; HAYANO et al. 2007). PCT may provide a way to measure tumor malignancy noninvasively, guide biopsies to the most malignant portion of the tumor, and assess response to treatment. However, further investigation is still necessary to validate such an approach.

### 9.4
### Controversies

The quantitative accuracy of the PCT CBF results is debated. PCT CBF results were demonstrated in a few small studies to be highly correlated with PET (KUDO et al. 2003) and xenon-CT (WINTERMARK et al. 2001b) quantitative values. As mentioned above, this however requires appropriate selection of accurate arterial input functions (WINTERMARK et al. 2007a).

The reproducibility of PCT post-processing has also not been fully validated. Software to analyze the PCT data is commercially available and relatively simple to use, although training is required. Results of initial investigations indicate that post-processing findings are reproducible between different operators (SANELLI et al. 2007a, 2007b). Another limitation of PCT is its limited anatomic coverage. We described above two alternative approaches to increase PCT coverage (two separate PCT boluses and the toggle-table technique). The limited coverage of PCT is becoming less and less of an issue with the advent of large coverage, whole-brain multidetector CT scanners. As a note, perfusion-weighted MRI is often advocated because it provides whole-brain coverage, but it can do so only at a cost. Indeed, on most scanners, either of a long time of repetition (2,000 ms), limiting the temporal resolution of the acquisition and the accuracy of the perfusion measurements, or of a low matrix size or large slice thickness or interslice gap, limiting the spatial resolution of the PWI maps, the limited coverage of PCT has been demonstrated *not* to be an obstacle when assessing the extent of a stroke for making treatment decision (WINTERMARK et al. 2005a).

### 9.5
### Conclusion

PCT is a very easy-to-use imaging technique to assess brain perfusion. Its main application is the evaluation of stroke patients, but clinical applications are quickly expanding to include assessment of patients with chronic cerebrovascular diseases, vasospasm, head trauma, and brain tumors. Several limitations, including mainly standardization and automation of the processing, remain to be addressed, hopefully in a close future.

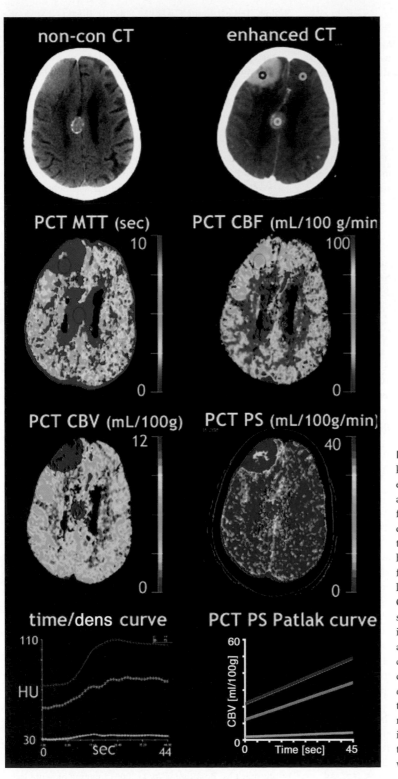

**Fig. 9.4.** An 83-year-old woman with known meningiomas presented in the emergency room with left-sided face, arm, and leg weakness of 1-day duration, following a seizure episode. The CT survey demonstrated two extra-axial masses containing calcifications and characterized by heterogeneous enhancement in the right frontal region and in the right parafalcine location, consistent with meningiomas. On PCT, these meningiomas demonstrated increased CBV and CBF, but also increased PS product. Increased permeability translated on the time-density curves into a large and rapid increase in density within the meningiomas (*red and orange curves*), without significant return to baseline compared to normal white matter (*green curve*). On the Patlak plot, increased permeability is responsible for the steep slope of the curves calculated within the meningiomas

# References

Awad IA, Carter LP, Spetzler RF, Medina M, Williams FC Jr (1987) Clinical vasospasm after subarachnoid hemorrhage: response to hypervolemic hemodilution and arterial hypertension. Stroke 18:365–372

Cenic A, Nabavi DG, Craen RA, Gelb AW, Lee TY (2000) A CT method to measure hemodynamics in brain tumors: validation and application of cerebral blood flow maps. AJNR Am J Neuroradiol 21:462–470

Cianfoni A, Cha S, Bradley WG, Dillon WP, Wintermark M (2006) Quantitative measurement of blood-brain barrier permeability using perfusion-CT in extra-axial brain tumors. J Neuroradiol 33:164–168

Clyde BL, Resnick DK, Yonas H, Smith HA, Kaufmann AM (1996) The relationship of blood velocity as measured by transcranial Doppler ultrasonography to cerebral blood flow as determined by stable xenon computed tomographic studies after aneurysmal subarachnoid hemorrhage. Neurosurgery 38:896–904; discussion 904–895

Detre JA, Samuels OB, Alsop DC, Gonzalez-At JB, Kasner SE, Raps EC (1999) Noninvasive magnetic resonance imaging evaluation of cerebral blood flow with acetazolamide challenge in patients with cerebrovascular stenosis. J Magn Reson Imaging 10:870–875

Eastwood JD, Alexander MJ, Petrella JR, Provenzale JM (2002) Dynamic CT perfusion imaging with acetazolamide challenge for the preprocedural evaluation of a patient with symptomatic middle cerebral artery occlusive disease. AJNR Am J Neuroradiol 23:285–287

Eastwood JD, Lev MH, Provenzale JM (2003) Perfusion CT with iodinated contrast material. AJR Am J Roentgenol 180:3–12

Gandhi D, Hoeffner EG, Carlos RC, Case I, Mukherji SK (2003) Computed tomography perfusion of sqamous cell carcinoma of the upper aerodigestive tract. Initial results. J Comput Assist Tomogr 27:687–693

Hayano K, Okazumi S, Shuto K, Matsubara H, Shimada H, Nabeya Y, Kazama T, Yanagawa N, Ochiai T (2007) Perfusion CT can predict the response to chemoradiation therapy and survival in esophageal squamous cell carcinoma: initial clinical results. Oncol Rep 18:901–908

Hirano T, Minematsu K, Hasegawa Y, Tanaka Y, Hayashida K, Yamaguchi T (1994) Acetazolamide reactivity on 123I-IMP single photon emission computed tomography in patients with major cerebral artery occlusive disease: correlation with positron emission tomography parameters. J Cereb Blood Flow Metab 14:763–770

Josephson SA, Dillon WP, Smith WS (2005) Incidence of contrast nephropathy from cerebral CT angiography and CT perfusion imaging. Neurology 64:1805–1806

Kaste M (2004) Reborn workhorse, CT, pulls the wagon toward thrombolysis beyond 3 hours. Stroke 35:357–359

Komiyama M, Nishikawa M, Yasui T, Sakamoto H (1997) Reversible pontine ischemia caused by acetazolamide challenge. AJNR Am J Neuroradiol 18:1782–1784

Kudo K, Terae S, Katoh C, Oka M, Shiga T, Tamaki N, Miyasaka K (2003) Quantitative cerebral blood flow measurement with dynamic perfusion CT using the vascular-pixel elimination method: comparison with H2(15)O positron emission tomography. AJNR Am J Neuroradiol 24:419–426

Lewis DH, Eskridge JM, Newell DW, Grady MS, Cohen WA, Dalley RW, Loyd D, Grothaus-King A, Young P, Winn HR (1992) Brain SPECT and the effect of cerebral angioplasty in delayed ischemia due to vasospasm. J Nucl Med 33:1789–1796

Mayberg MR, Batjer HH, Dacey R, Diringer M, Haley EC, Heros RC, Sternau LL, Torner J, Adams HP, Jr., Feinberg W et al. (1994) Guidelines for the management of aneurysmal subarachnoid hemorrhage. A statement for healthcare professionals from a special writing group of the Stroke Council, American Heart Association. Circulation 90:2592–2605

Nariai T, Suzuki R, Hirakawa K, Maehara T, Ishii K, Senda M (1995) Vascular reserve in chronic cerebral ischemia measured by the acetazolamide challenge test: comparison with positron emission tomography. AJNR Am J Neuroradiol 16:563–570

Roberts HC, Roberts TP, Lee TY, Dillon WP (2002a) Dynamic contrast-enhanced computed tomography (CT) for quantitative estimation of microvascular permeability in human brain tumors. Acad Radiol 9 (Suppl 2):S364–367

Roberts HC, Roberts TP, Lee TY, Dillon WP (2002b) Dynamic, contrast-enhanced CT of human brain tumors: quantitative assessment of blood volume, blood flow, and microvascular permeability: report of two cases. AJNR Am J Neuroradiol 23:828–832

Roberts HC, Roberts TP, Smith WS, Lee TJ, Fischbein NJ, Dillon WP (2001) Multisection dynamic CT perfusion for acute cerebral ischemia: the "toggling-table" technique. AJNR Am J Neuroradiol 22:1077–1080

Sanelli PC, Nicola G, Johnson R, Tsiouris AJ, Ougorets I, Knight C, Frommer B, Veronelli S, Zimmerman RD (2007a) Effect of training and experience on qualitative and quantitative CT perfusion data. AJNR Am J Neuroradiol 28:428–432

Sanelli PC, Nicola G, Tsiouris AJ, Ougorets I, Knight C, Frommer B, Veronelli S, Zimmerman RD (2007b) Reproducibility of postprocessing of quantitative CT perfusion maps. AJR Am J Roentgenol 188:213–218

Smith LM, Elkins JS, Dillon WP, Schaeffer S, Wintermark M (2008) Perfusion-CT assessment of the cerebrovascular reserve: a revisit to the acetazolamide challenges. J Neuroradiol 21:1441–1449

Tan JC, Dillon WP, Liu S, Adler F, Smith WS, Wintermark M (2007) Systematic comparison of perfusion-CT and CT-angiography in acute stroke patients. Ann Neurol 61:533–543

Wintermark M, Bogousslavsky J (2003) Imaging of acute ischemic brain injury: the return of computed tomography. Curr Opin Neurol 16:59–63

Wintermark M, Chiolero R, Van Melle G, Revelly JP, Porchet F, Regli L, Maeder P, Meuli R, Schnyder P (2006a) Cerebral vascular autoregulation assessed by perfusion-CT in severe head trauma patients. J Neuroradiol 33:27–37

Wintermark M, Chiolero R, van Melle G, Revelly JP, Porchet F, Regli L, Meuli R, Schnyder P, Maeder P (2004a) Relationship between brain perfusion computed tomography variables and cerebral perfusion pressure in severe head trauma patients. Crit Care Med 32:1579–1587

Wintermark M, Fischbein NJ, Smith WS, Ko NU, Quist M, Dillon WP (2005a) Accuracy of dynamic perfusion CT with deconvolution in detecting acute hemispheric stroke. AJNR Am J Neuroradiol 26:104–112

Wintermark M, Flanders AE, Velthuis B, Meuli R, van Leeuwen M, Goldsher D, Pineda C, Serena J, van der Schaaf I, Waaijer A, Anderson J, Nesbit G, Gabriely I, Medina V, Quiles A, Pohlman S, Quist M, Schnyder P, Bogousslavsky J, Dillon WP, Pedraza S (2006b) Perfusion-CT assessment of infarct core and penumbra: receiver operating characteristic curve analysis in 130 patients suspected of acute hemispheric stroke. Stroke 37:979–985

Wintermark M, Ko NU, Smith WS, Liu S, Higashida RT, Dillon WP (2006c) Vasospasm after subarachnoid hemorrhage: utility of perfusion CT and CT angiography on diagnosis and management. AJNR Am J Neuroradiol 27:26–34

Wintermark M, Lau BC, Chien J, Arora S (2007a) The anterior cerebral artery is an appropriate arterial input function for perfusion-CT processing in patients with acute stroke. Neuroradiology 50:227–236

Wintermark M, Maeder P, Thiran J-P, Schnyder P, Meuli R (2001a) Quantitative assessment of regional cerebral blood flows by perfusion CT studies at low injection rates: a critical review of the underlying theoretical models. Eur Radiol 11:1220–1230

Wintermark M, Maeder P, Verdeb FR, Thiran J-P, Valley J-F, Schnyder P, Meuli R (2000) Using 80 kVp versus 120 kVp in perfusion CT measurement of regional cerebral blood flows. Am J Neuroradiol 21:1881–1884

Wintermark M, Meuli R, Browaeys P, Reichhart M, Bogousslavsky J, Schnyder P, Michel P (2007b) Comparison of CT perfusion and angiography and MRI in selecting stroke patients for acute treatment. Neurology 68:694–697

Wintermark M, Reichhart M, Cuisenaire O, Maeder P, Thiran JP, Schnyder P, Bogousslavsky J, Meuli R (2002a) Comparison of admission perfusion computed tomography and qualitative diffusion- and perfusion-weighted magnetic resonance imaging in acute stroke patients. Stroke 33:2025–2031

Wintermark M, Reichhart M, Thiran JP, Maeder P, Chalaron M, Schnyder P, Bogousslavsky J, Meuli R (2002b) Prognostic accuracy of cerebral blood flow measurement by perfusion computed tomography, at the time of emergency room admission, in acute stroke patients. Ann Neurol 51:417–432

Wintermark M, Sesay M, Barbier E, Borbely K, Dillon WP, Eastwood JD, Glenn TC, Grandin CB, Pedraza S, Soustiel JF, Nariai T, Zaharchuk G, Caille JM, Dousset V, Yonas H (2005b) Comparative overview of brain perfusion imaging techniques. J Neuroradiol 32:294–314

Wintermark M, Thiran JP, Maeder P, Schnyder P, Meuli R (2001b) Simultaneous measurement of regional cerebral blood flow by perfusion CT and stable xenon CT: a validation study. AJNR Am J Neuroradiol 22:905–914

Wintermark M, van Melle G, Schnyder P, Revelly JP, Porchet F, Regli L, Meuli R, Maeder P, Chiolero R (2004b) Admission perfusion CT: prognostic value in patients with severe head trauma. Radiology 232:211–220

Yonas H, Pindzola RR, Meltzer CC, Sasser H (1998) Qualitative versus quantitative assessment of cerebrovascular reserves. Neurosurgery 42:1005–1010; discussion 1011–1002

Yonas H, Sekhar L, Johnson DW, Gur D (1989) Determination of irreversible ischemia by xenon-enhanced computed tomographic monitoring of cerebral blood flow in patients with symptomatic vasospasm. Neurosurgery 24:368–372

# MDCT in Neuro-Vascular Imaging

## 10

Dominik Morhard and Birgit Ertl-Wagner

CONTENTS

## ABSTRACT

New generations of multi detector row CT (MDCT) scanners offer previously unparalleled options in neurovascular imaging. Comprehensive stroke imaging with MDCT now usually includes perfusion CT and CT angiography. Modern techniques moreover also enable the retrieval of dynamic CT-angiographic data from the perfusion CT, if a perfusion of the entire brain is performed. Occlusions of the basilar artery can usually be readily diagnosed in the CT angiography. CT angiography of the cervicocranial arteries also allows to assess the degree of carotid artery stenoses and of possible intracranial stenoses. Newer scanner types lead to increasing sensitivity and specificity parameters for detecting intracranial aneurysm. Cerebrovenous thromboses can be diagnosed with a venous CT angiography of the brain. Even thromboses of small bridging and internal cerebral veins can usually be readily discerned.

## Background

In the early 1990s the first spiral CT scanners using only one detector row were introduced. With the advent of multi detector row CT scanners (MDCT) in 1998, larger scan volumes and an improved longitudinal resolution at a shorter scanning time was archived by simultaneous acquisition of multiple slices per gantry rotation. The acquisition of volume data using the spiral scanning technique was a ground-breaking step in CT development. With volume data sets it became for the first time possible to reconstruct images in any orientation along the patient axis (CRAWFORD and KING 1990; KALENDER et al. 1990) enabling applications like CTA and thereby

D. MORHARD, MD
Department of Clinical Radiology, Ludwig-Maximilians-University of Munich, Munich University Hospitals
Marchioninistrasse 15, 81377 Munich, Germany

B. ERTL-WAGNER, MD
Department of Clinical Radiology, Ludwig-Maximilians-University of Munich, Munich University Hospitals
Marchioninistrasse 15, 81377 Munich, Germany

revolutionizing non-invasive assessment (RUBIN et al. 1995). Also, three-dimensional reformations like MPR (multi planar reformations), MIP (maximum intensity projections), VRT (volume rendering technique) and SRT (surface rendering technique) could be attained from volume data sets (NAPEL et al. 1993).

In 2004, 32- to 64-slice CT systems were introduced establishing neurovascular CT-angiographic examinations in a submillimeter resolution and thereby enabling isotropic reformations and acquisitions in a strictly arterial phase (FLOHR et al. 2002a, b; ERTL-WAGNER et al. 2005). In 2008 the first 320-slice CT prototype system was introduced.

The first dual-source-CT was installed in 2006. Using two tubes and detectors mounted orthogonally, it became possible to acquire one axial image by a gantry rotation of 90° instead of 180° at single-source scanners. This cuts acquisition time by half, which is an important factors especially in cardiac imaging (FLOHR et al. 2006). It is also possible to run the two tubes at different voltages—the so-called dual-energy-CT-mode, e.g. with 140 and 80 kV—in order to obtain different attenuations for material decomposition (JOHNSON et al. 2007). This can

also be used for selective bone-removal or iodine quantification without motion-artefacts or misregistrations.

In addition to the fast-paced innovations of new scanners, new developments in post processing with semi-automatic quantifications of stenoses or bone-removal techniques had a pronounced influence on current clinical routine (ANDERSON et al. 1999; CHAPPELL et al. 2003). Modern neurovascular CTA as a non-invasive imaging modality is more and more replacing conventional diagnostic DSA (LELL et al. 2006; TOMANDL et al. 2006; HOH et al. 2004).

## 10.2
## Protocol Parameters for Neurovascular MDCT

As there are numerous different MDCT-systems on the market, a multitude of optimized scanning protocols are available for neurovascular imaging depending on the respective systems. Sample protocols for NECT are provided in Table 10.1, while sample protocols for CTA are shown in Table 10.2 (ERTL-WAGNER et al. 2004).

**Table 10.1.** Scan parameters: non-enhanced cranial CT

| Parameters | 4–8 detector row scanners | 10–20 detector row scanners | 32–64 detector row scanners |
|---|---|---|---|
| **Scanner protocol** | | | |
| Tube voltage (kV) | 120 | 120 | 120 |
| Rotation time (s) | 0.75 | 1.0 | 1.0 |
| Tube current time product (mAs) | 190–250 CDTIvol <60 | 190–250 CDTIvol <60 | 350 CDTIvol <60 |
| Collimation (mm) | 2.5 | 1.5 | 0.6 |
| Normalized pitch | 0.65–0.85 | 0.65–0.85 | 0.85 |
| Scan range | Sagittal suture to foramen magnum | | |
| Scan direction | Craniocaudal | | |
| **Reconstruction settings** | | | |
| Slice increment (mm) | Whole brain reconstructions: 5 or Split reconstructions: supratentorial: 8, and infratentorial: 3 | | |
| Slice thickness (mm) | Whole brain reconstructions: 5 or Split reconstructions: supratentorial: 8 and infratentorial: 3 | | |
| Kernel | Standard | | |

If a purely intracranial CT is to be performed, it should be kept in mind that most of the latest MDCT-systems do not allow the gantry to be tilted for spiral scanning. Therefore, the only option to keep the radiation-sensitive eye-lenses out of the radiation beam is by correcting the patient positioning (Fig. 10.1).

In addition, it needs to be considered that spiral CT scanning always includes a short area of overbeaming, i.e. a radiation exposure in front and at the end of the imaging scan range that exceeds the scan range, and an area of overranging to obtain additional data required for interpolation. Overbeaming depends on the diameter of the imaging beam, which correlates to the number of used detectors and the collimation. For instance, on a 64-detector row scanner only the inner 20 detectors can be used for imaging and therefore a smaller beam is used, reducing the area of overbeaming and overranging, but increasing scan time.

Modern MDCT scanners allow to cover long scan ranges with a single scan. This is advantageous for neu-

**Table 10.2.** Scan parameters: CTA

| Parameters | 4–8 detector row scanners | 10–20 detector row scanners | 32–64 detector row scanners | Dual-energy scanners |
|---|---|---|---|---|
| **Scanner protocol** | | | | |
| Tube voltage (kV) | 120 | 120 | 120 | Tube-A: 140 Tube-B: 80 |
| Rotation time (s) | 0.5 | 0.33–0.5 | 0.33 | 0.33 |
| Tube current time product (mAs) | 135–200 | 135–200 | 135–240 | Tube-A: 55 Tube-B: 230 |
| Collimation (mm) | 1–1.25 | 0.6–0.75 | 0.6 | 0.6 |
| Normalized pitch | 0.9–1 | 0.9–1 | 0.9–1.2 | 1.0 |
| Scan range | Intracranial scans: sagittal suture to foramen magnum Scans including extracranial vasculature: aortic arch to sagittal suture | | | |
| Scan direction | Caudocranial | Craniocaudal for standard scans in a late arterial phase, caudocranial for scanning in a explicit very early arterial phase (e.g. aneurysm visualization in therapy-planning) | | |
| **Reconstruction settings** | | | | |
| Slice increment (mm) | 1 | 0.6 | 0.4–0.5 | 0.4–0.5 |
| Slice thickness (mm) | 1.25 | 0.75–1 | 0.6–0.75 | 0.6–0.75 |
| Kernel | Standard CTA-kernel for cross-sectional MPR and MIP reformations (e.g. H20 for Siemens scanners), using softer kernels (e.g. H31 for Siemens scanners) for VRT or SRT reconstructions can provide more convenient results | | | |
| **Contrast agent injection protocol** | | | | |
| Concentration (mg iodine/ml) | 300–400 | | | |
| Volume (ml) | 80–120 | 80–100 | 80–100 | 80–100 |
| Injection rate (ml/s) | 3–4, monophasic injection | | | |
| Saline pusher (ml; ml/s) | 30; 3.0 | | | |
| Delay (s) | Automatic bolus detection at aortic arch plus 3–6 s if available, if not available 20 s for strict intracranial scans, 12–15 s for scans including extracranial vasculature | | | |

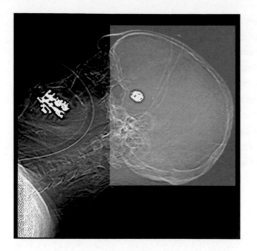

**Fig. 10.1.** Correct patient positioning for intracranial scans, *light box* indicates the scan volume, eye-lenses outside of scan volume. Note the titanium coils after endovascular coil embolization of an aneurysm at the anterior communication artery (ACoA)

rovascular CT, especially in stroke-imaging, as all supraaortic arteries can be visualized from their origin at the aortic arch to the circle of Willis including its branches. However, the easy availability and high quality of these long scan ranges can be tempting to cover longer scan ranges as indicated for the individual diagnostic evaluation and thereby increasing radiation dose. The scan ranges should always be individualized for the respective patient situation and limited to the diagnostically relevant area in order to protect radiation sensitive organs such as the thyroid gland and the lenses of the eye. If available, dose-modulation functions on the scanner side should always be used in cervical CTA in order to reduce the radiation dose at the upper and mid-cervical levels and to achieve enough dose at the lower cervical level, i.e. the shoulder region.

With modern MDCT scanners, the indications for sequential CT scanning—as opposed to spiral scanning—are usually limited to dynamic protocols such as perfusion CT (PCT) and to sequential scans of the infratentorial brain or skull base. Sequential scanning can reduce beam hardening artefacts and overbeaming; however, 3D-refomation options are limited.

For dynamic CT-perfusion, it is mandatory to prevent any motion of the patient's head during the entire scanning period, either by explicit instructions to the patient, or by effective fixation. For fixation in unconscious patients large patches covering the forehead and the headrest are preferable to hook-and-loop fasteners and cushions.

Sample scan parameters for CT-perfusion scanning are:

- Tube voltage 80 kV
- Tube current 120–240 mAs
- Rotation time 1 s
- Scanning time 40–45 s
- Start delay of 6 s

For application of 40–50 ml contrast agent at a flux of 5–10 ml/s, a central venous catheter or an 18-gauge injection catheter at the cubital vein is mandatory. Using a saline pusher at the same injection speed directly after contrast agent administration improves the quality of the arterial input function.

In 2007 a new imaging technique was introduced. During sequential perfusion acquisition the table moves in cranio-caudal direction periodically. This technique offers PCT scan ranges of 10 cm and more—independently of the width of the detector. Multiplanar reformations can be used analogous to "conventional" spiral scan data. Non-static cycle time settings can help to reduce radiation dose significantly, e.g. high temporal resolution in the first-pass-phase with 1–1.5 s scan interval for 20–30 s followed by lower temporal resolution with 3–4.5 s for 10–20 s in the second-pass phase. Large volume data sets acquired by broad detector CT (e.g. 320-slice-CT) or by sliding-table-technique can also be used to reconstruct angiograms out of the PCT data, if necessary even in different contrast phases, e.g. arterial or venous phase.

## 10.3
## Clinical Applications of Neurovascular MDCT

There are numerous applications and indications for neurovascular MDCT. These include comprehensive stroke imaging, evaluation of the extra- and intracranial vasculature of head and neck, as well as preoperative therapy planning. In this chapter we will focus on the most commonly used and on more specialized, but highly relevant neurovascular MDCT applications.

### 10.3.1
### Comprehensive Stroke Imaging

In most clinical settings, suspected ischemic or haemorrhagic stroke is the most frequent indication for emergency CT. CT is widely available and rapidly performed—these advantages are crucial parameters in stroke, where "time is brain". Even though modern MR imaging is a very valuable methods to evaluate early stroke, only a small number of specialized radiology/ neuroradiology departments offer stroke-MRI in a 24/7 time frame.

Historically, NECT was the only CT method available. Even in modern stroke MDCT, the evaluation always starts with standard NECT. NECT allows one to differentiate between hemorrhagic and ischemic stroke, and also to exclude many other differential diagnoses. In case of a subarachnoid haemorrhage (SAH), a subsequent intracranial CTA should be performed (see Sect. 10.3.4) (TOMANDL et al. 2003). If no haemorrhage or other obvious reasons for stroke-like symptoms are identified and contraindications for the administration of contrast medium are absent, the next step is usually

to perform a PCT followed by a CTA of brain and neck. As an alternative, some centres acquire the CTA prior to PCT in order to obtain better CTA results. There is an on-going discussion about the order of the administration of contrast agent for CTA and PCT. CT studies will have to prove whether the result of MR-perfusion studies showing no relevant influence regarding the order of MR-perfusion and MRA also pertain to PCT (RYU et al. 2006).

After performing CTA and NECT, it is important to evaluate any discrepancies between early stroke signs or visibly manifest infarction in NECT (Fig. 10.2a) and potential occlusions of vessels in CTA (Fig. 10.2b). It is therefore mandatory to check every segment of the intracranial arteries. Additional axial MIP reformations with a slice thickness of 5 mm and an increment of

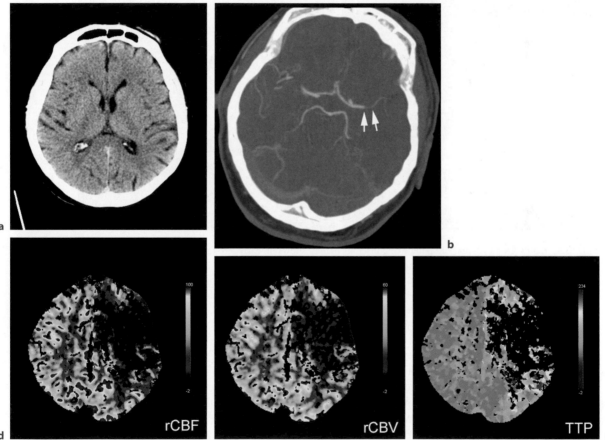

**Fig. 10.2.** **a** A 59-year old male patient with known colorectal cancer and acute hemiparesis. NECT 1 h after stroke-onset does not show any early stroke signs, hemorrhage or edema. **b** MIP reconstruction of intracranial CTA scan shows a stop of contrast agent (*arrows*) at the distal main stem of the left middle cerebral artery (MCA). **c** Dynamic perfusion-CT (PCT) analysis reveals subtotal restriction of cerebral blood flow (CBF) at the left frontal and parietal lobe. **d** Analogue to the CBF the cerebral blood volume (CBV) parameter map shows extreme loss of blood volume corresponding to a dysfunction of vessel auto-regulation, a sign for infarction. **e** Nearly no contrast agent delivery to the infarcted brain territory during the whole scan period (40 s) is shown at the Time-to-peak (TTP) parameter map

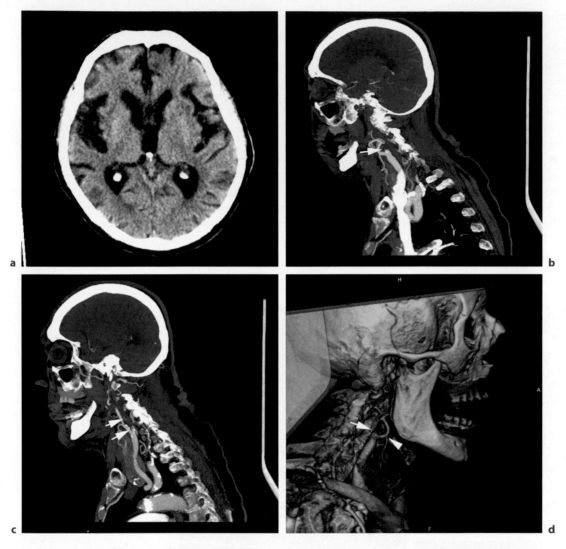

**Fig. 10.3.** **a** NECT of a 72-year old female unconscious patient shows no early stroke signs or hemorrhage. **b** Sagittal MIP of the CTA data set delineates proximal vessel occlusion (*arrow*) of the left internal carotid artery (ICA). **c** High-grade stenosis of the contra lateral (right) ICA with only weak contrast enhancement of the distal ICA (*arrows*), sagittal MIP. **d** VRT reconstruction of CTA data visualizes the occlusion of the left ICA (*arrow*) at the carotid bulb. Note the non-occluded external carotid artery (*arrowhead*). **e** (*see next page*)

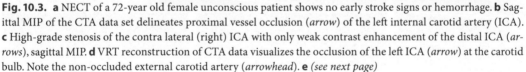

1 mm can provide a very convenient and fast overview of all cerebral vessels (ERTL-WAGNER et al. 2006). Most commonly, thrombembolic occlusions can be found in one of the middle cerebral arteries (MCA). In addition, potential hemodynamic stenoses or dissections need to be sought for. These are most commonly located in the proximal internal carotid artery (ICA) in close proximity to the carotid bulb (Fig. 10.3a–h). Other common locations for relevant stenoses are the proximal portion of the common carotid artery and the distal, intracranial part of the ICA. Dissections are often located at the ICA and at the vertebral arteries.

If the extent of a cerebral infarction appears to be less extensive in NECT than would be concordant to the territory of the occluded vessel, a perfusion analysis is indicated (if PCT has not already been acquired before) (Figs. 10.2c–e and 10.3e,f) (WINTERMARK 2005; KLOSKA et al. 2004). For perfusion CT (PCT), sequential slices are acquired in cine mode during an intravenous contrast injection, typically with a high flow rate of 5–10 ml/s and a scanning time of 40 s. By using PCT, it is possible to distinguish ischemic brain tissue ("tissue at risk", "penumbra") from infarction, thereby supporting therapeutic decision-making in regard to whether

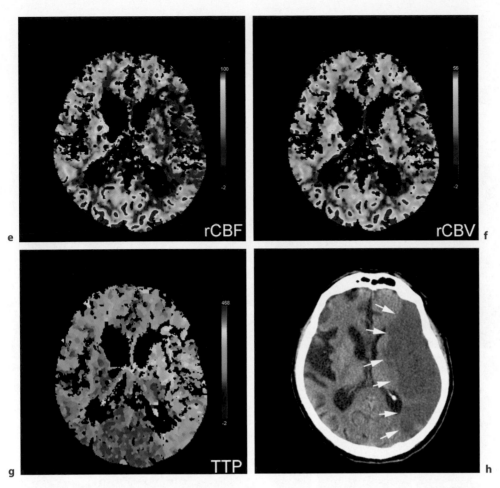

**Fig. 10.3.** *(continued)* **e** CBF shows a strong flow restriction at the left MCA territory, PCT. **f** CBV shows a mild reduction of blood volume at the left MCA territory as a sign for dysfunction of the auto-regulation of the vessel and infarction. **g** TTP visualizes the prolonged contrast agent delivery at left ICA territory as well as at the right (post-stenotic) ICA territory. No prolongation at the territories of the posterior cerebral arteries. **h** NECT follow up after two days of stroke-onset shows complete infarction of the left MCA territory *(arrows)*

a thrombolysis or mechanical recanalization may be of benefit to the patient.

Depending on the vendor of the scanner, mainly two different mathematical reconstruction models are used for analysing PCT—the maximum slope/gradient model (e.g. Siemens and Vitrea) and the deconvolution model (e.g. GE and Toshiba). Both models provide parameter maps of cerebral blood flow (CBF) and relative cerebral blood volume (rCBV). In addition, the time-to-peak (TTP, maximum slope model) or the mean-transit-time (MTT, deconvolution model) are shown.

In non-ischemic brain tissue, the CBF value is about 50–80 ml blood per 100 mg brain per minute. Flow reductions below 10–15 ml/100 mg/min usually lead to irreversible infarction after a few minutes. CBF val-

ues of 10–25 ml/100 mg/min tend to cause neurological dysfunction, but a complete recovery may occur, if normal levels of perfusion are restored within hours or days. CBV values reflect the extent of regional autoregulation. Regional CBV is usually increased at the penumbra as a result of vasodilatation to compensate for regional CBF lowering. Low or normal CBV values at regions with lowered CBF are normally predictive of irreversible infarction.

PCT can also aid in evaluating patients with a new onset of stroke symptoms and old infarctions in the patient's history or patients with multiple high-grade stenoses in different vessel territories (Fig. 10.4a–d).

There is a new theoretical approach for estimating perfused blood volume from CTA and NECT volume

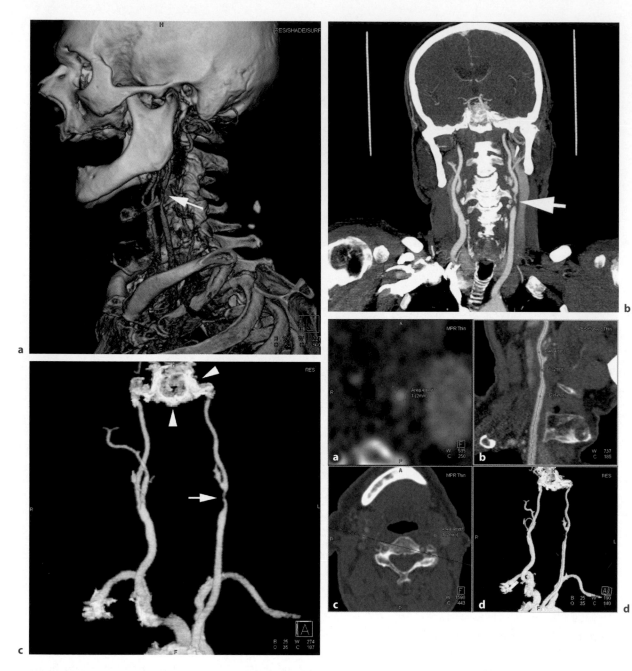

**Fig. 10.4. a** An 80-year old male patient with high-grade stenosis at the left carotid bulb. VRT reconstruction of the CTA dataset clearly delineates the stenosis (*arrow*). **b** Coronal thin-MIP reconstruction provides more detailed information about the stenosis (*arrow*). **c** SRT reconstruction after region-grow-based bone-removal. Aortic arch, subclavian arteries and extracranial carotid arteries remain visible. Vertebral arteries and distal segments of the external carotid artery have been removed by the bone-removal algorithm. Typical bone artefacts (*arrowheads*) at the infraclinoidal intracranial segments of both ICA after region-grow bone-removal. Stenosis of the left carotid bulb indicated by *arrow*. **d** Computer-aided vessel analysis (Syngo Advanced Vessel Analysis, Siemens Medical Solutions, Erlangen, Germany). MPR reconstruction in axial orientation to the vessel with threshold based diameter and area calculation of the vessel lumen (**a**). Stretched MPR view of the traced vessel showing the whole vessel in one image, marks indicate user-driven quantifications (**b**). Original axial CTA data (**c**). SRT reconstruction after bone-removal with vessel trace (**d**)

data, with a recent study showing promising results (KLOSKA et al. 2007); however, further evaluation of this technique is needed.

## 10.3.2
### Carotid Artery Stenosis

Carotid atherosclerosis is an important predisposing factor for ischemic stroke, and patients with high-grade stenosis of the carotid arteries are known to benefit from endarterectomy or stent-angioplasty. An exact determination of the degree of a carotid artery stenosis is crucial for therapeutic decision making (LELL et al. 2006). Several studies have demonstrated reliable results using MD-CTA compared to other imaging

techniques (CLEVERT et al. 2006; HACKLANDER et al. 2006; SILVENNOINEN et al. 2007; ERTL-WAGNER et al. 2004).

For evaluating carotid artery stenoses with MD-CTA, the scan range should include the aortic arch and the circle of Willis to ensure that stenoses at the origin of the CCA, at the carotid bulb and at the carotid siphon are reliably depicted (Fig. 10.4a,b). To avoid streak artefacts due to high contrast agent concentrations at the superior vena cava at the beginning of the injection, it is recommended to use a craniocaudal scan direction (DE MONYE et al. 2006).

For image analysis semi-automatic bone-segmentation/elimination algorithms can be used (Figs. 10.4c and 10.5a). There are different approaches to bone-elimination: The most commonly used algorithms

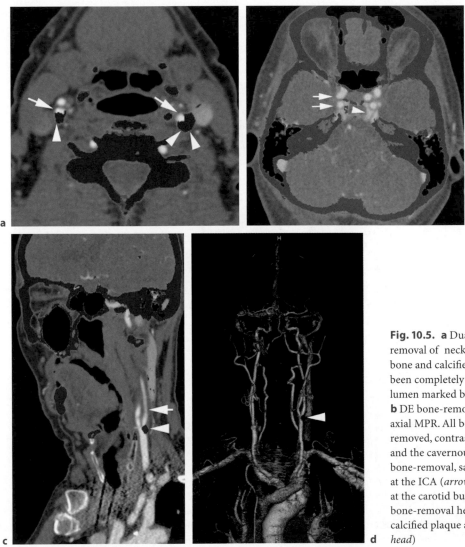

**Fig. 10.5. a** Dual-Energy (DE) bone-removal of neck-CTA, axial MPR. Note that bone and calcified plaques (*arrowheads*) have been completely removed. Stenotic vessel lumen marked by contrast agent (*arrows*). **b** DE bone-removal of CTA of the head, axial MPR. All bony structures have been removed, contrast agent at the ICA (*arrows*) and the cavernous sine (*arrowhead*). **c** DE bone-removal, sagittal MPR. Contrast agent at the ICA (*arrows*), removed calcified plaque at the carotid bulb (*arrowhead*). **d** VRT of DE bone-removal head and neck CTA. Removed calcified plaque at the carotid bulb (*arrowhead*)

rely on threshold-based region-growing techniques (Fig. 10.4c). These techniques can rapidly extract bone or vessels as long as there is a clear separation between both structures, e.g. in the cervical part of the carotid arteries. The major disadvantage of this method is that time-consuming manual corrections at the base of skull are oftentimes necessary, as region-grow-algorithm regularly fail in this region. In addition, the application of the algorithm on calcified plaques can result in excessive reduction of the residual lumen, thus exaggerating the degree of stenosis.

Alternatively, bone-subtraction algorithms exist that use either NECT volume data (TOMANDL et al. 2006) or dual-energy material decomposition (FLOHR et al. 2006, JOHNSON et al. 2007) to subtract bone from the CT-angiographic data (Fig. 10.5a–d). After the segmentation process, cross-sectional MPR images perpendicular to the vessel can be aligned automatically using a center-line function by a commercial vessel analysis tools. Optional corresponding VRT reformations and stretched vessel images (MPR) can provide anatomic orientations

(Fig. 10.4d). Manual or semi-automated measurements of the vessel lumen diameter or area can be performed on the basis of these cross-sectional images. When using semi-automated measurements, it is mandatory to check for common errors in lumen quantification, especially in cases of branching or neighbouring vessels and boundary identification in calcifications (BUCEK et al. 2007).

## 10.3.3
## Basilar Artery Occlusions

Although the majority of cerebral infarctions are located in the territories of the internal carotid arteries, 20% of cerebral ischemic infarctions involve tissue supplied by the vertebrobasilar circulation. Basilar artery occlusion is a life-threatening condition whose unfavourable spontaneous prognosis can only be improved by early detection and subsequent aggressive recanalization therapy (PFEFFERKORN et al. 2006).

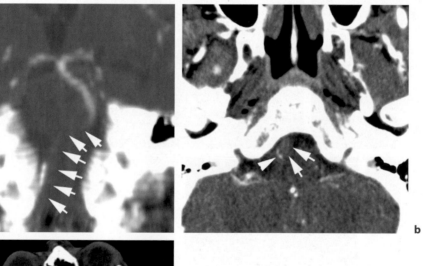

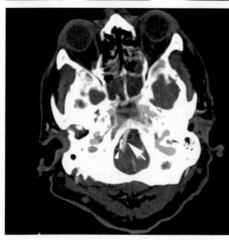

**Fig. 10.6.** **a** Basilar artery thrombosis. Coronal MIP reconstruction of a four-slice-CTA data set showing normal contrast enhancement at the top and the middle segment of the BA. Occluded lower BA and occluded V4-segment of the right VA (*arrows*). Note the calcified plaque at the VA. **b** Axial MPR showing the completely by thrombus occluded V4-segment of the right VA (*arrows*) at the level of the calcified plaque (*arrowhead*). **c** After thrombolysis follow-up 64-slice-CTA shows complete recanalisation of the former occluded V4-segment of the right VA (*arrow*), a high grade stenosis at the level of the calcified plaque (*arrowhead*) remains

In cases of suspected ischemia in the posterior circulation, CTA offers a swift and easy to perform imaging modality to rule out pathologies of the vertebrobasilar arteries. The scan range should include the level of the second cervical vertebra in order to include the passage of the vertebral arteries (VA) through the dura mater. In selected cases, a scan range including the entire vertebrobasilar circulation from the origin of the VA at the subclavian arteries provides additional information about potential pathologies of VA at the neck, such as dissections.

Additional sagittal and coronal or pseudo-coronal MIP reformations parallel to the clinoid provide excellent information about the basilar artery (Fig. 10.6a–c). Additional VRT after bone-subtraction may be useful to visualize stenosis.

## 10.3.4
## Intracranial Aneurysms

Acute subarachnoidal haemorrhage (SAH) following a rupture of a cerebral aneurysm is associated with a high mortality. The incidence of intracranial aneurysm is thought to be about 1.9%. CTA can be used for the emergency evaluation of SAH in order to determine the appropriate neurosurgical or endovascular intervention for cerebral aneurysms and as a non-invasive screening modality for patients with a familial predisposition for developing intracranial aneurysms. The gold-standard examination in SAH is still DSA. However, with modern MD-CTA techniques some authors now advocate MDCT as the primary method of choice to evaluate

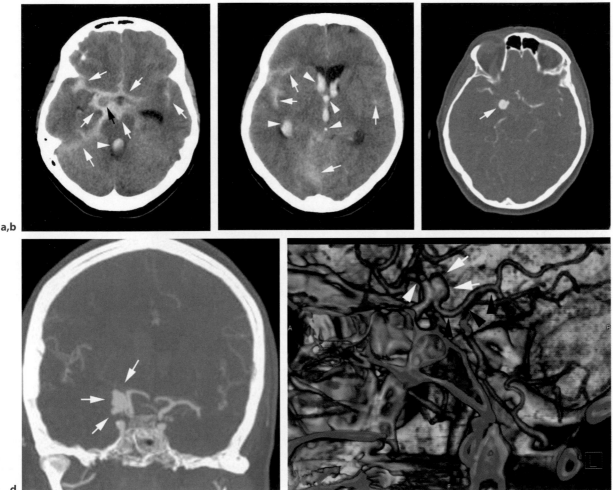

**Fig. 10.7. a,b** NECT of a patient with SAH (Fisher°4) with massive subarachnoidal haemorrhage at the Sylvian fissures, perimesencephalic and at the tentorium (*arrows*). Intraventricular blood clots (*arrowheads*) and aneurysm surrounded by SAH (*black arrow*). **c,d** CTA showing a large and roundly shaped aneurysm (*arrows*) at the posteriolateral wall of the right ICA, MIP. **e** VRT for treatment planning visualizes the localisation and orientation of the aneurysm

cerebral aneurysms (TIPPER et al. 2005; VILLABLANCA et al. 2002).

With the latest generation of MDCT it is possible to acquire CTA scan in a arterial phase without relevant contrast enhancement of the cerebral veins, thereby facilitating the evaluation of the intracavernous segments of the ICA much easier. If available, bone-subtraction is strongly recommended for evaluating the infraclinoid segments of the ICA (MORHARD et al. 2008). When evaluating a CTA in a patient with SAH (Fig. 10.7a,b), it is helpful to perform cross-sectional sliding-thin-slab MIP reformations (Fig. 10.7c,d). In addition, VRT can be used for 3D visualization in therapy planning (Fig. 10.7e).

In contrast to primarily diagnosing aneurysms with MDCT, follow-up of clipped or coiled aneurysms with CT angiography faces considerable challenges,

as surgical clips or coils usually cause significant beamhardening artifacts, thus altering the Hounsfield unit values in surrounding soft tissue and vessels (LELL et al. 2006).

### 10.3.5
### Cerebral Venous Thrombosis

About 1% of all acute strokes or stroke-like events are caused by cerebral venous thrombosis (CVT). Thromboses can be located in the intracranial dural sinuses, in the superficial cerebral veins or in the deep cerebral veins.

On NECT, patients with CVT often demonstrate venous infarctions (50%) with cortical/subcortical petechial haemorrhages and oedema. The so-called "cord

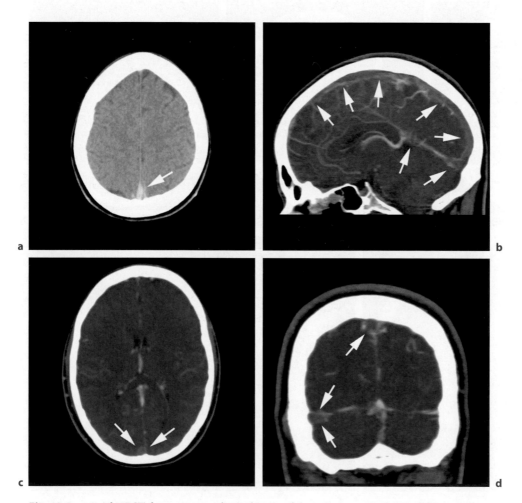

**Fig. 10.8.** **a** Axial NECT demonstrates a hyperdensity of the superior sagittal sinus (SSS, *arrow*), no contrast agent applied. **b** Sagittal MIP reconstruction of CTA delineating extensive thrombosis at the SSS, as well as at the straight sinus and the confluens sinuum (*arrows*). **c** CTA: empty triangle sign at the SSS (*arrows*) in the axial MIP. **d** CTA: empty triangle signs at the SSS and the right transverse sinus (*arrows*) in coronal MIP

sign" (Fig. 10.8a) reflects a more hyperdense dural sinus, which is filled with thrombotic material. The so-called "empty delta" or "empty triangle" sign (Fig. 18.8b–d) refers to enhancing dura surrounding non-enhancing thrombus. It can be found in 25%–30% of patients with CVT in CTA.

When reporting a CTA of the intracranial veins and sinuses it always needs to be considered that a large number of anatomic variants and arachnoidal granulations can mimic CVT.

Cerebral CT venography provides anatomical images of the intracranial venous circulation in a consistently high quality and can be used to rule out thrombosis and to preoperatively map venous structures in patients with a neoplasm (CASEY et al. 1996). CT venography is considered to be superior to MR venography in the identification of cerebral veins and dural sinuses and is at least equivalent in the diagnosis of dural sinus thrombosis (OZSVATH et al. 1997). A scan delay of 30–35 s after contrast administration usually leads to a combined arterial and venous contrast, which can be advantageous, when the symptomatology of the patient is not clear-cut and arterial pathologies are in the differential diagnosis.

# References

Anderson GB, Steinke DE, Petruk KC, Ashforth R, Findlay JM (1999) Computed tomographic angiography versus digital subtraction angiography for the diagnosis and early treatment of ruptured intracranial aneurysms. Neurosurgery 45:1315–1320; discussion 1320–1322

Bucek RA, Puchner S, Kanitsar A, Rand T, Lammer J (2007) Automated CTA quantification of internal carotid artery stenosis: a pilot trial. J Endovasc Ther 14:70–76

Casey SO, Alberico RA, Patel M, Jimenez JM, Ozsvath RR, Maguire WM, Taylor ML (1996) Cerebral CT venography. Radiology 198:163–170

Chappell ET, Moure FC, Good MC (2003) Comparison of computed tomographic angiography with digital subtraction angiography in the diagnosis of cerebral aneurysms: a meta-analysis. Neurosurgery 52:624–630; discussion 630–631

Clevert DA, Johnson T, Jung EM, Clevert DA, Flach PM, Strautz TI, Ritter G, Gallegos MT, Kubale R, Becker C, Reiser M (2006) Color Doppler, power Doppler and B-flow ultrasound in the assessment of ICA stenosis: Comparison with 64-MD-CT angiography. Eur Radiol 60(3):379–386

Crawford CR, King KF (1990) Computed tomography scanning with simultaneous patient translation. Med Phys 17:967–982

de Monye C, de Weert TT, Zaalberg W, Cademartiri F, Siepman DA, Dippel DW, van der Lugt A (2006) Optimization of CT angiography of the carotid artery with a 16-MDCT scanner: craniocaudal scan direction reduces contrast material-related perivenous artifacts. AJR Am J Roentgenol 186:1737–1745

Ertl-Wagner B, Bruning R, Hoffmann RT, Meimarakis G, Reiser MF (2004) [Diagnostic evaluation of carotid artery stenoses with multislice CT angiography. Review of the literature and results of a pilot study]. Radiologe 44:960–966

Ertl-Wagner BB, Bruening R, Blume J, Hoffmann RT, Mueller-Schunk S, Snyder B, Reiser MF (2006) Relative value of sliding-thin-slab multiplanar reformations and sliding-thin-slab maximum intensity projections as reformatting techniques in multisection CT angiography of the cervicocranial vessels. AJNR Am J Neuroradiol 27:107–113

Ertl-Wagner BB, Bruening R, Blume J, Hoffmann RT, Snyder B, Herrmann KA, Reiser MF (2005) Prospective, multireader evaluation of image quality and vascular delineation of multislice CT angiography of the brain. Eur Radiol 15:1051–1059

Ertl-Wagner BB, Hoffmann RT, Bruning R, Herrmann K, Snyder B, Blume JD, Reiser MF (2004) Multi-detector row CT angiography of the brain at various kilovoltage settings. Radiology 231:528–535

Flohr T, Bruder H, Stierstorfer K, Simon J, Schaller S, Ohnesorge B (2002a) New technical developments in multislice CT, part 2: sub-millimeter 16-slice scanning and increased gantry rotation speed for cardiac imaging. Rofo 174:1022–1027

Flohr T, Stierstorfer K, Bruder H, Simon J, Schaller S (2002b) New technical developments in multislice CT—Part 1: Approaching isotropic resolution with sub-millimeter 16-slice scanning. Rofo 174:839–845

Flohr TG, McCollough CH, Bruder H, Petersilka M, Gruber K, Suss C, Grasruck M, Stierstorfer K, Krauss B, Raupach R, Primak AN, Kuttner A, Achenbach S, Becker C, Kopp A, Ohnesorge BM (2006) First performance evaluation of a dual-source CT (DSCT) system. Eur Radiol 16:256–268

Hacklander T, Wegner H, Hoppe S, Danckworth A, Kempkes U, Fischer M, Mertens H, Caldwell JH (2006) Agreement of multislice CT angiography and MR angiography in assessing the degree of carotid artery stenosis in consideration of different methods of postprocessing. J Comput Assist Tomogr 30:433–442

Hoh BL, Cheung AC, Rabinov JD, Pryor JC, Carter BS, Ogilvy CS (2004) Results of a prospective protocol of computed tomographic angiography in place of catheter angiography as the only diagnostic and pretreatment planning study for cerebral aneurysms by a combined neurovascular team. Neurosurgery 54:1329–1340; discussion 1340–1342

Johnson TR, Krauss B, Sedlmair M, Grasruck M, Bruder H, Morhard D, Fink C, Weckbach S, Lenhard M, Schmidt B, Flohr T, Reiser MF, Becker CR (2007) Material differentiation by dual energy CT: initial experience. Eur Radiol 17(6):1510-1517

Kalender WA, Seissler W, Klotz E, Vock P (1990) Spiral volumetric CT with single-breath-hold technique, continuous transport, and continuous scanner rotation. Radiology 176:181–183

Kloska SP, Fischer T, Nabavi DG, Dittrich R, Ditt H, Klotz E, Fischbach R, Ringelstein EB, Heindel W (2007) Color-coded perfused blood volume imaging using multidetector CT: initial results of whole-brain perfusion analysis in acute cerebral ischemia. Eur Radiol 17(9):2352–2358

Kloska SP, Nabavi DG, Gaus C, Nam EM, Klotz E, Ringelstein EB, Heindel W (2004) Acute stroke assessment with CT: do we need multimodal evaluation? Radiology 233:79–86

Lell MM, Anders K, Uder M, Klotz E, Ditt H, Vega-Higuera F, Boskamp T, Bautz WA, Tomandl BF (2006) New Techniques in CT Angiography. Radiographics 26(Suppl 1):S45–62

Morhard D, Fink C, Becker C, Reiser MF, Nikolaou K (2008) Value of automatic bone subtraction in cranial CT angiography: comparison of bone-subtracted vs. standard CT angiography in 100 patients. Eur Radiol 18(5):974-982

Napel S, Rubin GD, Jeffrey RB Jr (1993) STS-MIP: a new reconstruction technique for CT of the chest. J Comput Assist Tomogr 17:832–838

Ozsvath RR, Casey SO, Lustrin ES, Alberico RA, Hassankhani A, Patel M (1997) Cerebral venography: comparison of CT and MR projection venography. AJR Am J Roentgenol 169:1699–1707

Pfefferkorn T, Mayer TE, Schulte-Altedorneburg G, Bruckmann H, Hamann GF, Dichgans M (2006) [Diagnosis and therapy of basilar artery occlusion]. Nervenarzt 77:416–422

Rubin GD, Dake MD, Semba CP (1995) Current status of three-dimensional spiral CT scanning for imaging the vasculature. Radiol Clin North Am 33:51–70

Ryu CW, Lee DH, Kim HS, Lee JH, Choi CG, Kim SJ, Suh DC (2006) Acquisition of MR perfusion images and contrast-enhanced MR angiography in acute ischaemic stroke patients: which procedure should be done first? Br J Radiol 79:962–967

Silvennoinen HM, Ikonen S, Soinne L, Railo M, Valanne L (2007) CT angiographic analysis of carotid artery stenosis: comparison of manual assessment, semiautomatic vessel analysis, and digital subtraction angiography. AJNR Am J Neuroradiol 28:97–103

Tipper G, U-King-Im JM, Price SJ, Trivedi RA, Cross JJ, Higgins NJ, Farmer R, Wat J, Kirollos R, Kirkpatrick PJ, Antoun NM, Gillard JH (2005) Detection and evaluation of intracranial aneurysms with 16-row multislice CT angiography. Clin Radiol 60:565–572

Tomandl BF, Hammen T, Klotz E, Ditt H, Stemper B, Lell M (2006) Bone-subtraction CT angiography for the evaluation of intracranial aneurysms. AJNR Am J Neuroradiol 27:55–59

Tomandl BF, Klotz E, Handschu R, Stemper B, Reinhardt F, Huk WJ, Eberhardt KE, Fateh-Moghadam S (2003) Comprehensive imaging of ischemic stroke with multisection CT. Radiographics 23:565–592

Villablanca JP, Jahan R, Hooshi P, Lim S, Duckwiler G, Patel A, Sayre J, Martin N, Frazee J, Bentson J, Vinuela F (2002) Detection and characterization of very small cerebral aneurysms by using 2D and 3D helical CT angiography. AJNR Am J Neuroradiol 23:1187–1198

Wintermark M (2005) Brain perfusion-CT in acute stroke patients. Eur Radiol 15(Suppl 4):D28–31

## 11

# Anatomy and Pathology
# of the Temporal Bone

Sabrina Kösling, Kerstin Neumann and Curd Behrmann

## CONTENTS

## ABSTRACT

Prerequisites for optimal radiological findings of the temporal bone are profound knowledge of the complex anatomy, a CT technique with the best local resolution, and a close cooperation with ENT colleagues. MSCT, with its resulting post-processing possibilities, clearly improves diagnostic safety. This chapter gives a short overview of: (1) anatomical structures that are relevant for the interpretation of CT images of the temporal bone, (2) technical points for achieving optimal multi-slice CT images of the temporal bone, and (3) the current importance of CT in the diagnostics of common and less common ear diseases in the context of other diagnostic methods.

## 11.1
## Introduction

The temporal bone is a region of difficult anatomy. Very subtle structures require an adequate imaging technique. Diverse diseases are often difficult to diagnose to their full extent by clinical methods alone. Of all the fields of otorhinolaryngology, imaging plays the most special role in the diagnostics of diseases of the temporal bone. Radiologists need to understand the questions of clinicians and their way of proceeding. This chapter starts with a summary of relevant anatomical structures for the analysis of CT images. In the following, the main points of the multi-slice CT (MSCT) technique are briefly mentioned. The main emphasis is put on the explanation of the current diagnostic importance of CT in different diseases.

S. Kösling, MD
Martin-Luther-Universität Halle-Wittenberg, Klinik für Diagnostische Radiologie, Ernst-Grube-Str. 40, 06097 Halle, Germany

K. Neumann, PD
Department of Otorhinolaryngology, University of Halle, Ernst-Grube-Str. 40, 06097 Halle, Germany

C. Behrmann, MD
Martin-Luther-Universität Halle-Wittenberg, Klinik für Diagnostische Radiologie, Ernst-Grube-Str. 40, 06097 Halle, Germany

## Anatomy

According to the embryological development, several parts can be differentiated in the temporal bone: the petrous, tympanic, and squamous parts, and the styloid process. The mastoid process is ventrally formed from the squamous part and dorsally from the petrous part.

Thin-sliced high-resolution CT visualises the bony two thirds of the external auditory canal, middle ear structures, the cell system, and bony canals of the inner ear very well. Often the drum is visible as a very fine line, but it is better assessed by otoscopy. The drum is not of direct radiological interest. A systematic analysis should include the following (Fig. 11.1):

1. Bony part of the external auditory canal. Scutum: spur at the cranial border of the external auditory

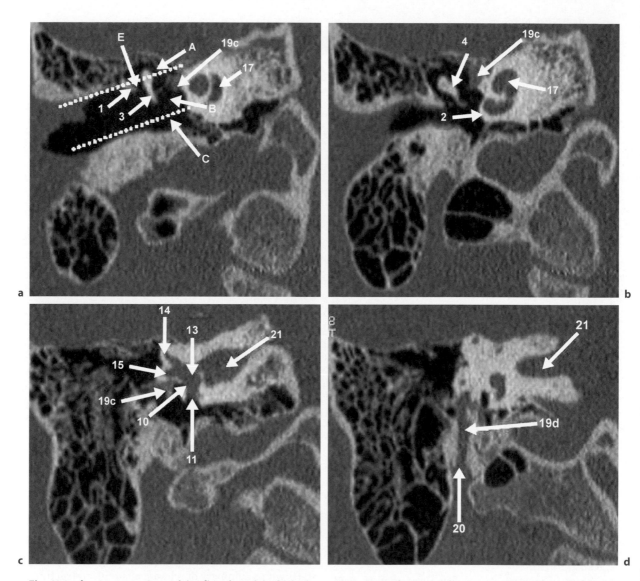

**Fig. 11.1a–h.** Anatomy. Coronal (**a–d**) and axial (**e–h**) high-resolution MPR of the temporal bone from ventral to dorsal (**a–d**) and cranial to caudal (**e–h**). Spaces: *A* Epitympanum, *B* mesotympanum, *C* hypotympanum, *D* mastoid antrum, *E* Prussak's space, *F* sinus tympani. *1* Scutum, *2* promontory, *3* malleus, *4* incus, *5* stapes, *6* incudomalleolar joint, *7* tensor tympani muscle, *8* stapedius m., *9* cochleariform process, *10* oval window, *11* round w., *12* auditory tube, *13* vestibule, *14* superior semicircular canal, *15* lateral s.c., *16* posterior s.c., *17* cochlea, *18* vestibular aqueduct, *19* facial nerve segments: *19a* labyrinthine, *19b* genicular fossa, *19c* tympanic, *19d* mastoid, *20* stylomastoid foramen, *21* internal auditory canal

meatus to the middle ear, which is essential for the diagnosis of cholesteatomas.

2. Middle ear. Spaces of the tympanic cavity: epitympanum, mesotympanum, hypotympanum, Prussak's space, sinus tympani; mastoid antrum. Promontory. Ossicles: malleus (caput, collum, manubrium), incus (corpus, short and long crus, lenticular process–often only partly visible), stapes–best visible on paraxial images (anterior and posterior crus, caput–

inconstantly visible, basis within the oval window), incudomalleolar joint, incudostapedial joint–inconstantly visible. Ligaments stabilise ossicles differently. In normal cases only some of them (especially the lateral ligament of the malleus) are visible on CT. Muscles: tensor tympani m.–its tendon is often visible between the cochleariform process and manubrium of the malleus, stapedius m.–within a small pit at the dorsal wall of the tympanic cavity. Cochle-

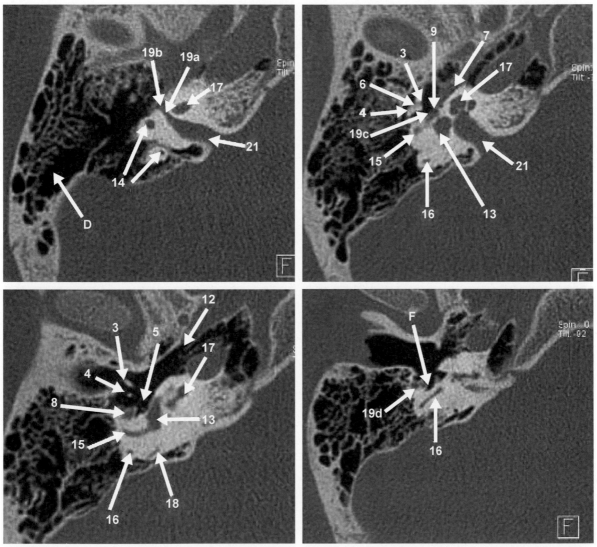

**Fig. 11.1a–h.** (*continued*) Anatomy. Coronal (**a–d**) and axial (**e–h**) high-resolution MPR of the temporal bone from ventral to dorsal (**a–d**) and cranial to caudal (**e–h**). Spaces: *A* Epitympanum, *B* mesotympanum, *C* hypotympanum, *D* mastoid antrum, *E* Prussak's space, *F* sinus tympani. *1* Scutum, *2* promontory, *3* malleus, *4* incus, *5* stapes, *6* incudomalleolar joint, *7* tensor tympani muscle, *8* stapedius m., *9* cochleariform process, *10* oval window, *11* round w., *12* auditory tube, *13* vestibule, *14* superior semicircular canal, *15* lateral s.c., *16* posterior s.c., *17* cochlea, *18* vestibular aqueduct, *19* facial nerve segments: *19a* labyrinthine, *19b* genicular fossa, *19c* tympanic, *19d* mastoid, *20* stylomastoid foramen, *21* internal auditory canal

ariform process–small osseous excrescence at the medial tympanic wall. Windows: oval (vestibular) w., round (cochlear) w. Auditory tube. Chorda tympani–the tympanic part is rarely visible as a fine line in the tympanic cavity near the manubrium mallei.

3. Cellulae mastoideae.
4. Inner ear: vestibule; semicircular canals: superior, lateral, posterior; cochlea–2½ turns (basal, middle, apical), modiolus; vestibular aqueduct; cochlear aqueduct.
5. Internal auditory canal: porus, fundus. Nerves within the internal auditory canal are not visible on CT images.
6. Facial nerve. The cisternal (within the cerebellopontine angle cistern) and canalicular (within the internal auditory canal) segment cannot be demonstrated on CT images. Well visible are the labyrinthine segment, genicular fossa = 1. knee, tympanic segment, 2. knee (= crossing from the tympanic to the mastoid segment), mastoid segment and stylomastoid foramen.

Furthermore, the analysis should include foramina and canals at the posterior and dorsal central skull base (jugular foramen, carotid canal, foramen lacerum, foramen ovale and spinosum, canalis n. hypoglossi) and as pseudofractures small sutures and canaliculi.

## 11.3
## Multi-Slice CT Technique

Temporal bone diagnostic requires the best local resolution. In the first place, this means a small slice thickness (0.3–1 mm), bone algorithm, and a high zoom (low field of view). In the majority of cases (cholesteatoma, trauma, malformation, otosclerosis, and post-operative diagnostics), the investigation is performed without intravenous injection of contrast medium and reconstruction of soft tissue images. Then a lower radiation exposure can be taken, but it cannot be as low as in low-dose CT of the paranasal sinuses because the increased image noise would not allow a sufficient visualisation of small details, especially of the stapes. Concrete values depend on the CT device used. The current limit lies at about 120 mAs. Due to exquisite post-processing possibilities, especially multi-planar reconstructions (MPR), a spiral modus should be chosen. Prerequisite for high quality MPR is a small increment (0.3 mm) and for 3D reconstructions the use of soft tissue data. Often, small details, such as the stapes, can be studied better by means of several oblique reconstructions. If contrast medium and soft window settings are needed (tumour, otitis externa necroticans, and inflammatory complications), radiation exposure has to be higher. For specific

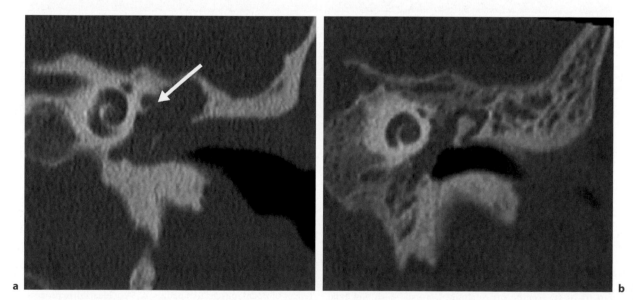

a                                                                                                      b

**Fig. 11.2a,b.** Inflammation. Coronal MPR. Secondary cholesteatoma of the middle ear (**a**) with completely opacified tympanic cavity, destructed ossicles, small erosions along the walls of the tympanic cavity, and at the canal tympanic facial nerve segment (*arrow*), protrusion of the drum, soft tissue masses in the external auditory canal, reduced mastoid pneumatisation.

The diagnosis was known at the time of CT. CT was performed to show the extent of the cholesteatoma. Otitis media chronica mesotympanalis (**b**). The tympanic cavity is opacified, too. The often reduced mastoid pneumatisation is not so pronounced in this case, there are no signs of bony destructions or erosions, and the drum is retracted

details the investigation protocols of the Head and Neck Working Group of the German X-Ray Society can be recommended.

## Pathology

### 11.4.1
### Inflammation

Imaging is seldom necessary for inflammations, which are the most common diseases of the temporal bone. In many acute and less severe chronic inflammations (e.g., many kinds of external otitis, glue ear, actue otitis media, and otitis media chronica mesotympanalis), clinical methods provide the needed therapeutic information.

CT indications are given in chronic aggressive inflammations, such as otitis externa necroticans, secondary cholesteatoma (Fig. 11.2a), and granulations of the middle ear. The task of CT is mainly the assessment of the extension of the inflammation, including bony destructions; it is not as often used for the presentation of the concrete diagnosis. For instance, it is often easier to differentiate an otitis media chronica mesotympanalis from a cholesteatoma by otoscopy than by CT. Cho-

lesteatoma and granulations may be indistinguishable on CT. Further indications are extracranial inflammatory complications, such as abscesses; for intracranial complications, MRI is preferred. If there are hints that an aggressive middle ear inflammation has spread into the inner ear or intracranially, MRI has to be performed additionally. Skull base osteomyelitis is a very rare inflammatory complication in which CT is indicative, but for the detection of the full amount of bone marrow involvement, MRI is needed. For differential diagnosis, CT signs of otitis media chronica mesotympanalis (Fig. 11.2b) and tympanosclerosis should be known. Possible calcifications developing in the course of labyrinthitis can only be identified by CT.

### 11.4.2
### Trauma

CT is the method of choice in clinically suspected fractures of the temporal bone. Fracture lines, fragment dislocation, and potential complications (inclusion of the facial nerve canal, carotid canal, and roof of the tympanic cavity) can be unequivocally detected. In routine work, the traditional differentiation into longitudinal, transverse (Fig. 11.3), and mixed fractures is used despite newer classifications. As a result, the damage to the

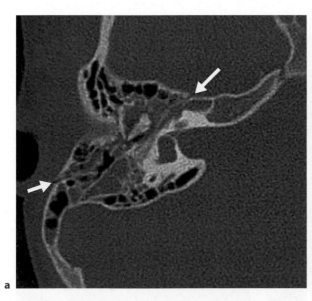
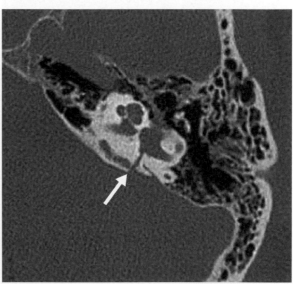

a                                                                                                                    b

**Fig. 11.3a,b.** Trauma. Axial MPR. Typical course of fracture lines (*arrows*) in a longitudinal (**a**) and transverse fracture (**b**). Opacities in the tympanic cavity and mastoid cells (**a**) are

bleedings after a trauma in first line. They occur more often in longitudinal fractures. In transverse fractures the labyrinth is usually involved, leading to a damage of inner ear function

middle (longitudinal fractures) or inner ear (transverse fractures) is explainable. MSCT and modern post-processing clearly increase the detection rate of traumatic ossicular chain lesions without reaching the diagnostic accuracy of tympanoscopy. If there is a fracture line in the carotid canal, vessel complications can be non-invasively identified by CTA. In single cases, MRI can be helpful in identifying the exact localisation of a facial nerve injury. The diagnosis of labyrinthine contusion can be indirectly made in cases of traumatically induced decrease or loss of inner ear function without detection of a fracture on CT.

## 11.4.3
## Tumour

Tumours are rare pathologies in the temporal bone. In the majority of cases they are benign–most commonly schwannomas and paragangliomas are found that have characteristic sites of origin. Both are slow growing. Schwannomas mostly occur in the cerebellopontine angle–a region where MRI is the preferred method.

Paragangliomas (glomus tympanicum and glomus jugulare tumours) have a high vascularisation. CT demonstrates the typical permeative osteolysis of glomus jugulare tumours–the only real differential diagnosis is a metastasis, but in contrast to glomus tumours, it shows rapidly progressive cranial nerve palsies. Con-

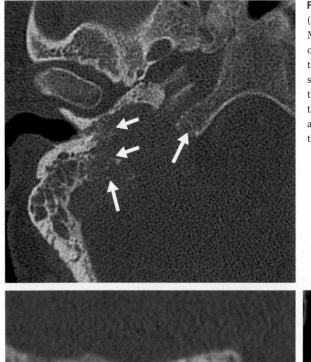

a

**Fig. 11.4a–c.** Tumour. Contrast-enhanced MSCT with axial (**a**), coronal (**b**) high-resolution MPR, and axial soft tissue MPR (**c**). Localisation, high vascularisation, permeative osteolysis (*arrow* in **a**), typical path of extension (middle ear, along the caudal and dorsal surface of the petrous bone) are highly suggestive of a glomus jugulare tumour. CT clearly visualises the extension in the carotid space and relationship to the internal carotid artery (**c**). The high age of this patient and very advanced extension of the tumour lead to a decision for radiotherapy

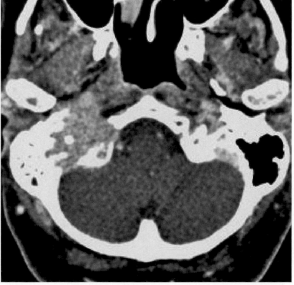

b                                                                                                   c

trast-enhanced MSCT with reconstruction in soft tissue and high-resolution algorithm is able to provide all the needed therapeutic information (presumptive diagnosis; extension within the temporal bone, into the posterior cranial fossa and/or the carotid and parapharyngeal space; relationship to the internal carotid artery) (Fig. 11.4).

The most common malignant tumour of the temporal bone is carcinoma with the main localisation in the external auditory canal. Clinically it is very difficult to differentiate from otitis externa neroticans; on imaging, the latter shows a more diffuse pattern. The diagnosis is made by histology. The main task of imaging is the exact description of the tumour extensions, including the relationship to the middle ear and facial nerve. If CT gives hints that the tumour is spreading intracranially, MRI should follow. On principle, CT should be chosen first in suspected tumours of the external auditory canal and middle ear as well as in presumed glomus jugulare tumours.

### 11.4.4
### Malformation

The incidence of malformations of the temporal bone is less than 1%. Malformations are characterised by a deviation from normal anatomical development and regular function. They can result from a developmental arrest, irregular embryogenesis, or from both because of spontaneous genetic mutations, genetic transmission, and exogenic factors, and may be found in syndromes. Due to different embryological tissue of origin and different times of development, typical and less typical combinations of malformed parts of the ear result. Combined external and middle ear malformations are common (Fig. 11.5), isolated middle ear malformations are less common than inner ear malformations, and combined malformations of the middle and inner ear are rarities.

CT has a high clarification rate in suspected malformations of the external and middle ear, including the detection of other causes for conductive hearing loss. Only in a few cases can no cause be found. The rate where imaging finds a morphological correlate in suspected inner ear malformation is clearly lower (about one fifth). CT is somewhat inferior in the detection of inner ear malformations compared to MRI.

Apart from the recognition of the malformation, CT plays an important role in the estimation of the degree of external and middle ear malformation and in providing the required morphological information for therapeutic planning. Malformed structures have to be described exactly in the radiological findings. The course of the facial nerve, the stapes, and windows are the most important ones in planned surgery to restore hearing.

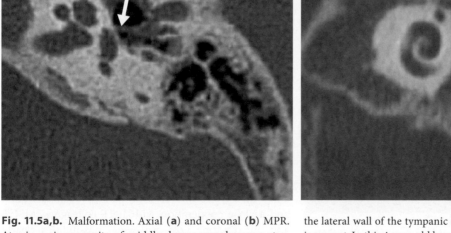

a

b

**Fig. 11.5a,b.** Malformation. Axial (**a**) and coronal (**b**) MPR. Atresia auris congenita of middle degree–membranous atresia (*star*) and stenosis of the external auditory canal (EAC), hypoplasia of the tympanic cavity, reduced mastoid pneumatisation, slightly dysplastic malleus (*arrow* in **b**), which is fixed at the lateral wall of the tympanic cavity. The stapes (arrow in **a**) is present. In this 4-year-old boy a congenital ear malformation was known due to deformed auricles. CT was performed to clarify the kind of EAC stenosis and assessment of the middle ear morphology

### 11.4.5
### Otosclerosis

Otosclerosis is an osteodystrophy of unknown aetiology in the enchondral labyrinthine capsule. Described demineralised areas (otospongiotic foci) occur that ossify later (otosclerotic foci). Most of them are very well detectable on CT. Commonly, they are localised near the oval window (Fig. 11.6), less commonly near the round window and around the cochlea and/or vestibular structures. According to the site of foci, fenestral, retrofenestral, and mixed forms are differentiated.

In the fenestral and mixed form, the diagnosis is made clinically. Nevertheless, CT appearance should be known for unclear cases and in patients with retrofenestral form. A very similar CT morphology as in the latter one can be found in Paget's disease, but these patients are normally older, and additional areas of the skull base are involved. If the patient is investigated in the pure otosclerotic stage and there are no hyperosteotic formations along the medial wall of the tympanic cavity, the diagnosis can be missed by CT.

### 11.4.6
### Postoperative CT

Usually postoperative imaging is merely performed in tumour patients, and then mostly as MRI. Postoperative

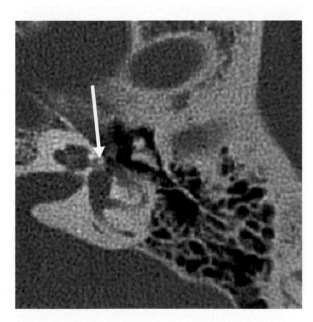

**Fig. 11.6.** Otosclerosis, fenestral type. Axial MSCT scan. Otospongiotic plaque at the fissula ante fenestram (*arrow*)–ventral of the oval window

CT of the temporal bone is mainly ordered because of suspected complications and residuum or recurrence of inflammation after mastoidectomy. After stapes surgery due to otosclerosis, the visualisation of the prosthesis can be required. For the correct interpretation of postoperative images, information about the underlying disease, the kind and time of operation, as well as information about current problems is needed. Radiologists have to be familiar with the main operative procedures–open and closed technique of mastoidectomy, tympanoplasty type III, including the nowadays often used prostheses for restoring hearing (partial and total ossicular replacement prostheses–PORP and TORP), and stapedoplasty–and with the normal postoperative CT.

After cholesteatoma surgery (the main indication for mastoidectomy), CT has been proven as a method with a high negative value if there is a completely air-filled cavity (Fig. 11.7a). In opacities the interpretation may be difficult. Sometimes the analysis of the margin is helpful; a small opacity with a smooth margin is a scar. Bony erosions may be pre-existent. Only the comparison with preoperative CT can clarify this problem. The tissue in a completely opacified cavity cannot be differentiated by CT (Fig. 11.7b). If such a differentiation is desired, which is not always the case, MRI can be recommended. Dislocation of prostheses after tympanoplasty is well demonstrable by CT. It occurs often in combination with recurrence of inflammation.

CT is the method of first choice in cases of persistent or renewed vertigo and/or hearing loss after insertion of stapes prostheses (Fig. 11.7c-d). It clearly reveals dislocations of prostheses into the middle ear or vestibule, scarring around the prosthesis, and the extent of otospongiotic foci. On coronal MPR or 3D visualisation, incus necrosis can be shown as a late complication. An air bubble at the prosthesis in the vestibule and/or a small fluid collection in the sinus tympani is an indirect sign for a perilymphatic fistula.

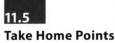

### Take Home Points

Prerequisites for optimal radiological findings of the temporal bone are profound knowledge of the complex anatomy, a CT technique with the best local resolution, and a close cooperation with ENT colleagues. MSCT and the resulting post-processing possibilities clearly improve the diagnostic safety.

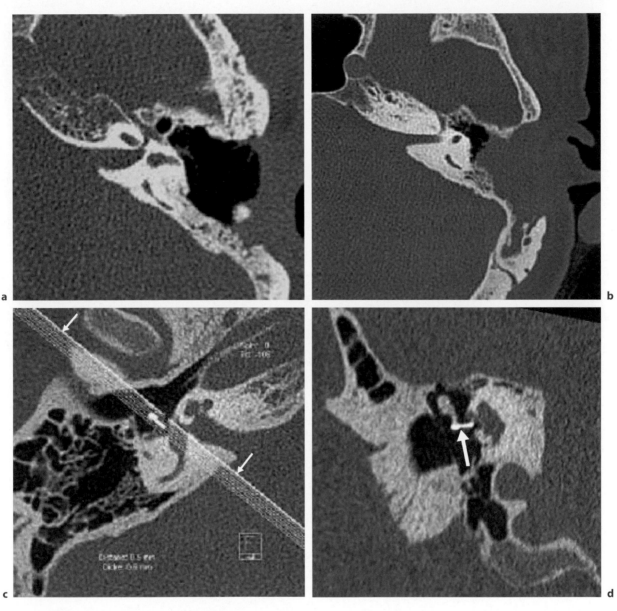

**Fig. 11.7a–d.** Postoperative CT. Axial MPR (**a-c**), paracoronal MPR (**d**). *Lines* in **c** show the slice orientation of **d**. Normal CT after open mastoidectomy (**a**). Nearly completely opacified cavity after open mastoidectomy (**b**) in which CT can demonstrate the extension of opacities and situation along the walls of the cavity, but it cannot clarify the kind of tissue that caused the opacities. CT after stapedotomy (**c, d**). The inserted prosthesis (*arrow* in **d**) does not exactly reach the level of the oval window, which is demanded in regular postoperative results

## References

Arbeitsgemeinschaft Kopf-Hals-Diagnostik der Deutschen Röntgengesellschaft. CT- und MRT-Protokolle. www.drg.de

AWMF online. Leitlinien der Deutschen Röntgengesellschaft. Radiologische Diagnostik im Kopf-Hals-Bereich. Schläfenbein. www.uni-duesseldorf.de/awmf/

Curtin HD, Som PM (2003) Head and neck imaging, 5th edn. Mosby, St Louis

Harnsberger HR, Wiggins RH, Hudgins PA et al. (2004) Diagnostic imaging, head and neck. Amirsys, Salt Lake City

Henrot P, Iochum S, Batch T et al. (2005) Current multiplanar imaging of the stapes. Am J Neuroradiol 26:2128-2133

Kösling S, Bootz F (2001) CT and MR imaging after middle ear surgery. Europ J Radiol 40:113-118

Schuknecht HF (1993) Pathology of the ear, 2nd edn. Lea & Febinger, Philadelphia

Sreepada GS, Kwartler JA (2003) Skull base osteomyelitis secondary to malignant otitis externa. Curr Opin Otolaryngol Head Neck Surg 11:315-23

Swartz J, Harnsberger HR (1998) Imaging of the temporal bone, 3rd edn. Thieme, Stuttgart New York

Ullrich G. Mueller-Lisse and Juergen Lutz

CONTENTS

### ABSTRACT

Pathologic lesions of the orbit continue to be a great challenge to the diagnostic radiologist. The complex anatomy of the orbit on the one hand and the multitude of disease entities that may affect the orbit on the other hand demand a simple, well-structured approach to diagnostic imaging. Subdividing the orbit into four (or five) distinct spaces, i.e., the eyeball, the intraconal space, the optic nerve, and the extraconal space (with some authors adding the conal space as a separate compartment), facilitates both the localization and characterization of orbital lesions and helps the ophthalmic surgeon to select the best approach to a lesion. Multidetector-row CT (MDCT), due to its thin collimation and resulting multiplanar image reformatting capabilities, has greatly improved the precision of CT imaging of orbital pathology. MDCT allows for multiplanar views of the bony orbital walls and their apertures, i.e., the optic foramen, the superior and inferior orbital fissures, and their respective affection by trauma, tumor, or inflammation. Inclusions of gas or air within the orbit indicate complications of facial trauma, inflammation of the paranasal sinuses, or head and neck tumors. However, due to the separation of the various soft tissue contents of the orbit by orbital fat tissue, MDCT also lends itself

U. G. MUELLER-LISSE, MD
MBA, Attending Radiologist, Associate Professor of Radiology, Health Care Management, Ludwig-Maximilians-University of Munich, Munich University Hospitals, Ziemssenstrasse 1, 80336 Munich, Germany

J. LUTZ, MD
Resident, Department of Clinical Radiology, Ludwig-Maximilians-University of Munich, Munich University Hospitals, Ziemssenstrasse 1, 80336 Munich, Germany

to the assessment of primary intra-orbital lesions or secondary affection of the orbit by lesions extending from the face, the neurocranium, the skull base, or distant primary malignancies.

## 12.1
### Introduction

Due to the complex anatomy of the human face and the close proximity of its structures to one another and to the neurocranium, the human orbit presents a great challenge to radiologists. The radiologist's task may be described as visualizing and seeing what ophthalmologists do not see with their own eyes and optical tools. While the majority of lesions affecting the eyelids, the conjunctiva, and the various structures of the eyeball are accessible by means of optical instruments, disease affecting the deeper structures of the orbit oftentimes does not reveal itself to such inspection. Proptosis may be the key clinical finding, and visual impairment the chief complaint of the patient. While trans-bulbar ultrasonography may disclose the source of the lesion, computed tomography (CT) and/or magnetic resonance imaging (MRI) help to detect, localize, characterize, and deter-

**Table 12.1.** Suggested protocols for scanning, image reconstruction, and image reformation in MDCT of the orbit, midface, and paranasal sinuses (modified and amended from: DAMMANN F (2006) Sinuses and facial skeleton. In: Bruening R, Kuettner A, Flohr T (eds) Protocols for multislice CT, 2nd edn. Springer, Berlin, Heidelberg, New York, pp 101–105

| Parameters | Number of CT detector rows | | |
|---|---|---|---|
| Scanner settings | 4–8 rows | 10–16 rows | 32–64 rows[1] |
| Tube voltage (KV) | 120 | 120 | 120 |
| Rotation time (s) | <1 | <1 | <1 |
| Tube current time product (mAs) | 20/200[2] | 20/90–200[2] | 20/90–200[2] |
| Pitch-corrected tube current time product (eff. mAs) | 20/220[2] | 20/140–200[2] | 20/140–200[2] |
| Collimation (mm) | 1.00–1.25 | 0.625–0.750 | 0.600–0.625 |
| Norm. pitch | 0.9 | 0.6–1.0 | 0.6–1.0 |
| Reconstruction increment (mm) | 0.6 | 0.5 | 0.5 |
| Reconstruction slice thickness (mm) | 1.00–1.25 | 0.75–1.00 | 0.60–0.75 |
| | | | |
| Convolution kernel | Bone, brain, soft tissue[3] | | |
| Scan range and direction (from-to) | Craniocaudal frontal sinus–maxilla (dental alveoli) | | |
| Reformations, required | Multiplanar (MPR) | | |
| Reformations, optional | Curved MPR, 3D volume rendering (VRT) | | |
| Contrast media application | Depends on clinical indication | | |

[1] MDCT scanners with 32-64 detector rows allow for restriction to 16–40 detector rows. Ideally, the number of rows should be selected such as to result in the lowest CTDIvol and effective dose for the scan

[2] Tube current settings exceeding 100 mAs should be restricted to tumorous or complex disease or complicated inflammatory disease, particularly when intravenous contrast media are administered. Unless particularly complicating, trauma or benign disease should be examined at low dose settings

[3] Selection of convolution kernels should be adapted to the clinical question. Complex disease of the orbit may require all three kernels, since it may affect facial bone, facial and orbital soft tissue, and brain matter

mine the extent and destructive properties of lesions of the orbit. Multidetector-row CT (MDCT) has greatly increased the speed and the spatial resolution of CT images, such that image reconstruction in any desirable plane and volume-rendering techniques may now help radiologists to assess lesions of the orbit (Table 12.1).

## 12.2
## Orbital Anatomy

### 12.2.1
### Orbital Confines

The orbit is defined as the anatomic space in the skull that contains the eyeball and its accessory organs. At the orbital apex, many nerves and blood vessels pass from the orbit into the cranial cavity and vice versa. The orbit is pyramidal in shape, with four bony walls narrowing posteriorly toward the apex.

- Superiorly, below the frontal sinus and the anterior cranial fossa, the orbital roof is shaped by the frontal and sphenoid bones.
- Medially, the bony orbit is confined by the ethmoid, lacrimal, sphenoid, and maxillary bones. The most anterior part of the medial wall of the orbit includes the nasolacrimal fossa, with the aperture of the nasolacrimal duct.
- Inferiorly, the orbital floor covers the top of the maxillary antrum and sinus. The orbital floor and the medial orbital wall are the weakest parts of the bony orbit. The orbital floor is shaped by the maxillary, zygomatic, and palatine bones.
- Laterally, the orbital wall includes parts of the zygomatic, sphenoid, and frontal bones and neighbors the temporalis fossa laterally and the middle cranial fossa posterolaterally.
- Anteriorly, the bony orbit ends in the orbital rim or entrance, which is the strongest part of the bony orbit. Covering or extending from the orbital entrance, the eyelid complex with its medial and lateral canthal tendons, the orbital septum, and the eyeball define the facial aspect of the orbit. The orbital septum is a thin, elastic membrane that separates the intra- and extra-orbital spaces and acts as an important barrier to disease (Fig. 12.1) (HINTSCHICH and ROSE 2005; AVIV and CASSELMAN 2005).

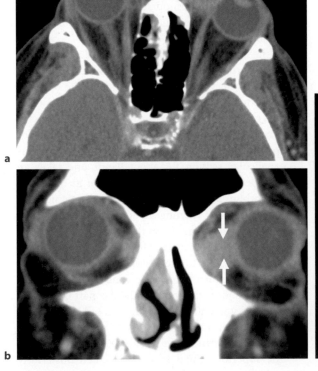

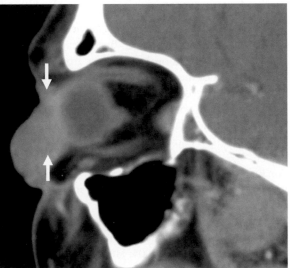

**Fig. 12.1a–c.** Squamous cell carcinoma of the upper and lower eyelid (*arrows*) displaces left eyeball laterally (**a**, axial MDCT image) but not superiorly or inferiorly (**b** and **c**, coronal and sagittal MDCT images). While the tumors extend from skin surface to conjunctiva, there is no evidence of intra-orbital extension. The orbital septum constitutes an important barrier that prevents disease to enter the orbit from the face

## 12.2.2
## Surgical and Radiological
## Spaces Within the Orbit

Inside the orbit, four surgical spaces may be distinguished, namely, the subperiosteal or extraperiosteal space, the extraconal space, the intraconal space, and the sub-Tenon's space.

- The subperiosteal space exists only when created surgically or filled in by a pathological process. It lies between the bony orbital walls and the periorbita. The periorbita is loosely attached to all bones of the orbit and to the orbital septum and consists of multiple connective tissue septa that separate the contents of the orbit from its bony confines.
- The extraconal space contains the oblique muscles of the eye, the trochlea, the motoric trochlear nerve, the sensory nerves, some blood vessels, orbital fat tissue, and the lacrimal gland. The lacrimal gland is the largest structure within the extraconal space and lies behind the orbital rim in the superotemporal quadrant of the orbit.
- The intraconal space is defined by the rectus muscles and their interconnecting septa. It contains the optic nerve, motor nerves, some blood vessels, and intraconal orbital fat tissue. Among the intraconal blood vessels, the ophthalmic artery, which branches off from the intracranial internal carotid artery, enters through the optic foramen. Near the orbital apex, the central retinal artery takes off from the ophthalmic artery and runs caudal to the optic nerve, whose dura mater it usually enters approximately 1 cm dorsal to the eyeball.
- The sub-Tenon's space is located between the eyeball and the anterior surface of Tenon's capsule, which separates the intra-orbital fat tissue from the posterior aspect of the eyeball. It is a potential space that can be enlarged by inflammatory fluid (as in posterior scleritis) or infiltrated by extraocular extension of intraocular tumors (as in uveal melanoma) (HINTSCHICH and ROSE 2005).

For the purposes of radiological cross-sectional image interpretation, the orbit may also be subdivided into four distinct spaces.

- The extraconal and intraconal spaces may be defined as above (MUELLER-FORELL and PITZ 2004; AVIV and MISZKIEL 2005; HINTSCHICH and ROSE 2005; LEMKE et al. 2006).
- Within the intraconal space, the optic nerve may be distinguished as an entity in its own right, since there are diseases that primarily affect the optic nerve and its meningeal covering without necessarily affecting other structures within the intraconal space to a similar degree (MUELLER-FORELL and PITZ 2004; LEMKE et al. 2006).
- The eyeball represents the fourth radiological space (MUELLER-FORELL and PITZ 2004), while the subperiosteal space only appears as a distinct compartment within the orbit at cross-sectional imaging when it is filled with pathologic fluid collections, such as pus or blood, or with pathologic tissue, such as tumor tissue.
- It has also been argued that the conal muscles, i.e., the superior, inferior, medial, and lateral rectus muscles of the orbit, along with their tendons and connective tissue layers, represent a space of their own (the "conal" space) and that this space may be affected by disease in its own right (AVIV and MISZKIEL 2005). However, this view is not shared by all authors.

## 12.2.3
## Orbital Foramina
## and Fissures and Their Contents

The bony confines of the orbit include various foramina and fissures that accommodate different neurovascular structures, which are essential for normal ocular function (Table 12.2).

- In the center of the orbital apex, medial to the superior orbital fissure, the optic foramen contains the optic nerve and its meninges and the ophthalmic artery. Starting at the optic chiasm, the optic nerve measures approximately 4 mm in diameter, extends intracranially toward the orbital canal for approximately 10 mm, passes through the intracanalicular section for about 9 mm, and takes an S-shaped curve toward the eyeball for its 30 mm of intraorbital length. Intraorbitally, the optic nerve is surrounded by meningeal dura mater, arachnoid, and pia mater layers from the optic foramen to the eyeball. The intracanalicular part of the optic nerve is immobile due to the fusion of the dura mater to the periosteum of the optic canal. This particular feature renders the intracanalicular part of the optic nerve vulnerable to the impacts of blunt trauma, hemorrhage, and edema (AVIV and CASSELMAN 2005; HINTSCHICH and ROSE 2005).
- The superior orbital fissure is located posteriorly and superiorly to the inferior orbital fissure, at the junction of the lateral wall and the roof of the orbit. It is subdivided into a lateral and a medial compart-

**Table 12.2.** Orbital foramina and fissures and their contents

| Foramen or Fissure | Contents |
| --- | --- |
| Optic foramen | II (optic nerve and accompanying meninges) |
| | Ophthalmic artery |
| Superior orbital fissure | III (superior and inferior division) |
| | IV |
| | V1 (lacrimal, frontal and nasociliary branches) |
| | VI |
| | Superior ophthalmic veins |
| Inferior orbital fissure | Infraorbital nerve and zygomatic branch (V2) |
| | Emissary veins between inferior ophthalmic vein and |
| | Pterygoid plexus |
| Lacrimal foramen/Hyrtl's canal | Lacrimal artery in meningo-lacrimal variant of the middle meningeal artery |
| Zygomatico-frontal foramen | Zygomatico-frontal artery (branch of lacrimal artery) and nerve (branch V2) |
| Ethmoidal foramina (ant./post.) | Anterior and posterior ethmoidal arteries and nerves |
| Supraorbital notch/foramen | Frontal and lacrimal nerve branches (V1) and vessels |
| Infraorbital groove/foramen | Infraorbital nerve (V2) and vessels |

Modified and amended from: Aviv RI, Casselman J (2005) Orbital imaging: Part 1. Normal anatomy. Clin Radiol 60:279–287 and Hintschich C, Rose G (2005) Tumours of the orbit. In: Neuro-oncology of CNS tumours. Tonn J (ed). Springer, Berlin, Heidelberg, New York, pp. 269-290

ment by the fibrous ring (Anulus tendineus) of Zinn, which is the origin of the orbital rectus muscles. The lateral compartment contains the lacrimal, frontal, and trochlear nerves, the anastomosis of the recurrent lacrimal and middle meningeal arteries, and the superior ophthalmic vein. The medial compartment contains the superior and inferior divisions of the oculomotor nerve, the nasociliary nerve, the abducens nerve, and the sympathetic nerves (Hintschich and Rose 2005).

- The supraorbital neurovascular bundle passes through a bony canal or notch in the superior orbital rim and contains the frontal and lacrimal branches of the ophthalmic division of the trigeminal nerve (V1) (Aviv and Casselman 2005; Hintschich and Rose 2005).

- The infraorbital neurovascular bundle enters the orbit through the inferior orbital fissure, passes through the infraorbital canal, and reaches the cheek through the infraorbital foramen (Fig. 12.2). The bundle contains fibers from the maxillary division of the trigeminal nerve (V2) and transmits sensation for the cheek, upper lid, and upper anterior teeth. The inferior orbital fissure measures approximately 20 mm in length and separates the orbital floor from the lateral wall. It contains fat tissue, the infraorbital nerve, and veins leaving the orbit for the pterygopalatine fossa (Hintschich and Rose 2005).

- The zygomatic neurovascular bundle passes through the infero-lateral aspect of the orbital wall, just posterior to the orbital rim (Aviv and Casselman 2005; Hintschich and Rose 2005).

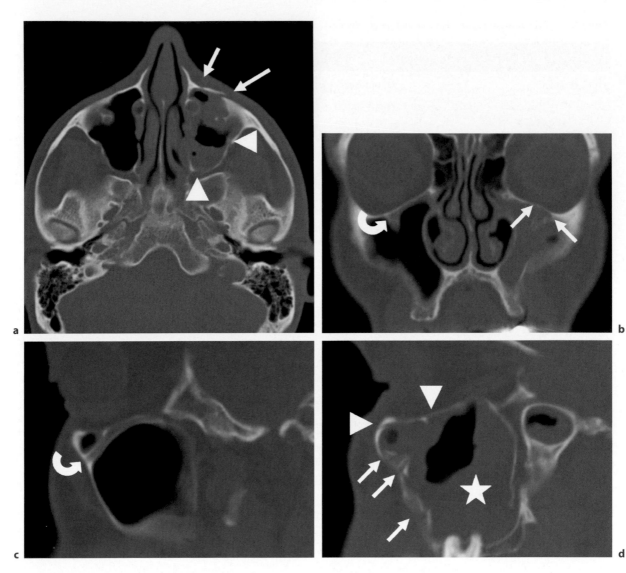

**Fig. 12.2a–d.** Fracture of the left orbital floor with associated fracture of the bony canal of the infraorbital nerve [*arrows* in axial (**a**), coronal (**b**), and sagittal (**d**) reformations] and fractures of the orbital floor (*arrowheads* in **d**) and the anterior, lateral, and posterior walls of the maxillary sinus (*arrowheads* in **a**,**b**). Hemorrhage within the maxillary sinus (*asterisk* in **d**) is a typical feature of orbital floor fracture. Normal course and appearance of the bony canal of the infraorbital nerve is demonstrated in **b** and **c** (*curved arrows*)

<table>
<tr><td>12.3</td></tr>
</table>

## Orbital Tumors and Tumor-Like Lesions

### 12.3.1
### Tumors of the Eyeball

In most instances, cross-sectional imaging will not be required when dealing with diseases of the eyeball. However, retinoblastoma, choroideal melanoma, choroideal hemangioma, and metastasis may be visualized by means of MDCT or MRI (Aviv and Miszkiel 2005).

### 12.3.1.1
### Retinoblastoma

Retinoblastoma represents the most common malignant intra-ocular tumor in children under the age of 5 years, with up to 90% of intra-ocular malignancies.

It derives from neuroectodermal cells of the retina and presents clinically with strabism, leukocoria, and, perhaps, pain. While primarily being diagnosed by visual means, retinoblastoma may present with characteristic calcifications within an intraocular mass at CT. MRI allows to determine intra- and extra-ocular tumor extension and the presence of bilateral or trilateral (including pinealoma) tumor or intra-cranial metastasis. Differential diagnosis includes persistent hyperplastic primary vitreous body and Coats' disease (MUELLER-FORELL and PITZ 2004).

### 12.3.1.2
### Melanoma

Melanoma represents the most common malignant intra-ocular tumor in adults, with a mean age at diagnosis of 53 years. Melanoma of the eyeball (uveal melanoma) affects the choroideal layer in approximately 85% of cases and is rarely found in the ciliary body (approximately 9%) or in the iris (approximately 6%). Intra-ocular melanoma is more often nodular than diffuse in its growth pattern, such that it can be detected by means of cross-sectional imaging. MRI demonstrates intra-ocular melanoma better than CT. At MRI, uveal melanoma shows with intermediate to high signal intensity on unenhanced T1-weighted and proton density-weighted images, low signal intensity on T2-weighted images, and strong enhancement after intravenous contrast administration. Disruption by intra-ocular melanoma of Bruch's membrane may cause tumor extension into the orbit. The differential diagnosis of intra-ocular melanoma includes hemangioma or nevus of the choroideal layer, choroideal amotion, neurofibroma, disciform degeneration of the macula, and metastasis of other tumors (MUELLER-FORELL and PITZ 2004).

### 12.3.1.3
### Other Tumor-Like Lesions of the Eyeball

Choroideal hemangioma is a congenital, vascularized hamartoma that is predominantly found in middle-aged adults affected by neuro-cutaneous syndromes. CT and MRI demonstrate a well-defined, lenticular lesion of high signal intensity on both unenhanced T1-weighted and T2-weighted MR images and of high CT density, respectively, which shows high uptake of intravenously administered contrast media. In patients with von-Hippel-Lindau disease (VHL), the differential diagnosis includes capillary hemangioma (MUELLER-FORELL and PITZ 2004).

Choroideal osteoma is a rare, benign, ossifying tumor predominantly found in women in their 3rd decade of life. It has been described at MRI as showing high signal intensity on unenhanced T1-weighted images, low signal intensity on T2-weighted MR images, and high uptake of intravenously administered contrast media (MUELLER-FORELL and PITZ 2004).

### 12.3.2
### Intraconal Tumors

Cross-sectional imaging may be of considerable help to detect, localize, characterize, and distinguish various tumors and tumor-like lesions of the orbit.
- Typical intraconal tumors include schwannoma and neurofibroma of cranial nerves, while lymphoma and metastasis of extra-orbital tumors may be found in both the intraconal and the extraconal space.
- Among vascular diseases that may clinically appear as tumor-like lesions, there are capillary and cavernous hemangioma, orbital vein anomaly, venous-lymphatic malformation, orbital vein thrombosis, and carotid-cavernous fistula. When large, vascular lesions oftentimes are not confined to one orbital space alone, and they may extend to extra-orbital locations of the head and neck (FLIS and CONNOR 2005).

### 12.3.2.1
### Tumors of Peripheral Nerves

Approximately 4% of all intra-orbital tumors affect peripheral portions of cranial nerves, which may be either intraconal or extraconal (see above, Sect. 12.2.2). Among those tumors, the majority are either schwannoma or plexiform neurofibroma, affecting the motor branches of the third, fourth, and sixth cranial nerve or the sensory branches of the fifth cranial nerve. At cross-sectional imaging, schwannoma is usually well delineated and round to ovoid in shape, with intermediate to high contrast uptake. Schwannoma may be intraconal or extraconal in location. Neurofibroma tends to be irregular in shape and oftentimes appears to be infiltrating into orbital fat (MUELLER-FORELL and PITZ 2004). At unenhanced MRI, both neurofibroma and schwannoma are usually hypointense on T1-weighted and hyperintense on T2-weighted images (AVIV and MISZKIEL 2005). At both MRI and CT, neurofibroma and schwannoma show very high contrast uptake (MUELLER-FORELL and PITZ 2004; AVIV and MISZKIEL 2005).

#### 12.3.2.2
#### Lymphoma

Lymphoma accounts for approximately 55% of all malignant orbital tumors. Predominant subgroups of lymphoma found in the orbit include B-cell lymphoma, low-grade non-Hodgkin's lymphoma, and MALT (mucosa-associated lymphatic-tissue) lymphoma. Patients with a diagnosis of orbital lymphoma are frequently over 50 years old and complain of proptosis (which is most frequently unilateral), displacement of the eyeball, limitations of ocular motility, and, eventually, decrease of visual acuity. At cross-sectional imaging, orbital lymphoma is usually well delineated, non-encapsulating, and round or lobular in shape. However, orbital lymphoma may occasionally be infiltrative, without a definitive intra-orbital mass (MUELLER-FORELL and PITZ 2004). Lymphoma may affect one or several orbital structures or spaces. Isolated affection by lymphoma of the lacrimal gland is frequently seen, and lymphoma may even affect individual rectus muscles of the orbit (AVIV and MISZKIEL 2005).

#### 12.3.2.3
#### Tumor-Like Vascular Lesions

Various vascular lesions of the orbit may appear to be tumor-like at cross-sectional imaging. In particular, hemangiomas of the orbit have also been referred to as "vascular tumors" and should be distinguished from lymphangioma, venous-lymphatic malformations, and arterio-venous malformations (AVIV and Miszkiel 2005).

- Cavernous hemangioma (also referred to as "varicose hemangioma") is a venous malformation (FLIS and CONNOR 2005) that is predominantly found in adults (MUELLER-FORELL and PITZ 2004). Cavernous hemangiomas are frequently intraconal and cause a slowly progressing, painless proptosis that may be accompanied by modest visual impairment when the optic nerve is compressed or stretched. At cross-sectional imaging, cavernous hemangiomas usually present as well-delineating, round or ovoid, tumor-like lesions that may contain phleboliths and usually spare the orbital apex (MUELLER-FORELL and PITZ 2004; AVIV and MISZKIEL 2005). However, cavernous hemangiomas may cause remodeling of orbital bone and may even involve an intra-osseous component, which is most frequently fronto-parietal (FLIS and CONNOR 2005). The differential diagnosis of cavernous hemangioma of the orbit includes orbital venous anomaly (orbital varix), hemangio-

pericytoma, fibrous histiocytoma, and neurinoma (MUELLER-FORELL and PITZ 2004).

- Orbital venous anomaly (orbital varix) refers to abnormally dilated intraorbital veins. Clinically, orbital venous anomaly presents with intermittent or variable proptosis, which is influenced by changes in systemic intravascular pressure (e.g., during Valsalva maneuver) and transmits to intraorbital veins because the latter do not have venous valves. At cross-sectional imaging, a well-delineating, intraconal lesion of triangular shape may be seen, which is pointed toward the orbital apex. The most important differential diagnosis of orbital venous anomaly is cavernous hemangioma (MUELLER-FORELL and PITZ 2004; AVIV and MISZKIEL 2005).

- Venous lymphatic malformation (also known as "lymphangioma") is a term that describes a spectrum of low-flow vascular malformations that ranges from predominantly venous to predominantly lymphatic (AVIV and MISZKIEL 2005). FLIS and CONNOR (2005) distinguish between capillary venous malformation, lymphatic malformation, and combined venous and lymphatic malformation. Venous lymphatic malformation affects children and young adults and is frequently located at the head and neck. When it affects the orbit (intra- or extraconally, or both) or periorbital facial soft tissues, spontaneous hemorrhage within the venous lymphatic malformation may cause sudden proptosis, impaired ocular motility, compression of the optic nerve, and periorbital tissue swelling. At cross-sectional imaging, venous lymphatic malformation presents as a multilobular or infiltrative, hardly encapsulating mass that may include calcifications. Contrast uptake is usually intermediate. The most important differential diagnosis in children is rhabdomyosarcoma (MUELLER-FORELL and PITZ 2004).

- Carotid-cavernous-sinus fistula (CCF) involves high-flow or low-flow arterio-venous shunting of blood from the cavernous segment of the internal carotid artery to the cavernous sinus, which may occur spontaneously or post-traumatically. Increased blood pressure within the cavernous sinus forces venous blood back into the superior orbital vein and causes venous congestion of the orbit. Associated clinical findings include pulsating exophthalmus, dilated episcleral veins, and chemosis. Secondary manifestations of CCF are glaucoma, papillary edema, ophthalmoplegia, and pain. Cross-sectional imaging may demonstrate the extent of vascular dilation within and around the orbit. Digital subtraction angiography may demonstrate the fistula and allows for radiological intervention and therapy (Mueller-Forell and Pitz 2004; Flis and Connor 2005).

### 12.3.3
### Tumors of the Optic Nerve

Although the optic nerve is demonstrated by trans-bulbar ultrasonography, it is more precisely depicted along its entire course by means of MDCT or MRI. Tumors affecting the optic nerve, such as glioma and meningeoma, are demonstrated by both MRI and CT. Often it will be helpful to apply both modalities, particularly when trying to determine the exact extent of the tumor prior to surgery. It is crucial to determine if and how far the optic nerve canal is involved and if disease spreads further into the neurocranium (Mueller-Forell

2004; Hintschich and Rose 2005). Surgical access routes and associated rates of success and morbidity may differ (Hintschich and Rose 2005).

### 12.3.3.1
### Glioma of the Optic Nerve

Glioma of the optic nerve accounts for approximately two thirds of all primary tumors of the optic nerve, is oftentimes diagnosed at young age, i.e., in children and young adults, and grows intra-neurally and intra-axially. There is an association between glioma of the optic nerve and type-1-neurofibromatosis (NF1), which may include perineural and arachnoidal gliomatosis (Mueller-Forell and Pitz 2004). However, glioma of the optic nerve may be divided into a form with a child-

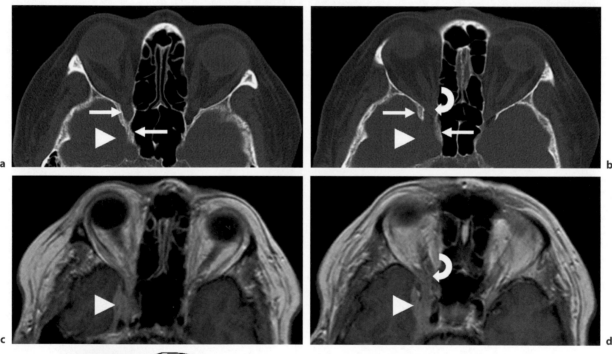

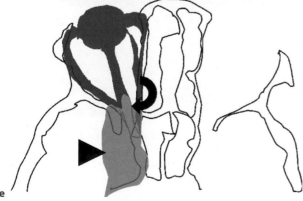

**Fig. 12.3a–e.** Sphenoid bone meningeoma on unenhanced axial MDCT images in bone window (**a** and **b**), contrast-enhanced axial T1-weighted MR images (**c** and **d**), and schematic overlay of MDCT and MR imaging findings (**e**). Meningeoma (*arrowheads*) extends from temporal cavity along cavernous sinus into optic nerve canal and compresses optical nerve (*curved arrows*). MDCT demonstrates permeation by meningeoma of major wing of sphenoid bone, with widening and structural irregularity of affected bony septa (*arrows*)

hood onset, with a variable but largely indolent course and histological features of a low-grade astrocytoma, usually of a pilocytic type, and an adult form, which is clinically aggressive, associated with a high mortality, and has histological features of an anaplastic astrocytoma or glioblastoma multiforme (Aviv and Miszkiel 2005). Although most gliomas are located in the optic nerve, some also involve the optic chiasm. In turn, only about 7% of pilocytic astrocytomas exclusively involve the optic chiasm, while 46% touch the optic chiasm and the hypothalamus (Mueller-Forell 2004). While CT may demonstrate marked contrast enhancement, glioma of the optic nerve demonstrates with high signal intensity on T2-weighted MR images and marked en-

hancement after intravenous administration of contrast media on T1-weighted MR images. The differential diagnosis includes meningeoma, metastasis, sarcoidosis, idiopathic inflammatory disease of the orbit, and optic nerve neuritis (Mueller-Forell and Pitz 2004).

### 12.3.3.2
### Meningeoma
### of the Optic Nerve Sheath Complex

Meningeoma of the optic nerve sheath complex is a benign, extra-axial tumor entity that is predominantly found in adults, with a mean age of approximately 40

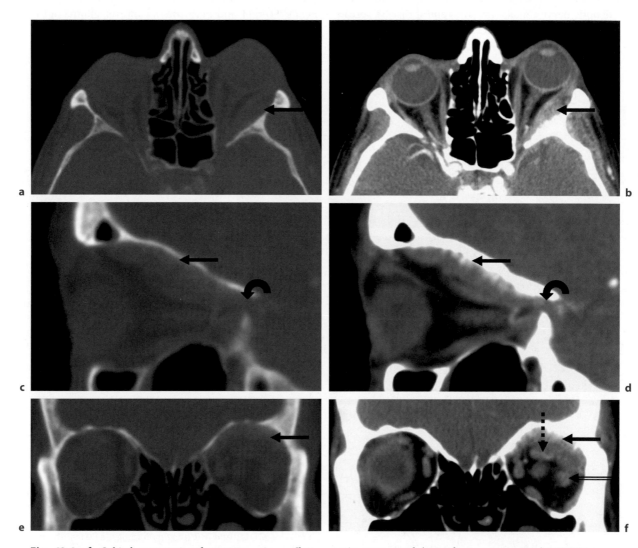

**Fig. 12.4a–f.** Orbital metastasis of prostate cancer affects major wing of sphenoid bone and extraconal compartment of orbit, with bony spiculae extending into the intra-orbital soft tissue mass (*arrows*). Metastasis causes proptosis of left eyeball (axial MDCT images, **a** and **b**), compression of optic nerve in optic nerve canal (*curved arrows* in sagittal MDCT images, **c** and **d**), inferior displacement of superior rectus muscle (dotted *arrow* in coronal MDCT image **f**), and medial displacement of lateral rectus muscle (*double-lined arrow* in coronal MDCT images **f**)

years, and affects women more frequently than men (MUELLER-FORELL and PITZ 2004, AVIV and MISZKIEL 2005). Meningeoma of the optic nerve sheath complex constitutes approximately 3% of all orbital tumors. When found bilaterally (approximately 5% of cases), optic nerve sheath meningeoma is usually associated with type-2-neurofibromatosis (NF2), radiotherapy, or meningeomatosis. Primary affection of the optic nerve by meningeomas arising from arachnoid cells within the leptomeninges or, very rarely, from arachnoid rest cells inside the orbit, should be distinguished from secondary orbital involvement by meningeoma from an intracranial source, such as an intraosseous meningeoma involving the greater wing of the sphenoid bone (Fig. 12.3), which extends from the neurocranium into the orbit (AVIV and MISZKIEL 2005). Clinically, meningeoma of the optic nerve is characterized by slowly progressive loss of vision and unilateral proptosis. The growth pattern may be diffuse, fusiform, or excentric. Since there is no blood-brain barrier, meningeoma shows very high uptake of contrast media at cross-sectional imaging. On T2-weighted MR images, meningeoma demonstrates with an intermediate to high signal. At times, it may be difficult at cross-sectional imaging to distinguish between excentric meningeoma of the optic nerve and cavernous hemangioma (MUELLER-FORELL 2004, MUELLER-FORELL and PITZ 2004, LEMKE et al. 2006).

## 12.3.4
## Extraconal Tumors and Tumor-Like Lesions

In tumors of the extraconal compartment, cross-sectional imaging not only helps to detect, localize, and characterize lesions, but also to determine whether the disease originates in the extraconal compartment or extends into it from elsewhere. A range of benign and malignant tumors as well as metastases may affect the extraconal compartment, which includes the lacrimal gland and lacrimal canal. Involvement of the orbit with metastasis is usually extraconal, involving retrobulbar fat, orbital bone, or the lacrimal gland. However, the conal muscles may be primarily involved. Common primary malignancies in cases of orbital metastasis include cancers of the breast, lung, stomach, thyroid, kidney, or prostate, and melanoma (Fig. 12.4). In neuroblastoma of childhood, the orbit is a common site for metastasis (AVIV and MISZKIEL 2005). At cross-sectional imaging of extraconal tumors and tumor-like lesions, it is particularly helpful to obtain images in several planes of view, i.e., by means of multiplanar reformatting at MDCT.

## 12.3.4.1
## Rhabdomyosarcoma

Rhabdomyosarcoma is the most common soft tissue tumor of the orbit in children under the age of 15 years. Clinically, rhabdomyosarcoma of the orbit is characterized by rapidly progressive proptosis, a decrease of ocular motility, and unilateral ptosis. Cross-sectional imaging reveals a well-delineating tumor whose density or signal intensity is similar to intra-orbital muscles on unenhanced images and increases markedly after intravenous contrast administration. The differential diagnosis includes venous lymphatic malformation, lymphoma, intra-orbital neuroblastoma, and idiopathic inflammatory disease of the orbit (MUELLER-FORELL and PITZ 2004).

## 12.3.4.2
## Various Extraconal Tumors and Tumor-Like Vascular Lesions

- Hemangiopericytoma is an encapsulating tumor that tends to erode adjacent bony structures and markedly takes up contrast media (MUELLER-FORELL and PITZ 2004).
- Olfactory neuroblastoma or esthesioneuroblastoma is found at the frontobasis as a paramedian tumor structure that may extend from the nasal cavity into the orbit (MUELLER-FORELL and PITZ 2004).
- Sinonasal malignomas or metastases may occur in various primary tumor entities, but are most frequently associated with carcinoma, metastatic breast cancer, and metastatic prostate cancer (MUELLER-FORELL and PITZ 2004).
- Langerhans-cell histiocytosis may affect the extraconal compartment of the orbit. At cross-sectional imaging, its density or signal intensity resembles grey brain matter, while contrast uptake is very high (MUELLER-FORELL and PITZ 2004).
- Hamartoma of the inner angle of the eye reveals itself to CT due to the presence within the tumor-like lesion of fat tissue and bony matter (MUELLER-FORELL and PITZ 2004).
- Capillary hemangioma has been referred to as a vascular tumor when it presents in the orbit and has been known as "port wine stain" when it presents extra-orbitally at the head and neck (FLIS and CONNOR 2005). Capillary hemangioma is an inborn lesion predominantly found in small children that shows a tendency toward spontaneous involution up to the 5th year of life. However, capillary hemangioma may displace other orbital contents

and impede vision when spreading out extensively within the orbit. At cross-sectional imaging, capillary hemangioma of the orbit appears as a tumor-like, lobular structure with irregular margins and very high uptake of contrast media (MUELLER-FORELL and PITZ 2004).

- Orbital vein thrombosis may occur by itself or as a sequel of thrombosis of the cavernous sinus. It presents as an intravenous mass and most frequently involves the superior orbital vein. The most important cross-sectional imaging features include dilated venous vessels and lack of contrast enhancement. Additional findings on unenhanced scans are increased density at CT and variable appearance at MRI, which depends on the age of the blood clot and associated degradation of hemoglobin (MUELLER-FORELL and PITZ 2004).

### 12.3.4.3
### Various Tumors of the Lacrimal Gland

- Congenital dermoid cysts are painless, slow-growing tumor-like lesions that contain fat tissue, integumental appendages, and exocrine glands. Cross-sectional imaging demonstrates a well-delineating, round or oval, encapsulating lesion of the upper lateral quadrant of the orbit that contains fat and calcifications and may leave an impression in adjacent bony structures. At diffusion-weighted MR imaging, congenital dermoid cysts show very high signal intensity (MUELLER-FORELL and PITZ 2004).
- Benign pleomorphic adenoma of the lacrimal gland is a slow-growing tumor that displaces the eyeball inferiorly and medially. Cross-sectional imaging shows a well-delineating, encapsulating lesion

of heterogeneous density or signal intensity, due to its myxoid, chondroid, and mucinous contents (MUELLER-FORELL and PITZ 2004).

- Malignant adenoid-cystic carcinoma of the lacrimal gland presents clinically with a hard and painful nodule of the lateral upper eyelid and demonstrates at cross-sectional imaging as a poorly delineating, nodular tumorous structure with erosion of adjacent bony structures (MUELLER-FORELL and PITZ 2004).
- Various lymphatic lesions may affect the lacrimal gland, including reactive lymphoid hyperplasia, MALT lymphoma, malignant non-Hodgkin lymphoma and other malignant lymphomas (Fig. 12.5). They present as slowly growing, tumorous lesions of the upper eyelid that displace the eyeball caudally and are accompanied by visual impairment and redness of the conjunctiva. Lymphatic lesions of the lacrimal gland present at cross-sectional imaging as infiltrative masses with soft contours that adapt to surrounding structures, but may infiltrate bone when they are malignant. They are of homogenous internal density or signal intensity and demonstrate with high contrast uptake. At unenhanced MRI, lymphatic lesions of the lacrimal gland show with high signal intensity on T1-weighted images and low signal intensity on T2-weighted images (MUELLER-FORELL and PITZ 2004).

### 12.4
### Orbital Trauma

Trauma may affect any compartment of the orbit, either alone or in combination with other compartments and

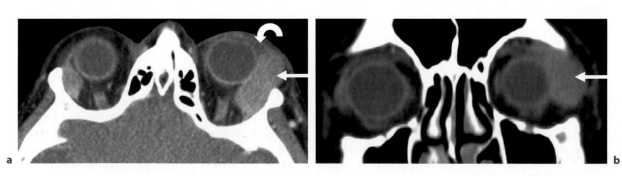

**Fig. 12.5a,b.** Lymphoma of the lacrimal gland (arrows) presents as homogenously enhancing mass with gross enlargement of the gland, medial displacement of the eye bulb, and edema of the upper eyelid (curved arrow) on axial (**a**) and coronal (**b**) contrast-enhanced MDCT images

extraorbital structures. MDCT, with its multi-planar image reformatting options, is the method of first choice in finding X-ray-attenuating foreign bodies within the eyeball and surrounding structures, determining the extent and degree of injury to orbital soft tissue contents, and to detect, localize, and characterize fractures and associated hemorrhage and air inclusions. In particular, when ophthalmoscopy is impaired, e.g., by extreme swelling of the eyelid, CT may rapidly and accurately visualize the full extent of the injury (MUELLER-FORELL and PITZ 2004).

Since the orbital floor and the lamina papyracea represent the weakest structures of the bony orbit (see above, Sect. 12.2.1), they are most frequently involved in fractures affecting the orbit. Typically, a blow-out fracture of the bony orbit disrupts continuity of the infraorbital canal, injures the infraorbital neurovascular bundle (see above, Sect. 12.2.3, and Fig. 12.2), and results in hemorrhage within the adjacent maxillary sinus. When hemorrhage is limited to the immediate surroundings of the infraorbital canal, it oftentimes presents as a "hanging drop" in a space of its own, between the bony orbital floor and the mucosal lining of the maxillary sinus. Rarely, and mostly in association with trauma of high impact or great force, orbital fractures affect the orbital roof, the lateral wall, or even the bony anterior rim of the orbit (see above, Sect. 12.2.1).

Traumatic lesions of neural structures within or surrounding the orbit seldom occur without associated bony or soft tissue injury to the orbit. They are most frequently associated with complex trauma to the face or the frontal neurocranium (MUELLER-FORELL and PITZ 2004). MDCT and MRI are particularly useful to demonstrate the acute and chronic features of complex facial and neurocranial injury, and to visualize affection of the optic nerve canal (LINNAU et al. 2003).

Traumatic injury to the eyeball may occur alone or in conjunction with more extensive facial trauma, and may be due to blunt or penetrating injury. MDCT is applied when facial periorbital edema is too strong to allow for visual inspection of the eyeball or when there is suspicion or evidence of bony involvement or presence of foreign bodies (MUELLER-FORELL and PITZ 2004).

## 12.5
## Orbital Inflammatory Disease

Orbital inflammatory disease may be either non-infectious or infectious and may affect one or more orbital spaces.

### 12.5.1
### Idiopathic Inflammation of the Orbit

Idiopathic inflammation of the orbit may be diffuse with affection of all orbital spaces or locally confined with affection of one space or one particular structure within the orbit. Clinically, idiopathic inflammation of the orbit presents with proptosis, which is oftentimes unilateral.

- Diffuse idiopathic inflammation of the orbit shows with findings at CT and MRI that are non-specific, with high contrast uptake of inflamed structures, infiltration of orbital fat tissue, and inflammation with edema of intraorbital muscles and tendons. As a differential diagnosis, autoimmune hyperthyroidism (Morbus Basedow, Grave's disease, associated with endocrine orbitopathy or EO, see below, Sect. 12.6) does not affect intra-orbital tendons.

- Posterior scleritis is a special, locally confined type of idiopathic inflammation of the orbit, which presents clinically with slowly progressive, painful proptosis. Cross-sectional imaging shows diffuse thickening of the sclera and inflammation of adjacent tissue, with marked contrast uptake. As differential diagnoses, nodular scleritis does not show with contrast uptake, while uveal melanoma does take up contrast media, but usually delineates well (MUELLER-FORELL and PITZ 2004).

### 12.5.2
### Infectious Disease of the Orbit

- In children, infectious disease of the orbit frequently is a complication of paranasal sinusitis.

- Subperiosteal abscess may occur when the infection enters the bony orbit through fissures and apertures, such as the entry or exit sites of neurovascular bundles through the medial orbital wall. Although the periosteum of the orbit or periorbita is a tough layer that is loosely attached to and covers much of the orbit, it includes apertures at the optic canal, superior orbital and inferior orbital fissure, where it fuses with the dura mater, and anteriorly to the orbital rim and lacrimal sac fossa. Fusion of the periorbita with the dura mater implies that there is potential continuity between the subperiosteal space and the epidural space (AVIV and MISZKIEL 2005). Subperiosteal abscess is one disease entity that may create a subperiosteal space in its own right (see Sect. 12.2.2). Its continuity with the extradural space, in turn, explains complications, such as epidural brain abscess and intracranial spread of infection, which may also progress to meningitis, subdural or parenchymal abscess (Aviv and Miszkiel 2005). Other entry sites into the orbit include the orbital septum, whose barrier layer of periorbita needs to be penetrated to allow for spread of infection from the preseptal region (Aviv and Miszkiel 2005).

- Preseptal cellulitis is a bacterial infection of the skin and subcutaneous tissue that may proceed into the orbit. Complications of infectious disease of the orbit include orbital abscess, epidural or subdural abscess of the neurocranium, purulent meningitis, and thrombosis of the cavernous sinus (Mueller-Forell and Pitz 2004).

- A mucocele develops when mucous is retained in a cyst-like structure within an inflamed paranasal sinus. It turns into a pyocele when superinfected. Inflammatory lesions of the paranasal sinuses may develop primarily, when a paranasal sinus ostium is occluded, or secondarily, as a sequel of trauma, surgery, or neoplasia. By growth and pressure, or by inflammation, mucoceles and pyoceles may extend from the paranasal sinuses into the orbit (Fig.12.6). Cross-sectional imaging demonstrates a crescent-shaped tumor-like lesion that sharply delineates and may erode adjacent bony structures; pyoceles show with ring-shaped contrast enhancement along their contours (Mueller-Forell and Pitz 2004).

- Extension of dental abscess to distant areas of the head and neck leads to orbital infection of odontogenic origin in just over 1% of cases (Blake et al. 2006).

## 12.6
### Endocrine Orbitopathy

Dysthyroid endocrine orbitopathy (EO) or "thyroid eye disease" is the most common disorder affecting the orbit, usually presents in middle-aged women, and represents the most frequent cause of unilateral or bilateral proptosis in adults (Mueller-Forell and Pitz 2004; Aviv and Miszkiel 2005). EO is predominantly associated with autoimmune hyperthyroidism, which is also referred to as Morbus Basedow or Grave's disease (Mueller-Forell and Pitz 2004), but the orbitopathy may precede thyroid disease or occur with euthyroid or hypothyroidism (Aviv and Miszkiel 2005). EO is associated with edema of all structures of the orbit. The hallmarks of EO, however, are spindle-shaped edema of the intra-orbital muscles, which leaves out the tendons, and enlargement of the intra-orbital fat tissue (Fig. 12.7) (Mueller-Forell and Pitz 2004; Aviv and Miszkiel 2005). Muscular edema usually is most pronounced in the medial and inferior rectus muscles. Oftentimes, both eyes are affected to a similar degree (Mueller-Forell and Pitz 2004). Edematous muscles may cause apical crowding and venous congestion. The inflammatory response may extend into the intraorbital fat and result in streaking within the fat, which has been referred to as "dirty fat" (Aviv and Miszkiel 2005). As a complication of intra-orbital edema in EO, the optic nerve may be compressed such that there is visual impairment. A complication of muscular edema is fibrosis of the intra-orbital muscles, with the clinical consequence of impaired ocular motility. Cross-sectional imaging demonstrates the pattern and degree of EO. MDCT in particular, with its multiplanar reformatting capabilities, shows the affection of individual intra-orbital muscles and of the intra-orbital fat tissue with edema. The imaging differential diagnosis of EO includes orbital lymphoma, orbital metastasis of extra-orbital primary malignancies, carotid-cavernous fistula (CCF), and idiopathic inflammation of the orbit (Mueller-Forell and Pitz 2004).

## 12.7
### Summary

Pathologic lesions of the orbit remain a great challenge to the diagnostic radiologist. The complex anatomy of the orbit on the one hand and the multitude of disease entities that may affect the orbit on the other hand demand a simple, well-structured approach to diagnostic imaging. Subdividing the orbit into four (or five) distinct spaces, i.e., the eyeball, the intraconal space, the optic nerve, and the extraconal space (with some authors adding the conal space as a separate compartment), facilitates both the localization and characterization of orbital lesions and helps the ophthalmic surgeon to select the best approach to a lesion. Multidetector-row CT (MDCT), due to its thin collimation and resulting multiplanar image reformatting capabilities, has greatly improved the precision of CT imaging of orbital pathology. MDCT allows for multiplanar views of the bony orbital walls and their apertures, i.e., the optic foramen, the superior and inferior orbital fissures, and their respective affection by trauma, tumor, or inflammation. Inclusions of gas or air within the orbit indicate complications of facial trauma, inflammation of the paranasal sinuses, or head and neck tumors. However, due to the separation of the various soft tissue contents of the orbit by orbital fat tissue, MDCT also lends itself to the assessment of primary intra-orbital lesions or secondary affection of the orbit by lesions extending from the face, the neurocranium, the skull base, or from distant primary malignancies.

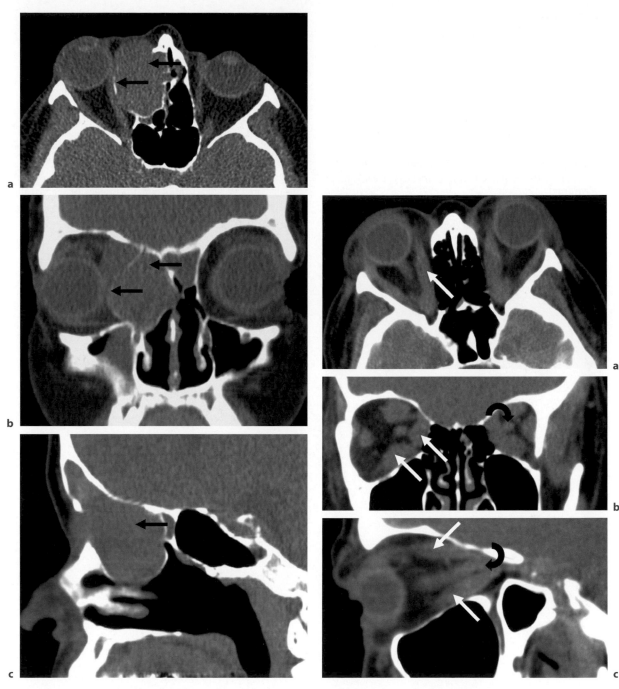

**Fig. 12.6a–c.** Large mucocele extends from right ethmoid sinus into right orbit and displaces both lamina papyracea and right eyeball laterally, anteriorly, and inferiorly (*arrows* in **a**, axial, **b**, coronal, and **c**, sagittal MDCT images). Clinical symptoms include proptosis, double vision, and dry eye due to inability to close the eyelids of the affected eye

**Fig. 12.7a–c.** Endocrine orbitopathy (EO) is among the most common causes for proptosis. Axial (**a**), coronal (**b**) and sagittal (**c**) MDCT images of the orbit demonstrate severe bilateral thickening of intra-orbital muscles, which is usually most pronounced in the medial and inferior rectus muscles (*arrows*), leaves out the tendons, and may result in optic nerve compression at the aperture of the optical nerve canal (*curved arrows*). Hypertrophy of intra-orbital fat tissue is another feature typical of EO

# References

Aviv RI, Casselman J (2005) Orbital imaging: Part 1. Normal anatomy. Clin Radiol 60:279–287

Aviv RI, Miszkiel K (2005) Orbital imaging: Part 2. Intraorbital pathology. Clin Radiol 60:288–307

Blake FAS, Siegert J, Wedl J, Gbara A, Schmelzle R (2006) The acute orbit: Etiology, diagnosis, and therapy. J Oral Maxillofac Surg 64:87-93

Dammann F (2006) Sinuses and facial skeleton. In: Bruening R, Kuettner A, Flohr T (eds) Protocols for multislice CT, 2nd edn., Springer, Berlin, Heidelberg, New York, pp 101-105

Flis CM, Connor SE (2005) Imaging of head and neck venous malformations. Eur Radiol 15:2185–2193

Hintschich C, Rose G (2005) Tumours of the orbit. In: Neuro-oncology of CNS tumours. Tonn J (ed). Springer, Berlin, Heidelberg, New York, pp 269-290

Lemke AJ, Kazi I, Felix R (2006) Magnetic resonance imaging of orbital tumors. Eur Radiol 16:2207–2219

Linnau KF, Hallam DK, Lomoschitz FM, Mann FA (2003) Orbital apex injury: trauma at the junction between the face and the cranium. Eur J Radiol 48:5–16

Mueller-Forell W, Pitz S (2004) Orbital pathology. Eur J Radiol 49:105–142

Mueller-Forell W (2004) Intracranial pathology of the visual pathway. Eur J Radiol 49:143–178

# Dental CT: Pathologic Findings in the Teeth and Jaws

Bernhard Sommer

## CONTENTS

B. Sommer, MD
Center of Diagnostic Radiology Munich Pasing, Pippingerstrasse 25, 81245 Munich, Germany

**ABSTRACT**

The introduction of high-resolution, multislice computed tomography (HRCT) has opened new inquiries from dentists, oral surgeons, and orthodontists. HRCT is ideal for diagnosis of osteolytic and inflammatory disease, odontogenic and non-odotogenic cysts and tumors, traumatic injuries of the teeth and jaw, postoperative complications, including implants, deeply rooted unerupted wisdom teeth, especially relative to the mandibular canal, orthodontia, and ENT questions, including dentogenic sinusitis, antrostomy, midface fractures, and developmental anomalies. Experiences in this new field are reported.

## 13.1 Introduction

Computed tomography (CT) for dental diagnosis was begun with a single-slice technique. The quality of these images, especially of reconstructions, was limited by long scanning times yielding artifacts due to respiration and swallowing. Critical improvement was achieved with multislice, spiral, high-resolution CT (HR CT) with short scanning time, high quality, and very thin slices. The HR thin slices allowed high quality reconstruction in various planes.

CT images, which formerly were used only for volumetric mesurements in difficult cases of implant planning, now provided images with valuable additional information. High quality images are attainable with astonishingly low radiation doses due to the high contrast of jaw bones and teeth (COHNEN et al. 2002;

Lenglinger et al. 1999). New clinical questions have arisen from the new information in the last few years. We have been performing dental CT scans in our offices for 15 years. In the first few years, these scans were exclusively for the planning of implants. Scans for questions not involving dental implants have increased to more than 35 percent of our dental workload in recent years. We now perform about 900 dental CT examinations per year, and the number is increasing.

## 13.2
## Scanning Technique

All scans are performed with a multislice CT Lightspeed Ultra by GE Medical Systems. Scan parameters are: 120 KV, 20 mA for children, 60–80 mA for adults, SD 0,65 mm, pitch 2, and FOV 13. The scan starts from the biting level of the teeth and extends to the lower edge of the chin or to the middle of the maxillary sinuses for mandibular or maxillary examinations, respectively. Processing and reformatting are performed on an Advantage Windows 4.1, GE Medical Systems workstation, with the Dentascan program, or interactively on a PACS workstation with the program Efilm from the firm Merge Healthcare.

## 13.3
## Anatomy and Terminology

Knowledge of dental anatomy and terminology is a prerequisite for understanding colleagues' questions and for communication. The method of counting teeth is characterized by two numbers. The first number is for the quadrant, beginning with one for the upper right and then proceeding clockwise to four for the lower right. The second number describes the corresponding tooth from one to eight in each quadrant. One stands for the first incisor, three for the canine, and eight for the wisdom tooth. For deciduous teeth, the quadrant numbers five to eight are used in the same order instead of quadrants one to four. The terms frontal and occipital, ventral and dorsal are not used in dental radiology. Here the terms mesial for frontal and distal for occipital are substituted. The terms lingual or, in the case of the maxilla, also palatinal are used for orientation in the oral cavity. The side facing the cheek or the lips is called buccal, vestibular, or, in the case of the incisors, labial. The chewing area of the tooth is called occlusal, and the area facing the neighboring tooth approximal. The alveole is the term for the tooth socket in the jaw; the alveolar crest is the top edge of the jaw (Figs. 13.1 and 13.2).

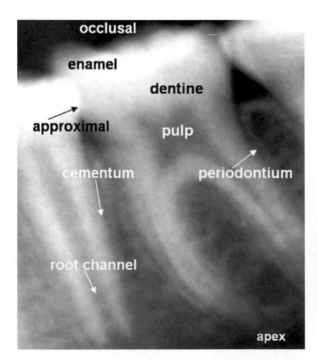

**Fig. 13.1.** Tooth anatomy

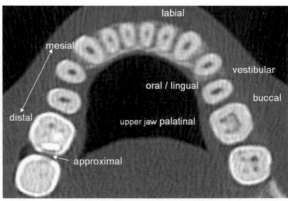

**Fig. 13.2.** Localization terminology

## 13.4
## Clinical Questions

### 13.4.1
### Cystic or Osteolytic Lesions

The following are classed as osteolytic or cystic processes: inflammatory osteolytic diseases of the teeth, odontogenic cystic (epithelial) lesions without internal structures, nonodontogenic cysts, pseudocysts, and regional osteopenia.

The differential diagnosis for these areas is complex. Only the most common cases will be presented.

### 13.4.1.1
### Inflammatory Diseases of the Teeth

Differentiation must be made between *parodontal and endodontal inflammation* (Abrahams et al. 2001). These findings are not, as a rule, the primary reason for the CT examination. The radiologist is, however, often confronted with these diseases within the framework of other questions, such as implant plans or paranasal sinus CT scans, and should comment on them in the report. Both types of inflammation result in bone resorption.

*Parodontal diseases* begin with gingivitis and progress to resorption at the enamel/cementum border along the periodontal ligament and along the root of the tooth in the alveole. The resulting periodontal pockets must be described with their relationship to neighboring teeth, their furcal spreading, i.e., between the roots, and their relationship to the mandibular canal or maxillary sinus. CT images are clearly superior to conventional methods when judging parodontal diseases (Fig. 13.3).

*Endodontal diseases* develop in patients with caries followed by pulpitis. The infection follows the root canal and exits at the apical foramina. Endodontal disease may also follow dental treatment by root canal filling. We will consider periapical parodontitis, periapical granuloma, and periapical cysts. These conditions are often caused by symptomless inflammation in nonvital teeth. Granulomas are, as a rule, round, periapical lytic zones with a diameter less than 1 cm. They may or may not have a sclerotic border. Larger periapical lesions with a diameter of more than 1 cm are more likely to be cystic caseated granulomas and can spread enormously. They occur in the maxilla more often than in the mandible. The radiologist is confronted by them often during CT examination of the paranasal sinuses (Figs. 13.4 and 13.5b).

### 13.4.1.2
### Odontogenic Cystic Lesions of Epithelial Origin

Odontogenic cysts include follicular cysts or dentigerous cysts, keratocysts, residual cysts, and ameloblastoma. Follicular cysts (or dentigerous cysts) are the most common noninflammatory cysts. They can be found surrounding the crowns of unerupted teeth, most often around the unerupted third mandibular molars, followed by the upper and lower canine and upper wisdom teeth. The distance between the crown and the wall of the cyst should be wider than 3 mm; otherwise, it is the normal follicle around the unerupted crown. The size of such follicular cysts can vary greatly and can spread widely (Fig. 13.5a). They are most common during the 2nd decade. They can expand bone and displace neighboring teeth or cause root resorption due to pressure.

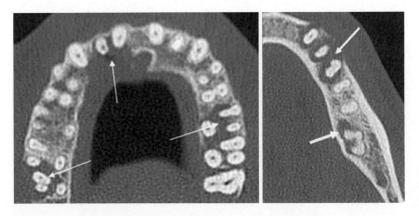

**Fig. 13.3.** Parodontal inflammations in two patients. Axial views of periodontal pockets

**Fig. 13.4.** Endodontal inflammations. *Patient A* with periapical granulomas in area 26 surrounding all three roots. In direct contact with these, periapical inflammatory bone resorption mucous swelling of the bottom of the maxillary sinus, typical for dentogenic sinus disease. *Patient B* with a very small periapical granuloma around the distal buccal root of tooth 27 after incomplete root filling. Only the other two roots are filled completely

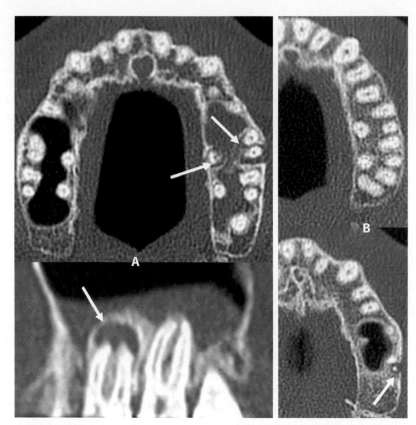

**Fig. 13.5a,b.** *Patient A* with large follicular cyst around unerupted tooth 18. *Patient B* with huge periapical cyst arising from treated tooth 21 by canal filling. Both patients were referred by ENT doctors for sinus disease

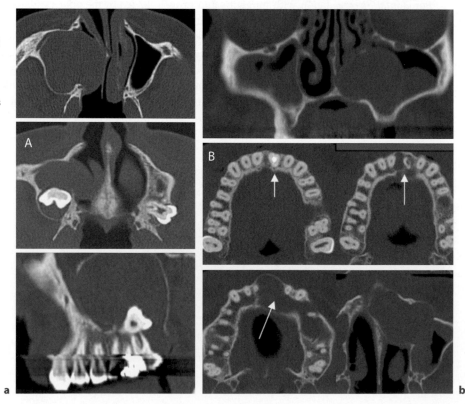

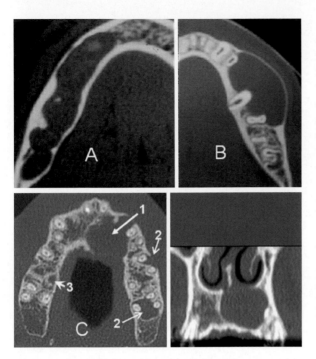

**Fig. 13.6.** Three patients with keratocysts. *Patient A* with a huge keratocyst along the whole right mandible below all the roots. *Patient B* with a keratocyst along the teeth 34, 35 and 36 with cortical expansion and thinning and *patient C* with a frontal keratocyst in the left upper jaw (*1*), additional parodontal inflammatory pockets (*2*), and extraction sockets (*3*)

Keratocysts are primarily a flaw in the development of the dental lamina. Therefore, they are not located near the crown of the tooth, like follicular cysts, but rather between the roots. They can spread widely and tend to recur. Serial examinations are, therefore, advisable. More often they arise in the mandible than in the maxilla. They frequently press on the roots of other teeth and lead to root resorption. Their edges are smooth or undulant. They occur most frequently in the 3rd and 4th decades, similar to ameloblastoma (Fig. 13.6).

Residual cysts are the remains of radicular cysts that can continue to grow after the corresponding tooth has been extracted.

Ameloblastomas develop from odontogenic epithelium. Most are benign, but have an aggressive local growth. Radiologically, they can appear monocystic or polycystic, resembling soap bubbles. The monocystic ameloblastomas are similar to follicular cysts. About half of ameloblastomas develop out of such follicular cysts (SCHOLL et al. 1999). The bubble-like forms are common in the mandible, mostly around the third molar, with 20 percent in the maxilla, where they are usually unicameral. Their edges are always clear, and they grow slowly with thinning and deformation of the cortex. They can displace the mandibular canal. The most common age is the 4th and 5th decades (Fig. 13.7).

### 13.4.1.3
### Nonodontogenic Cysts

These include fissural cysts, such as nasopalatinal cyst or incisive canal cyst arising in the incisive canal, and midpalatal cysts of infants.

### 13.4.1.4
### Pseudocysts

These include:
- Juvenile bone cysts, also solitary traumatic hemorrhagic bone cysts, occur mostly in the mandible in the vicinity of the lateral teeth; they spread into the interdental cavity without displacement or root resorption.
- Stafne cyst is also called lingual salivary gland inclusion defect. This defect is due to the displacement of a salivary gland on the lingual side of the mandible (Fig. 13.8).

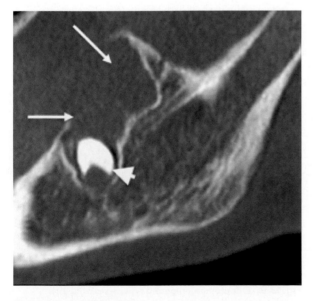

**Fig. 13.7.** Ameloblastoma

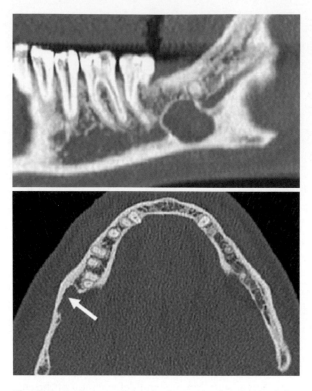

**Fig. 13.8.** Stafne cyst. Lingual salivary gland inclusion defect of the mandible

### 13.4.1.5
### Regional Osteopenia

Especially in the mandible, the spongiosa pattern in older patients can be reduced regionally and can mimic an osteolytic tumor in panoramic views. The mandibular canal may no longer be identified. By CT, the rarification of the spongiosa can be clarified as a systemic process relatively easily and differentiated from neoplasm.

### 13.4.2
### Hyperdense Lesions and Tumors

This group includes odontogenic tumors, osteogenic tumors and metastases, and tumor-like lesions.

### 13.4.2.1
### Odontogenic Tumors
### with Hyperdense Internal Structure

Ameloblastomas and myxomas are not relevant here because they are osteolytic diseases. They are included in the differential diagnosis of cystic processes. Benign tumors include odontomas, odontogenic fibromas and fibromyxomas, and cementomas. Very rare malignant forms are also reported.

Odontomas are not true neoplams, but a hamartomatous developmental fault of the dental lamina (DUNFEE et. al. 2006). They represent the most common group of odontogenic benign lesions. The WHO differentiates between complex odontomas and compound types.

The compound form has recognizable parts of the teeth with dentine or enamel and displays high differentiation. Most compound odontomas are in the vicinity of an impacted tooth. The most common location is the anterior portion of the maxilla. Complex odontomas have amorphous calcifications, either in the region of the lower wisdom teeth or near the posterior region of the maxilla (Fig. 13.9).

Odontogenic fibromas are rare, unilocular, benign lesions of fibrous tissue. Radiologically, they show thin, well-defined hyperdense margins and are more common in the maxilla than in the mandible. They can be found in any age group and show a female predilection (Fig. 13.10). The following subtypes belong to the group of the cementoma:

• *The cementoblastoma* grows around the apex of a root in the region of a molar or premolar, with or without a thin surrounding lucent area. It arises from cementoblasts and shows a decreased transparency periapically early in its development. It may be multiple and, in contrast to the periapical cemental dysplasia, occur more frequently adjacent to the mandibular molars. Later, they show increasing density. Patients are usually in their 3rd decade (Fig. 13.10a).

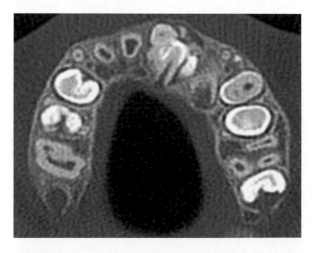

**Fig. 13.9.** Odontoma, compound type, 8-year-old girl

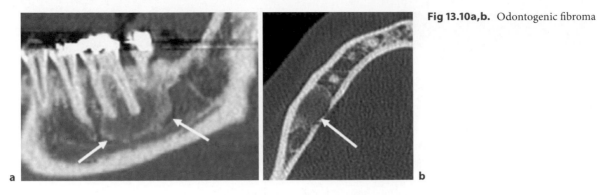

**Fig 13.10a,b.** Odontogenic fibroma

- *Periapical cemental dysplasia* occurs most often in the region of the incisors of the mandible, especially in middle-aged women. The findings probably represent reactive periapical decreased density that can later reverse to increased density and thus appears as a mixed image of lucency and opacity. In most cases, there is no need for treatment. Synonyms are periapical cementoma or periapical cementoosseous dysplasia. (Sciubba et al. 2001) (Fig. 13.10b).

### 13.4.2.2
### Osteogenic Tumors and Metastases

These are not described further in this article.

### 13.4.2.3
### Tumor-Like Lesions

Only the following are named here:
- Fibrous dysplasia with a ground-glass homogenous opacity of the spongiosa and thinning or expansion of the cortex arises more often in the maxilla than the mandible (Fig. 13.11). Others include ossifying fibroma, giant cell granuloma, osteoma, Paget's disease, and cartilaginous lesions.

### 13.4.3
### Conditions After Trauma,
### Especially After Jaw or Tooth Fracture

HR CT contributes to diagnosis when a fracture of the jaw is suspected in cases of skull base or midface frac-

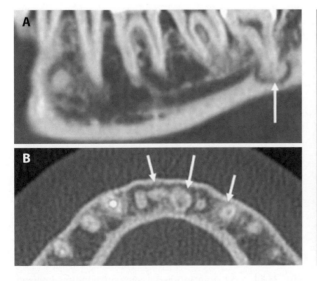

**Fig. 13.11.** *Patient A*, cementoblastoma with periapical opaque mass with a thin radiolucent rim in a molar tooth. *Patient B*, periapical cemental dysplasia

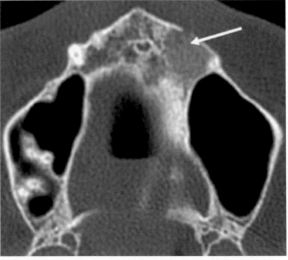

**Fig 13.12.** Fibrous dysplasia in a young woman complaining of constant tickling in her upper cheek. Exams done by ENT doctor and dentist were without any result

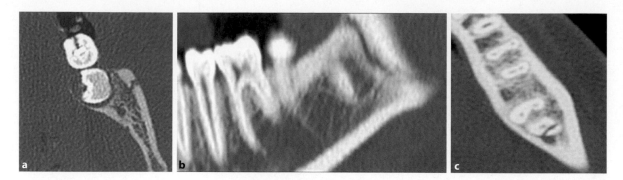

**Fig. 13.13a–c.** Image **a** and **b** mandibular fracture; image **c** dental root fracture

ture. These sometimes hairline fractures in the jaw or near the temporomandibular joint can easily be over-looked in panoramic images or cannot be seen at all due to the oval form of the jaw. Vertical root fractures of a tooth can be easily overlooked with conventional im-ages when the line of the fracture is slanted or frontal, but they are usually easy to detect by CT (GAHLEITNER et al. 2003) (Fig. 13.13).

### 13.4.4
### Postoperative Complications

This group includes patients with suspected:
- Osteomyelitis and periimplantitis (infection adja-cent to implants);
- Nerve lesions with anesthesia of the alveolar inferior nerve or lingual nerve;
- Remnants of roots after tooth extraction;
- Root dislocation in the maxillary sinuses;
- Antrostomy with an oroantral fistula;
- Patients with postoperative new or continuing pain;
- Forensic and insurance questions.

HR CT is also appropriate to identify osteomyelitis or periimplantitis. Nuclear bone scans are nonspecific for a long time after surgery and useless. MRI also shows a nonspecific long-term edema postoperatively with in-creased contrast enhancement inconsistent with resolu-tion of changes in the spongiosa (Fig. 13.14).

After implant surgery on the mandible with a per-sisting numbness, an early CT can prove the extent of the injury of the mandibular canal. In some cases, CT demonstrates the mandibular canal has been only mini-mally touched at the roof or tangentially. After prompt consultation with the surgeon, the implants could be left in such cases and the anesthesia allowed to resolve spontaneously. The paresis in these cases was probably due to intracanalicular bleeding with increased pressure on the infraalveolar nerve. In some cases, the oral sur-geon may elect to turn back the implant slightly after the operation, especially when the CT has been performed immediately postoperatively. However, when the im-plant was straight in the canal or the drilling hole could be seen as a defect on the bottom of the canal, then a severe nerve injury has to be assumed (Fig. 13.15). Se-vere postoperative pain and swelling in the floor of the mouth were found in the case of cortical perforation of an implant on the lingual side of the lower jaw accompa-nied by bleeding into the soft tissue of the mouth floor

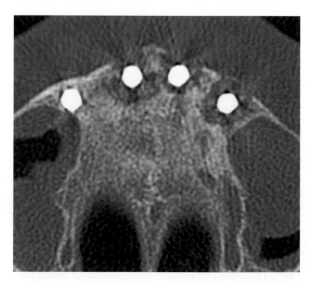

**Fig. 13.14.** Peri-implantitis, lucency surrounding implants several weeks after surgery

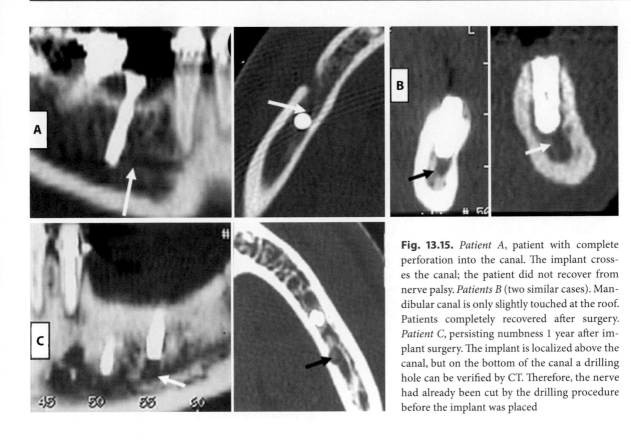

**Fig. 13.15.** *Patient A*, patient with complete perforation into the canal. The implant crosses the canal; the patient did not recover from nerve palsy. *Patients B* (two similar cases). Mandibular canal is only slightly touched at the roof. Patients completely recovered after surgery. *Patient C*, persisting numbness 1 year after implant surgery. The implant is localized above the canal, but on the bottom of the canal a drilling hole can be verified by CT. Therefore, the nerve had already been cut by the drilling procedure before the implant was placed

(Fig. 13.16A). Perforation of a submucosal implant into the floor of the nasal cavity caused new postoperative rhinorrhea, which could not be otherwise explained. The patient was sent for CT on her own insistence (Fig. 13.16B).

Suspected root remnants can be easily recognized due to the typical dentine density and the central neurovascular channel (Fig. 13.17A). Root remnants can also be demonstrated in the maxillary sinus.

An antrostomy with oroantral fistula, a connection between the oral cavity and the maxillary sinus, can be identified through the HR vertical reconstructions of the maxillary sinus floor (Fig. 13.17B). Prompt telephone notification of the dentist or oral surgeon and documentation in the report before discussion with the patient are essential in cases of iatrogenic complication. Optimal information on the operation is a condition for the correct interpretation of these critical findings.

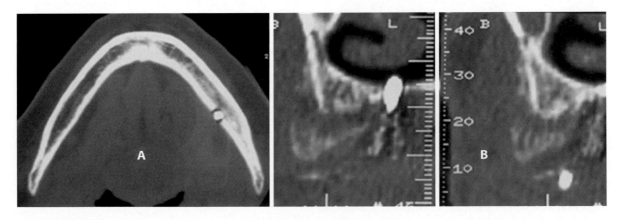

**Fig. 13.16.** *Patient A*, implant perforation of the lingual corticalis; patient suffered from pain and swelling in the mouth floor. *Patient B*, postoperatively patient complained of persistent dripping nose due to perforation of the nasal floor

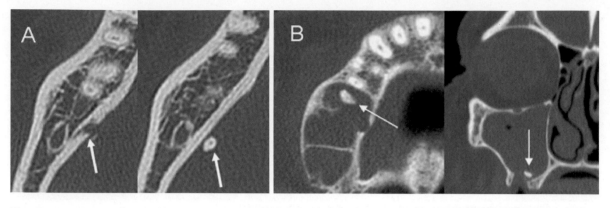

**Fig. 13.17.** *Patient A*, after tooth 48 extraction control X-ray demonstrates some density suspicious for root remains. Operative investigation could not find any remains, so patient came to rule out salivary gland stone. CT demonstrates clearly the perforation of lingual corticalis and some root remains orally. *Patient B*, perforation of sinus floor with displaced root remains in the maxillary sinus and oro-antral communication after extraction of tooth 17

### 13.4.5
### Deeply Rooted, Unerupted Wisdom Teeth

CT is helpful when extraction of an unerupted wisdom tooth is planned and where the mandibular canal crosses the roots of the wisdom teeth, i.e., the roots reach deeper than the mandibular canal. In these cases, it is helpful for the surgeon to know whether the canal runs along the roots on the lingual or the buccal side, or whether the canal meanders through the roots. These cases are liked least by the surgeons. With the knowledge of the path of the nerve, the extraction can be planned with less risk of paresis of the inferior alveolar nerve.

In the case of an interfurcal path of the nerve, i.e., a path between the roots, many dentists decide to refer the patient to an oral surgeon. The analysis of the mandibular canal is, in our experience, best made using the primary axial slices interactively on the workstation.

Beginning distally from the wisdom tooth, the mandibular canal is identified and then followed through the slices along the wisdom tooth. The determination of the pathway is, in most cases, relatively easy. The deformation of the channel on the lingual or buccal side of the roots is sometimes considerable, and sometimes the channel runs only slit-like within the cortex (Fig. 13.18A, B, C).

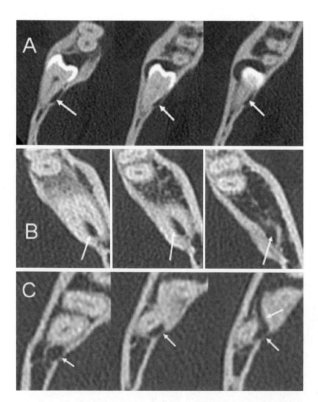

**Fig.13.18.** *Patient A*, mandibular canal passes the wisdom tooth on the lingual side. *Patient B*, nerve canal passes straight between the roots. *Patient C*, nerve canal meanders between the roots from lingual side between the roots to the buccal side

### 13.4.6
### Orthodontic Problems

Requests from orthodontists have become frequent in recent years. Panoramic jaw images of children are confusing at first glance and require a basic knowledge of

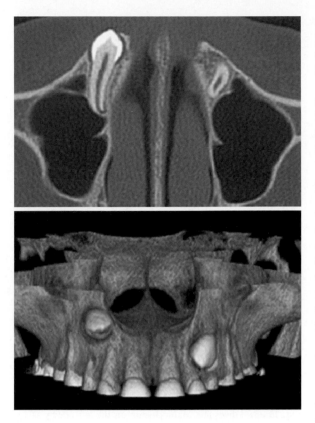

**Fig. 13.19.**  Unerupted eye teeth 13 and 23

tooth development. Initially, it is advisable to contact the orthodontist directly to understand the problems and to establish a common language to describe localization disorders.

For children and young adults, we have adjusted the examination technique to reduce the CT dose to only 20 mAS for 0.6-mm slice thickness with a pitch of 2. The field of measurement should be limited to the necessary region.

After primary axial slices, we perform coronal reconstructions in a semicircle along the curve of the jaw. We may also create oblique reconstructions in selected cases. Additionally, in most of these cases we use stereoscopic images and document them in the cranial, caudal, and both lateral views. All images are stored on a CD, and the most important are printed. The additional views on the CD allow the interested orthodontist to work out further positions individually.

Other orthodontic problems:

- Unerupted canine teeth without position change (Fig. 13.19);
- Narrow jaw, with unerupted tooth or teeth, to help decide which tooth should be extracted to make room for remaining unerupted teeth;
- Surplus teeth, e.g., mesiodentes (Fig. 13.20);
- Possible root resorption by neighboring teeth (Fig. 13.21);
- Unsuccessful orthodontic treatment without movement of the teeth;
- Tooth dysplasia, twin teeth, or root anomalies (Fig. 13.22);
- Suspicion of ankylosis;
- Jaw and facial deformations (Fig. 13.23)

With this last point, we are encroaching on otorhinolaryngology, which is beyond the scope of this article.

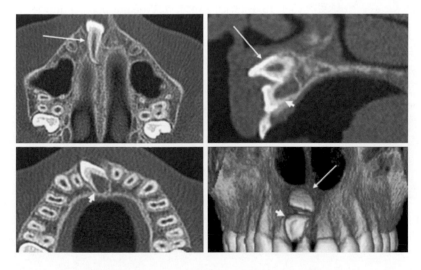

**Fig. 13.20.**  Surplus mesiodens (short arrow) between first incisor (long arrow) above and milk incisor below

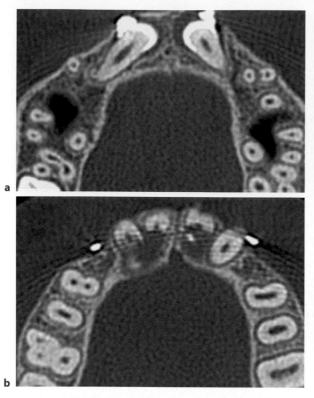

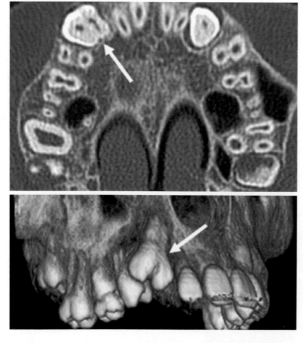

**Fig. 13.21a,b.** Root resorption of both incisors (arrows in **b**) by unerupted eye teeth (**a**) on both sides

**Fig. 13.22.** Blocked twin tooth 13. By CT the differentiation of a real twin tooth from two teeth projecting only on each other was possible

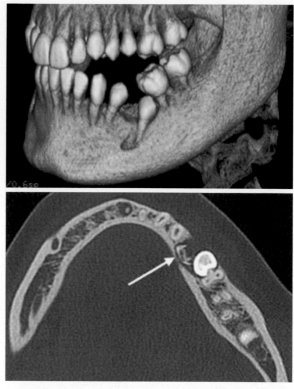

**Fig. 13.23.** Lower jaw. Malocclusion on the *left side* by asymmetry of the lower jaw due to a surplus unerupted tooth in area 35; one of them was destroyed by caries; the other one is blocked against tooth 36

## 13.4.7
## Borderline ENT Examinations for Chronic Sinus Diseases

Many of the examples demonstrate the relationship of dental problems to the maxillary sinuses (Figs. 13.4–13.6, 13.12, 13.17). CT of the maxilla and teeth can deliver important information for our ENT colleagues about sinus disease, root disease, displaced root remnants, antrostomy, and fistulas. HR CT is also unrivaled after trauma with midface and jaw fractures and developmental anomalies, such as cleft palate.

Roots of teeth should be checked routinely during CT examinations for paranasal sinuses. The radiologist should be especially attentive if patients report sinus or cheek problems and previous consultations with ENT colleagues or dentists were nonproductive.

Since the introduction of the multislice CT, we have performed all paranasal sinuses CT scans axially, including the maxilla, and thus have avoided dental artifacts when reconstructing the images in coronal and sagittal planes. This technique automatically includes the maxillary teeth and discloses clinically inapparent inflammations of the teeth and dentogenic reasons for sinus diseases (Figs. 13.4 and 13.5B). We evaluated 641 paranasal sinus CTs and found a frequency of dental inflammatory root diseases in 61 patients (9.5 percent).

**13.5**

## Experiences Made in Cooperation with Dentists, Dental Surgeons, and Orthodontists

- Radiological diagnosis of dental problems is not included in most radiology residencies. Because of the independent radiological images made by dentists, dental surgeons, and orthodontists, there is no necessity for it. Multislice CT is a valuable additional method in difficult cases of implants and in the case of unclear panoramic findings. Positive experiences have led to new and complex demands on the radiologist from dentists and surgeons in this innovative area.
- The great variety of new queries and the possibilities of differential diagnosis require initial investment of time from the radiologist when cooperating with colleagues in this unfamiliar area.
- Knowledge of dental terminology is critical.
- It is necessary to have a basic knowledge in the interpretation of panoramic images to understand problem areas.
- A collection of basic literature on dental radiology with image atlases (PASLER et al. 2000; SITZMANN et al. 2000; THIEL et al. 2001) and articles on dental CT are prerequisite.
- It is very helpful to have a basic knowledge of the embryology and development of the teeth, especially to be able to interpret cystic, tumorous, or pseudotumorous processes in the jaw.
- Initially, it is advisable to discuss the expectations and clinical queries with referring colleagues; this will often require many telephone calls.
- When examining children, the radiologist must be aware of the radiation dose and minimize it as much as possible. It is advisable to have an established protocol for children and not to leave decisions to the technologist.
- Inviting interested dentists and oral surgeons to workshops fosters mutual understanding of the problems endemic to each group.
- By informing referring implant surgeons, we have, in the case of questionable nerve injury during implant operation, insured that patients with palsies

are sent to CT as soon as possible. The patients are scanned without an appointment, and the referring doctor is informed by telephone immediately.

- To reduce telephone queries, it is helpful to have a dedicated form for the dental CT with the following questions:
  - Implant planning?:
    - With planning prosthesis and special markings?
    - Without a prosthesis?
    - Is a complete evaluation desired with reconstructions, prints, CD, and report?
    - Are image data on a CD to be integrated in another external planning program?
    - Which planning program do you use? (There are different technical requirements for each of them.)
  - Clarification of unerupted teeth? Which?
  - Clarification of an unclear X-ray finding (panoramic views or images of teeth should be available) with a description of the problem.
  - Orthodontic query with a comprehensive description.

## References

Abrahams JJ (2001) Dental CT imaging: A look at the jaw. Radiology 219:334–345

Cohnen M, Kemper J, Möbes O, Pawelzik J, Mödder U (2002) Radiation dose in dental radiology. Eur Radiol 12:634 – 637

Dunfee BL, Sakai O, Pistey R, Gohel A (2006) Radiologic and pathologic characteristics of benign and malignant lesions of the mandible. Radiographics 26:1757–1768

Gahleitner A, Watzek G, Imhof H (2003) Dental CT: imaging technique, anatomy and pathologic conditions of the jaws. Eur Radiol 13:366–376

Lenglinger FX, Muhr T, Krennmair G (1999) Dental-CT: Untersuchungstechnik, Strahlenbelastung und Anatomie. Der Radiologe 39:1027–1034

Pasler FA, Visser H (2000) Zahnmedizinische Radiologie Farbatlanten der Zahnmedizin Band 5. Thieme, Stuttgart

Scholl RJ, Kellett HM, Neumann DP, Lurie AG (1999) Cysts and cystic lesions of the mandible: Clinical and radiologic-histopathologic review. Radiographics 19:1107–1124

Sciubba JJ, Fantasia JE, Kahn LB (2001) Tumors and cysts of the jaw. Atlas of tumor pathology, 3rd series, fascicle 29. AFIP, Washington

Sitzmann F, Benz C., Düker J, Hardt N, Hirschfelder U, Rother UJ, Spitzer WJ (2000) Zahn-, Mund- und Kiefererkrankungen, Atlas der bildgebenden Diagnostik. Urban & Fischer, Munich

Thiel HJ, Haßfeld S (2001) Schnittbilddiagnostik in MKG-Chirurgie und Zahnmedizin. Thieme, Stuttgart

# Anatomy and Corresponding Oncological Imaging of the Neck

14

Juergen Lutz, Ullrich G. Mueller-Lisse and Lorenz Jäger

## CONTENTS

14.1 **Introduction** *178*

14.2 **Paranasal Sinuses
and Nasopharynx** *181*
14.2.1 Anatomy *181*
14.2.2 Oncological Imaging
of Sinonasal Masses *181*

14.3 **Oral Cavity and Oropharynx** *182*
14.3.1 Anatomy *182*
14.3.2 Oncological Imaging
of Oral Masses *185*

14.4 **Hypopharynx and Larynx** *187*
14.4.1 Anatomy *187*
14.4.2 Imaging of Hypopharyngeal
and Laryngeal Masses *187*

**References** *190*

## ABSTRACT

High-resolution (HR) multislice computed tomography (MSCT) has become the essential tool for the evaluation of malformations, trauma, and especially tumors of the midface and head and neck region. Important for an adequate evaluation of pathologic findings in the head and neck region is a profound knowledge of the organization of the anatomic compartments and their neighboring relation. Therefore, CT scanning of different head and neck regions should be fitted for the special needs of the anatomic region under investigation, for example, particular adjusted protocols for the evaluation of the larynx. The rapid technical improvement of MSCT in recent years has made CT the first-choice imaging modality in many clinical conditions. The thinner slice collimation with improved anatomic detail visualization, the considerably reduced scanning time, and the possibility to calculate multiplanar reconstructions (MPR) from the scanned volume data set have contributed to the ascent of CT scanning in head and neck oncology. Especially helpful is the ability of cross-sectional imaging to reveal pathologic conditions that are not detectable by endoscopy or in the setting of staging underestimated due to submucosal spread. The aim of this article is to provide protocol suggestions for MSCT of the head and neck regions on the basis of a tailored review of the most important anatomic structures and their pathologic conditions.

J. Lutz, MD
Department of Clinical Radiology, Ludwig-Maximilians-University of Munich, Munich University Hospitals, Ziemssenstrasse 1, 80336 Munich, Germany

U. G. Mueller-Lisse, MD, MBA
Department of Clinical Radiology, Ludwig-Maximilians-University of Munich, Munich University Hospitals, Ziemssenstrasse 1, 80336 Munich, Germany

L. Jäger, MD, PD
Diagnostisches Zentrum Garmisch Partenkirchen, Partnachstrasse 65, 82467 Garmisch Partenkirchen, Germany

## Introduction

The anatomy of the face and the neck is always a challenge to clinicians and radiologists. Many small, but critical structures pass from the brain through the neck to the thoracic region. Complex anatomic structures and regions, such as the facial skeleton, the paranasal sinuses, the deep spaces of the neck, and the larynx, require a profound knowledge of the different neighboring cervical structures and compartments. This un-

derstanding is crucial for the radiologist to be able to choose the appropriate imaging modalities, communicate the findings precisely to the clinician, and generate a valuable differential diagnosis. The purpose of this chapter is to describe regional distinctions of the head and neck anatomy and their characteristic pathologic lesions and to offer state-of-the-art protocols for multislice spiral computed tomography (MSCT) for the evaluation of the head and neck.

In this chapter we try to summarize the special MSCT scan protocols dependent upon the different anatomic regions and their needs. The MSCT protocols

**Table 14.1.** Trauma protocol: Scan und reconstruction parameters for MSCT of midface and paranasal sinuses (mAs above 100 for the diagnosis of malignant disease). Additional convolution kernels are necessary for tumor evaluation and i.v. contrast administration. Sagittal and coronal multiplanar reconstructions are mandatory

| Scan parameters | 16 slice | 64 slice |
| --- | --- | --- |
| Scan range | Frontal sinus/mandibula | Frontal sinus/mandibula |
| Tube voltage (kV) | 120 | 120 |
| Tube current time product (mAs) | 40/160 | 40/160 |
| Rotation time (s) | <1 | <1 |
| Pitch | 0.8 | 0.8 |
| Collimation (mm) | 0.625 | 0.625 |
| Recon increment (mm) | 0.5 | 0.5 |
| Kernel | Bone | Bone |
| Reconstructions slice thickness (mm) | 0.75 | 0.75 |

**Table 14.2.** Tumor protocol: Scan und reconstruction parameters for MSCT of nasopharynx, oropharynx (including oral cavity), and hypopharynx. Blood parameters about renal (creatinin) and thyroid (TSH) function should be obtained before i.v. contrast application. The scan range should be chosen from the skull base till the aortic arch to evaluate intracranial tumor spread or suspect lymphoid node stations. Sagittal and coronal multiplanar reconstructions (MPRs) are mandatory. Delay can be varied for more highly vascularized tumors to achieve good contrast

| Scan parameters | 16 slice | 64 slice |
| --- | --- | --- |
| Scan range | Frontal sinus/aortic arch | Frontal sinus/aortic arch |
| Tube voltage (kV) | 120 | 120 |
| Tube current time product (mAs) | 180 | 180 |
| Rotation time (s) | 0.75 | 0.75 |
| Pitch | 1–1.5 | 1–1.5 |
| Collimation (mm) | 1.25 | 0.625 |
| Recon increment standard (mm) | 2 | 2 |
| Recon slice thickness  standard (mm) | 3 | 3 |

**Table 14.2.** (*continued*) Tumor protocol: Scan und reconstruction parameters for MSCT of nasopharynx, oropharynx (including oral cavity), and hypopharynx. Blood parameters about renal (creatinin) and thyroid (TSH) function should be obtained before i.v. contrast application. The scan range should be chosen from the skull base till the aortic arch to evaluate intracranial tumor spread or suspect lymphoid node stations. Sagittal and coronal multiplanar reconstructions (MPRs) are mandatory. Delay can be varied for more highly vascularized tumors to achieve good contrast

| Scan parameters | 16 slice | 64 slice |
|---|---|---|
| Scan range | Frontal sinus/aortic arch | Frontal sinus/aortic arch |
| Kernel 1 | Standard | Standard |
| Kernel 2 | Bone | Bone |
| Recon increment bone (mm) | 1.0 | 0.6 |
| Recon slice thickness | | |
| bone (mm) | 1.5 | 0.75–1 |
| Contrast media | | |
| Volume (ml) | 100 | 100 |
| Mg iodine/ml | 300 | 300 |
| Injection rate (ml/s) | 2 | 2 |
| Delay (s) | 50-70 | 50-70 |

**Table 14.3.** Tumor protocol: Scan und reconstruction parameters for MSCT of the larynx and hypopharynx. Blood parameters about renal (creatinine) and thyroid (TSH) function should be obtained before i.v. contrast application. The acquisition should be performed in breath technique. Thin sagittal and coronal multiplanar reconstructions (MPRs) are also mandatory

| Scan parameters | 16 slice | 64 slice |
|---|---|---|
| Scan range | Mandibula/jugulum | Mandibula/jugulum |
| Tube voltage (kV) | 120 | 120 |
| Tube current time product (mAs) | 220 | 220 |
| Rotation time (s) | 0.5 | 0.5 |
| Pitch | 1.0-1.5 | 1.0-1.5 |
| Collimation (mm) | 0.625 | 0.625 |
| Recon increment (mm) | 0.5 | 0.5 |
| Recon slice thickness (mm) | 0.75–1.0 | 0.75–1.0 |
| Kernel | Standard | Standard |
| Contrast media | | |
| Volume (ml) | 100 | 100 |
| Mg iodine/ml | 300 | 300 |
| Injection rate (ml/s) | 3 | 3 |
| Delay (s) | Arterial / 70 | Arterial / 70 |

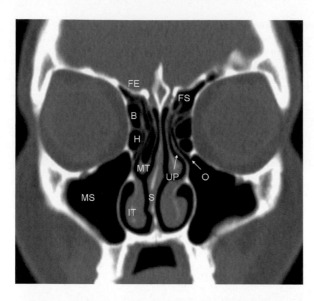

**Fig. 14.1.** MSCT with coronal multiplanar reconstruction of the midface. Key structures of the sinuses and the osteomeatal complex: *FE*, fovea ethmoidales; *UP*, uncinate process; *FS*, frontal sinus; *MS*, maxillary sinus; *O*, ostium of maxillary sinus; *B*, ethmoid bulla; *H*, inferior "Haller" cell; *IT*, inferior turbinate; *MT*, middle turbinate; *S*, septum

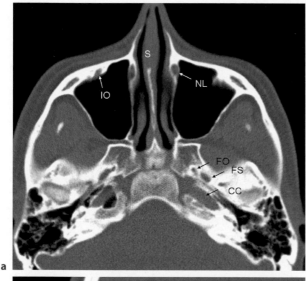

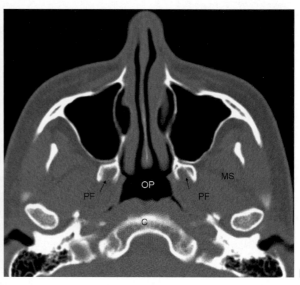

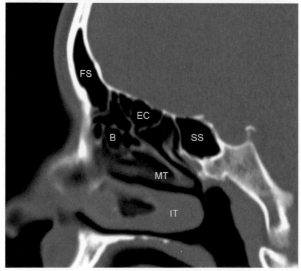

**Fig. 14.2a–c.** MSCT images showing important anatomic landmarks of the midface and adjacent structures. **a** Axial MSCT image at the plane of the corpus of the sphenoid bone: *NL*, nasolacrimal duct; *S*, nasal septum; *IO*, infraorbital canal; *FO*, foramen ovale; *FS*, formanen spinosum; *CC*, carotid canal. **b** Axial MSCT image at the plane of the clivus: *C*, clivus; *OP*, oropharynx; *MS*, masticator space; *PF*, pterygopalatine fossa. **c** Sagittal MDCT image in the midline through the frontal recess: *B*, ethmoid bulla; *FS*, frontal recess; *EC*, ethmoid cells; *SS*, sphenoid sinus; *IT*, inferior turbinate; *MT*, middle turbinate

for the paranasal sinuses and the nasopharynx are separated because, for the sake of completeness, the possibility of a low dose protocol for the evaluation of the sinuses and the facial skeleton should be mentioned. Table 14.1 shows the MSCT scan and reconstruction protocol suggested for the paranasal sinuses and Table 14.2 shows the MSCT scan and reconstruction protocol suggested for the nasopharynx and MSCT scan and the reconstruction protocol suggested for the oral cavity and the oropharynx; Table 14.3 shows the MSCT scan and reconstruction protocol for the hypopharynx and the larynx.

## 14.2
## Paranasal Sinuses and Nasopharynx

### 14.2.1
### Anatomy

The region of the paranasal sinus and nasal cavity is subject to a wide range of detailed anatomic findings and a variety of different lesions. The normal anatomic variation and the different appearance of sinonasal masses make good anatomic knowledge mandatory. Essential anatomic structures of the sinuses are the ostiometal complex, the frontal recess, and the spheno-ethmoid recess (Fig. 14.1).

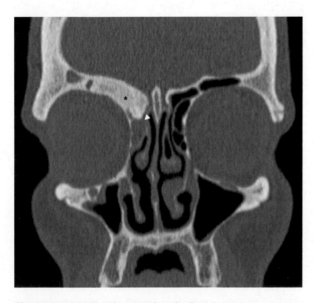

**Fig. 14.3.** MSCT with coronal multiplanar reconstruction using a bone algorithm of the midface. The CT shows a characteristic osteoma (*asterisks*) of the right frontal sinus (Δ). This is a benign intrasinus mass of osseous origin

The osteomeatal complex is the decussation of different structures such as the anterior ethmoid, the frontal sinus, and the maxillary mucus drainage. Of special importance is the uncinate process (MAROLDI et al. 2004). Another crucial landmark is the pterygopalatine fossa, a narrow space between the pterygoid process and the vertical process of the palatine bone, which comprise the pterygopalatine ganglion, part of the maxillary nerve (LANDSBERG and FRIEDMAN 2001) (Fig. 14.2). Histologically, the paranasal sinus and nasal cavity are lined by ciliated columnar epithelium that harbors mucinous and serous glands (Fig. 14.3).

### 14.2.2
### Oncological Imaging
### of Sinonasal Masses

Malignant tumors of the paranasal sinuses and the nasal cavity comprise only 3% of all malignancies of the head and neck region. There is some essential information for imaging sinonasal malignancies. Despite the anatomic diversity, there is some prevalence of the origin of neoplasms. About 75% arise from the maxillary sinus, and about 25% arise primarily in the nose or the ethmoid sinus (TIWARI et al. 2000). Comprising up to 80% of these masses, the most common malignancy of the sinonasal area is squamous cell carcinoma (Fig. 14.4). Up to now, no direct link to cigarette smoking has been found. However, nickel and thorotrast exposures are thought to be risk factors for the development of squamous cell carcinoma. Not to be forgotten, human papilloma virus may have a role in the malignant transformation of inverted papilloma to squamous cell carcinoma. Other entities are malignancies arising from the surface epithelium or seromoucous glands, such as adenocarcinoma, over 50% of which can also be found in the maxillary sinus. Within the head and neck region, the most common site is the sinonasal melanoma (Fig. 14.5).

The most common clinical signs for most of these tumors are symptoms of medical refractory chronic sinusitis, and, dependent on size and location, additional signs of unilateral nasal obstruction and epistaxis. The relevant areas to evaluate in imaging tumors of the maxillary sinus include the posterior wall of the maxillary sinus, the pterygopalatine fossa, and the floor of the orbit. Especially the posterior spread in the pterygopaltine fossa and a possible perineural tumor spread are crucial information for surgical planning and are associated with a poorer prognosis. Initially, high-resolution computed tomography (CT) with i.v. contrast can demonstrate replacement of fat in the fossa, associated with

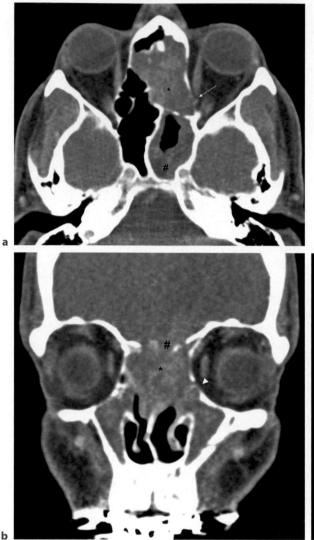

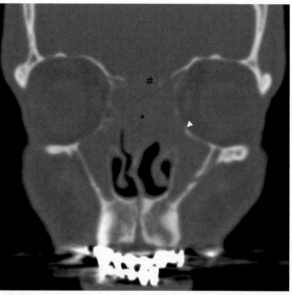

**Fig. 14.4a–c.** Squamous cell carcinoma of the ethmoid sinuses. **a** Enhanced axial MSCT image shows an expansile, enhancing mass in the anterior ethmoid cells (*) and bulging into the left orbit (*white arrow*). Mucosal thickening in the sphenoid sinus (#). **b** Enhanced MSCT as coronal MPR (*standard tissue kernel*) showing the inhomogenous mass in the ethmoid sinus (*) with suspicious destruction of the cribriform plate (#) and infiltration of the anterior cranial fossa. **c** Coronal MPR (bone kernel) confirms the bony destruction of the superior nasal turbinate (*) and the cribriform plate (#) as well as thinning of the medial orbital wall (Δ)

information about destruction of palatine bony structures. Additional information about the integrity of the walls of the orbit can be achieved with MSCT. The distortions of the orbital walls occur frequently because of maxillary and ethmoidal neoplasms. Similar to orbital bone invasion, bone destruction of the skull base is excellently demonstrated by CT with sagittal and coronal multi-planar-reconstructions (MPRs). Especially for the evaluation of the thin bony region between the ethmoid roof, the cribriform plate, and the anterior cranial fossa, sagittal MPRs with a thin bone reconstruction kernel are mandatory. CT with multi-planar reconstructions is the most reliable imaging modality to diagnose fat and bone invasion, although, especially for oncologic imaging of the sinuses, MRI is superior in soft tissue invasion (e.g., perineural tumor spread and intracerebral edema) and should be used additionally for pre-therapeutic staging.

## 14.3
## Oral Cavity and Oropharynx

### 14.3.1
### Anatomy

#### Oral Cavity

The anatomic details of the oral cavity contain the floor of the mouth, centrally located, the anterior two thirds of the tongue (the posterior one third belongs to the oropharynx), the lips, and the oral vestibule (SMOKER 2003). The oral cavity lies anterior to the oropharynx and is separated posteriorly by the soft palate, the anterior tonsillar pillars, and circumvillate papillae (of the tongue). The tongue consists of two kinds of muscula-

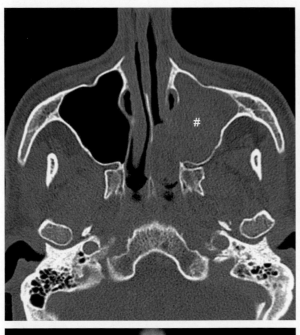

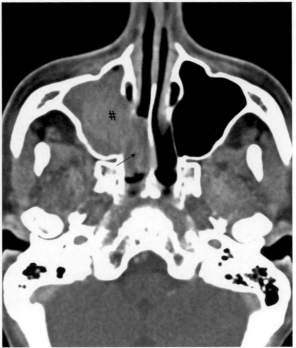

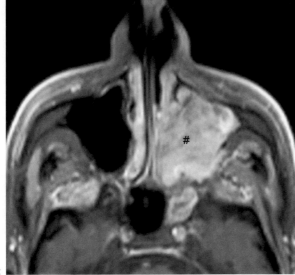

**Fig. 14.5a–c.** Melanoma of the left maxillary sinuses. **a** Enhanced axial MSCT image depicts an enhancing mass in the left maxillary sinus (#). The tumor has grown through the medial wall of the maxillary sinus and reached the nasal cavity (*black arrow*). **b** Axial MSCT image (thin bone reconstruction) demonstrating the melanoma (#) filling the maxillary sinus without bony reaction of the anterior or lateral wall. **c** Axial T1-weighted fat-saturated spin echo image after contrast (gadolinum) administration showing an inhomogenous enhancing mass (#) of the sinus with bright, hyperintense areas of melanin, typical for melanoma

ture: the intrinsic muscles (longitudinal, transverse, and vertical fibers) and the extrinsic muscles (palatoglossus, genioglossus, hyoglossus, and styloglossus muscles). The hard palate and the superior alveolar ridge are the superior, the mylohyoid muscle (floor of the mouth), constitutes the inferior border. The lateral borders are the cheeks (Fig. 14.6).

Within the oral cavity lies the submandibular, the submental, and the sublingual space. The submandibular space is located between the hyoid bone and the mylohoid muscle and contains the submandibular glands, lymph nodes, and the facial artery and vein. The sublingual space, which is not encapsulated by its own fascia, communicates posteriorly with the submandibular space and contains the sublingual gland, the submandibular duct, the hypoglossal and facial nerve, as well as the facial artery and vein. The retromolar region, a region posterior to the last molar, and the pterygomandibular raphe, a fibrous band extending from the mandible to insert into the pterygoid process, are common anatomic crossroads of tumor spread (SMOKER 2003; LENZ et al. 2000).

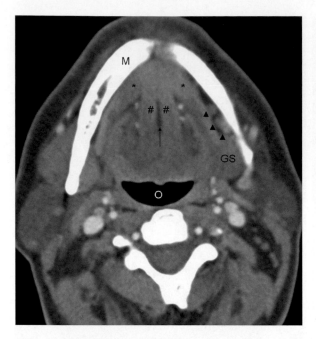

**Fig. 14.6.** Axial MSCT image of the floor of the mouth at the level of the mandible. The pharyngeal mucosal space of the oropharynx (O). The base of the tongue with the genioglossus muscle (#) and the middle lingual septum (*black arrow*). The mylohyoid muscle (*) separates the submandibular space containing the submandibular gland (*GS*) laterally (*black arrowheads*), ramus mandibulae (*M*)

### Oropharynx

The oropharynx can be described as a three-dimensional structure bounded anteriorly by the anterior pillars of the pharyngeal fauces (the palatoglossus muscle), the circumvallate papillae (sulcus terminales), or the junction of the hard and soft palates. Posterior and lateral boundaries are formed by the muscular pharyngeal wall (superior and middle constrictor muscles). The superior extent is the level of the hard palate. The extension inferiorly reaches the level of the base of the tongue or level of the hyoid. The oropharynx is further subdivided into five areas. These include the lateral pharyngeal walls, tonsillar regions, posterior wall, base of the tongue, and soft palate. Beneath the mucosal compartments, the oropharynx is surrounded laterally and posteriorly by fascial compartments. These spaces are the retropharyngeal, and bilaterally, the parapharyngeal spaces. These are potential routes of per continuitatem tumor growth or spread of infections reaching until the mediastinum. Histogically, the oropharynx is lined by a non-keratinizing stratified squamous epithelium.

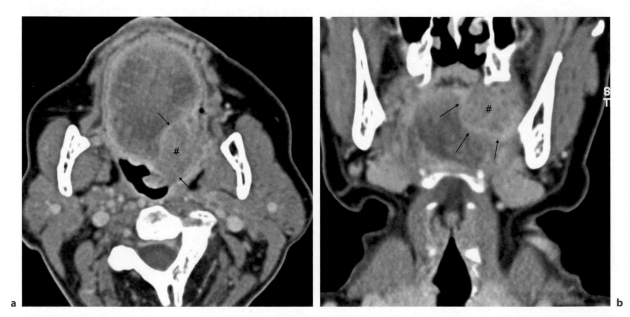

a                                                                                                          b

**Fig. 14.7a,b.** Squamous cell carcinoma of the tongue base. **a** Enhanced axial MSCT image clearly demonstrates an enhancing mass at the lateral tongue (#). The mass shows delineation to the surrounding tissue medially (*white arrow*) and bulging towards the oropharyngeal mucosal surface (*black arrow*). **b** Coronal MPR of the same patient showing the cranio-caudal extent of the tumor within the intrinsic muscles of the tongue (# and *black arrow*)

## 14.3.2
## Oncological Imaging of Oral Masses

Malignant tumors of the oropharynx, the floor of the mouth, and the oral cavity represent about 2–5% of all malignancies. Overall, the most common type of oral cancer is squamous cell carcinomas (SCCa) (Fig. 14.7). They account for more than 90% of all oral malignant lesions. The underlying alterations may be genetically determined or are thought to be caused by prolonged exposure to factors such as tobacco and alcohol (MEYERS 1996). Other neoplasms are minor salivary gland tumors (e.g., adenocarcinomas) that preferentially spread along nerves. Additional entities are lymphomas and, very rarely, sarcomas. In childhood, rhabdomyosarcoma is the most frequent malignant mass of this area (LENZ et al. 2000). One type of differential diagnosis of enhancing masses of the oral cavity is an infectious mass-demanding process, especially abscess formation (Fig. 14.8). Abscess of odontogenic origin is very common.

Oral cavity cancers can be subdivided into the following areas: the buccal and gingival mucosa, the upper alveolus and lower alveolus, the hard palate, the tongue, and the floor of mouth.

The choice of imaging modality is determined by answering critical clinical questions: precise tumor location, submucosal and potential neurovascular spread, and lymph node and cortical bone invasion. Crucial for the prognosis of the patient's outcome is the location and size of the early metastasizing into regional lymph nodes. Depending on the size and infiltration into surrounding connective tissue, surgical treatment with or without radiation is the appropriate approach.

Common sites for squamous cell carcinomas are the buccal mucosa where the lateral walls of the buccal cavity are preferred. The tumor can spread along the submucosa and can erode the adjacent alveolar or mandibular ridge. Especially for tumor of this entity, CT can detect early mucosal masses and associated indirect signs. So about 85% of all squamous cell carcinomas show contrast enhancement; the others are only apparent through their demanding of space (LENZ 2000).

If the squamous cell carcinomas arise in the floor of the mouth, they commonly arise in the anterior third and most spread medially.

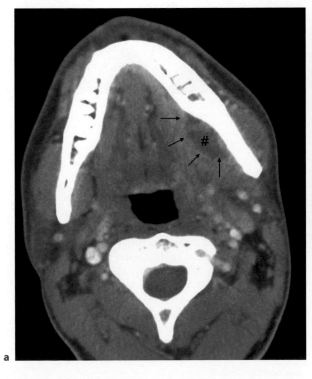

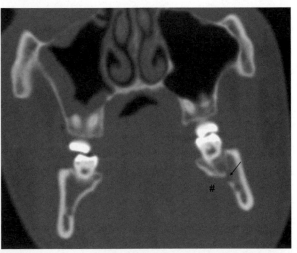

**Fig. 14.8a,b.** Odontogenic abscess formation of the floor of the mouth. **a** Axial enhanced MSCT with rim enhancing mass (*black arrow*), with hypodense center (#) adjacent to the mandible. **b** Coronal MPR (bone algorithm) detects cortical disconnection at the lingual aspect of the tooth (region 38) and contact to the root tip

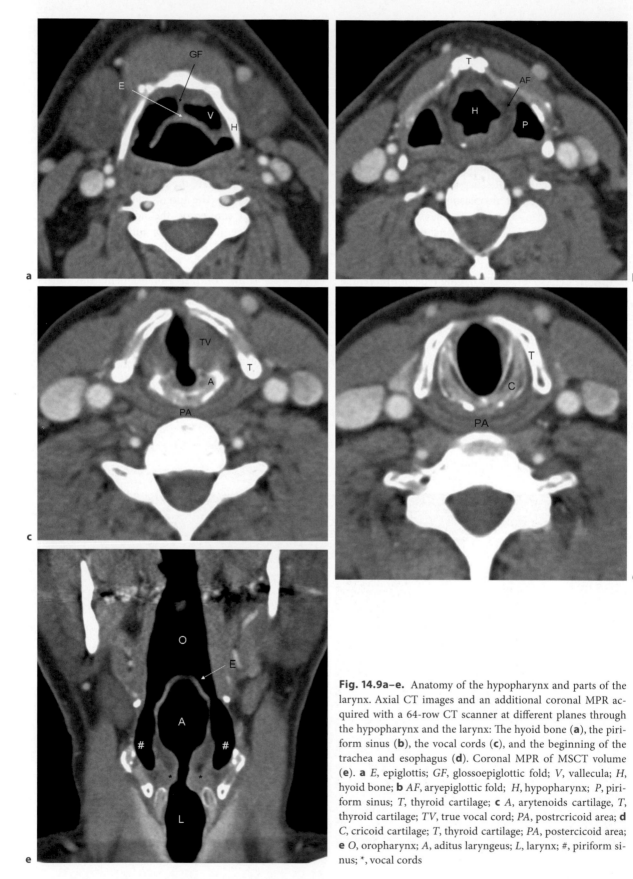

**Fig. 14.9a–e.** Anatomy of the hypopharynx and parts of the larynx. Axial CT images and an additional coronal MPR acquired with a 64-row CT scanner at different planes through the hypopharynx and the larynx: The hyoid bone (**a**), the piriform sinus (**b**), the vocal cords (**c**), and the beginning of the trachea and esophagus (**d**). Coronal MPR of MSCT volume (**e**). **a** *E*, epiglottis; *GF*, glossoepiglottic fold; *V*, vallecula; *H*, hyoid bone; **b** *AF*, aryepiglottic fold; *H*, hypopharynx; *P*, piriform sinus; *T*, thyroid cartilage; **c** *A*, arytenoids cartilage, *T*, thyroid cartilage; *TV*, true vocal cord; *PA*, postrcricoid area; **d** *C*, cricoid cartilage; *T*, thyroid cartilage; *PA*, postercicoid area; **e** *O*, oropharynx; *A*, aditus laryngeus; *L*, larynx; #, piriform sinus; *, vocal cords

## 14.4
## Hypopharynx and Larynx

### 14.4.1
### Anatomy

#### Hypopharynx

The hypopharynx can be described as the link between the oropharynx and the esophagus. It is the caudal continuation of the pharyngeal mucosa space and the most inferior portion of the pharynx (WYCLIFFE et al. 2007). It extends from the hyoid bone to the lower margin of the cricoid cartilage. The hypopharynx can be divided into three sub-regions: the piriform sinus, the posterior pharyngeal wall, and the post-cricoid region (Fig. 14.9).

The paired piriform sinus is the anterolateral recess of the hypopharynx. They extend cranio-caudaly from the pharyngoapiglottic fold to the lower margin of the cricoid cartilage, centered laterally to the inner surface of the thyroid cartilage and medially to the aryepiglottic folds. The apex of the sinus is the inferior margin at the level of the true vocal cords. With 65% to 85% occurrence, the piriform sinus is the most common area of all hypopharyngeal masses arising.

The posterior wall consists of the inferior continuation of the posterior orophayryngeal mucosal wall (HARNSBERGER 1995). About 20% of carcinomas of the hypopharynx arise in this area (BECKER 2004).

The post-cricoid region is the anterior wall of the inferior hypopharynx and the posterior wall of the larynx. It is the link between the larynx and the hypopharynx. It extends from the cricoarytenoid joints to the cricopharyngeos muscle inferiorly.

#### Larynx

A thorough understanding of basic laryngeal anatomy is essential for the accurate diagnosis and staging of malignant laryngeal tumors. Towards this aim and the defined purpose of this chapter, we kindly refer the reader to excellent text books and review articles dealing with the detailed anatomy of the larynx. The detailed, very complex anatomy of the larynx and accompanying laryngeal structures would by far extend the context of this chapter. Therefore, we explain the three clinically important levels of the larynx and try to highlight the most important anatomical landmarks with the appropriate regional distinctions for oncological imaging.

On principle, two horizontal planes divide the larynx into the three regions of the supraglottis, glottis and subglottis. The first (cranial) plane extends horizontally through the apex of the two laryngeal ventricles. The second plane is located about 1 cm caudally to the first. Here, the supraglottic larynx is the region that lies cranial to the first, with the superior border of the supraglottis as the tip of the epiglottis. Within this plane lies the upper arytenoids cartilage (Figs. 14.9). The plane of the glottis is the level between the two mentioned planes and includes the anterior and posterior commissure. Finally, the most caudal level, the subglottis, is the region below the lowest plane and the cricoid cartilage (ZINREICH 2002).

### 14.4.2
### Imaging of Hypopharyngeal and Laryngeal Masses

#### Hypopharynx

Hypopharyngeal cancers are most often squamous cell carcinoma and have the worst prognosis of all head and neck cancers (WYCLIFFE et al. 2007). These tumors tend to present with early nodal metastasis and surrounding tissue invasion at diagnosis due to the unspecific and late onset of clinical symptoms. Especially distant metastasis is more common in hypopharyngeal cancers than in any other head and neck masses (HARNSBERGER 1995). Overall, the 5-year survival rate is extremely poor and ranges between about 25%–40% (WYCLIFFE et al. 2007). Etiologically, there is a strong association with alcohol and tobacco use in western countries.

On a cellular level, most masses arise from the epithelial layer of the mucous membrane and are predominantly (about 95%) squamous cell carcinoma. Other entities, which comprise less than 5% of all masses, are carcinomas of the minor salivary gland, basal cell carcinoma, and spindle cell carcinomas.

The goals of imaging hypopharyngeal cancers are similar to cancer imaging in other neck areas. Contrast-enhanced MSCT is often the first imaging modality to delineate the tumor extent by contrast enhancement and invasion of fat or muscle tissue. CT (as well as MRI) can give crucial information, additional to clinical examination, about staging and the status of important landmarks, such as infiltration of parapharyngeal fat and cartilage or midline invasion.

Due to the advent of new generation MSCT scanners, high-resolution image volumes can be obtained in a few seconds. Further, more detailed coronal and sagittal MPR can be reconstructed. Especially in the area of the hypopharynx and the bordering larynx, reduction in scan time can minimize swallowing artifacts and enhance image quality.

The three subtypes of hypopharyngeal cancer have distinct characteristics, which can be important to know for correct staging:

Tumors of these regions all spread through the muscles of the hypopharyngeal wall. The lateral wall piriform sinus masses tend to spread laterally to the oropharyx and the base of the tongue as well as the me-

dially located masses anteriorly to the supraglottic and glottic larynx (WYCLIFFE et al. 2007).

Tumors of the posterior pharyngeal wall extend through the hypopharynx to the posterior oropharyngeal wall (JONES and STELL 1991). They usually appear as asymmetrical thickening of the posterior wall. The postcricoid masses are very rare, but show a growth pattern anteriorly invading the posterior cricoarytenoid muscle and spreading submucosally towards the cricoid cartilage, the trachea, or the esophagus.

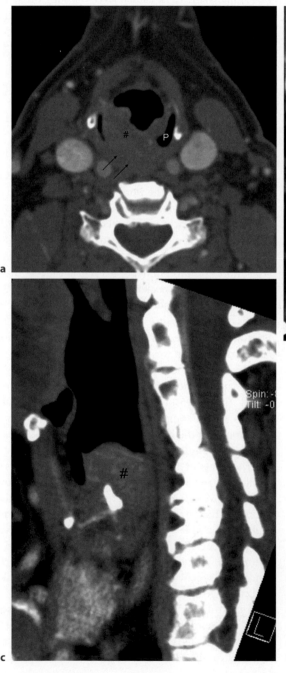

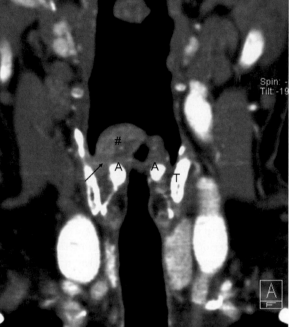

Fig. 14.10a–c. MSCT image demonstrating a supraglottic carcinoma of the right aryepiglottic fold. **a** Contrast-enhancing mass in the right aryepiglottic fold (#). The right piriform sinus is compressed by the mass (*P*). Extension to the pharyngeal wall (*arrow*). **b** The craniocaudal extension (#), the relation to the arytenoid (*A*) and the thyroid cartilage (*T*), as well as the aryepiglottic fold (*arrow*) are observed in the coronal reconstruction. **c** Additional sagittal reconstruction (MPR) delineating the mass (#) in anterior-posterior direction

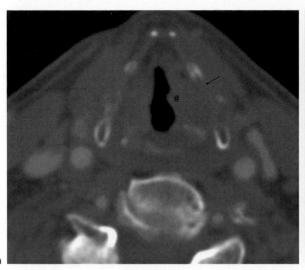
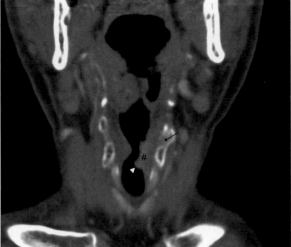

a

b

**Fig. 14.11a,b.** Glottic carcinoma at the level of the vocal cords. **a** Axial MSCT contrast-enhancing glottic neoplastic mass (#) invasion of the left paraglottic space due to a ventricular mass. The tumor mass erodes the medial aspect of the thyroid carti-lage (*arrow*). **b** The coronal MPR demonstrates, additional to the glottic mass (#), a subglottic part of the tumor extension (*arrowhead*). Cartilaginous disruption of the thyroid cartilage (*arrow*)

Overall squamous cell carcinoma of the hypopharynx has a relatively poor prognosis, with up to 75% of patients having metastases to cervical lymph nodes at initial presentation. Another challenge for the radiologist is the detection of tumor recurrence. Especially in the hypopharyngeal region, the regional recurrence rate is the highest in the neck region with 38% and distant metastasis with 11% (WYCLIFFE et al. 2007).

### Larynx

Due to the complex anatomy of the laryngeal structures and the constitution on covering the whole neck, we refer the to dedicated and excellent books and review articles dealing with the anatomy of the larynx (ZINNREICH 2002; BECKER 2004). Laryngeal tumors are classified by their location in one of three distinct anatomic regions: the supraglottis, the glottis, and subglottis. This classification not only provides information regarding the exact location, but also the extension pattern, the progression of the disease, and the expected response to treatment. Additional, the widely used TNM staging system for laryngeal cancers is organized on the basis of these three anatomic regions (SOM and CURTIN 2003). According to hypopharyngel malignant tumors, over 90% of laryngeal tumors are squamous cell carcinoma (BECKER 2004). Carcinomas of the larynx arise in 30%

in the supraglottic region, 65% in the glottis, and about 5% in the subglottis.

*Supraglottic tumors* have a reported incidence of about 60–70%. Clinical signs such as hoarseness and change in voice can be the first suspicion. Axial CT images as well as MRI scans can provide an excellent overview of this region and give additional information to endoscopy. Supraglottic masses originating from the epiglottis primarily invade the pre-epiglottic space. As well as masses arising from the false cord, the laryngeal ventricles or aryepiglottic fold primarily infiltrates the paraglottic space. The diagnostic clue on axial images is the enhancing mass and the replacement of hypodense fat tissue by tumor tissue. Additional sagittal reconstructions (MPR) can excellently delineate the infiltration of the pre-epiglottic space. CT and MRI provide a good illustration of tumor infiltration in this anatomic region and show high sensitivities. The primarily lymphatic spread is directed towards the superior jugular lymph nodes and is very common (ZINREICH 2002). Axial scan range should always include the tip of the lung (Fig. 14.10).

*Glottic carcinoma* is the most common form of laryngeal cancer and is usually diagnosed in very early stages due to the typical hoarseness caused by vocal cord masses. In addition to the primary diagnostic tool, the endoscopy, the role of cross-sectional imaging is the determination of growth pattern and submucosal

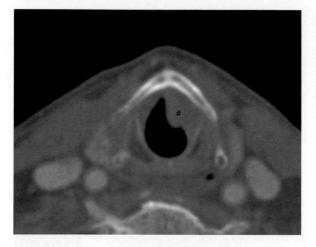

**Fig. 14.12.** Small subglottic carcinoma (#) with partial obstruction of the trachea on an axial MSCT image

thyroid gland. Lymph node metastasis is much more common than in glottic carcinoma, and cross-sectional imaging is not only to define the exact extent, but also the nodal status of the para- and pretracheal nodes (BECKER 2004). The upper mediastinal region should be included in the scan range when imaging patients with suspected subglottic carcinomas (Fig. 14.12).

## References

Becker M (2004) The larynx. In: Valvassouri G, Mafee M, Becker M (eds) Imaging of the head and neck. Thieme, New York, Stuttgart

Harnsberger HR (1995) Handbook of head and neck imaging, 2nd edn. Mosby, St Louis

Jones AS, Stell PM (1991) Squamous carcinoma of the posterior pharyngeal wall. Clin Otolaryngeol Allied Sci 16:462–465

Landsberg R, Friedman M (2001) A computed-assisted anatomical study of the nasofrontal region. Laryngoscope 111:2125–2130

Lenz M, Grees H, Baum U et al. (2000) Oropharynx, oral cavity, floor of the mouth: CT and MRI. Eur J Radiol 33:203–215

Myers JN (1996) Molecular pathogenesis of squamous cell carcinoma of head and neck. In: Myers EN, Syuen JY (eds) Cancer of head and neck. WB Saunders, Philadelphia

Som PM, Curtin HD (2003) Head and neck imaging, 4th edn. Mosby, St Louis

Smoker WRK (2003) The oral cavity. In: Som PM, Curtin HD (eds) Head and neck imaging, 5th edn. Mosby, St Louis, pp 1377–1464

Tiwari R, Hardillo JA, Mehta D et al. (2000) Squamous cell carcinoma of maxillary sinus. Head Neck 22:164–169

Wycliffe ND, Grover RS, Kim PD et al. (2007) Hypopharyngeal cancer. Top Magn Reson Imaging 18:243–258

Zinreich SJ (2002) Imaging in laryngeal cancer: computed tomography, magnetic resonance imaging, positron emission tomography. Otolaryngol Clin N Amer 35:971–991

spread. Glottic tumors typically arise from the anterior half of the vocal cords and spread into the anterior commissure (BECKER 2004). The contralateral cord, the paraglottic space, and the thyroarytenoid muscle are important landmarks to delineate until the tumor reaches the anterior commissure. Deep submucosal subglottic spread is very common and especially difficult to diagnose. Therefore, the axial and coronal planes are necessary so as not to underestimate the tumor size. However, nodal metastasis from vocal cord tumors is rare, and the radiographic examination should include the lower neck up to the sinuses (Fig. 14.11).

*Subglottic carcinoma* is a very rare entity with an incidence of about 1.5% (ZINREICH 2002). Nevertheless, this subtype of laryngeal cancer has the worst prognosis and is highly malignant. The carcinoma of the subglottic region tends to spread to the trachea or invade the

# Cardiovascular Imaging

# Noninvasive Coronary Artery Imaging

15

Hatem Alkadhi and Paul Stolzmann

## CONTENTS

## ABSTRACT

Recent technological advances in MDCT enabled the introduction of the noninvasive technique for the routine workup of the coronary arteries in daily clinical practice. Patients with a low to intermediate likelihood of coronary artery disease (CAD) and having equivocal findings at electrocardiogram (ECG) or stress tests are the optimal candidates to undergo noninvasive coronary imaging with CT. In order to gain high diagnostic accuracy, the CT scanner system should provide high temporal and spatial resolutions. This is necessary to compensate for motion of the coronary arteries and to allow for multiplanar reformations without artifacts. The CT data need to be synchronized to the simultaneously recorded ECG, and both retrospective ECG gating or prospective ECG triggering can be used for data acquisition and reconstruction. When implementing the technique of ECG pulsing for reducing the radiation dose, flexible adjustments of the pulsing widths at different heart rates are recommended. With regard to the image quality, the dependency on the average heart rate and variability decreases with the increasing temporal resolution of the CT system. When using 64-slice CT, average heart rate and heart rate variability should be diminished through the foregoing administration of β-blockers. With dual-source CT, a reduction of heart rate and variability is no longer necessary. Severe arterial wall calcification still hamper the diagnostic capabilities of CT, even when using the most recent technology. With every new CT scanner generation, the robustness increases, while the rate of nondiagnostic coronary artery segments decreases.

H. Alkadhi, MD
Associate Professor, Section Head–Body Computed Tomography, Institute of Diagnostic Radiology, University Hospital Zurich, Raemisstrasse 100, 8091 Zurich, Switzerland

P. Stolzmann, MD
Institute of Diagnostic Radiology, University Hospital Zurich, Raemisstrasse 100, 8091 Zurich, Switzerland

## Introduction

Coronary artery disease (CAD) is recognized as the leading cause of mortality in the Western world (THOM et al. 2006). Over the past decades, conventional catheter coronary angiography (CCA) has been the only accepted gold standard method for clinical imaging of CAD. However, CCA is cost-extensive and results in inconvenience to the patients, and is associated with a small but distinct procedure-related morbidity (1.5%) and mortality (0.15%) (ZANZONICO et al. 2006). Moreover, the accuracy of CCA is severely hampered by a significant intra-observer as well as interobserver variability in defining the stenoses degree of up to 50% (GALBRAITH et al. 1981; WHITE et al. 1984), which is underlined by a poor correlation with postmortem coronary pathology (VLODAVER et al. 1973; ARNETT et al. 1979).

In 2002, about 2 million conventional CCA procedures were performed in Europe alone (MAIER et al. 2005). Interestingly, only a third of these were subsequently followed by a percutaneous intervention, which indicated that CCA was mostly used as a purely diagnostic tool. The associated economic burden and the inconvenience to patients have prompted an intensive search for alternative, noninvasive means for coronary artery imaging (ACHENBACH et al. 2001). In fact, over the last 5 years, we have witnessed an impressive growth of the literature on noninvasive techniques for the assessment of CAD. In particular, the introduction of MDCT scanners having a submillimeter spatial resolution and subsecond gantry rotation times has revolutionized the field of cardiac imaging by enabling a "direct" noninvasive imaging of the coronary arteries.

With 16-slice CT, early results for the noninvasive assessment of the coronary arteries were promising. However, it was not until the introduction of 64-slice CT that noninvasive CT coronary angiography could be fully integrated into daily routine clinical practice (LESCHKA et al. 2005; RAFF et al. 2005; MOLLET et al. 2005; LEBER et al. 2005). This was fascilitated by the high temporal and spatial isotropic resolutions of these systems, which enabled robust cardiac imaging with a considerably reduced number of nonevaluable coronary segments.

As a result of these technical advances, the Task Force on the Management of Stable Angina Pectoris of the European Society of Cardiology has recently recommended the performance of CT coronary angiography in patients having a stable angina, a low pretest probability of CAD, and an inconclusive exercise ECG or stress imaging test (Fox et al. 2006). The American Heart Association (AHA) has recently stated that, particularly if the symptoms, age, and gender of a patient suggest a low to intermediate pretest probability of hemodynamically relevant stenoses, ruling out these stenoses by CT coronary angiography may be clinically useful and may help to avoid invasive CCA (BUDOFF et al. 2006). Finally, a consensus paper of various international radiological and cardiovascular societies has noted the use of CT coronary angiography to be appropriate in patients with chest pain having an intermediate pretest probability of CAD and an uninterpretable ECG or who are unable to exercise (HENDEL et al. 2006).

Nevertheless, despite of these numerous improvements in CT scanner technology, a number of factors still have rendered some examinations nondiagnostic. In particular, motion artifacts of coronary segments occurred, particularly at higher heart rates, and led to a decline in the diagnostic performance of the noninvasive technique (LESCHKA et al. 2005; RAFF et al. 2005; MOLLET et al. 2005; LEBER et al. 2005). Consequently, a heart-rate reduction using either oral or intravenous β-receptor antagonists in order to achieve a heart rate lower than 65 or even 60 beats per minute (bpm) was considered necessary for coronary imaging with 64-slice CT.

Because of these still-existing limitations, further CT scanner technology developments ensued. As a result, the dual-source 64-slice CT scanner was introduced. This CT system offers a high temporal resolution of 83 ms in a monosegment reconstruction mode, which has dispensed the necessity for administering β-blocking medication for heart rate reduction prior to CT coronary angiography (ACHENBACH et al. 2006; JOHNSON et al. 2006; SCHEFFEL et al. 2006).

This chapter provides a summary of knowledge that has accumulated over the past years with respect to noninvasive imaging of coronary arteries with MD CT.

## Technical Issues

In order to freeze an image of the beating heart, the imaging modality should provide high temporal resolution. This is necessary to compensate for motion of the coronary arteries, which demonstrate a complex and nonuniform movement pattern within and across the different coronary arteries, as well as within the different parts of the cardiac cycle (ACHENBACH et al. 2000). At heart rates below 80 bpm, the diastolic phase represents that phase of the cardiac cycle with the least coronary motion, whereas at heart rates above 80 bpm, motion during the systolic phase is equal or even below that during diastole. Thus, data reconstruction must be synchronized to the cardiac cycle that is performed through simultaneous recording of the patient's ECG. After data acquisition, the ECG will be synchronized with the acquired raw data for image reconstruction.

In addition to high temporal resolution in combination with ECG synchronization, high spatial resolution is needed to resolve the tiny coronary segments. This spatial resolution should enable the visualization of the various coronary segments that run in different directions both within and through the imaging plane. Coronary artery segments range from a few millimeters in diameter at their origin to submillimeters along their course. For diagnostic imaging of the coronary segments, the spatial resolution of the system should be isotropic in order to allow for multiplanar reformations in any arbitrary planes. These requirements of a high temporal and a high isotropic spatial resolution with regard to coronary imaging were fulfilled since the introduction of 64-slice CT.

## 15.2.1
## Phase Synchronization

Retrospective ECG gating represents the most commonly used technique of data reconstruction in CT coronary angiography examinations. With this mode, the X-ray tube runs in a helical or spiral fashion continuously around the patient. With use of the recorded ECG signal, image reconstruction is performed retrospectively, and the interval can be freely chosen. The major advantage of retrospective ECG gating represents the fact that theoretically, any desired phase of the cardiac cycle can be reconstructed. This can be particularly important in patients with higher or irregular heart rates. The disadvantage of the retrospective ECG gating mode is the associated increased radiation dose that results from the continuous and non-overlapping acquisition of data. Because of the radiation dose issue of retrospective ECG gating, the technique of ECG controlled tube current modulation, or ECG pulsing technique, has been introduced (Jakobs et al. 2002). With this technique, the tube output is raised to the nominal level within every cardiac cycle during a limited interval in the diastolic phase where data are most likely to be reconstructed. During the remaining part of the cardiac cycle, the tube output is reduced to approximately 25% by a corresponding decrease of the tube current. This results in radiation doses reductions of up to 47% as compared with continuous scanning with a uniform tube current.

Another technique for phase synchronization is the prospective ECG triggering or step-and-shoot mode technique. This technique is widely used for the quantification of the coronary calcium burden (calcium scor-

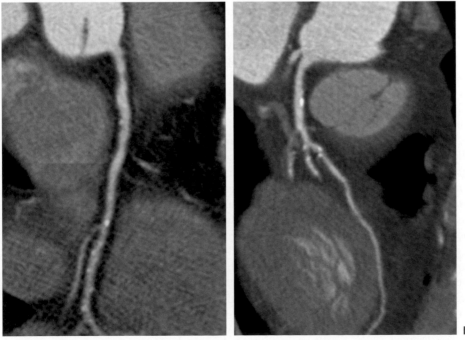

**Fig. 15.1a–d.** Dual-source CT coronary angiography in a 49-year-old man with a single episode of atypical chest pain. Scanning was performed with in the step-and-shoot mode (mean heart rate 66 bpm). Curved multiplanar reformations of the right coronary artery (**a**), left anterior descending artery (**b**), and the left circumflex artery. (**c,d** *see next page*)

a

b

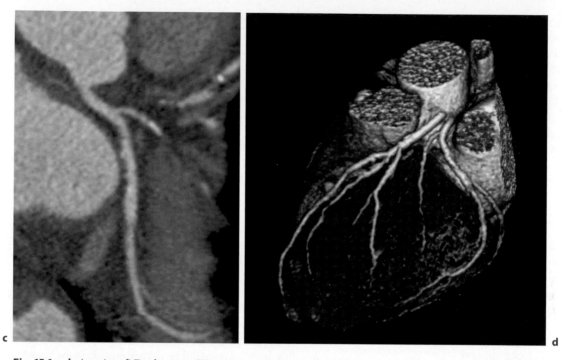

c                                                                                          d

**Fig. 15.1a–d.** (*continued*) Dual-source CT coronary angiography in a 49-year-old man with a single episode of atypical chest pain. Scanning was performed with in the step-and-shoot mode (mean heart rate 66 bpm). Curved multiplanar reformations of the right coronary artery (**a**), left anterior descending artery (**b**), and the left circumflex artery (**c**) demonstrate some eccentric calcified plaques, but no significant stenosis. The volume rendered image (**d**) shows the separate origin of the left anterior descending and left circumflex artery from the left sinus of Valsalva. Estimated effective radiation dose of this examination was 0.9 mSv

ing) (BUDOFF et al. 2006). However, a recent experimental study has brought into attention this low-dose technique also for CT coronary angiography (HSIEH et al. 2006). In the step-and-shoot mode, data is only acquired at predefined time points of the cardiac cycle when the data acquisition is considered relevant. The table remains stationary, and only the gantry rotates around the patient. The X-ray tube is turned on at an a priori chosen time interval from the last monitored R–R (waves) peak. Then, the table is translated to the next bed position, and the scanner acquires more projections. This cycle repeats until the entire scan length of the heart is covered. An increasing number of detectors allow larger volume coverage per gantry rotation, which decreases the required breath hold time. The major advantage of scanning in the step-and-shoot mode is a low radiation exposure through shortening of the X-ray on time (Fig. 15.1). On the other hand, higher and irregular heart rates prevent the use of this technique for CT coronary angiography, because of the predefined nature of reconstruction interval selection.

## 15.2.2
## Data Reconstruction

The minimum data that is required to reconstruct a CT image is 180° of one gantry rotation with single-source CT and 90° with dual-source CT. These data may be reconstructed either utilizing monosegment or multiple-segment reconstruction techniques (MCNITT-GRAY 2002).

With monosegment reconstructions, the time needed to complete a half rotation in single-source CT or a quarter rotation in dual-source CT determines the temporal resolution of the scanner. The gantry rotation time is defined as the time that is required to complete one full rotation (360°) of the X-ray tube and detector elements around the subject. If the gantry rotation time is 500 ms, then the temporal resolution is little greater than half the gantry rotation time and equals between 270 and 280 ms, with monosegment reconstructions (it is not exactly 500 ms/2 because the fan beam angle has to be considered too). In order to improve further the temporal resolution of the scanners, the gantry rotation times were made increasingly faster. Actual commercially available CT scanners have maximum gantry rotation times of 330 ms. However, high accelerations of the rotating gantry result in considerable centrifugal forces of up to 28 g, which have prevented the development of even faster gantry rotation times.

The dual-source CT scanner overcomes the limitations with respect to the high but limited gantry rotation time by introducing a second X-ray tube and corresponding detector that is mounted with an offset of 90° to the rotating gantry (FLOHR et al. 2006). With this configuration, only a quarter rotation is required (90° plus the fan beam angle) for reconstructing cardiac CT images resulting in a temporal resolution of 83 ms.

Another software approach to further increase the temporal resolution of single-source CT scanners represents the multiple-segment reconstruction algorithms. The basic principle behind these algorithms is that the scan projection data required to reconstruct an axial slice are selected from segmental scans obtained during sequential heart cycles at the same z-position, opposite to the monosegment reconstruction, in which data from only a single heartbeat is used. Usually, up to four segments can be sampled, which results in an increased temporal resolution by the factor of four. HERZOG et al. (2007) has investigated the use of the multisegment reconstruction technique of 64-slice CT for heart rates higher than 65 bpm, and showed an improvement of overall image quality when compared with the monosegment algorithm. On the other hand, the diagnostic accuracy for the diagnosis of CAD was not improved when compared with the monosegment technique. The disadvantage of multisegment reconstruction techniques is that any misregistration results in a degradation of the image quality by introducing blurring artifacts. Thus, its use is limited in patients with variable heart rates and with interheartbeat variability of the coronary artery position. Finally, the necessity of lower pitch factors for multisegment reconstructions that prolong the data acquisition time result in an increase in the radiation dose delivered to the patient (FLOHR et al. 2001; WINTERSPERGER et al. 2006).

## 15.2.3
## Reconstruction Phases

Coronary artery motion shows a biphasic pattern of rapid movement; the maximum of motion is observed during the ventricular contraction at early to mid-systole and during rapid filling in early diastole (ACHEN-BACH et al. 2000, LU et al. 2001; HUSMANN et al. 2007). During isovolumetric relaxation at mid-diastole and during mid- to late systole, coronary motion is relatively quiescent. With increasing heart rates, the minimum mid-diastolic velocity increases, while the width of the mid-diastolic velocity trough successively decreases and eventually disappears. At heart rates greater than approximately 80 bpm, the lowest velocities in systole are lower than the lowest velocities in diastole.

The motion of the left anterior and left circumflex artery follows the motion of the left ventricle; therefore, the best reconstruction interval is in mid-diastole, at 50%–80% of the R–R interval, when the left ventricle is relatively quiescent. In contrast, the contraction of the right atrium is causative for the motion of the right coronary artery. Thus, reconstructions are best at late systole and early diastole, at 30%–60% of the R–R interval, representing a time interval with the right atrium being relatively free of motion. Since the diastole shortens more than the systole with increasing heart rates, imaging of the right coronary artery in late systole and early diastole is less prone to motion artifacts when shortening of the diastole occurs.

These heart rate-dependent variations in reconstruction phases must be taken into account when implementing the technique of ECG pulsing for radiation dose reduction. Accordingly, flexible adjustments of the pulsing width with different heart rates are necessary. LESCHKA et al. (2007) recently gave recommendations concerning the narrowest time window required for reconstructing data sets with diagnostic image quality, depending on the heart rate, in order to keep the radiation dose as low as possible. At heart rates below 60 bpm, the ECG pulsing window should be from 60 to 70%, between 60 and 70 bpm from 60 to 80%, between 70 and 80 bpm from 55 to 80%, and at heart rates above 80 bpm from 30 to 80% of the R–R interval.

## 15.3
### Image Quality

## 15.3.1
### Average Heart Rate

A significant inverse correlation between average heart rate and image quality has been observed with both 4-slice and 16-slice CT. HONG et al. (2001) found with 4-slice CT that image quality was significantly decreased in each coronary artery, with increasing average heart rate. HOFFMANN et al. (2005) found with 16-slice CT, a

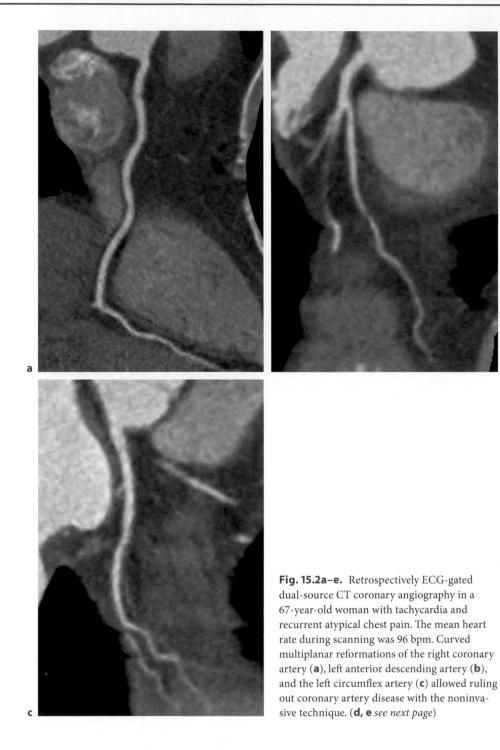

**Fig. 15.2a–e.** Retrospectively ECG-gated dual-source CT coronary angiography in a 67-year-old woman with tachycardia and recurrent atypical chest pain. The mean heart rate during scanning was 96 bpm. Curved multiplanar reformations of the right coronary artery (**a**), left anterior descending artery (**b**), and the left circumflex artery (**c**) allowed ruling out coronary artery disease with the noninvasive technique. (**d, e** *see next page*)

negative correlation between overall image quality and the average heart rate. LESCHKA et al. (2006) found with 64-slice CT that the image quality for the left circumflex artery showed a weak dependence on the average heart rate, but no correlation was found for the right coronary, the left main coronary, and the left anterior descending arteries, and for all coronary segments to-gether. ACHENBACH et al. (2006) were the first to report on a series of patients who underwent dual-source CT coronary angiography without heart rate control. The authors showed that 98% of all coronary artery segments could be depicted with diagnostic image quality and with no motion artifacts. Later on, JOHNSON et al. (2006) published the data in patients undergoing dual-

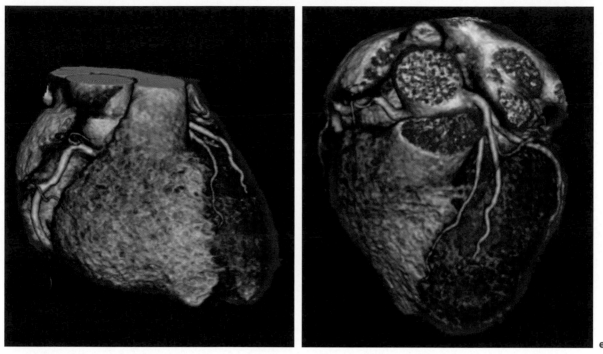

d                                               e

**Fig. 15.2a–e.** (*continued*) Retrospectively ECG-gated dual-source CT coronary angiography in a 67-year-old woman with tachycardia and recurrent atypical chest pain. The mean heart rate during scanning was 96 bpm. . The volume-rendered images (**d, e**) demonstrate the excellent image quality of the examination, despite a high heart rate during scanning

source CT coronary angiography demonstrating the preservation of diagnostic image quality even at higher heart rates.

MATT et al. could show with dual-source CT that no significant correlation was present between the average heart rate and the image quality of each coronary artery and for the overall image quality of all coronary segments. In this study, the entire coronary artery tree could be visualized with diagnostic image quality in all patients with a mean heart rate less than 65 bpm, whereas in patients with heart rates above 65 bpm, 98% of the coronary segments could be visualized with a diagnostic image quality.

These results indicate that the dependency of image quality on the average heart rate decreases with the increasing temporal resolution of the CT scanners. Another conclusion from these studies is that until the use of 64-slice CT for noninvasive coronary imaging, the administration of β-receptor antagonists is advisable when the heart rate exceeds a certain threshold (60 or 65 bpm). With dual-source CT, heart rate control through the use of beta-blockers is no longer required (Fig. 15.2).

## 15.3.2
## Heart Rate Variability

The variability in heart rate during scanning has been repetitively suggested to have a negative effect on image quality (HONG et al. 2001), however, was not investigated with either 4-slice or 16-slice CT. With 64-slice CT, increasing heart rate variability could be identified as the major determinant of image quality degradation for all coronary arteries and for the overall image quality of all segments (LESCHKA et al. 2006). In this study, a two-segment reconstruction algorithm at heart rates greater than 65 bpm was used. With dual-source CT employing a monosegment reconstruction technique, heart rate variability was no longer affecting the overall image quality in any segment, the right coronary artery, or the left anterior descending artery, but there was a significant correlation between heart rate variability in the left circumflex artery (MATT et al. 2007).

With intercycle variability in the heart rate, the commonly applied relative ECG-gated image reconstruction technique (i.e., performing reconstructions at a certain percentage of the R–R interval) does not generate images in exactly corresponding cardiac phases. This is because the different functions within one cardiac cycle shorten or prolong non-proportionally with different heart rates (HUSMANN et al. 2007).

Therefore, it appears that the dependency of image quality on heart rate variability decreases with the increasing temporal resolution of the CT scanners. But more importantly, the study results indicate that the use of monosegment reconstruction algorithms that do not merge data from adjacent heartbeats in different cardiac phases is advantageous for coronary imaging. When using 64-slice CT for coronary imaging, heart rate variability should be diminished through the use of β-blockers (LESCHKA et al. 2006). With dual-source CT, reduction of heart rate variability through the administration of β-blockers is no longer necessary (MATT et al. 2007).

### 15.3.3
### Vessel Wall Calcifications

Vessel wall calcifications may deteriorate the visualization of the coronary artery lumen through the effect of blooming. The blooming artifact results in an artificial obscuring of the vessel lumen, causing an overestimation of the degree of stenosis. This overestimation leads to false-positive findings that are associated with a decline in the specificity and positive

predictive value of the examination. With 64-slice CT, RAFF et al. (2005) reported a considerable decline in diagnostic accuracy in patients with Agatston scores >400. ONG et al. (2006) compared the accuracy of 64-slice CT coronary angiography in patients having minimal to mild calcifications, with patients having moderate to heavy calcifications. For patients with minimal to mild calcifications, 93% of the segments were considered evaluative, with high specificity of 98% and high negative predictive value of 99%. In contrast, in patients with moderate to heavy calcifications, the rate of evaluative segments decreased to 87%, and the specificity and negative predictive value were significantly lower. Therefore, the authors concluded that 64-slice CT can accurately detect stenosis in coronary arteries with minimal to mild calcifications, but becomes less reliable when the calcium score is high.

### 15.4
### Diagnostic Performance

Table 15.1 lists the results of recent publications that have analyzed the diagnostic performance of  detection in patients referred for diagnostic coronary angiography, using CT in comparison to the reference standard modality invasive CCA.

**Table 15.1.** Per-segment and per-patient-based sensitivity, specificity, positive (*PPV*) and negative predictive value (*NPV*) of CT coronary angiography as compared to CCA

| 64-Slice CT | Analysis | Number | Sensitivity (%) | Specificity (%) | PPV (%) | NPV (%) | Heart rate (bpm)[a] |
|---|---|---|---|---|---|---|---|
| LESCHKA et al. 2005 | Segment-based | 1,005 | 94 | 97 | 87 | 99 | 66±15 |
| | Patient-based | 67 | 100 | 100 | 100 | 100 | |
| RAFF et al. 2005 | Segment-based | 935 | 86 | 95 | 66 | 98 | 65±10 |
| | Patient-based | 70 | 95 | 90 | 93 | 93 | |
| MOLLET et al. 2005 | Segment-based | 725 | 99 | 95 | 76 | 100 | 58±7 |
| | Patient-based | 51 | 100 | 92 | 97 | 100 | |
| LEBER et al. 2005 | Segment-based | 798 | 64 | 97 | 83 | 93 | 62±13 |
| | Patient-based | 45 | 88 | 85 | 88 | 85 | |

[a]Values are means±standard deviations

[b]Agatston score <142 (68 patients)

[c]Agatston Score >142 (66 patients)

**Table 15.1.** (*continued*) Per-segment and per-patient-based sensitivity, specificity, positive (*PPV*) and negative predictive value (*NPV*) of CT coronary angiography as compared to CCA

| 64-Slice CT | Analysis | Number | Sensitivity (%) | Specificity (%) | PPV (%) | NPV (%) | Heart rate (bpm)[a] |
|---|---|---|---|---|---|---|---|
| PUGLIESE et al. 2005 | Segment-based | 494 | 99 | 96 | 78 | 99 | 58±6 |
| | Patient-based | 35 | 100 | 90 | 96 | 100 | |
| ONG et al., 2006 | Segment-based[b] | 748 | 85 | 98 | 77 | 99 | 62±9 |
| | Segment-based[c] | 726 | 78 | 98 | 86 | 96 | 62±9 |
| SCHUIJF et al. 2006 | Segment-based | 842 | 85 | 98 | 82 | 99 | 60±11 |
| | Patient-based | 60 | 94 | 97 | 97 | 93 | |
| ROPERS et al. 2006 | Segment-based | 1,083 | 93 | 97 | 56 | 100 | 59±9 |
| | Patient-based | 81 | 96 | 91 | 83 | 98 | |
| EHARA et al. 2006 | Segment-based | 884 | 90 | 94 | 89 | 95 | 72±13 |
| | Patient-based | 67 | 98 | 86 | 98 | 86 | |
| NIKOLAOU et al. 2006 | Segment-based | 923 | 82 | 95 | 72 | 97 | 61±9 |
| | Patient-based | 68 | 97 | 79 | 86 | 96 | |
| MEIJBOOM et al. 2006 | Segment-based | 1,003 | 94 | 98 | 65 | 100 | 60±8 |
| | Patient-based | 70 | 100 | 92 | 82 | 100 | |
| MÜHLENBRUCH et al. 2006 | Segment-based | 726 | 87 | 95 | 75 | 98 | 70±14 |
| | Patient-based | 51 | 98 | 50 | 94 | 75 | |
| **Dual-source CT** | | | | | | | |
| SCHEFFEL et al. 2006 | Segment-based | 420 | 96 | 98 | 86 | 99 | 70±14 |
| | Patient-based | 30 | 93 | 100 | 100 | 94 | |
| LEBER et al. 2007 | Segment-based | 1,216 | 90 | 98 | 81 | 99 | 73 |
| | Patient-based | 88 | 95 | 90 | 74 | 99 | |
| JOHNSON et al. 2007 | Segment-based | 473 | 88 | 98 | 78 | 99 | 68 |
| | Patient-based | 35 | 100 | 89 | 89 | 100 | |
| HEUSCHMID et al. 2007 | Segment-based | 663 | 96 | 87 | 61 | 99 | 65±14 |
| | Patient-based | 51 | 97 | 73 | 90 | 92 | |
| LESCHKA et al. 2007 | Segment-based | 1,001 | 95 | 96 | 79 | 99 | 68±13 |
| | Patient-based | 80 | 97 | 87 | 88 | 97 | |

[a]Values are means±standard deviations

[b]Agatston score <142 (68 patients)

[c]Agatston Score >142 (66 patients)

**Table 15.1.** (*continued*) Per-segment and per-patient-based sensitivity, specificity, positive (*PPV*) and negative predictive value (*NPV*) of CT coronary angiography as compared to CCA

| Dual-source CT | Analysis | Number | Sensitivity (%) | Specificity (%) | PPV (%) | NPV (%) | Heart rate (bpm)[a] |
|---|---|---|---|---|---|---|---|
| WEUSTINK et al. 2007 | Segment-based | 1498 | 95 | 95 | 75 | 99 | 68±11 |
| | Patient-based | 100 | 99 | 87 | 96 | 95 | |
| ROPERS et al. 2007 | Segment-based | 1343 | 90 | 98 | 79 | 99 | 64±13 |
| | Patient-based | 100 | 98 | 82 | 80 | 98 | |
| ALKADHI et al. 2008 | Segment-based | 2059 | 96 | 96 | 76 | 99 | 68±12 |
| | Patient-based | 150 | 97 | 87 | 83 | 98 | |
| SCHEFFEL et al. 2008* | Segment-based | 1803 | 97 | 97 | 84 | 99 | 59±6 |
| | Patient-based | 120 | 100 | 93 | 94 | 100 | |

[a]Values are means±standard deviations

[b]Agatston score <142 (68 patients)

[c]Agatston Score >142 (66 patients)

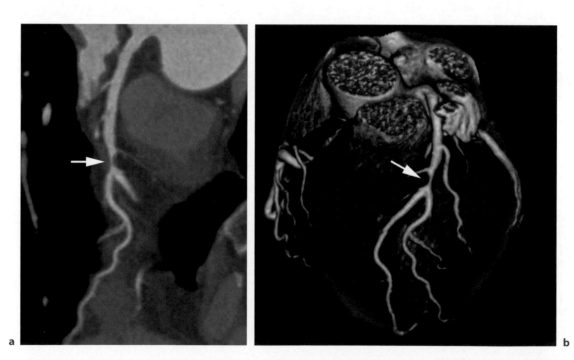

**Fig. 15.3a–c.** Retrospectively ECG-gated dual-source CT coronary angiography in a 56-year-old man with recurrent atypical chest pain and an inconclusive stress test. The mean heart rate during scanning was 68 bpm. Curved multiplanar reformation along the centerline of the left anterior descending artery demonstrates a high-grade stenosis (*arrow*) caused by a noncalcified plaque (**a**). The volume-rendered image (**b**) similarly demonstrates the site of the stenosis (*arrow*). (**c** see next page)

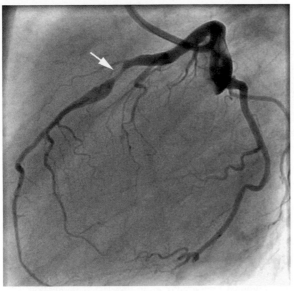

c

**Fig. 15.3a–c.** (*continued*) Retrospectively ECG-gated dual-source CT coronary angiography in a 56-year-old man with recurrent atypical chest pain and an inconclusive stress test. The mean heart rate during scanning was 68 bpm. The volume-rendered image (**b**) similarly demonstrates the site of the stenosis (*arrow*). Invasive CCA (**c**) confirms the findings from CT (*arrow*)

## 15.4.1
## Diagnostic Performance of 16-Slice and 64-Slice CT

In a recently published meta-analysis (HAMON et al. 2007), the pooled diagnostic performance for the detection of significant stenoses of the coronary artery tree improved with 64-slice CT when compared with 16-slice CT. This was the case with regard to the sensitivity on a per-segment based analysis. The highest improvement with 64-slice CT when compared with 16-slice CT was the significant increase in specificity from 69 to 90% and the increase in the positive predictive value from 79 to 93%. Thus, 64-slice CT performs more accurately as compared with 16-slice CT in the determination of healthy individuals.

Furthermore, the rate of nondiagnostic or excluded segments decreased with 64-slice CT as compared with 16-slice CT, potentially reducing the need for conventional catheter angiography, due to an improved spatial resolution and shorter acquisition times. In conclusion, 64-slice CT provides—when compared with 16-slice

CT—an increased clinical feasibility with fewer non-evaluable coronary artery segments and leads to a significant increase in specificity and positive predictive value (HAMON et al. 2007).

## 15.4.2
## Diagnostic Performance of Dual-Source CT

SCHEFFEL et al. (2006) demonstrated a high diagnostic performance for the diagnosis of CAD with dual-source CT as compared with CCA (Fig. 15.3). The authors included a patient population with extensive calcifications and in whom no heart rate control using β-blocker medication prior to CT was performed. One of the most important results of that study was that high diagnostic performance could be maintained even in the subgroup of patients with a heart rate of greater than 70 bpm. Nondiagnostic segments were present in 1.4% of the segments and were most frequently due to extensive calcifications rather than to motion. Another important study finding was that the diagnostic accuracy was even high in the subgroup of patients having a high calcium burden, with an Agatston score of more than 400. Considering the spatial resolution of dual-source CT is the same as that of the foregoing single-source 64-slice CT scanner, this reduction in coronary calcification dependency indicates that the blooming artifact is often superimposed by additional motion artifacts, which can now be minimized with the higher temporal resolution of the dual-source CT scanner. These results could be confirmed in several subsequent studies investigating larger patient populations (LEBER et al. 2007, HEUSCHMID et al. 2007, JOHNSON et al. 2007 ; LESCHKA et al. 2007, WEUSTINK et al. 2007, ROPERS et al. 2007, ALKADHI et al. 2008). Importantly, heart-rate reduction through the administration of β-blockers prior to CT was not used in any of these studies. Finally, high diagnostic performance could also be demonstrated for low-dose cardiac CT in the step-and-shoot mode in patients with regular heart rates up to 70 bpm (SCHEFFEL et al. 2008).

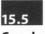

## Conclusion

High temporal resolution in combination with high isotropic spatial resolution of 64-slice single- and dual-source CT enables robust coronary imaging. This is paralleled by an excellent diagnostic performance of the noninvasive technique. Patients with a low to intermediate likelihood of CAD and having equivocal findings at ECG or stress tests are the optimal candidates to undergo noninvasive coronary imaging with CT.

## References

Achenbach S, Daniel WG (2001) Noninvasive coronary angiography—an acceptable alternative? N Engl J Med 345:1909–1910

Achenbach S, Ropers D, Holle J et al. (2000) In-plane coronary arterial motion velocity: measurement with electron-beam CT. Radiology 216:457–463

Achenbach S, Ropers D, Kuettner A et al. (2006) Contrast-enhanced coronary artery visualization by dual-source computed tomography—initial experience. Eur J Radiol 57:331–335

Alkadhi H, Scheffel H, Desbiolles L, et al. (2008) Dual-source computed tomography coronary angiography: influence of obesity, calcium load, and heart rate on diagnostic accuracy. Eur Heart J 29:766–776

Arnett EN, Isner JM, Redwood DR et al. (1979) Coronary artery narrowing in coronary heart disease: comparison of cineangiographic and necropsy findings. Ann Int Med 91:350–356

Budoff MJ, Achenbach S, Blumenthal RS et al. (2006) Assessment of coronary artery disease by cardiac computed tomography: a scientific statement from the American Heart Association Committee on Cardiovascular Imaging and Intervention, Council on Cardiovascular Radiology and Intervention, and Committee on Cardiac Imaging, Council on Clinical Cardiology. Circulation 114:1761–1791

Flohr T, Ohnesorge B (2001) Heart rate adaptive optimization of spatial and temporal resolution for electrocardiogram-gated multislice spiral CT of the heart. J Comput Assist Tomogr 25:907–923

Flohr TG, McCollough CH, Bruder H et al. (2006) First performance evaluation of a dual-source CT (DSCT) system. Eur Radiol 16:256–268

Fox K, Garcia MA, Ardissino D et al. (2006) Guidelines on the management of stable angina pectoris: executive summary: the Task Force on the Management of Stable Angina Pectoris of the European Society of Cardiology. Eur Heart J 27:1341–1381

Galbraith JE, Murphy ML, Desoyza N (1981) Coronary angiogram interpretation: interobserver variability. JAMA 240:2053–2059

Hamon M, Morello R, Riddell JW, Hamon M (2007) Coronary arteries: diagnostic performance of 16- versus 64-section spiral CT compared with invasive coronary angiography—meta-analysis. Radiology 245:720–731

Hendel RC, Patel MR, Kramer CM et al. (2006) ACCF/ACR/SCCT/SCMR/ASNC/NASCI/SCAI/SIR 2006 appropriateness criteria for cardiac computed tomography and cardiac magnetic resonance imaging: a report of the American College of Cardiology Foundation Quality Strategic Directions Committee Appropriateness Criteria Working Group, American College of Radiology, Society of Cardiovascular Computed Tomography, Society for Cardiovascular Magnetic Resonance, American Society of Nuclear Cardiology, North American Society for Cardiac Imaging, Society for Cardiovascular Angiography and Interventions, and Society of Interventional Radiology. J Am Coll Cardiol 48:1475–1497

Herzog C, Nguyen SA, Savino G et al. (2007) Does two-segment image reconstruction at 64-section CT coronary angiography improve image quality and diagnostic accuracy? Radiology 244:121–129

Heuschmid M, Burgstahler C, Reimann A et al. (2007) Usefulness of noninvasive cardiac imaging using dual-source computed tomography in an unselected population with high prevalence of coronary artery disease. Am J Cardiol 100:587–592

Hoffmann MH, Shi H, Manzke R et al. (2005) Noninvasive coronary angiography with 16-detector row CT: effect of heart rate. Radiology 234:86–97

Hong C, Becker CR, Huber A et al. (2001) ECG gated reconstructed multi-detector row CT coronary angiography: effect of varying trigger delay on image quality. Radiology 220:712–717

Hsieh J, Londt J, Vass M et al. (2006) Step-and-shoot data acquisition and reconstruction for cardiac x-ray computed tomography. Med Phys 33:4236–4248

Husmann L, Leschka S, Desbiolles L et al. (2007) Coronary artery motion and cardiac phases: dependency on heart rate—implications for CT image reconstruction. Radiology 245:567–576

Jakobs TF, Becker CR, Ohnesorge B et al. (2002) Multislice helical CT of the heart with retrospective ECG gating: reduction of radiation exposure by ECG controlled tube current modulation. Eur Radiol 12:1081–1086

Johnson TR, Nikolaou K, Busch S et al. (2007) Diagnostic accuracy of dual-source computed tomography in the diagnosis of coronary artery disease. Invest Radiol 42:684–691

Johnson TR, Nikolaou K, Wintersperger BJ et al. (2006) Dual-source CT cardiac imaging: initial experience. Eur Radiol 16:1409–1415

Leber AW, Johnson T, Becker A et al. (2007) Diagnostic accuracy of dual-source multi-slice CT coronary angiography in patients with an intermediate pretest likelihood for coronary artery disease. Eur Heart J doi:10.1093/eurheartj/ehm294

Leber AW, Knez A, von Ziegler F et al. (2005) Quantification of obstructive and nonobstructive coronary lesions by 64-slice computed tomography: a comparative study with quantitative coronary angiography and intravascular ultrasound. J Am Coll Cardiol 46:147–154

Leschka S, Alkadhi H, Plass A et al. (2005) Accuracy of MSCT coronary angiography with 64-slice technology: first experience. Eur Heart J 26:1482–1487

Leschka S, Wildermuth S, Boehm T et al. (2006) Noninvasive coronary angiography with 64-section CT: effect of average heart rate and heart rate variability on image quality. Radiology 241:378–385

Leschka S, Scheffel H, Desbiolles L et al. (2007) Combining Dual-Source Computed Tomography Coronary Angiography and Calcium Scoring: Added Value for the Assessment of Coronary Artery Disease. Heart doi:10.1136/hrt.2007.124800

Leschka S, Scheffel H, Desbiolles L et al. (2007) Image quality and reconstruction intervals of dual-source CT coronary angiography: recommendations for ECG pulsing windowing. Invest Radiol 42:543–549

Lu B, Mao SS, Zhuang N et al. (2001) Coronary artery motion during the cardiac cycle and optimal ECG triggering for coronary artery imaging. Invest Radiol 36:250–256

Maier W, Abay M, Cook S et al. (2005) The 2002 European registry of cardiac catheter interventions. Int J Cardiol 113:299–304

Matt D, Scheffel H, Leschka S et al. (2007) Dual-source CT coronary angiography: image quality, mean heart rate, and heart rate variability. AJR Am J Roentgenol 189:567–573

McNitt-Gray MF (2002) AAPM/RSNA Physics Tutorial for Residents: Topics in CT. Radiation dose in CT. Radiographics 22:1541–1553

Mollet NR, Cademartiri F, van Mieghem CA et al. (2005) High-resolution spiral computed tomography coronary angiography in patients referred for diagnostic conventional coronary angiography. Circulation 112:2318–2323

Ong TK, Chin SP, Liew CK et al. (2006) Accuracy of 64-row multidetector computed tomography in detecting coronary artery disease in 134 symptomatic patients: influence of calcification. Am Heart J 151:1323, e1321–1326

Raff GL, Gallagher MJ, O'Neill WW, Goldstein JA (2005) Diagnostic accuracy of noninvasive coronary angiography using 64-slice spiral computed tomography. J Am Coll Cardiol 46:552–557

Ropers U, Ropers D, Pflederer T, et al. (2007) Influence of heart rate on the diagnostic accuracy of dualsource computed tomography coronary angiography. J Am Coll Cardio 50:2393–2398

Scheffel H, Alkadhi H, Leschka S, et al. (2008) Low-Dose CT Coronary Angiography in the Step-and-Shoot Mode: Diagnostic Performance. Heart

Scheffel H, Alkadhi H, Plass A, et al. (2006) Accuracy of dual-source CT coronary angiography: first experience in a high pretest probability population without heart rate control. Eur Radiol 16:2739–2747

Thom T, Haase N, Rosamond W et al. (2006) Heart disease and stroke statistics—2006 update: a report from the American Heart Association Statistics Committee and Stroke Statistics Subcommittee. Circulation 113:e85–e151

Vlodaver Z, Frech R, Van Tassel RA, Edwards JE (1973) Correlation of the antemortem coronary arteriogram and the postmortem specimen. Circulation 47:162–169

Weustink AC, Meijboom WB, Mollet NR, et al. (2007) Reliable high-speed coronary computed tomography in symptomatic patients. J Am Coll Cardio 50:786–794

White CW, Wright CB, Doty DB et al. (1984) Does visual interpretation of the coronary arteriogram predict the physiologic importance of a coronary stenosis? N Engl J Med 310:819–824

Wintersperger BJ, Nikolaou K, von Ziegler F et al. (2006) Image quality, motion artifacts, and reconstruction timing of 64-slice coronary computed tomography angiography with 0.33-second rotation speed. Invest Radiol 41:436–442

Zanzonico P, Rothenberg LN, Strauss HW (2006) Radiation exposure of computed tomography and direct intracoronary angiography: risk has its reward. J Am Coll Cardiol 47:1846–1849

## 16

# Technical Innovations in Cardiac and Coronary MSCT

Martin H. K. Hoffmann

## CONTENTS

## ABSTRACT

The current evolution of CT is driven by cardiac imaging. Reliable and robust diagnostic performance for this application is crucially dependent on temporal resolution. Very different approaches are taken by the major vendors. Rotational time is unanimously accelerated and has currently arrived at 270 msec per rotation, but today's scanners barely meet the requirement of 65 msec per image at higher heart rates.

Another industry focus relates to the detector with more and more rows added. A complete cardiac dataset can nowadays be acquired in less than 6 sec with detector sizes > 8 cm in z-direction. This renders the method less susceptible to arrhythmia and heart rate variations. The best, currently available, solution operates at a detector size of 16 cm covering the heart at a single rotation, albeit compromising on temporal resolution.

The technical evolution has also realized that dose exposure needs to be decreased substantially for a widespread application. This has culminated in a trend away from spiral acquisitions to prospective axial rotations. This allows to reduce dose exposure by as much as 80%.

Provided that the current speed of technical improvements will persist it is foreseeable that most invasive angiograms will be replaced in the upcoming years. CT equipped with future detector technology has the potential to become the prime imaging modality for cardiovascular medicine.

M. H. K. Hoffmann, MD
Klinik für Diagnostische und Interventionelle Radiologie, Unikliniken Ulm, Steinhoevelstrasse 9, 89075 Ulm, Germany

## Basic Rationale

The state of the art of CT is constantly improving. Today, new scanner generations with improved technology are being introduced every 1–2 years, a pace that is foreseeably persisting, if not accelerating. The current driving force behind this rapid evolution of technology is CAD, the number one disease entity with the highest ranking incidence and mortality. CT-based coronary angiography has emerged as a reliable, noninvasive test to rule out CAD in symptomatic patients (De Feyter et al. 2007). The method is still associated with major limitations, but has been met with great enthusiasm, and its use worldwide is increasing rapidly. MDCT for noninvasive coronary angiography is appealing because it has the potential to replace invasive coronary angiography and could become a cornerstone diagnostic tool for clinical decision-making.

Before MDCT coronary angiography can become a reliable alternative to invasive coronary angiography, however, several problems must be resolved. The most important obstacle to the use of MDCT coronary angiography (MDCT-CA) is severe coronary calcification, which either prevents assessment of the integrity of the underlying coronary lumen or, because of its "blooming" effect, leads to overestimation of coronary stenosis severity. The same holds true for in-stent imaging with blooming artifacts even more pronounced around dense metallic structures such as stent struts.

In addition, the presence of arrhythmias or unstable sinus rhythm precludes the use of MDCT-CA, because the technique requires data to be obtained from the same phase of several cardiac cycles (6–10 heartbeats) for the reconstruction of coronary images.

A third concern is the fact that MDCT-CA is associated with relatively high X-ray radiation exposure (15–20 mSv; Earls et al. 2008; Klass et al. 2008). Substantial reductions are mandatory before a widespread use can be safely advocated.

Finally, improvement in temporal resolution to less than 50 ms (currently 83–135 ms with newest CT scanners) to reduce motion artifacts is desirable, but extremely difficult to achieve because such an improvement requires peak tube output power not available with current technology.

The aforementioned shows that substantial further improvements are required before MDCT-CA may compete for the standard of reference in CAD imaging, replacing 2D coronary angiography based upon catheterization techniques. Correction of these limitations will require a substantial amount of time, effort, and technical innovation.

## Today's State of the Art and Its Limitations

A prerequisite to understand the current evolution of technology designed for cardiac CT is the knowledge of its current limitations in lieu of the multifaceted possibilities. This chapter therefore focuses on four typical applications for cardiac CT: (1) initial diagnostic workup of suspected CAD (confined to a low to intermediate pretest likelihood group to rule out disease), (2) follow-up of patients after coronary artery bypass graft (CABG) procedures to assess graft patency, (3) valve imaging (a new application made possible by constantly improving temporal resolution), and (4) the strongholds of cardiac CT to visualize the proximal parts of the coronary tree to identify anomalies or other infrequent entities.

### 16.2.1
### Rule-Out CAD

MDCT-CA is currently considered to be a useful technique to rule out the presence of clinically significant CAD (stenosis with >50% diameter obstruction) only in symptomatic patients who are at intermediate pretest risk of CAD (Meijboom et al. 2007). A normal coronary CT scan in symptomatic patients reliably rules out clinically significant CAD; these patients do not require further diagnostic procedures and can be safely discharged. These statements are deducted from a persistently high negative predictive value shown in multiple single-center and a few multicenter comparison trials referencing CT findings systematically to catheterization angiography (Hamon et al. 2006). In addition to that first prospective, outcome studies confirm the strong prognostic value of a CT scan negative for disease (Pugliese et al. 2006; Gilard et al. 2007).

The widespread application suffers from improving but still insufficient temporal resolution. Most researchers therefore agree that a reduction in heart rate to lengthen the rest phase of the coronary tree is needed, even using the latest editions of scanner technology.

The novice user may wonder why such a limited indication scenario is constructed for noninvasive CT coronary angiography. An unrestricted indication of the method is limited by low spatial resolution. Exact delineation of densely calcified or metallic structures is gradually improved by technological advances but persistently inaccurate. MDCT-CA oversizes the calcified plaque or the metallic stent strut. This artificially reduces the size of the adjacent contrast filled lumen. False-positive findings are therefore produced, resulting in a low positive predictive value.

The algorithm applied in most institutions today is therefore utilizing CT in a gate-keeping function (Hoffmann et al. 2005). A negative finding safely excludes the patient from further workup. A positive finding is used to transfer the patient either to functional diagnostic procedures to test for perfusion defects or to transfer the patient to catheterization angiography.

Very low-risk patients are not good candidates for CT imaging due to the risk of contrast and radiation exposure. Cardiac CT imaging based on the current standard of retrospective helical acquisitions is associated with a radiation dose exposure of 15 mSv (three times the average exposure rate of conventional catheterization angiography), precluding use of the method for asymptomatic patients.

The application of the method for symptomatic patients with a high pretest probability is not indicated for two reasons. A patient with an acute coronary syndrome should be taken to the catheterization laboratory directly in order to offer a timely and direct possibility of transluminal interventions. But for patient with stable angina and high probability, increasing evidence indicates that transluminal intervention does not reduce the rate of future cardiac events in comparison to medical therapy. This has fueled a quest for a noninvasive accurate luminogram to stratify differential therapy options. The demand could be served by CT if the above-outlined restrictions could be overcome.

## 16.2.2
## Post-CABG Follow-Up

Patients after CABG may suffer either from acute and early or chronic and late occlusion of bypass grafts. The graft vessels are subjected to less motion during the cardiac cycle than is the coronary tree proper. This allows visualizing of the graft pedicles even at high heart rates. On average, catheterization procedures have to administer a lot more contrast volume to visualize all coronary bypass grafts compared with CT. This constitutes a good indication for cardiac CT imaging (Marano et al. 2007).

But the clinical utility of post-CABG CT imaging could be substantially augmented if the distal anastomosis and the target vessel could be reliably assessed.

Along the evolution of technology from 4 to the 64 detector rows, much progress is achieved in terms of reliable access to the distal anastomosis. The proximal vessels though are usually vastly calcified. This constitutes a shortcoming for accurate luminal evaluation, but is perceived by some cardiac surgeons as a benefit allowing identification of suitable target vessels prior to surgery (Simon et al. 2007).

## 16.2.3
## Valve Imaging

The rapidly improving temporal resolution provided by recent scanner generations has rendered functional imaging along the cardiac cycle feasible. CT is certainly not the first-line modality for global ventricular function assessments but may serve as a good second-line option for patients with pacemakers and intracardial defibrillators (Orakzai et al. 2006). Global left ventricular (LV) functional parameters measured with MDCT have been found to be in good agreement with results of cine MRI (Belge et al. 2006; Juergens et al. 2008).

Aortic valve evaluations may utilize both increasing temporal resolution and the susceptibility for calcified structures inherent to CT imaging. Studies have shown very promising results to measure the aortic valve area (Pouleur et al. 2007). The comparison of results generated with CT was highly correlated with MR and transesophageal echocardiogram (TEE)-derived direct planimetry of aortic valve area. Amazingly, CT imaging of valves can be done with relatively low temporal resolution (200 ms in the study of Pouleur et al. [2007]). The average duration of a systolic contraction is 300 ms, which compares unfavorably to the 200 ms generated by CT at a low rotational speed of 400 ms. But the time during which the aortic valve remains fully open averages 297±40 ms. This is within the range of the temporal resolution of most MDCT scanners used for cardiac imaging today. The issue for valve imaging in contrast to global ventricular assessments is not to capture the right heart phase but to minimize residual motion blurring the accurate delineation of the aortic valve leaflet. The pathologic condition of aortic stenosis with substantially reduced valve leaflet motion works in favor of MDCT at this end.

Transcutaneous aortic valve replacements emerge as a bail-out option for nonsurgical candidates. The procedure is based on a stent mounted bioprosthetic valve that unfolds in aortic position after balloon valvuloplasty. One of the risks associated with this procedure is to push calcified patches located on the native valve leaflets into coronary flow, obstructing positions in the sinuses of Valsalva. Therefore, most of the researchers involved in trans-cutaneous valve procedures deem a cardiac CT mandatory for the selection of patients.

## 16.2.4
## Coronary Anomalies and the Coronary Ostium

Catheterization angiography relies on the proximal insertion of a catheter tip into the ostium of the proximal coronary artery. Contrast agents are then injected directly via this catheter. This constitutes a limitation readily apparent in clinical routine for the detection of ostial left main disease. Most of the cases are identified indirectly either by a steep pressure drop measured during the insertion process, indicating occlusive size of the catheter in relation to the stenosed ostium, or by a missing back-flush of contrast medium into the aortic root, prevented by surrounded plaque material encroaching upon the lumen size. These restrictions do not apply for CT imaging and are therefore regarded as a stronghold of the method in clinical routine.

The predominance of coronary anomalies is composed of abnormal branching patterns of the proximal segments. CT is therefore used in many instances of suspected coronary anomalies after catheterization angiography to verify or supplement suspected findings. The supplemental function includes visualizing abnormal branches that could either not be reached by the catheter tip during the catheterization procedure or were not at all detected. For this application, CT offers the only way to assess the peripheral parts of that particular branch. Hence, all the restrictions apply as mentioned in the section on initial CAD workup.

Another indication for CT after catheterization angiography that is requested with increasing frequency is the delineation of occluded segments. The 2D projections generated in the catheterization laboratory (cath lab) are prone to so-called foreshortening effects. At certain projections, the segment of interest may be artificially shortened and partially not visualized at all. This effect holds the risk of false-negative findings. The effect is well known, and the propensity of false-negative findings produced by 2D angiography films has been shown in comparison to intravascular ultrasound studies (Topol and Nissen 1995).

The clinical utility generated for coronary CT in relation to the foreshortening effect is twofold. CT datasets are used in the cath lab for navigation of the C-arm to produce angulations with minimal foreshortening ratios. Planned recanalization of chronically occluded segments is one application utilizing CT for navigation purposes. Another clinical scenario utilizing the same algorithm is the verification of positive CT findings in the cath lab. Interventionalists familiar with CT imaging acquire nonstandard angulations in order to prevent foreshortening to produce false-negative 2D projections.

## 16.3
## Extrapolation of the Continuous Evolutionary Process

The evolution in CT technology over nearly two decades has been impressive. Single-slice helical CT was introduced in 1989. It was another 10 years before 4-slice CT was introduced. After that, it took only 3 years until the release of 16-slice CT, and another 2 years until the release of 64-slice CT. The next step was dual-source CT, which was introduced only 1 year after 64 detector rows became commercially available. Today, we experience a new situation with the community of vendors providing a diversity of different approaches. CT scanners with a dedicated cardiac functionality of 2008 have a bandwidth of detector sizes ranging from 2 cm (32 detector rows) up to 16 cm (320 detector rows) and range from a rotational speed of 350 ms to 270 ms.

In the era of 4-detector row CT, cardiac applications were at a level of proof-of-concept, with very few centers involved. Although a very high interest was noted, artifacts and other pitfalls caused significant problems in the majority of patients. Sixteen-detector-row scanners were the first to introduce the method and reveal the clinical potential. Still, most clinical studies were published by investigators from just a few selected institutions. Multicenter data available for 16-detector-row-based coronary angiography show a substantially compromised robustness that limits clinical utility to a selected range of patients (Garcia et al. 2006).

Sixty-four detector row scanners made cardiac CT a viable clinical tool for medical practice around the world. Clinical comparison studies referenced against catheterization-based coronary angiography report persistently high levels of sensitivity and specificity. A limited application for the initial workup of CAD was defined according to the persistently high negative predictive value. But restrictions still apply, namely a substantial amount of segments of the coronary tree still rendered with residual motion or blooming artifacts and hence, compromised diagnostic image quality.

Another persistent restriction is identifiable in most of the exclusion criteria for major cardiac CT studies: heart rate variations and arrhythmia cannot be tolerated by current technology. This is due to the helical acquisition with a detector width small compared with the z-axis length of the organ of interest (typical length of the heart is 12–15 cm). The final dataset is composed of acquisitions conducted over multiple heartbeats. But not a single beat is like the other, with myriad of physiologic regulatory mechanisms constantly fine-tuning the strength and length of a cardiac cycle. The current evolution of CT technology for cardiac applications is therefore concentrated on increasing the temporal resolution to reduce motion artifacts and to acquire the dataset from a single heartbeat in order to reduce inhomogeneities induced by multiple heart beats.

## 16.3.1
### The Benefit of More Detector Rows

The benefit of very large detectors is easily deductable from the aforementioned. A detector covering the full z-axis width of the heart would allow capturing the morphologic coronary angiogram from a single cardiac cycle. Functional datasets could be obtained either from very few successive or just only one heartbeat. This would render both morphologic and functional imaging much less susceptible for artifacts induced by arrhythmic contractions. The clinical potential of such a scanner is huge, provided sufficient spatial and temporal resolution is granted. The technological restraints preventing such a machine today are centered on the X-ray-emitting tube. A 16-cm detector rotating with a speed of more than 300 ms per rotation requires an extremely high peak tube output in order to acquire noiseless images. Current "large-area" detector models have therefore been restricted in terms of rotational speed at 350 ms. Very high rotational speed for cardiac CT is up to now only achievable at a maximum detector width of 8 cm.

Another major benefit of large area detectors is the acquisition of images in axial mode rather than in helical fashion; this is much more dose efficient. This benefit is available utilizing much smaller detector width in a stepping fashion as outlined in Sect. 16.5.2.

## 16.3.2
### How Much Temporal Resolution Do We Need?

One of the most important questions for the daily practice of cardiac CT is how much temporal resolution is required for robust imaging at any arbitrary heart rate. Very few studies are available to address this issue. Most of the available literature is focused on MRI-based coronary morphologic imaging. WANG et al. (1999) have measured the length of the coronary rest period, using biplane conventional angiography with a high frame rate. The shortest rest period was found both for the left and right coronary artery at higher heart rates was 66 ms. Jahnke et al. in a similar study conducted in 2006 found the rest period to be as short as 20 ms for the right coronary artery (RCA) and 48 ms for the left coronary artery (LCA). Probably the most intriguing finding of both studies is the high patient-to-patient variability and low linear correlation of duration of rest period and heart rate. Different conclusions for MR and CT imaging have to be drawn from these data. Whereas in a larger patient population the duration of the rest period does not well correlate with absolute heart rate, the individual patient's rest period does significantly lengthen with the lowering of heart rate induced by the application of β-blockers.

This finding explains why the CT scanners used today with inadequate temporal resolution achieve reasonable results in some patients with higher heart rates. Some patients with high heart rates render sufficiently long rest periods to accomplish motion artifact-free images. For the robust and reliable acquisition, much higher temporal resolutions are required than are available on today's platforms.

Averaging the results of the relevant literature, it may be postulated that the required temporal resolution for reliable cardiac imaging is in the range of 65 ms (WANG et al. 1999; SHECHTER et al. 2005; JAHNKE et al. 2006). The amount of residual motion allowed within this rest period is in the range of 1 mm; lower thresholds require much more temporal resolution. This is so far not achieved by any available CT scanner platform, with the most efficient available technology acquiring a complete dataset in a temporal window of 83 ms. It is therefore foreseeable that even with the latest technology, reliable coronary imaging results will only be achieved with lengthening of rest periods induced by medications (as, e.g., β-blockers or Procoralan) that lower the heart rate.

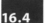

## 16.4
### The High-Density Dilemma

The sensitivity of cardiac CT for the attenuation of material with high Z-numbers allows the detection of calcium even on a noncontrasted scan acquisition. This

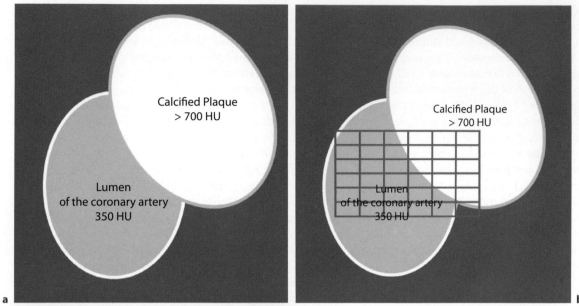

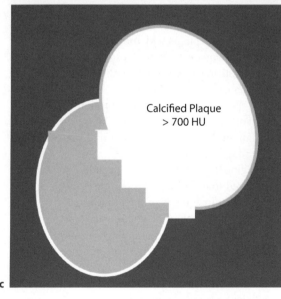

**Fig. 16.1a–c.** Illustration of the partial volume-averaging artifact. **a** Simulated cross-section of a coronary artery with a calcified plaque. The dense plaque structure shows positive remodeling (outbound growth pattern). The lumen is not significantly narrowed. The coronary artery lumen is filled with a high concentration of iodine (350 HU). **b** The grid represents the maximum voxel size available for CT imaging (e.g., 0.4-mm voxel length). **c** All voxels that partially contain high-density calcium are registered as high-density objects for image reconstruction. The calcified plaque is represented with artificial enlargement and a stair-stepping artifact on the CT image (smoothed later on by filtering)

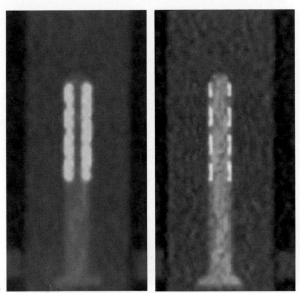

a    b

**Fig. 16.2a,b.** In-stent lumen imaging. **a** Imaging of a stent phantom acquired on a conventional 16-detector-row scanner with a voxel size of 1 mm. A conventional cobalt–chromium alloy bare metal stent (Multi-Link Vision Rx Coronary Stent System, Boston Scientific, Gatwick, Mass.) with thin struts (0.08 mm) is used. **b** The same stent as in **a** is visualized with a fourfold-better spatial resolution (voxel size of 0.25 mm), utilizing a flat-panel detector. (Modified according to MAHNKEN et al. 2005)

principle founds the basis for calcium scoring. Contrast-enhanced scanning conducted for the purpose of noninvasive coronary angiography, on the other hand, suffers substantially from the artifacts induced by both metallic stent struts and densely calcified plaques. It is readily apparent in the schematic drawing of Fig. 16.1 that the blooming artifact induced by all high-attenuation objects is due to partial volume averaging. The phenomenon is well defined for conventional CT imaging, and alleviation of the shortcoming has been proven by an increase in spatial resolution (Fig. 16.2). But a substantial increase in spatial resolution requires exponentially increasing radiation dose exposure in order to keep image noise at a constant level (PROKOP 2003). This precludes conventional CT technology to achieve a solution for low-dose diagnostic CT angiography.

One option for the accurate delineation of the vessel lumen versus the calcified plaque would be to evaluate images at a higher window center setting. A prerequisite to achieve this is to fill the vessel lumen with higher amounts of iodine. The Hounsfield-unit density of the vascular lumen should be close to the window center in order to accomplish accurate border definition. In other words, the contrast density within the coronary vessel lumen should be increased. The clinical benefit of this principle has been shown for the detection of hemodynamically significant stenoses in the epicardial vessels (CADEMARTIRI et al. 2006a,b). But various researchers

have questioned the potential of this approach (BECKER et al. 2003) and recommend an intraluminal contrast attenuation value of 250 HU should not be exceeded.

A soft plaque at the initial stage of calcification may have an overall density of less than 400 HU. Should we now fill the vascular lumen with more than 400 HU of iodine contrast, some of the calcified structures adjacent to the lumen might be obscured and undiscernible from lumen territory on cross-sectional cuts (Fig. 16.3). This may potentially result in false-negative findings on coronary angiograms, which would constitute a worst-case scenario for the current clinical application of the modality.

Fortunately, the typical atherosclerotic lesion initially calcifies in the outer plaque layers (Figs. 16.3d, 16.4). The low-density calcification is separated from the lumen by a soft tissue layer, with low attenuation values. The soft tissue layer vanishes with progression of plaque calcification, and the calcification sits right on top of the lumen. But at this stage of disease progression, the density of the calcification almost invariably attenuates at much higher values than those of the contrasted lumen (Fig. 16.3b). The accuracy of stenosis detection is therefore maintained even at high iodine concentrations equivalent to low-density calcifications on the majority of coronary angiograms. The aforementioned statement is deducted from clinical practice and awaits vigorous scientific testing.

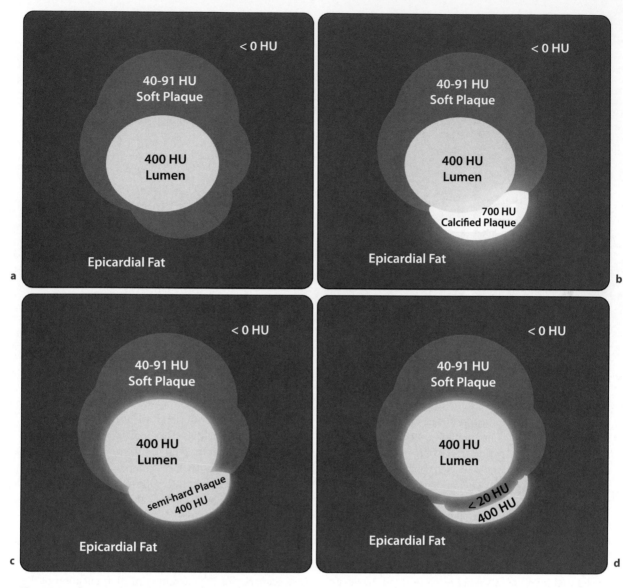

**Fig. 16.3a–d.** Hypothetical density of lumen versus plaque on representative cross-sections. **a** The coronary lumen (filled with an iodine contrast agent at 400 HU) is surrounded by soft plaque and epicardial fat. The problem zone in this situation is the delineation of soft plaque versus epicardial fat. **b** Part of the soft plaque structures are densely calcified. The calcified plaque with a density of 700 HU is oversized due to partial volume averaging, but delineation against the lumen is not compromised by contrast issues. **c** For a hypothetical plaque structure at an initial stage of calcification (Hounsfield units equivalent to lumen at 400 HU) a false-negative detection ensues. The plaque and lumen structures cannot be separated due to equivalent density. This relation triggered the postulation that lumen opacification should not be higher than 250 HU. **d** Initial plaque calcifications in clinical practice tend to occur in the outer layers of the plaque structure. The calcification with a density equivalent to the lumen is separated from the lumen by an interposition of soft plaque components. This allows safe identification and hence prevents false-negative readings

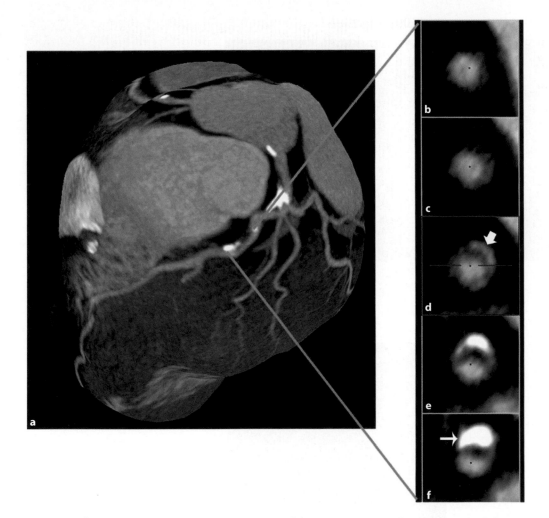

**Fig. 16.4a–f.** Cross-sections of a mixed plaque on a 64-detector-row scanner. **a** 3D Global view in left anterior oblique projection shows a mixed plaque located on the left anterior descending artery (LAD). Enlarged successive cross-sections (**b–f**) represent different parts of the plaque structure. **b** Soft components are barely contrasted against the surrounding epicardial fat. **c** and **d** Low-density calcifications (*thick arrow*) appear at the outer medial or advential layers of the plaque structure and are separated from the lumen (same density as plaque calcification) by a layer of soft plaque components. This prevents false-negative readings as outlined in Fig. 16.3. **e, f** Densely calcified plaque components (*thin arrow*) are readily apparent as bright structures on the cross-sections

In other words, the above-constructed potential for false-negative readings lingers within the concept of high-attenuation contrast application and cannot be satisfactorily solved by conventional CT technology. A potential solution for the dilemma may be offered by spectral CT utilizing the additional information contained in the spectrum of X-ray photons emitted by regular tube designs.

### 16.4.1
### Basic Principle of Spectral CT

The energy source used for conventional X-ray CT imaging is operating based on the bremsstrahlung principle. A continuous spectrum of X-ray photons is emitted and filtered before exposure of the scanned object. After passage through tissue, the energy spectrum of a poly-

**Mathematical Chest/Heart Phantom**

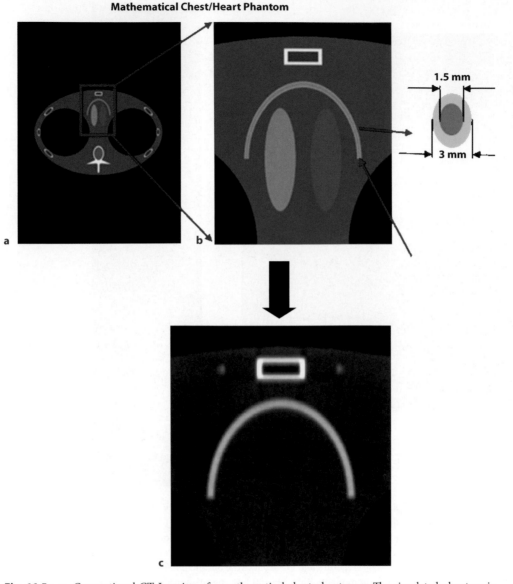

**Fig. 16.5a–c.** Conventional CT Imaging of a mathematical chest phantom. **a** The simulated phantom is composed of rib structures, sternum, and spine. The cardiac structures are represented by a left ventricle (bright elliptical structure) and a right ventricle (low-density elliptical structure) and a semicircular coronary artery. The coronary artery wall is homogenously calcified (white bands on enlarged *inset* **b**). The total diameter of the coronary artery amounts to 3 mm with a residual lumen of 1.5 mm, surrounded by calcified plaque (enlarged diagram on the *left*). The coronary artery lumen is contrasted with a contrast agent at a regular clinical density (250 HU). **c** Conventional CT imaging of the enlarged region as represented in **b** will not be able to discriminate the calcified plaque components from the contrasted lumen

chromatic beam of X-rays contains valuable information about the elemental composition of the absorber. Conventional X-ray systems or X-ray CT systems, equipped with scintillator detectors, operate in integrating mode. They are largely insensitive to the spectral information contained in different X-ray photons, since the detector output is proportional to the energy fluence integrated over the whole spectrum (Fig. 16.5).

One first approach to utilize the information contained in the polychromatic beam is to measure two different energy levels separately. This can be achieved with either tube voltage switching or layered detectors (as described in detail in Chap. 4) (CARMI et al. 2005). The method has great potential for material separation in the high-density domain, and first clinical results are very encouraging (JOHNSON et al. 2007). But the application for cardiac purposes is thus far limited by the phase shift inherent in most approaches or hampered by inefficient dose utilization. Another far more sophisticated approach exploiting the full potential of energy-dependent imaging is spectral CT (ROESSL and PROKSA 2007).

The method is based on so-called photon-counting detectors. Spectral CT is designed to detect K-edge discontinuities. K-edges occur in the element-specific photoelectric cross-section. X-ray photons are counted by the detector and sorted in energy bins representing preselected partial bandwidths of the full spectrum. Material differentiation in the high-density domain is fully accomplished by this approach. In order to apply this method for routine clinical imaging, completely different detector technology has to be developed. Today's technology provides only low count rates for spectral detectors and it is therefore not realistic to predict clinically usable products within the next 5 years.

## 16.4.2
## The Unobscured 3D Luminogram

To achieve a perfect noninvasive 3D luminogram of the coronary tree, we would need a visualization unobscured by high-density overlay (as, e.g., calcium or metal). This may either be achieved by the material separation approaches described for dual energy imaging (see Chap. 4 for details) or be accomplished by acquiring contrast-only images. Spectral imaging may be adapted to acquire several images below and above specific K-edges (Fig. 16.6). Subsequent subtraction (or more mathematically correct de-convolution) of images around the K-edge removes all tissue from the dataset except for the element characterized by the K-edge (Fig. 16.6). This allows generating contrast-only images for compounds with high Z-numbers. Iodine with a K-edge at 33.2 keV is not suited for such an endeavor. The vast majority of X-ray photons at this energy level are completely absorbed within the human body structure. This renders detection of residual photons on the detector side impossible and only contributes to artifacts as beam hardening and photon starvation. Gadolinium, though originally designed for MRI imaging, is well visualized by conventional CT and exhibits better attenuation characteristics than iodine. It is not widely used clinically because concentrations much higher than those routinely applied for MRI imaging would not be

needed. Gadolinium is much better suited for spectral CT, with a K-edge discontinuity occurring at 50.2 keV. This is both well inside the energy regime relevant for medical imaging and is sufficiently high enough to render the thorax penetrable for the majority of emitted photons. Other agents that may be considered in the future include gold (K-edge = 80.7 keV) and bismuth (K-edge = 90.8 keV).

The deconvolution (or simply subtraction) of images adjacent to the K-edge of the contrast agent of interest allows visualization the lumen, without any overly. This concept has first been shown in simulation studies and subsequently been realized on a prototype scanner. First clinical proof-of-concept papers have shown the feasibility to separate gadolinium from stent struts and calcium in phantom studies (FEUERLEIN et al. 2008).

The generated images reveal a lot of image noise so far (Fig. 16.7). This is due to a limited count rate of the photon-counting detectors, but further technical improvements to address this issue are expected. It may be possible in the near term future to combine higher count rate detectors, with a miniaturization that allows producing a very small and efficient detector elements, allowing image acquisition at dose exposure levels comparable to conventional CT. The individual detector element would be smaller than the voxel size reconstructed for medical imaging. With such an approach, beam hardening is no longer an issue. Partial volume averaging on the other hand prevails, but correction algorithms may utilize the very small individual detector element used for spectral detectors.

Spectral CT could therefore have a major impact on the clinical value of CT coronary angiography. Without beam hardening artifacts, in-stent lumens become accessible and with partial volume averaging, reduced both vessel lumens adjacent to stent struts and densely calcified plaques are more accurately delineated (FEUERLEIN et al. 2008). Overall, two new application scenarios could be feasible: one is the follow-up of patients after percutaneous coronary interventions with stent implantation; the other is the evaluation of patients with known CAD or calcified vessels. Spectral detector technology may promote CT to become the primary tool for CAD imaging (ROESSL and PROKSA 2007; FEUERLEIN et al. 2008).

## 16.4.3
## Potential for Plaque Imaging

Conventional integrating CT offers a first step in plaque component visualization and differentiation. Many studies have been published to establish density thresholds

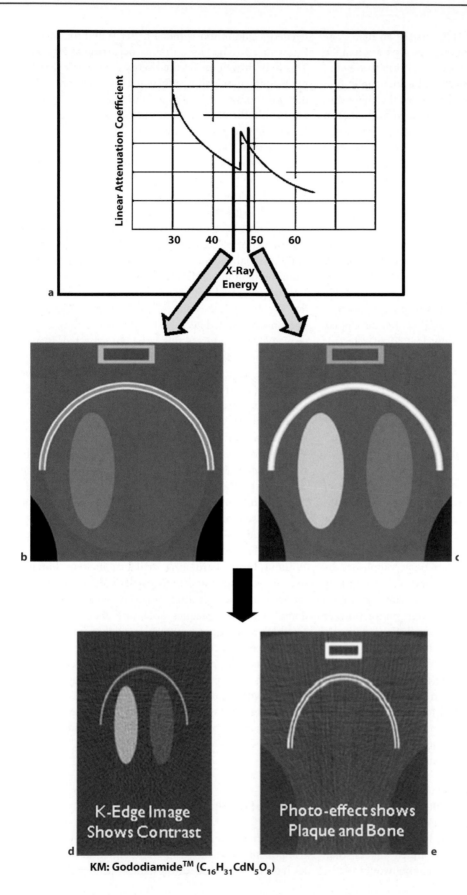

**Fig. 16.6a–e.** Spectral CT imaging. **a** Two energy bins are placed adjacent to the K-edge discontinuity of gadolinium (used as a contrast agent for the phantom as in Fig. 5). **b** This allows to reconstruct virtual images at 47 and 53 keV (**b**, **c**), respectively. **d**, **e** After deconvolution of the dataset gadolinium, K-edge images show contrast agent only without any surrounding high-density components (**d**). The photo-effect deconvolution is best suited to isolate calcified structures (**e**)

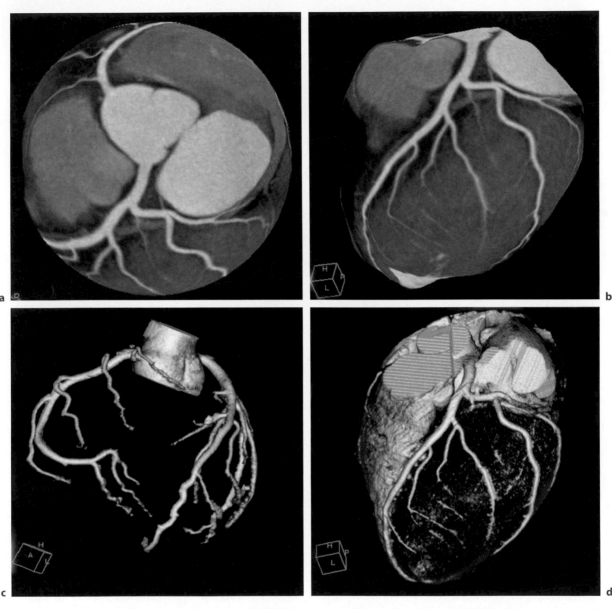

**Fig. 16.7a–d.** Representative coronary angiogram with PGA. **a, b** 3D Global views at different projection angles. No disease is apparent in the left and right coronary arteries. Volume renderings of the same dataset with coronary tree isolation (**c**) and surrounding cardiac structures (**d**). The dataset was acquired with prospectively gated axial acquisition at a total dose exposure of 3.5 mSv

for the differentiation of calcified, fibrous, and lipidic plaque components. But the discrimination of lipid and fibrous components failed, and in clinical practice only two components are reported, calcified and soft. Initially, one study was published that blamed partial volume averaging due to insufficient spatial resolution to be responsible for the failure of soft component differentiation (CADEMARTIRI et al. 2005). But today, evidence accumulates that the soft plaque components represent the active plaque structures. The soft structures are vascularized and a rapid wash-in of contrast is thought supplied by advential vasa vasorum (HALLIBURTON et al. 2006). This explains why a contrast-enhancement-based approach is predisposed to fail.

In this context, spectral CT could theoretically offer differentiation tools for lipid and fibrous components.

Fat-containing structures were found to increase in attenuation with increasing photon energy; this is opposing to higher density structures as, e.g., iodine contrast. However, a proof-of-concept for the differentiation of lipid versus fibrous tissue is still lacking.

The more relevant potential of spectral CT technology for the application of plaque imaging is contrast associated. Future applications may utilize two simultaneously injected contrast agents. One with a K-edge of, e.g., 50 keV (like gadolinium) is used for luminal opacification, the other with a K-edge of 90 keV (e.g., bismuth) is coupled to a receptor avidly binding to the endothelial surface of a vulnerable plaque. Both contrast agents would be apparent on different deconvolution images of the same dataset and could be secondarily superimposed using colored overlay as available for PET–CT postprocessing. The sensitivity of the plaque specific contrast compound will be a couple of orders lower than PET sensitivity. But ease of use and availability may allow a more widespread clinical application at a lower dose exposure.

## 16.5
## Dose Exposure

Since the advent of noninvasive coronary angiography utilizing CT, the clinical value of the modality has almost never been questioned. Criticism has concentrated on the very high dose exposure of CT imaging per se (BRENNER and HALL 2007) and cardiac CT imaging especially (EINSTEIN et al. 2007). As allude to in Sect. 16.4, the currently achieved spatial resolution of modern MDCT scanners is high, but it is not high enough for the imaging of small structures like the distal branches of the epicardial vessels. Noninvasive coronary angiography could easily utilize a lot more spatial resolution for in-stent lumen imaging and accurate delineation of calcified plaque structures.

In order to quantify dose exposure for the individual patient, most scanner consoles offer an estimated value prior to the initiation of the scan and after completion present an accumulated value for the examination. Values used on scanner consoles are not displayed in familiar effective dose values but rather encrypted in a dose length product (DLP). But the DLP value can easily be converted to familiar effective dose values by simple multiplication with a $k$ factor. The $k$ factor used to estimate the effective dose in cardiac CT is that used for the chest CT, 0.017 mSv/mGy·cm (BONGARTZ et al. 1999). Other $k$ factors apply to different body regions.

### 16.5.1
### Retrospective Helical Acquisition

Retrospective gating without any "dose saving" measures is not ideally suited for cardiac imaging. This is simply due to the fact that cardiac imaging requires phase or cardiac cycle correlation. If phase correlation is coupled with another cyclic process like the rotation of the scanner gantry, then one cyclic process has to wait for the other. In other words, helical CT imaging with ECG registration has to guarantee that the rotating CT gantry will capture at least one complete cardiac cycle at any given $z$-axis position. This results in a tremendous reduction of the acquisition speed or a very low pitch setting. Without any tube current modulation or other measures to reduce the dose exposure, this would result in a huge amount of redundant tissue exposure. Only a fraction of this dataset (centered on the phase of interest) is subsequently used for image reconstruction.

### 16.5.2
### Prospective Axial Acquisition

Prospective axial acquisitions have been completely replaced by spiral or helical acquisitions for most of the CT applications. In the era of single row detectors, this has been the only way to rapidly obtain larger $z$-axis coverage. For larger detectors (e.g., beyond 4 cm, with at least 64 detector rows,) this restriction does no longer apply. The stacked axial acquisition of a defined volume length as the heart can be done in four to five steps in most cases. This amounts to a total of 8–10 cardiac cycles with every other cardiac cycle used for gantry propagation along the $z$-axis (Fig. 16.8). This approach is far more dose efficient than is the above-described retrospectively gated helical acquisition. It is furthermore much less affected by ectopic premature beats than the continuously propagated helical scan is (Fig. 16.9). The prospectively gated axial (PGA) scan can be stopped on the spot to wait for the preventricular contraction (PVC) to pass and commence only at the reinitiating of regular sinus rhythm (KLASS et al. 2008). The continuous helical scan can only be truncated by the cycles located around the premature beat in a process called ECG editing. For cases with extensive occurrence of PVC, this may easily result in $z$-banding due to insufficient datasets for complete reconstructions. In summary, a prospectively acquired scan with a large detector versus a regular helical acquisition with retrospective gating reduces the dose exposure by a factor

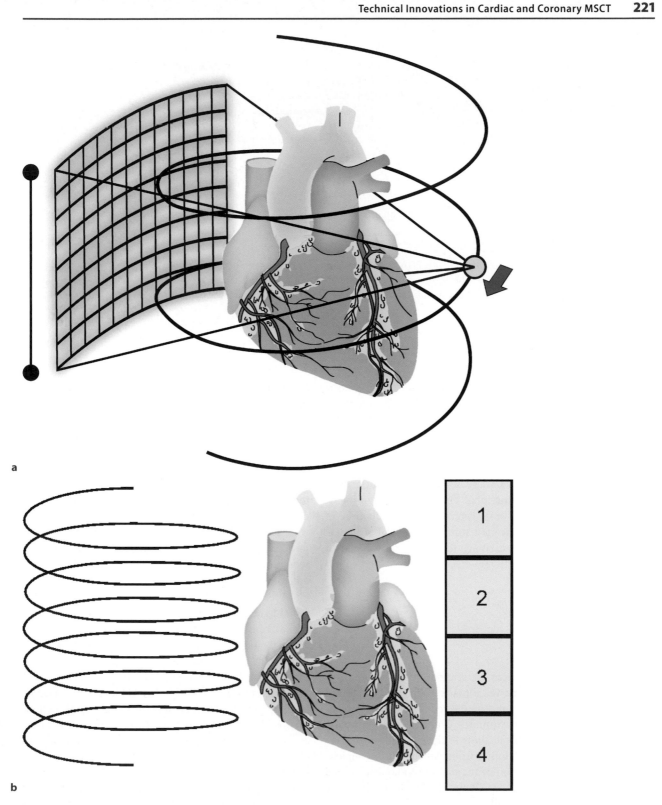

a

b

**Fig. 16.8a,b.** Helical versus axial acquisition. **a** A detector with a total *z*-axis coverage of less than 16 cm needs to be propagated along the heart in order to cover the volume of interest for coronary angiographic imaging. **b** This can be achieved either conventionally with a helical acquisition as on the *left* or in a stepping fashion with prospective triggering as on the *right*. For a given detector width of 4 cm, four to five steps are required to cover the heart from the aortic root down to the diaphragm

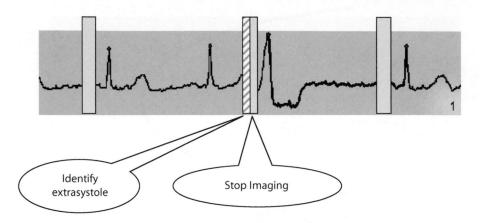

**Fig. 16.9.** Arrhythmia correction with PGA. Axial acquisitions may be combined with algorithms detecting arrhythmia. The scan can be stopped temporarily to prevent image acquisition during premature beats. Acquisition is subsequently completed at the reoccurrence of sinus rhythm

of 3 and additionally is more suited to address heart rate variations and arrhythmia. It is therefore foreseeable that with the advent of larger detectors beyond 64-detector rows, helical acquisitions will no longer be the standard mode for cardiac scanning (EARLS et al. 2008).

One major disadvantage of axial acquisition techniques is that a functional cine sequence cannot be reconstructed. This may preclude the evaluation of noncoronary cardiac structures. The helical scan will therefore remain first choice for additional valvular or ventricular imaging.

## 16.6
## Conclusion

Tremendous advances in scanner technology introduced in the recent years made cardiac CT a clinical reality. Automated software has reduced image postprocessing time to a few minutes. Coronary tree extraction allows obtaining projections of the CT dataset that resemble the views familiar from catheterization angiography. But application of the method today is confined to a selected range of patients. This is due to the many restrictions that prevail.

The current industry focus is to provide sufficient temporal resolution and coverage. The best performance achieved with clinically available technology allows reconstructing cardiac images in a temporal window of

83 ms. This almost matches the required threshold of 65 ms postulated by a few studies quantifying the rest period of the coronary tree.

In addition, another trend is already visible: full $z$-axis length coverage of the heart is provided in either a single or less than two to four axial rotations by latest scanner releases. This may add sufficient robustness to the acquisition to handle arrhythmia and variable heart rates. The rapidly growing detector size is associated with substantial reductions in dose exposure required for a complete coronary angiographic acquisition. Dose reductions in the range of 80% become available without compromises in image quality.

With all the achievements realized so far, one restriction becomes more and more prevalent: insufficient spatial resolution generates partial volume averaging artifacts and hence produces a high-density dilemma. Both stent struts and calcified plaques appear larger than they are on conventional CT images. One clinically available option to alleviate the problem is dual energy imaging. But the material differentiation of this method in the high-density domain is very limited. A much more sophisticated approach that has the potential to obviate high-density over-sizing artifacts is spectral CT. First proof-of-concept scanner setups have been realized in the research laboratories, but many innovations more technical are needed to render the method suitable for clinical application.

It is therefore predictable that coronary heart disease will continue to drive a rapid evolution of CT technology for many years to come.

# References

Becker CR, Hong C, Knez A, Leber A, Bruening R, Schoepf UJ, Reiser MF (2003) Optimal contrast application for cardiac 4-detector-row computed tomography. Invest Radiol 38:690–694

Belge B, Coche E, Pasquet A, Vanoverschelde JL, Gerber BL (2006) Accurate estimation of global and regional cardiac function by retrospectively gated multidetector row computed tomography: comparison with cine magnetic resonance imaging. Eur Radiol 16:1424–1433

Bongartz G, Golding SJ, Jurik AG, Leonardi M, van Meerten EvP (1999) European guidelines on quality criteria for computed tomography [EUR 16262 EN]. Office for Official Publications of the European Communities, Luxembourg

Brenner DJ, Hall EJ (2007) Computed tomography—an increasing source of radiation exposure. N Engl J Med 357:2277–2284

Cademartiri F, Mollet NR, Runza G, Bruining N, Hamers R, Somers P, Knaapen M, Verheye S, Midiri M, Krestin GP, de Feyter PJ (2005) Influence of intracoronary attenuation on coronary plaque measurements using multislice computed tomography: observations in an ex vivo model of coronary computed tomography angiography. Eur Radiol 15:1426–1431

Cademartiri F, de Monye C, Pugliese F, Mollet NR, Runza G, van der Lugt A, Midiri M, de Feyter PJ, Lagalla R, Krestin GP (2006a) High iodine concentration contrast material for noninvasive multislice computed tomography coronary angiography: iopromide 370 versus iomeprol 400. Invest Radiol 41:349–353

Cademartiri F, Mollet NR, Lemos PA, Saia F, Midiri M, de Feyter PJ, Krestin GP (2006b) Higher intracoronary attenuation improves diagnostic accuracy in MDCT coronary angiography. AJR Am J Roentgenol 187:430–433

Carmi R, Naveh G, Altman A (2005) Material separation with dual-layer CT. IEEE Nuclear Science Symposium Conference Record 4:1876–1878

De Feyter PJ, Meijboom WB, Weustink A, Van Mieghem C, Mollet NR, Vourvouri E, Nieman K, Cademartiri F (2007) Spiral multislice computed tomography coronary angiography: a current status report. Clin Cardiol 30:437–442

Earls JP, Berman EL, Urban BA, Curry CA, Lane JL, Jennings RS, McCulloch CC, Hsieh J, Londt JH (2008) Prospectively gated transverse coronary CT angiography versus retrospectively gated helical technique: improved image quality and reduced radiation dose. Radiology. Radiology 246:742–753

Einstein AJ, Henzlova MJ, Rajagopalan S (2007) Estimating risk of cancer associated with radiation exposure from 64-slice computed tomography coronary angiography. JAMA 298:317–323

Feuerlein S, Roessl E, Proksa R, Klass O, Jeltsch M, Rasche V, Brambs H-J, Hoffmann MH, Schlomka JP (2008) Multi-energy photon counting K-edge imaging: potential for improved luminal depiction in vascular imaging. Invest Radiol (in press)

Garcia MJ, Lessick J, Hoffmann MH (2006) Accuracy of 16-row multidetector computed tomography for the assessment of coronary artery stenosis. JAMA 296:403–411

Gilard M, Le Gal G, Cornily JC, Vinsonneau U, Joret C, Pennec PY, Mansourati J, Boschat J (2007) Midterm prognosis of patients with suspected coronary artery disease and normal multislice computed tomographic findings: a prospective management outcome study. Arch Intern Med 167:1686–1689

Halliburton SS, Schoenhagen P, Nair A, Stillman A, Lieber M, Murat Tuzcu E, Geoffrey Vince D, White RD (2006) Contrast enhancement of coronary atherosclerotic plaque: a high-resolution, multidetector-row computed tomography study of pressure-perfused, human ex-vivo coronary arteries. Coron Artery Dis 17:553–560

Hamon M, Biondi-Zoccai GG, Malagutti P, Agostoni P, Morello R, Valgimigli M (2006) Diagnostic performance of multislice spiral computed tomography of coronary arteries as compared with conventional invasive coronary angiography: a meta-analysis. J Am Coll Cardiol 48:1896–1910

Hoffmann MH, Shi H, Schmitz BL, Schmid FT, Lieberknecht M, Schulze R, Ludwig B, Kroschel U, Jahnke N, Haerer W, Brambs HJ, Aschoff AJ (2005) Noninvasive coronary angiography with multislice computed tomography. JAMA 293:2471–2478

Jahnke C, Paetsch I, Achenbach S, Schnackenburg B, Gebker R, Fleck E, Nagel E (2006) Coronary MR imaging: breath-hold capability and patterns, coronary artery rest periods, and beta-blocker use. Radiology 239:71–78

Johnson TR, Krauss B, Sedlmair M, Grasruck M, Bruder H, Morhard D, Fink C, Weckbach S, Lenhard M, Schmidt B, Flohr T, Reiser MF, Becker CR (2007) Material differentiation by dual energy CT: initial experience. Eur Radiol 17:1510–1517

Juergens KU, Seifarth H, Range F, Wienbeck S, Wenker M, Heindel W, Fischbach R (2008) Automated threshold-based 3D segmentation versus short-axis planimetry for assessment of global left ventricular function with dual-source MDCT. AJR Am J Roentgenol 190:308–314

Klass O, Jeltsch M, Feuerlein S, Brunner H, Nagel HD, Walker M, Brambs H-J, Hoffmann MH (2008) Prospectively-Gated Axial CT Coronary Angiography: Preliminary Experiences with a Novel Low-Dose Scan Technique. Invest Radiol (submitted)

Mahnken AH, Seyfarth T, Flohr T, Herzog C, Stahl J, Stanzel S, Kuettner A, Wildberger JE, Gunther RW (2005) Flat-panel detector computed tomography for the assessment of coronary artery stents: phantom study in comparison with 16-slice spiral computed tomography. Invest Radiol 40:8–13

Marano R, Liguori C, Rinaldi P, Storto ML, Politi MA, Savino G, Bonomo L (2007) Coronary artery bypass grafts and MDCT imaging: what to know and what to look for. Eur Radiol 17:3166–3178

Meijboom WB, van Mieghem CA, Mollet NR, Pugliese F, Weustink AC, van Pelt N, Cademartiri F, Nieman K, Boersma E, de Jaegere P, Krestin GP, de Feyter PJ (2007) 64-slice computed tomography coronary angiography in patients with high, intermediate, or low pretest probability of significant coronary artery disease. J Am Coll Cardiol 50:1469–1475

Orakzai SH, Orakzai RH, Nasir K, Budoff MJ (2006) Assessment of cardiac function using multidetector row computed tomography. J Comput Assist Tomogr 30:555–563

Pouleur A-C, le Polain de Waroux J-B, Pasquet A, Vanoverschelde J-LJ, Gerber BL (2007) Aortic Valve Area Assessment: Multidetector CT Compared with Cine MR Imaging and Transthoracic and Transesophageal Echocardiography. Radiology 244:745–754

Prokop M (2003) Multislice CT: technical principles and future trends. Eur Radiol 13 Suppl 5:M3–M13

Pugliese F, Mollet NR, Runza G, van Mieghem C, Meijboom WB, Malagutti P, Baks T, Krestin GP, deFeyter PJ, Cademartiri F (2006) Diagnostic accuracy of noninvasive 64-slice CT coronary angiography in patients with stable angina pectoris. Eur Radiol 16:575–582

Roessl E, Proksa R (2007) K-edge imaging in x-ray computed tomography using multi-bin photon counting detectors. Phys Med Biol 52:4679–4696

Shechter G, Resar JR, McVeigh ER (2005) Rest period duration of the coronary arteries: implications for magnetic resonance coronary angiography. Med Phys 32:255–262

Simon AR, Baraki H, Weidemann J, Harringer W, Galanski M, Haverich A (2007) High-resolution 64-slice helical-computer-assisted-tomographical-angiography as a diagnostic tool before CABG surgery: the dawn of a new era? Eur J Cardiothorac Surg 32:896–901

Topol EJ, Nissen SE (1995) Our preoccupation with coronary luminology: the dissociation between clinical and angiographic findings in ischemic heart disease. Circulation 92:2333–2342

Wang Y, Vidan E, Bergman GW (1999) Cardiac motion of coronary arteries: variability in the rest period and implications for coronary MR angiography. Radiology 213:751–758

## 17

# Assessment of Coronary Artery Stents by Coronary CT Angiography

David Maintz and Harald Seifarth

## CONTENTS

**ABSTRACT**

Stents reduce the acute risk of a coronary intervention and reduce the risk of restenosis afterwards. Today, stent placement is the most frequently performed coronary revascularization treatment. CT represents a possible noninvasive method for the detection of in-stent restenosis, but in the presence of stents imaging, it is impeded by artifacts. Therefore, coronary CT angiography for the evaluation of stents is a controversial topic. Knowledge of the clinical background of the patient, stent type, location of the stent, scanner technology, scan protocols, and image reconstruction methods are crucial to define an indication for the exam and to correctly interpret scan results.

D. Maintz, MD
Associate Professor, Department of Clinical Radiology, University of Muenster, Albert-Schweitzer-Strasse 33, 48149 Münster, Germany

H. Seifarth, MD
Department of Clinical Radiology, University of Muenster, Albert-Schweitzer-Strasse 33, 48149 Münster, Germany

## 17.1
## Background Information on Coronary Stents

### 17.1.1
### Epidemiology

Percutaneous coronary stent placement has become the preferred coronary revascularization strategy in most countries. Ninety-one percent of discharges with angioplasty were reported to have a stent inserted (Rosamond et al. 2008). Approximately 620,000 coronary stent procedures have been performed in the United States in the year 2008, compared to 469,000 coronary bypass procedures (in 261,000 patients).

### 17.1.2
### Coronary Artery Stent Types

Coronary artery stents are wire mesh tubes used to prop open an artery. They may be classified according to their modus of application (self-expandable or balloon expandable), their geometry (slotted tube, monofilament, multicellular, modular, or helical–sinusoidal), or the material they are made of (stainless steel, tantalum, cobalt alloy, platinum, nitinol, titanium, magnesium, or other). The material is the most important determinant of the radio-opacity of stents (atomic number, e.g., magnesium is 12, titanium is 22, chromium is 24, steel is 26, cobalt is 27, nickel is 28, and tantalum is 73). Steel is by far the stent material most frequently used, and is followed by cobalt alloys. The metallic mesh may have a covering (e.g., phosphorylcholine, carbon) or not (bare-metal stents [BMS]). Coverings may contain drugs that are eluded over time to prevent neo-intimal proliferation (drug-eluting stents [DES]). The most frequent antiproliferative substances in use are sirolimus (Cypher, Cordis, Johnson & Johnson) or paclitaxel (Taxus, Boston Scientific). In the last couple of years, DES have experienced a rapid increase over BMS. However, implantation rates vary regionally, mainly because of reasons related to reimbursement. In the United States, Portugal, and Switzerland, DES penetration rates exceed 80%, while in Germany DES and BMS are approximately equal (REMMELL et al. 2007).

### 17.1.3
### Stent Restenosis and Thrombosis

For BMS, in-stent restenosis rates have been reported ranging from 11 to 46% after 6 month (ANTONIUCCI et al. 1998). The need to treat restenosis with repeated percutaneous or surgical revascularization procedures was 14% for BMS (WILLIAMS et al. 2000).

DES have reduced the occurrence of restenosis and the need of repeated revascularization procedures by 50–70% (MOSES et al. 2003; STONE et al. 2004). One of the current concerns about DES is the increase of delayed in-stent thrombosis manifesting more than 30 days after stent implantation. This "late" manifestation of stent thrombosis may be related to delayed endothelialization of the stent and typically occurs when antiplatelet therapy is discontinued.

The length of an implanted stent is associated with an increased risk of both stent thrombosis and stent restenosis.

### 17.2
### CT of Coronary Stents

### 17.2.1
### Beam Hardening and "Blooming"

A combination of beam hardening and partial-volume artifacts causes artificial thickening of the stent struts during CT, the so-called blooming of stents. This blooming is responsible for the artificial lumen narrowing of stents. The magnitude of artifacts and consequently, the degree of lumen narrowing, depends on the type of stent, the stent diameter, and various scan and reconstruction parameters.

### 17.2.2
### CT Imaging Features Affecting Image Quality

#### 17.2.2.1
#### Contrast Enhancement

High-contrast enhancement of the coronary vessels is a prerequisite for coronary CTA, especially when coronary stents are to be evaluated. High contrast is crucial for stent imaging because sharper convolution kernels are used, which inherently produce noisier images, and at the same time, the window needs to be widened for evaluation decreasing the contrasts. High-contrast material concentration in the coronary vessels is achieved by using appropriate contrast material, by optimizing contrast material injection parameters, and by adequately timing the contrast material bolus using bolus tracking or a test bolus.

#### 17.2.2.2
#### Motion

Residual cardiac motion should be completely absent when performing coronary CTA for stent evaluation. While residual motion negatively affects all coronary CT exams, metal-related artifacts are especially increased. ECG gating, gantry rotation speed, heart rate, etc., apply as for all cardiac CT exams.

### 17.2.2.3
### Convolution Filters

The use of a dedicated, sharp convolution kernel (characterized by the presence of a relatively large proportion of high frequencies in the modulation–transfer curve and at the same time, less "overshoot" in the low-frequency region compared with conventional kernels) allows a significant decrease in the severity of blooming artifacts at the edges of high-attenuating structures. The positive effect of stent-dedicated kernels has been reported in a variety of studies (MAHNKEN et al. 2004; MAINTZ et al. 2003c; SEIFARTH et al. 2005) and can be appreciated in Fig. 17.1.

### 17.2.2.4
### Display Techniques and Window Settings

Maximum intensity projections or volume rendering techniques may be helpful to show the location of a coronary stent (Fig. 17.2). For the clinical evaluation of the coronary artery stent lumen, multiplanar reformations (MPR) of the data volume are needed. MPR are obtained in at least two orientations, longitudinal and perpendicular to the stent axis, to properly assess for the presence and, if positive, the degree of a stenosis.

The blooming artifacts can be decreased by widening the CT window compared with standard settings. However, the window may only be widened to a certain

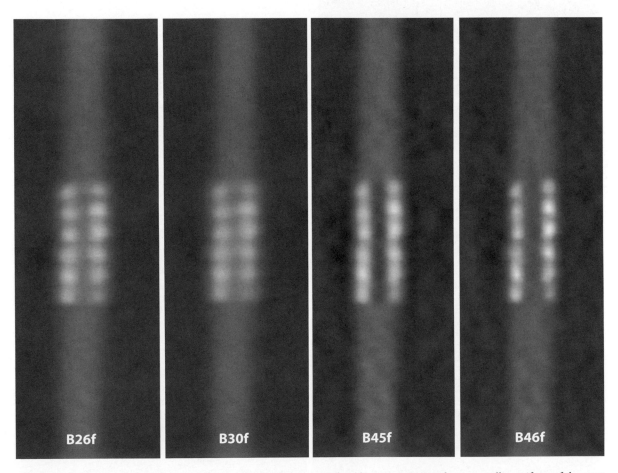

**Fig. 17.1.** The effect of different convolution kernels. Comparison of four different reconstruction protocols. Exemplary through-plane reformations of the PRO-Kinetic stent. The B26f kernel is a smooth kernel for cardiac applications, B30f is a standard medium-smooth kernel, B45f is a standard medium kernel, and B46f is a medium-sharp stent-dedicated kernel (all kernels by Siemens, Forchheim, Germany). Note artificial lumen narrowing due to metallic artifacts of the stent struts, almost equivalent in the B26f and B30f reconstructions. A medium kernel (B45f) increases the visible lumen diameter, but the stent lumen has an artificially low density. The use of a stent-dedicated kernel (B46f) combines good the lumen visibility and realistic lumen attenuation

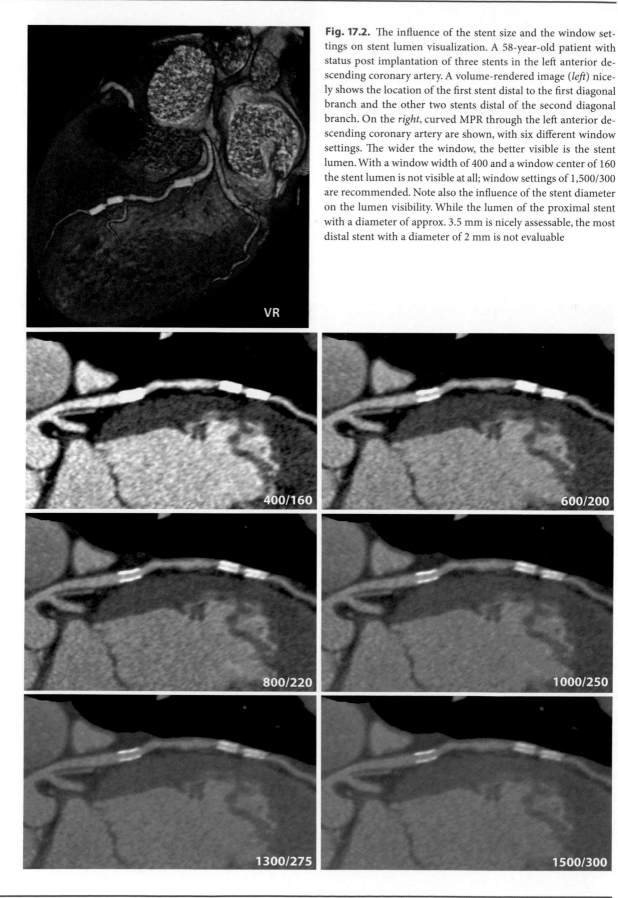

**Fig. 17.2.** The influence of the stent size and the window settings on stent lumen visualization. A 58-year-old patient with status post implantation of three stents in the left anterior descending coronary artery. A volume-rendered image (*left*) nicely shows the location of the first stent distal to the first diagonal branch and the other two stents distal of the second diagonal branch. On the *right*, curved MPR through the left anterior descending coronary artery are shown, with six different window settings. The wider the window, the better visible is the stent lumen. With a window width of 400 and a window center of 160 the stent lumen is not visible at all; window settings of 1,500/300 are recommended. Note also the influence of the stent diameter on the lumen visibility. While the lumen of the proximal stent with a diameter of approx. 3.5 mm is nicely assessable, the most distal stent with a diameter of 2 mm is not evaluable

degree to prevail enough contrast to evaluate lumen stenoses. Typically, a window setting with a window width of 1,500 HU and window center of 300 HU is used for stent evaluation (Fig. 17.2). Often it is advisable to "play" with the window settings.

## Stent Features Affecting CT Image Quality

### 17.3.1
### Stent Type

More than 100 different coronary stent types are known. Many of them are still available; others have been suspended but can still be found in patients that were treated in the past. Stents can be composed of different material. Most products are made from stainless steel. Cobalt–chromium is another material used frequently. Tantalum and nitinol (nickel–titanium alloy) are also being used but less frequently. Stents from biodegradable materials such as magnesium are being evaluated in phase III studies. The degree of artifacts produced by stents from different materials depends largely on the atomic number of the material. Consequently, tantalum causes the strongest artifacts, followed by steel, cobalt–

chromium, and nitinol. Magnesium stents exhibit only minor artifacts. Some stents bear radio-opaque markers at the stent ends. These markers can cause additional artifacts, superimposing the stent lumen at the ends. Besides the underlying material, the appearance of steel stents varies depending on the individual design. Figure 17.3 demonstrates the variation of the appearance of 8 different coronary artery stents. A large number of different coronary artery stents has been evaluated by Maintz et al. (2006). In that publication CT images of 68 coronary stents can be found.

### 17.3.2
### Stent Location and Size

The diameter of the stent is another important factor influencing the lumen visibility. The larger the stent diameter, the higher the visible percentage of the lumen. Stents with a diameter of ≥3 mm can often be evaluated (Gilard et al. 2005). Figure 17.3 demonstrates good lumen visibility of a 3.5-mm stent in the left anterior descending artery (LAD), while a 2-mm stent more distally is unevaluable. In a study by Schuijf et al. (2004), 28% of stents with a diameter ≤3 mm, but only 10% of stents with a diameter >3 mm were unevaluable. Stent implantation in the left main (LM) and proximal LAD/proxi-

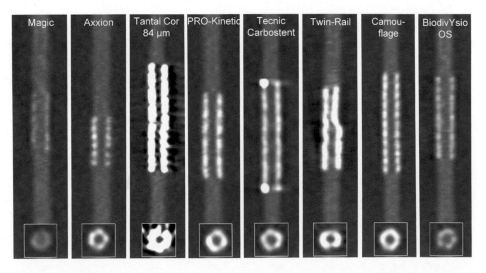

**Fig. 17.3.** Appearance of eight different coronary stents in DSCT. Longitudinal (*top*) and perpendicular (*small inserts on bottom*) reformations of in vitro experiments with eight different coronary stents. Note the variability of artifact magnitude, depending on the stent type. The Magic stent made from a magnesium alloy shows almost no artifacts and unrestricted lumen visibility, while severe blooming artifacts of the Tantal Cor stent make stent lumen assessment impossible. The Tecnic Carbostent exhibits radio-opaque markers at the stent ends. The Twin-Rail has a lumen diameter in part of 3 mm and in part of 1.5 mm, designed for vessel branches

mal left circumflex coronary artery (CCA) provides the best-case scenario for the use MDCT in the detection of in-stent restenosis. This is because of the relatively large stent diameters (usually approximately 3.9 mm in the LM), the fact that scan orientation is parallel to the stent axis and the relatively low motion in this area. Excellent results in patient studies confirm these considerations: in a series of 114 patients with 131 proximal stents (3.25 mm) CHABBERT et al. (2006) found lumen evaluability in 121 stents (92.4%) and correct identification of in-stent restenosis in 91.7% (prevalence of restenosis 22.5%), using 16-slice CT. GILARD et al. (2005) were able to evaluate the stent lumen of LM coronary stents (average diameter 3.9 mm) in 27/29 cases and to identify 4/4 in-stent restenoses. Identification of neo-intimal hyperplasia with lumen reduction of less than 35% was not possible in this 16-slice MDCT study.

VAN MIEGHEM et al. (2006) evaluated a large collective of patients with left main coronary stents using 16-slice CT ($n = 27$) or 64-slice CT ($n = 43$). All 10 of 70

**Table 17.1.** Literature overview on patient studies evaluating coronary artery stents using different CT scanner generations. The number of examined patients and stents is given; the diagnostic performance for the detection of stent restenosis and the percentage of stented segments that had to be excluded because of inferior image quality

| Scanner | Patients ($n$) | Stents ($n$) | Sensitivity (%) | Specificity (%) | PPV (%) | NPV (%) | Accuracy (%) | Excluded (%) |
|---|---|---|---|---|---|---|---|---|
| DSCT | | | | | | | | |
| PUGLIESE et al. 2007 | 100 | 178 | 94 | 92 | 77 | 98 | | 0 |
| 64-slice CT | | | | | | | | |
| CADEMARTIRI et al. 2007 | 182 | 192 | 95 | 93 | 63.3 | 99.3 | | 7.3 |
| DAS et al. 2007 | 53 | 110 | 96.9 | 88 | 77.5 | 98.5 | 91 | 0 |
| CARRABBA et al. 2007 | 41 | 87 | 84 | 97 | 92 | 97 | 96 | 0 |
| SCHUIJF et al. 2007 | 50 | 76 | 100 | 100 | | | | 14 |
| CARBONE et al. 2008 | 55 | 88 | 75 | 86 | | | | 28 |
| VAN MIEGHEM et al. 2006 | 74[a] | 162 | 100 | 91 | 67 | 100 | 93 | 5.4 |
| RIXE et al. 2006 | 64 | 102 | 86 | 98 | | | | 42 |
| EHARA et al. 2007 | 81 | 125 | 91 | 93 | 77 | 98 | | 12 |
| ONCEL et al. 2007 | 30 | 39 | 89 | 95 | 94 | 90 | | 0 |
| RIST et al. 2006 | 25 | 46 | 75 | 92 | 67 | 94 | 89 | 2 |
| 40-slice CT | | | | | | | | |
| GASPAR et al. 2005 | 65 | 111 | 88.9 | 80.6 | 47.1 | 97.4 | | 0 |
| 16-slice CT | | | | | | | | |
| SCHUIJF et al. 2004 | 22 | 68 | 78 | 100 | | | | 23 |
| CADEMARTIRI et al. 2005 | 51 | 76 | 83 | 98 | 83 | 97 | | 2.6 |
| GILARD et al. 2006 | 143[b] | 232 | 86 | 100 | 100 | 99 | | 46 |
| CHABBERT et al. 2006 | 134 | 145 | 92 | 67 | 43 | 97 | | 16.6 |
| KEFER et al. 2006 | 50 | 69 | 67 | 98 | | | 90 | 0 |

[a] $n = 27$ were scanned on a 16-slice CT

[b] Numbers given for fraction of stents larger than 3 mm in diameter

in-stent restenoses were correctly identified. However, there were also five false-positive results (sensitivity of 100%, specificity of 91%).

## Results of Stent Imaging with Different CT Scanners

Electron-beam CT (EBCT) enabled exact localization of coronary stents and indirect evaluation of stent patency by cine loop evaluation and time-attenuation curve analysis (Mohlenkamp et al. 1999; Pump et al. 1998, 2000; Schmermund et al. 1998). However, EBCT has been replaced by MDCT at most sites, mainly because of limitations in spatial resolution.

First results of coronary stent imaging using four-slice MDCT revealed that reliable lumen assessment was not possible due to severe blooming artifacts in vitro and in vivo (Mahnken et al. 2004; Kruger et al. 2003; Maintz et al. 2003a,b). Sixteen-slice MDCT systems with increased spatial and temporal resolution as well as optimized reconstruction algorithms improved general image quality and stent accessibility. Depending on stent type, scanner hardware, and convolution kernel, artificial lumen narrowing ranged from 20 to 100% (Mahnken et al. 2004; Maintz et al. 2003c). In a clinical study by Gilard et al. (2006), the lumen visibility depended on the stent diameter: on average, 64% (126/190 stents) were visible; of stents with a diameter >3 mm, 81% were visible, but only 51% of stents with a diameter ≤3 mm were visible. Likewise, restenosis detection sensitivity and specificity were 54 and 100% for small stents ≤3 mm, and 86% and 100% for larger stents >3 mm.

Sixty-four-slice MDCT and dual-source CT represent state-of-the-art technology for coronary stent assessment. However, detection rates of in-stent restenoses vary in several studies (Table 17.1). Rist et al. (2006) report a sensitivity and specificity of 75 and 92% for the detection of significant in-stent disease. In a larger study with 102 coronary stents (Rixe et al. 2006), sensitivity and specificity for the detection of stenoses were 86 and 98%, but only 58% were evaluable regarding lumen visibility. In another study, the detection rate of in-stent stenosis was 100%, and 86% of stents were evaluable (Schuijf et al. 2007). Only one study on dual-source CT for detecting in-stent restenosis has been published yet (Pugliese et al. 2007): 100 patients with chest pain after coronary stenting were investigated by dual-scan CT (DSCT)-CA. There were 178 stented lesions. Thirty-nine of 100 (39%) patients had angiographically proven restenosis. Sensitivity, specificity, positive predictive value (PPV), and negative predictive value (NPV) of DSCT-CA, calculated in all stents, were 94, 92, 77, and 98%, respectively. In stents ≥3.5 of mm (*n* = 78), sensitivity, specificity, PPV, NPV were 100%; in 3-mm stents (*n* = 59), sensitivity and NPV were 100%, specificity was 97%, PPV was 91%; in stents ≤2.75 mm (*n* = 41), sensitivity was 84%, specificity was 64%, PPV was 52%, and NPV was 90%. Nine stents ≤2.75 mm were not interpretable. The authors conclude that DSCT-CA performs well in the detection of in-stent restenosis. Although DSCT-CA leads to frequent false positive findings in smaller stents (≤2.75 mm), it reliably rules out in-stent restenosis irrespective of stent size.

## References

Antoniucci D, Valenti R, Santoro GM et al. (1998) Restenosis after coronary stenting in current clinical practice. Am Heart J 135:510–518

Cademartiri F, Mollet N, Lemos PA et al. (2005) Usefulness of multislice computed tomographic coronary angiography to assess in-stent restenosis. Am J Cardiol 96:799–802

Cademartiri F, Schuijf JD, Pugliese F et al. (2007) Usefulness of 64-slice multislice computed tomography coronary angiography to assess in-stent restenosis. J Am Coll Cardiol 49:2204–2210

Carbone I, Francone M, Algeri E et al. (2008) Noninvasive evaluation of coronary artery stent patency with retrospectively ECG-gated 64-slice CT angiography. Eur Radiol 18:234–243

Carrabba N, Bamoshmoosh M, Carusi LM et al. (2007) Usefulness of 64-slice multidetector computed tomography for detecting drug eluting in-stent restenosis. Am J Cardiol 100:1754–1758

Chabbert V, Carrie D, Bennaceur M et al. (2006) Evaluation of in-stent restenosis in proximal coronary arteries with multidetector computed tomography (MDCT). Eur Radiol 17:1452–1463

Das KM, El-Menyar AA, Salam AM et al. (2007) Contrast-enhanced 64-section coronary multidetector CT angiography versus conventional coronary angiography for stent assessment. Radiology 245:424–432

Ehara M, Kawai M, Surmely JF et al. (2007) Diagnostic accuracy of coronary in-stent restenosis using 64-slice computed tomography: comparison with invasive coronary angiography. J Am Coll Cardiol 49:951–959

Gaspar T, Halon DA, Lewis BS et al. (2005) Diagnosis of coronary in-stent restenosis with multidetector row spiral computed tomography. J Am Coll Cardiol 46:1573–1579

Gilard M, Cornily JC, Rioufol G et al. (2005) Noninvasive assessment of left main coronary stent patency with 16-slice computed tomography. Am J Cardiol 95:110–112

Gilard M, Cornily JC, Pennec PY et al. (2006) Assessment of coronary artery stents by 16 slice computed tomography. Heart 92:58–61

Kefer JM, Coche E, Vanoverschelde JL, Gerber BL (2006) Diagnostic accuracy of 16-slice multidetector-row CT for detection of in-stent restenosis vs detection of stenosis in nonstented coronary arteries. Eur Radiol 17:87–96

Kruger S, Mahnken AH, Sinha AM et al. (2003) Multislice spiral computed tomography for the detection of coronary stent restenosis and patency. Int J Cardiol 89:167–172

Mahnken AH, Buecker A, Wildberger JE et al. (2004) Coronary artery stents in multislice computed tomography: in vitro artifact evaluation. Invest Radiol 39:27–33

Maintz D, Grude M, Fallenberg EM, Heindel W, Fischbach R (2003a) Assessment of coronary arterial stents by multislice-CT angiography. Acta Radiol 44:597–603

Maintz D, Juergens KU, Wichter T, Grude M, Heindel W, Fischbach R (2003b) Imaging of coronary artery stents using multislice computed tomography: in vitro evaluation. Eur Radiol 13:830–835

Maintz D, Seifarth H, Flohr T et al. (2003c) Improved coronary artery stent visualization and in-stent stenosis detection using 16-slice computed-tomography and dedicated image reconstruction technique. Invest Radiol 38:790–795

Maintz D, Seifarth H, Raupach R et al. (2006) 64-slice multidetector coronary CT angiography: in vitro evaluation of 68 different stents. Eur Radiol 16:818–826

Mohlenkamp S, Pump H, Baumgart D et al. (1999) Minimally invasive evaluation of coronary stents with electron beam computed tomography: in vivo and in vitro experience. Catheter Cardiovasc Interv 48:39–47

Moses JW, Leon MB, Popma JJ et al. (2003) Sirolimus-eluting stents versus standard stents in patients with stenosis in a native coronary artery. N Engl J Med 349:1315–1323

Oncel D, Oncel G, Karaca M (2007) Coronary stent patency and in-stent restenosis: determination with 64-section multidetector CT coronary angiography-initial experience. Radiology 242:403–409

Pugliese F, Weustink AC, Van Mieghem C et al. (2007) Dual-source coronary computed tomography angiography for detecting in-stent restenosis. Heart doi:10.1136/hrt.2007

Pump H, Moehlenkamp S, Sehnert C et al. (1998) Electron-beam CT in the noninvasive assessment of coronary stent patency. Acad Radiol 5:858–862

Pump H, Mohlenkamp S, Sehnert CA et al. (2000) Coronary arterial stent patency: assessment with electron-beam CT. Radiology 214:447–452

Remmel M, Hartmann F, Harland LC, Schunkert H, Radke PW (2007) Rational use of drug-eluting stents: a comparison of different policies. Crit Pathw Cardiol 6:85–89

Rist C, von Ziegler F, Nikolaou K et al. (2006) Assessment of coronary artery stent patency and restenosis using 64-slice computed tomography. Acad Radiol 13:1465–1473

Rixe J, Achenbach S, Ropers D et al. (2006) Assessment of coronary artery stent restenosis by 64-slice multi-detector computed tomography. Eur Heart J 27:2567–2572

Rosamond W, Flegal K, Furie K et al. (2007) Heart disease and stroke statistics, 2008 update. A report from the American Heart Association Statistics Committee and Stroke Statistics Subcommittee. Circulation 117:e25–e146

Schmermund A, Rensing BJ, Sheedy PF, Bell MR, Rumberger JA (1998) Intravenous electron-beam computed tomographic coronary angiography for segmental analysis of coronary artery stenoses. J Am Coll Cardiol 31:1547–1554

Schuijf JD, Bax JJ, Jukema JW et al. (2004) Feasibility of assessment of coronary stent patency using 16-slice computed tomography. Am J Cardiol 94:427–430

Schuijf JD, Pundziute G, Jukema JW et al. (2007) Evaluation of patients with previous coronary stent implantation with 64-section CT. Radiology 245:416–423

Seifarth H, Raupach R, Schaller S et al. (2005) Assessment of coronary artery stents using 16-slice MDCT angiography: evaluation of a dedicated reconstruction kernel and a noise reduction filter. Eur Radiol 15:721–726

Stone GW, Ellis SG, Cox DA et al. (2004) A polymer-based, paclitaxel-eluting stent in patients with coronary artery disease. N Engl J Med 350:221–231

Van Mieghem CA, Cademartiri F, Mollet NR et al. (2006) Multislice spiral computed tomography for the evaluation of stent patency after left main coronary artery stenting: a comparison with conventional coronary angiography and intravascular ultrasound. Circulation 114:645–653

Williams DO, Holubkov R, Yeh W et al. (2000) Percutaneous coronary intervention in the current era compared with 1985—the National Heart, Lung, and Blood Institute Registries. Circulation 102:2945–2951

# Acute Chest Pain

Joachim-Ernst Wildberger

**18**

## CONTENTS

### ABSTRACT

Vascular emergencies play an important role amongst the various differential diagnoses for acute chest pain. Pulmonary embolism, acute aortic syndromes as well as acute coronary artery disease have to be considered. The latest scanner technology available (> 64-slice multi-detector-row spiral CT platforms) allows for a straight-forward work-up in the emergency situation. A dedicated triage based on a sophisticated clinical assessment, however, ist required.

## 18.1
## Introduction

Acute chest pain is one of the major clinical emergency conditions. Various differential diagnoses have to be considered, some of them are potentially life-threatening. CT assessment for vascular pathologies of the chest can be split up into three major categories. Pulmonary embolism, acute aortic syndromes and coronary artery disease (CAD) require a rapid, reliable and effective diagnostic pathway allowing for an immediate therapeutic decision thereafter. A simple and objective cross-sectional modality should ideally be available on a 24/7 basis.

Latest multi-detector-row spiral computed tomography (MDCT) scanners are able of such an "one-stop-strategy". Cardiac imaging can be incorporated into established examination standard operating procedures for non-cardiac vascular and non-vascular imaging of chest disorders. This approach can be summarized with the buzzword "triple rule-out™" (Gallagher and Raff 2008).

At first, it should be checked whether a CT angiography (CTA) of the coronaries is technically feasible with

J.-E. Wildberger, MD

Professor, Department of Radiology, University Hospital Maastricht, P.O. Box 5800, 6202 AZ Maastricht, The Netherlands

the equipment available. If so, referring physician and radiologist should discuss what kind of exam is clinically essential, especially in terms of radiation protection. An ECG-synchronization of the data set is a prerequisite for the evaluation of the coronary arteries. A differentiated approach utilizing MDCT for emergency conditions in so called "chest pain units" is under evaluation in many centres.

## 18.2
### Acute Pulmonary Embolism

Due to its mostly unspecific clinical presentation, pulmonary embolism (PE) is often referred to as the great masquerader and remains a diagnostic challenge (WILDBERGER et al. 2005). Accordingly, distinct diagnostic algorithms are needed to assist the general clinical assessment (e.g. using the Wells score; WELLS et al. 2000) and to optimise the use of diagnostic tests, especially in an emergency department setting. CTA is an appropriate initial test in patients with intermediate and high-clinical suspicion of PE under emergency conditions (RYU et al. 2001). In patients with a low clinical probability of PE, the most cost-saving strategy involves plasma D-dimer assessment, a degradation product of cross-linked fibrin (PERRIER et al. 2004). In the CT work-up, however, there is no diagnostic need for an ECG-synchronization of the data set, as this clinical question is safely answered by MDCT (SCHOEPF et al. 2005; BRITISH THORACIC SOCIETY STANDARDS OF CARE COMMITTEE PULMONARY EMBOLISM GUIDELINE DEVELOPMENT GROUP 2003). Already 4-detector-row platforms have proven excellent negative predictive values. Despite the direct visualization of thrombi and emboli, also secondary findings can be delineated. These include areas of decreased density as well as consolidated areas localized within the lung parenchyma (GHAYE et al. 2002). Right heart failure can be indirectly assessed by an enlargement of the right heart chambers (QUIROZ et al. 2004) as well as straightening of the interventricular septum and bowing into the left ventricle (HE et al. 2006).

## 18.3
### Acute Aortic Syndromes

MDCT has become the first-line imaging test in the assessment of acute aortic syndromes. A sudden onset of tearing and ripping chest discomfort can be summarized as the classic clinical presentation. Poorly regulated hypertension and soft-tissue disorders like Marfan´s disease are common underlying causes for the development of intramural hematoma, aortic dissection as well as aortic aneurysms and rupture. MDCT is nowadays referred to as the gold standard for the non-invasive clarification of these problems. The 4-detector-row CT platforms already allow for a combined assessment of the thoracic and abdominal aorta within a single breath-hold, therefore necessitating just a single contrast medium delivery.

The diagnostic work-up of the ascending aorta, however, may remain a formidable task. Here, ECG-gating minimizes transmission of cardiac motion. For 4-detector-row and 16-detector-row CT scanner, the increase in scan time will limit the overall scan range. Therefore, a differentiation is warranted, e.g. utilizing ECG-synchronization for Stanford A dissection, while a dissection originating in descending aorta (Stanford B) might be diagnosed with a "standard" (sub-)millimeter collimated MDCT protocol. The quality and speed of CTA is superior to other imaging modalities, and it is also cheaper and less invasive. CTA of the aorta has proven to be superior in diagnostic accuracy to conventional arteriography in several applications (YU et al. 2007).

## 18.4
### Acute CAD

A combined assessment of the lung parenchyma, the vasculature of the chest as well as a depiction of the heart and the coronaries can be done with the latest scanner technology available (256-detector-row, 320-detector-row CT per rotation; dual-source technology) (RYBICKI et al. 2008; FLOHR et al. 2006). From today´s standpoint, significant coronary stenosis can also be safely excluded using 64-detector-row MDCT platforms with retrospective ECG-gating. For 64-detector-row scanners, the use of beta-blockers is still needed to bring down the heart rate of the patient, as the temporal resolution is still not sufficient for imaging of unselected patients (ACHENBACH et al. 2008). Heart rates of 60–65 bpm are suggested to achieve good image quality. This premedication will limit the options under emergency conditions, as this might be time-consuming, and several contraindications have to be taken into account.

Patients with an intermediate pre-test likelihood for a CAD are especially of major interest (LEBER et al. 2007). Recently, a dedicated graduated scheme was published in a consensus statement of the North American Society of Cardiac Imaging and the European Society of Cardiac Imaging (Stillman et al. 2007). Hence, MDCT is especially valuable in the exclusion of CAD in patients with a normal and non-specific laboratory testing in combination with a negative ECG (Fig. 18.1). On the other hand, it should also be stressed that CTA of the coronaries does not add important information in patients with a high pre-test likelihood and known CAD (Meijboom et al. 2007).

In general, the contrast material application should be adapted according to the differential diagnoses that have to be addressed: On the one hand, an opacification of the pulmonary arteries is needed for the exclusion of pulmonary embolism. On the other hand, optimal density values are needed for the arterial vessels (aorta, coronaries) as well. This optimization might be the most crucial part of the entire exam, as quite complex contrast regimens have been inaugurated.

Generally speaking, a moderate to high iodine delivery rate (IDR) is needed for CTA of the chest. Therefore, 1.5–2.0 g iodine/s should be administered intravenously. The contrast medium delivery has to be maintained for a longer time, as an opacification of the pulmonary circulation and the systemic circulation is needed at the same time. Dual-head power injectors, individual adaptation of the contrast delivery

(test bolus methodology, bolus-tracking [ROI in the ascending aorta]) and a scanner-based adaptation of the overall injection duration according to the CTA acquisition time guarantee a robust regimen even under emergency conditions. Advanced protocols include biphasic and even triphasic contrast medium protocols for this "one-stop-shop" approach (Johnson et al. 2007; Litmanovitch et al. 2008). A high-flow IDR in combination with a larger overall volume (130 mL @ 370 mg iodine and 160 mL @ 300 mg iodine) have been advocated (Johnson et al. 2008b). Medication directly on the CT-table with glyceryl trinitrates (GLN) s.l. (sublingual application) might be added for vasodilatation during the scan procedure (Achenbach et al. 2008). A caudo-cranial scan direction is favourable for optimal results (Johnson et al. 2008b). Patients should be instructed to hold their breath after mild inspiration in order to avoid a Valsalva-effect and a split enhancement within the pulmonary vasculature. Transient interruption of contrast of the pulmonary arteries represents a flow-related phenomenon associated with an increased inferior vena cava contribution to the right side of the heart (Wittram and Yoo 2007).

In summary, modern MDCT equipment allows for a robust and straight-forward diagnostic work-up for acute chest pain in the emergency situation. The latest scanner technology guarantees a diagnostic examination quality without pre-medication even in acutely ill

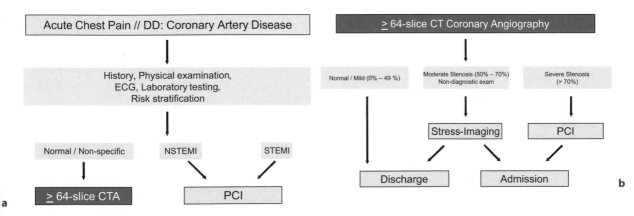

**Fig. 18.1. a** Pathway for patients with acute chest pain, in which CAD is one potential differential diagnosis. In case of a well-known CAD and a high pre-test likelihood, a percutaneous catheter intervention (PCI) should be performed. In case of non-specific symptoms, a MDCT angiography of the coronaries is technically feasible for the exclusion of CAD. **b** According to the results of the coronary MDCT angiography, the patient can be discharged (exclusion of relevant CAD) or should be treated (proof of hemodynamically relevant stenoses). In indeterminate cases as well as in non-conclusive exams, additional stress-testing is recommended (modified from: Stillman AE et al. (2007) Use of multi-detector computed tomography for the assessment of acute chest pain: a consensus statement of the North American Society of Cardiac Imaging and the European Society of Cardiac Radiology. Eur Radiol 17:2196–2207)

patients with high heart rates (ACHENBACH et al. 2008). Using DSCT, overall sensitivity rates for the cause of chest pain of 98% as well as a 100% negative predictive value for coronary stenoses have been reported (JOHNSON et al. 2008a). In order to avoid an overutilization of this method, precise indications for its use will have to be determined (WHITE 2007). A dedicated triage after a sophisticated clinical assessment is required especially in younger patients due to radiation safety necessities.

Further studies will prove whether this clinical pathway is also cost-effective in the long run, as patients with a negative MDCT/DSCT scan can be discharged directly from the emergency ward without further diagnostics (and therapy).

# References

Achenbach S, Anders K, Kalender WA (2008) Dual-source cardiac computed tomography: image quality and dose considerations. Eur Radiol 18:1188–1198

British Thoracic Society Standards of Care Committee Pulmonary Embolism Guideline Development Group (2003) British Thoracic Society guidelines for the management of suspected acute pulmonary embolism. Thorax 58:470–483

Flohr TG, McCollough CH, Bruder H, Petersilka M, Gruber K, Süss C, Grasruck M, Stierstorfer K, Krauss B, Raupach R, Primak AN, Küttner A, Achenbach S, Becker C, Kopp A, Ohnesorge BM (2006) First performance evaluation of a dual-source CT (DSCT) system. Eur Radiol 16:256–268

Gallagher MJ, Raff GL (2008) Use of multidetector-row CT for the evaluation of emergency room patients with chest pain: the so-called "triple rule-out". Catheter Cardiovasc Interv 71:92–99

Ghaye B, Remy J, Remy-Jardin M (2002) Non-traumatic thoracic emergencies: CT diagnosis of acute pulmonary embolism: the first 10 years. Eur Radiol 12:1886–1905

He H, Stein MW, Zalta B, Haramati LB (2006) Computed tomography evaluation of right heart dysfunction in patients with acute pulmonary embolism. J Comput Assist Tomogr 30:262–266

Johnson TR, Nikolaou K, Wintersperger BJ, Fink C, Rist C, Leber AW, Knez A, Reiser MF, Becker CR (2007) Optimization of contrast material administration for electrocardiogram-gated computed tomographic angiography of the chest. J Comput Assist Tomogr 31:265–271

Johnson TR, Nikolaou K, Becker A, Leber AW, Rist C, Wintersperger BJ, Reiser MF, Becker CR (2008a) Dual-source CT for chest pain assessment. Eur Radiol 18:773–780

Johnson TR, Nikolaou K, Becker CR (2008b) Vascular: extended chest pain protocol. In: Seidensticker P, Hofmann L (eds) Dual source CT imaging. Springer; Berlin Heidelberg New York, ISBN 978-3-540-77601-7, pp 132–139

Leber AW, Johnson T, Becker A, von Ziegler F, Tittus J, Nikolaou K, Reiser M, Steinbeck G, Becker CR, Knez A (2007) Diagnostic accuracy of dual-source multi-detector-row CT-coronary angiography in patients with an intermediate pretest likelihood for coronary artery disease. Eur Heart J 28:2354–2360

Litmanovitch D, Zamboni GA, Hauser TH, Lin PJ, Clouse ME, Raptopoulos V (2008) ECG-gated chest CT angiography with 64-MDCT and tri-phasic IV contrast administration regimen in patients with acute non-specific chest pain. Eur Radiol 18:308–317

Meijboom WB, van Mieghem CA, Mollet NR, Pugliese F, Weustink AC, van Pelt N, Cademartiri F, Nieman K, Boersma E, de Jaegere P, Krestin GP, de Feyter PJ (2007) 64-detector-row computed tomography coronary angiography in patients with high, intermediate, or low pretest probability of significant coronary artery disease. J Am Coll Cardiol 50:1469–1475

Perrier A, Roy PM, Aujesky D, Chagnon I, Howarth N, Gourdier AL, Leftheriotis G, Barghouth G, Cornuz J, Hayoz D, Bounameaux H (2004) Diagnosing pulmonary embolism in outpatients with clinical assessment, D-dimer measurement, venous ultrasound, and helical computed tomography: a multicenter management study. Am J Med 116:291–299

Quiroz R, Kucher N, Schoepf UJ, Kipfmueller F, Solomon SD, Costello P, Goldhaber SZ (2004) Right ventricular enlargement on chest computed tomography: prognostic role in acute pulmonary embolism. Circulation 109:2401–2404

Rybicki FJ, Otero HJ, Steigner ML, Vorobiof G, Nallamshetty L, Mitsouras D, Ersoy H, Mather RT, Judy PF, Cai T, Coyner K, Schultz K, Whitmore AG, Di Carli MF (2008) Initial evaluation of coronary images from 320-detector row computed tomography. Int J Cardiovasc Imaging 24:535–546

Ryu JH, Swensen SJ, Olson EJ, Pellikka PA (2001) Diagnosis of pulmonary embolism with use of computed tomographic angiography. Mayo Clin Proc 76:59–65

Schoepf UJ, Savino G, Lake DR, Ravenel JG, Costello P (2005) The age of CT pulmonary angiography. J Thorac Imaging 20:273–279

Stillman AE, Oudkerk M, Ackerman M, Becker CR, Buszman PE, de Feyter PJ, Hoffmann U, Keadey MT, Marano R, Lipton MJ, Raff GL, Reddy GP, Rees MR, Rubin GD, Schoepf UJ, Tarulli G, van Beek EJ, Wexler L, White CS (2007) Use of multidetector computed tomography for the assessment of acute chest pain: a consensus statement of the North American Society of Cardiac Imaging and the European Society of Cardiac Radiology. Eur Radiol 17:2196–2207

Wells PS, Anderson DR, Rodger M, Ginsberg JS, Kearon C, Gent M, Turpie AG, Bormanis J, Weitz J, Chamberlain M, Bowie D, Barnes D, Hirsh J (2000) Derivation of a simple clinical model to categorize patients probability of pulmonary embolism: increasing the models utility with the SimpliRED D-dimer. Thromb Haemost 83:416–420

White CS (2007) Chest pain in the emergency department: potential role of multidetector CT. J Thorac Imaging 22:49–55

Wildberger JE, Mahnken AH, Das M, Küttner A, Lell M, Günther RW (2005) CT imaging in acute pulmonary embolism: diagnostic strategies. Eur Radiol 15:919–929

Wittram C, Yoo AJ (2007) Transient interruption of contrast on CT pulmonary angiography: proof of mechanism. J Thorac Imaging 22:125–129

Yu T, Zhu X, Tang L, Wang D, Saad N (2007) Review of CT angiography of aorta. Radiol Clin North Am 45:461–483

# The Role of Cardiac Computed Tomography in Cardiac Surgery

ALEXANDER LEMBCKE

19

## CONTENTS

A. LEMBCKE, MD
Department of Radiology, Charité, University Medicine Berlin,
Charitéplatz 1, 10117 Berlin, Germany

### ABSTRACT

Electrocardiogram-synchronized multidetector computed tomography (MDCT) allows for a comprehensive assessment of the heart that facilitates planning and performing surgical procedures. MDCT permits for a high-resolution three-dimensional visualization of cardiac structures along with a simultaneous evaluation of cardiac function. Used for the preoperative work-up MDCT enables the non-invasive evaluation of the coronary arteries. With its high negative predictive value MDCT can often exclude the presence of significant coronary artery stenoses, for example in patients scheduled for cardiac valve surgery. Additional applications include the assessment of the great thoracic vessels, the evaluation of the cardiac valves and the visualization and differential diagnosis of cardiac masses. The use of MDCT in the postoperative follow-up comprises the evaluation of coronary bypass grafts with excellent accuracy for the detection of bypass graft occlusions and stenoses. MDCT also enables the detection of complications after heart transplantation such as graft vasculopathy. In addition, MDCT is a valuable imaging tool for planning of redo cardiothoracic surgery in order to avoid potential life-threatening intraoperative complications.

## 19.1
## Introduction

Substantial technological advances in data acquisition and data processing leading to an improved spatial and temporal resolution have established a central role for multi-detector-row computed tomography (MDCT) in the evaluation of the operative cardiac patient.

## 19.2
## Noninvasive Coronary Artery Imaging in Cardiac Surgery

Several studies have demonstrated a fairly high sensitivity and specificity of MDCT for detecting significant stenoses, primarily in patients with intermediate pre-test probability, low heart rate, and low calcium score (ABDULLA et al. 2007; SUN et al. 2007; JANNE D'OTHEE et al. 2007; SUN et al. 2006; HAMON et al. 2006). In patients scheduled for non-coronary cardiac surgery, preoperative management usually requires invasive coronary angiography to evaluate the presence of concomitant coronary atherosclerosis and to detect significant coronary artery stenoses. A few investigations exist that demonstrated the value of noninvasive coronary angiography by MDCT as an alternative imaging method for the preoperative evaluation of the coronary arteries. In a series of patients with aortic valve stenosis, GILARD et al. (2006) found a sensitivity, specificity, and positive and negative predictive value (PPV and NPV, respectively) of 100%, 80%, 55%, and 100%, enabling invasive coronary angiography to be avoided in 80% of patients. However, in 20% of patients assessment of the vessel lumen by MDCT was prevented due to heavy calcifications (Agatston score >1,000). In contrast, LAISSY et al. (2007) found a sensitivity, specificity, and PPV and NPV of only 85%, 93%, 85%, and 98%, respectively, and TANAKA et al. (2007) found a sensitivity and specificity of only 89% and 80%, respectively, for detection of coronary artery stenoses in patients with aortic valve stenosis.

A similar investigation was performed by SCHEFFEL et al. (2007) for a group of patients with aortic valve regurgitation. In this study, sensitivity, specificity, PPV, and NPV of 100%, 95%, 87%, and 100%, respectively, were found. Preoperative invasive coronary angiography could have avoided in 70% of patients, while unnecessary invasive procedures would have been in only 4%.

In patients who have undergone cardiac transplantation coronary artery vasculopathy of the donor heart remains the major limitation to long-term survival. Some authors have investigated the diagnostic value of coronary artery calcium measurements for the early detection of graft vasculopathy (KNOLLMANN et al. 2000; LUDMAN et al. 1999; RATLIFF et al. 2004). However, the results of these studies were not conclusive, and therefore the value of coronary artery calcium measurements remains questionable in heart transplant recipients. Recent investigations suggest that noninvasive coronary angiography by MDCT is more reliable for the detection of a transplant coronary artery disease. For a group of heart transplant recipients, SIGURDSSON et al. (2006) found a sensitivity, specificity, PPV, and NPV of 94%, 79%, 65%, and 97%, respectively, and ROMEO et al. (2005) a sensitivity, specificity, PPV, and NPV of 83%, 95%, 71%, and 95%, respectively, for the detection of coronary artery stenosis in the transplanted heart. In contrast, PICHLER et al. (2008) observed a sensitivity and specificity of 70% and 70%, respectively, with to a high number of patients with non-assessable coronary artery segments. However, PPV and NPV in this study were 88% and 97%, respectively, confirming the potential of MDCT for the exclusion of significant transplant coronary artery disease.

## 19.3
## Coronary Artery Anomalies

The three-dimensional, high-detailed anatomic information provided by cardiac MDCT allows for a precise assessment of patients with known or suspected coronary artery anomalies. Numerous reports in the literature have demonstrated the accuracy of MDCT for detecting and characterizing of coronary artery anomalies (DODD et al. 2007; KIM et al. 2006; MANGHAT et al. 2005). Although MDCT has some intrinsic limitations (radiation exposure, intravenous contrast media administration), it is therefore regarded as an excellent non-invasive tool for clinical decision-making (i.e., the need for surgical intervention) and as part of the diagnostic workup in individuals with anomalous coronary arteries.

## 19.4
## Imaging in Coronary Artery Bypass Surgery

The implantation of coronary artery bypass grafts has revolutionized the treatment of patients with coronary artery disease and now represents the most frequent procedure performed in cardiac surgery. However, despite surgical revascularization, there remains a certain risk of ischemic symptoms in the postoperative period. An occlusion rate for saphenous vein bypass grafts of 50% has been described 15 years after surgery (FITZGIBBON et al. 1996). In patients with recurrent ischemic symptoms, conventional coronary angiography is therefore often required to diagnose potential bypass graft stenosis and to evaluate the progression of coronary atherosclerosis in the native coronary arteries. However, asymptomatic patients are not routinely examined by conventional angiography due to the associated risks and costs. MDCT may therefore play an

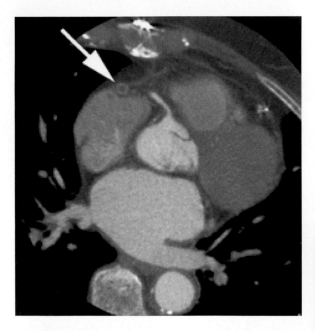

**Fig. 19.1.** A 56-year-old man who underwent coronary artery bypass grafting using a PTFE-graft. MDCT shows complete occlusion of the bypass (*arrow*)

important role as an alternative imaging method for the timely detection of bypass graft disease, although a routine screening by MDCT cannot be recommended due to radiation dose concerns. The latest MDCT scanner generations have substantially improved detail resolution, enabling excellent visualization of the entire bypass graft including the site of the distal anastomosis. In addition, the frequency and severity of artifacts, especially the occurrence of heavy streak artifacts caused by metal clips along the bypass graft, were significantly reduced. Using conventional angiography as the gold standard, the recent literature has described excellent results for the detection of bypass graft occlusion with sensitivities and specificities approaching 100% (Jones et al. 2007; Hamon et al. 2008). However, in a clinical setting it might be reasonable to not only evaluate the patency of the bypass graft, but also the presence of stenoses in the bypass graft or the native coronary arteries. This is often more difficult, especially in vessels with a smaller caliber or arteries with severe calcifications. However, with its high negative predictive value, MDCT can practically exclude significant graft disease, avoiding needless conventional angiography (Figs. 19.1 and 19.2). Based on the diameter measurements of an occluded venous bypass graft, MDCT may also allow for non-invasive differentiation between acute and chronic bypass graft occlusion as demonstrated earlier for electron-beam computed tomography (Enzweiler et al. 2003). This

could help in terms of clinical decision making and may prevent unnecessary re-canalization procedures after bypass surgery. Whereas MDCT is an efficient imaging method in the postoperative follow-up, its role in the preoperative diagnostic workup before coronary artery bypass surgery has not yet been well established. However, a few studies suggest that MDCT may accurately identify the target vessel for bypass surgery and may provide useful additional data on coronary morphology (for example, the extent of coronary calcifications) not obtained by conventional coronary angiography (Simon et al. 2007).

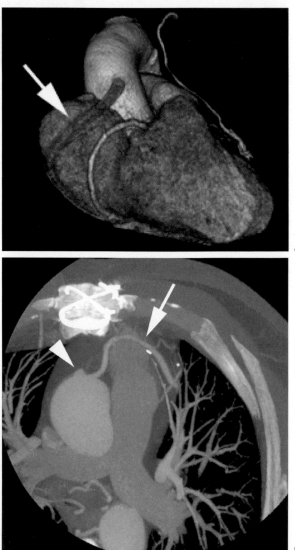

**Fig. 19.2a–c.** A 62-year-old man after coronary artery revascularization using two saphenous vein bypass grafts. MDCT clearly demonstrates the direct retrosternal course of a patent bypass vessel (*arrow*). The second bypass is occluded (*arrowhead*)

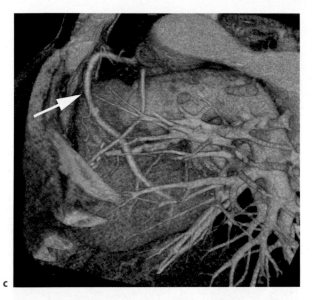

c

**Fig. 19.2a–c.** (*continued*) A 62-year-old man after coronary artery revascularization using two saphenous vein bypass grafts. MDCT clearly demonstrates the direct retrosternal course of a patent bypass vessel (*arrow*). The second bypass is occluded (*arrowhead*)

## 19.5
## Imaging for
## Planning Operative Perfusion Techniques

In patients with significant atherosclerosis, direct cannulation of the thoracic aorta for cardiopulmonary

bypass is associated with a substantial risk of cerebral embolism (MORINO et al. 2000; VAN DER LINDEN et al. 2001). In addition, an extensive circumferential calcification of the thoracic aorta (so-called porcelain aorta) represents a technical challenge for the cardiac surgeon, especially when aortic valve replacement of coronary artery bypass grafting is indicated (Fig. 19.3). Imaging by MDCT can accurately describe the site and extent of calcifications of the aortic valve and may therefore provide important information to be used for therapeutic decision making and definition of the surgical strategy evaluation.

## 19.6
## Imaging before Reoperative Cardiac Surgery

Cardiac reoperations are associated with a significantly higher risk than the initial procedure (SALOMON et al. 1990). Median sternotomy is a blind procedure that may result in injury of cardiac and extra-cardiac structures located adjacent to the posterior side of the sternum, such as the right ventricle, saphenous vein bypass grafts, the ascending aorta, and internal mammaria arteries. A close proximity of the right ventricle to the anterior chest wall is often caused by adhesions that form after previous surgery. Postsurgical adhesions may also cause migration of saphenous bypass grafts resulting in a retrosternal position with the risk of injury at re-sternotomy (Fig. 19.2). Thus, the assessment of the

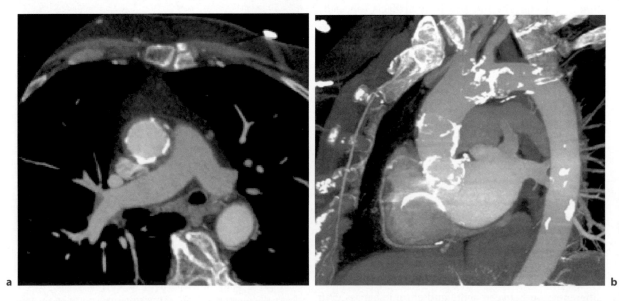

a                                                                                                                                          b

**Fig. 19.3a,b.** A 52-year-old man who was referred for aortic valve replacement due to high-grade stenosis. MDCT visualizes extensive circumferential calcifications in the entire thoracic aorta ("porcelain aorta")

anatomic relationship of the cardiac chambers, great thoracic arteries, and coronary artery bypass grafts to the chest wall in general, and the sternum in particular, is of utmost importance before reoperative cardiac surgery. Modification of surgical planning based on the preoperative assessment in MDCT may therefore help to prevent intraoperative complications and reduce perioperative mortality.

## 19.7
## Imaging in Heart Valve Surgery

### 19.7.1
### Aortic Valve Surgery

In patients with suspected aortic valve stenosis, a definite decision for surgery is generally based on the presence of symptoms in combination with a significant reduction of the aortic valve orifice area (AVA) during systole (BONOW et al. 2006). Different imaging modalities are currently in use to determine the aortic valve orifice area, but all have their own strengths and limitations. Invasive transvalvular pressure gradient measurements at cardiac catheterization were evaluated in numerous scientific studies and proved to be valuable in clinical practice for quantifying the aortic valve orifice area. However, cardiac catheterization is an invasive procedure associated with certain risks, especially when crossing the stenotic aortic valve (OMRAN et al.

2003). In addition, the Gorlin formula used at cardiac catheterization for quantifying the aortic valve orifice area has many well-described theoretical and practical limitations, which may result in inaccuracies in a variety of certain hemodynamic conditions (TURI 2005). In contrast, transthoracic echocardiography is a completely non-invasive and cost-efficient procedure that is relatively easy to handle and quick to perform. Echocardiography has been shown to be adequate to estimate the degree of stenosis in the majority of patients and is therefore widely used in the everyday clinical routine, maybe reducing the need for an invasive examination. However, echocardiography also has several well-known limitations, particularly a considerable variability depending on the quality of the patient's sonication conditions as well as the examiners level of expertise. Despite the good agreement between echocardiography and cardiac catheterization demonstrated in several experimental studies, there are numerous potential sources of error that may lead to significant discrepancies in AVA calculations, posing a dilemma in clinical decision making. Therefore, additional evaluation by direct visualization and planimetry of the AVA is often recommended. This can be done either by transesophageal echocardiography, magnetic resonance imaging, or alternatively by MDCT (Fig. 19.4). Recently published studies have also demonstrated a good reliability of planimetric AVA measurements by MDCT as compared with transesophageal echocardiography as well as magnetic resonance imaging (ALKADHI et al. 2006, 2006; BAUMERT et al. 2005). When comparing planimetric

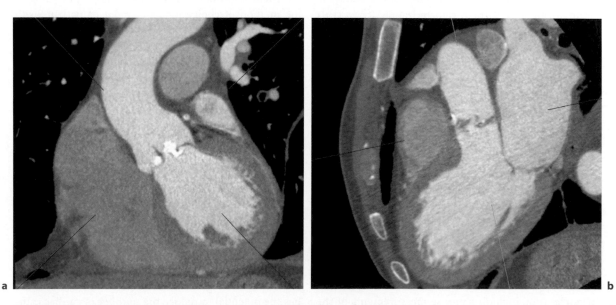

**Fig. 19.4a–d.** A 57-year-old man with bicuspid aortic valve. MDCT confirms heavy valvular calcifications and demonstrated a narrowed aortic valve orifice indicating severe valvular stenosis (**a–c**) (*see next page*)

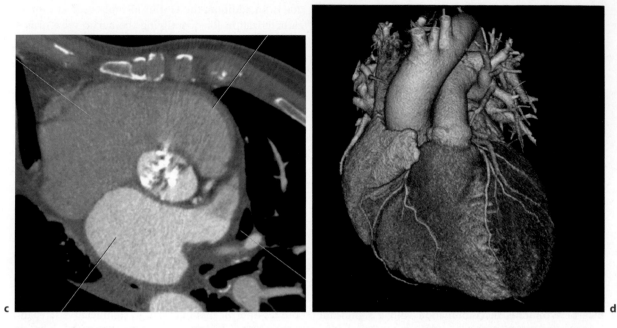

**Fig. 19.4a–d.** (*continued*) A 57-year-old man with bicuspid aortic valve. MDCT confirms heavy valvular calcifications and demonstrated a narrowed aortic valve orifice indicating severe valvular stenosis (**a–c**), but normal coronary arteries (**d**)

measurements of the anatomic AVA (obtained with MDCT, magnetic resonance imaging, or transesophageal echocardiography) with calculations of the hemodynamic effective AVA (using the continuity equation at transthoracic Doppler echocardiography or using the Gorlin formula at cardiac catheterization) (ALKADHI et al. 2006; DEBL et al. 2005). The difference between the actual anatomic AVA and the hemodynamic effective AVA can be explained by the fact that blood tends to flow through the center to the anatomic orifice. In addition, the planimetrically measured anatomic AVA represents a measurement at the time of maximal valve opening, whereas the calculated hemodynamic effective AVA represents an integration of measurements throughout the duration of valve opening.

Recent investigations also suggest that direct planimetric measurement of the aortic valve orifice area during diastole area provides useful additional information on the presence and severity of aortic valve regurgitation (Fig. 19.5). In addition, MDCT also provides important morphologic information on the aortic valve (bicuspid vs. tricuspid valve; severity of calcifications) and enables an exact three-dimensional visualization of the aortic root, including precise measurements of the aortic root diameters, which is of particular interest for

the cardiac surgeon with regard to therapeutic decision making (for example, with regard to the decision if aortic valve surgery should be performed with additional aortic root replacement or not).

There is no doubt that echocardiography remains the method of choice for assessment of patients with suspected aortic valve disease. However, MDCT may provide additional useful information when echocardiographic results are questionable due to poor sonication conditions, when echocardiographic findings do not match the clinical data, or if there is discordance between the quantitative data of echocardiography and cardiac catheterization. Moreover an additional planimetric evaluation of the aortic valve by MDCT may be useful in patients with borderline values at echocardiography or simply to confirm the diagnosis prior to surgery.

Used for preoperative risk assessment, MDCT at the same time allows for quantification of left ventricular function and noninvasive direct assessment of the coronary arteries (see above). With its high negative predictive value, MDCT might therefore be a suitable tool to exclude significant coronary artery stenosis and has the potential to reduce the number of cardiac catheterizations routinely performed to exclude concomi-

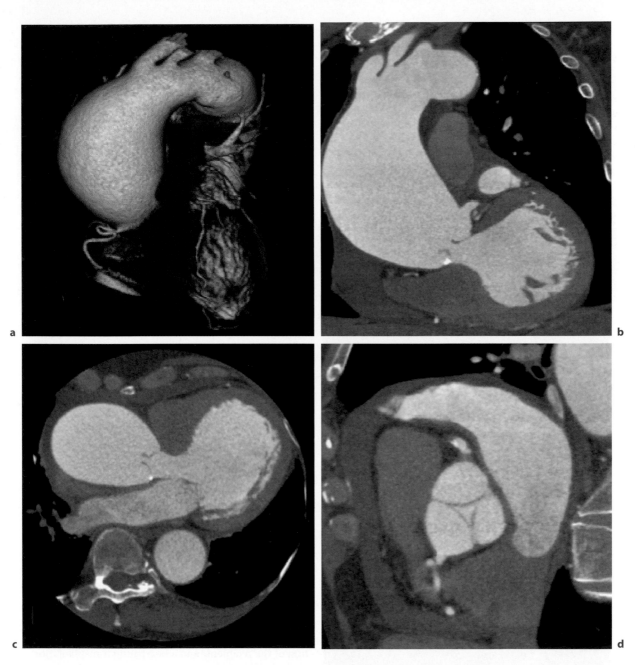

**Fig. 19.5a–d.** A 49-year-old man with an ascending aortic aneurysm. MDCT demonstrates the aortic geometry (**a–c**) and also depicts incomplete adaptation of the valvular cusps during diastole, indicating valvular regurgitation (**d**)

tant coronary disease in patients scheduled for surgery. Although initial results are promising, it must be borne in mind that these patients often have severely calcified coronary arteries that may considerably impair visualization of the vascular lumen. Moreover, the high image quality required for adequate evaluation of the coronary arteries is often achieved only if hemodynamically active drugs are administered, which may pose a risk, especially in patients with aortic valve disease at the stage of decompensation.

### 19.7.2
### Surgery of the Mitral Valve, Tricuspid Valve, and Pulmonary Valve

Only a few reports exist that deal with the accuracy of MDCT for detecting and quantifying mitral valve disease, i.e., mitral valve regurgitation and/or stenosis (ALKADHI et al. 2006; MESSIKA-ZEITOUN et al. 2006) (Fig. 19.6). Very little information is available on the usefulness of MDCT for the diagnosis of pulmonary valve and tricuspid valve disease. Thus, the value of MDCT in diseases of the mitral valve, pulmonary valve, and tricuspid valve is still unclear, and echocar-

diography remains the method of choice for a comprehensive assessment of valve disease, including the evaluation of directional blood flow, transvalvular flow velocity, and pressure gradient requirements. However, MDCT may provide useful information about chamber and valvular structure and function in patients with restricted acoustic windows and/or persistent diagnostic uncertainty.

## 19.8
## Surgery in Congestive Heart Failure

Despite substantial advances in pharmacological therapy, congestive heart failure (CHF) remains one of the most frequent causes of hospitalization and death worldwide. To increase the life expectancy and improve quality of life by relieving symptoms in patients with advanced, refractory CHD, surgical options are warranted. Therefore, treatment of CHF is currently the fastest growing segment of cardiac surgery, and a number of new options have been added to the therapeutic spectrum in the last years. MDCT may provide useful information regarding the morphology of the entire heart, including the coronary arteries, and may also provide data on left and right ventricular function that are pertinent to heart failure patients in cardiac surgery.

### 19.8.1
### Cardiac Transplantation

Cardiac transplantation is the ultimate therapeutic option in end-stage CHF. Orthotopic cardiac transplantation is the surgical technique of choice, whereas heterotopic cardiac transplantation is performed primarily when there is high resistance in the pulmonary circulation of the recipient (and a heart-lung transplantation is impossible), the donor heart is too small, or in selected cases with acute but potentially reversible heart failure. In orthotopic transplantation the donor heart is joined to the recipient's atria, aorta, and pulmonary artery. In heterotopic transplantation, the donor heart is implanted into the right thoracic cavity and anastomosed with the recipient's heart in a complex manner in such a way that the donor heart takes over most of left ventricular output, while the recipient's heart continues to ensure right ventricular output.

Noninvasive coronary angiography by MDCT enables the early detection of coronary allograft vascul-

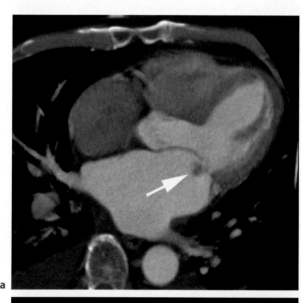

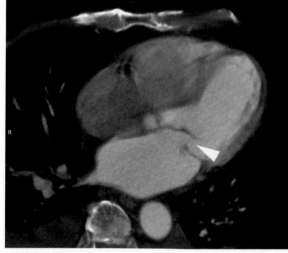

**Fig. 19.6a,b.** A 75-year-old woman with mitral valve endocarditis. MDCT detects a valvular vegetation (**a**, *arrow*) and prolapse of the posterior valve leaflet (**b**, *arrowhead*)

opathy (see above). MDCT also allows for a simultaneous assessment of myocardial function and geometry of the cardiac chambers, the morphology of the cardiac valves, and great thoracic vessels in a single scan. In addition, MDCT permits visualization of adjacent structures, such as the mediastinum, lungs, pleura, and chest wall. Thus, in the same examination MDCT also may allow the detection or exclusion of other non-cardiac, transplantation-related complications in the early or late stage after surgery. Complications include mediastinal or pulmonary bleeding, pneumo-thorax or pneumo-mediastinum, malignancies, or infection. These complications are usually associated with the surgical intervention itself, an endomyocardial biopsy, or long-term immunsuppressive medication (KNISELY et al. 2007; BOGOT et al. 2007; FERENCIK et al. 2007).

## 19.8.2
## Mechanical Cardiac Assist Devices

For long-term circulatory support in patients with advanced CHF (mostly as bridge-to-transplantation or bridge-to-recovery, rarely as destination therapy), a mechanical left ventricular assist device (LVAD) is often required, which decreases the left ventricular afterload by creation of a cardioaortic bypass through which the blood is directly pumped from the left ventricle into the aorta. In these patients MDCT not only allows for identification of the exact position of the cannula tip of the assist device, but may also allow for the detection of local complications associated with device implantation, such as intra/cardiac thrombosis, mediastinal, pericardial, or pleural fluid or air accumulations as well as mediastinal or pulmonary infections (JAIN et al. 2005; KNOLLMANN et al. 1999; KNISELY et al. 1997).

## 19.8.3
## Dynamic Cardiomyoplasty

This procedure consists in mobilizing a flap of the latissimus dorsi muscle, which is wrapped around the dilated heart and stimulated electrically. Its aim is to prevent further ventricular dilation by external stabilization, which is also known as "girdling effect," and to improve myocardial performance during systole by active compression. However, since the significance of its beneficial effects remains unclear, dynamic cardiomyoplasty has not yet become a standard surgical procedure and is today only used in selected cases. A frequent problem associated with dynamic cardiomyoplasty is lipoma-

tous involution of the muscle flap. Cardiac MDCT can identify atrophy and fatty replacement of the skeletal muscle. Moreover, cardiac MDCT may help to visualize the postoperative morphology and to quantify the functional status of the heart, especially in patients with restricted acoustic windows.

## 19.8.4
## Passive Cardiac Constraint (the CorCap Cardiac Support Device)

This type of passive external support has been introduced recently and is still undergoing worldwide clinical trials. In this technique, a compliant synthetic mesh rather than an actively stimulated muscle flap is wrapped around both ventricles and attached near the atrioventricular sulcus. This technique aims at preventing further ventricular dilation and at supporting myocardial function based on the "girdling effect." Following device implantation the thickness of the ventricular pericardium at MDCT slightly increases, but remains in the normal physiologic range. Abnormal thickening of the pericardium at MDCT may be a sign of a pericardial fibrous reaction, which may cause constrictive physiology. Other possible local complications that can be depicted by MDCT include paracardial adhesions and scar formations.

## 19.8.5
## Left Ventricular Reduction Surgery Using Partial Left Ventriculectomy (the Batista Procedure) or Aneurysmal Resection with Endoventricular Patch Plasty (the Dor Procedure)

The principle of left ventricular reduction according to Batista is to improve myocardial wall tension by reducing ventricular size based on Laplace's law. This is done by direct resection of a variable myocardial portion (partial left ventriculectomy) from the anterior, lateral, or posterior wall. In most patients having undergone this procedure, a circumscribed scar is visualized at the site of the ventriculotomy. In patients with left ventricular aneurysms, linear aneurysmal resection in which the aneurysmal sac is incised and the vital myocardium approximated by simple linear suture has become rare. The most widely used alternative technique is the Dor procedure where the aneurysm is incised and plicated by a purse-string suture around its neck. The remaining defect is covered with a synthetic patch over which the plicated sac is closed. Modifications of this procedure are now also used for reconstruction of a dilated, malformed left ventricle even when no aneurysm is present.

MDCT provides detailed three-dimensional information on the geometry of the left ventricle, including the exact location and dimension of the aneurysm. Three-dimensional models of the heart based on MDCT data sets may help the surgeon to assess the ideal resection lines and to determine the residual ventricular size and shape after a reconstructive procedure (Jacobs et al. 2008).

### 19.8.6
### Mitral Valve Surgery

Mitral regurgitation is a typical complication of dilated heart disease in which backflow of the blood from the ventricle into the atrium further contributes to the excessive volume load and progression of the disease. Mitral valve replacement or repair is thus one of the most common operations in advanced cardiac failure and is performed either alone or in combination with other procedures. While MDCT does not allow visualization of the regurgitant jet, it can provide basic information on the morphology of the valve structures and movement of the leaflets (Fig. 19.7).

### 19.8.7
### Cardiac Masses

MDCT has a high accuracy in detecting cardiac masses, but its ability to provide the final diagnosis of a cardiac tumor is sometimes limited. However, MDCT can give useful information on the exact location, dimension, and extent of the mass and may support the differential diagnosis based on typical imaging features (Grebenc et al. 2000; van Beek et al. 2007; Araoz et al. 2000) (Fig. 19.8). Nevertheless, the final diagnosis in a suspected cardiac tumor is generally based on patient's symptoms and history (especially if known concomitant cardiac or non-cardiac diseases are present), the location of the mass, and the specific imaging findings on echocardiography, as well as magnetic resonance imaging and MDCT. In the context of the preoperative workup, MDCT may be particularly helpful in planning tumor resection because it provides real three-dimensional anatomic information on the target area together with all structures at risk during surgery (such as coronary arteries with an intra-myocardial course or overlying fat tissue, papillary muscles, and the atrioventricular valves) (Jacobs et al. 2008).

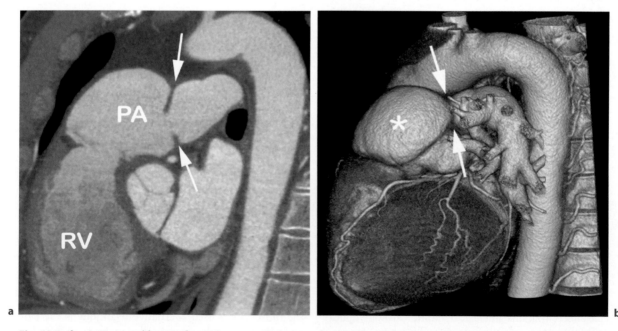

a    b

**Fig. 19.7a,b.** A 49-year-old man who underwent pulmonary valve replacement 2 years ago in the context of the Ross procedure. MDCT images clearly visualize a circumscribed membrane-like stenosis (*arrows*) and a large aneurysm (*asterisk*) in the pulmonary artery (*PA*). There is moderate dilatation and muscular hypertrophy of the right ventricle (*RV*)

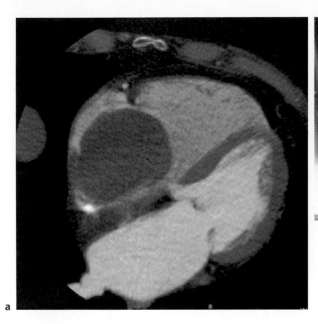

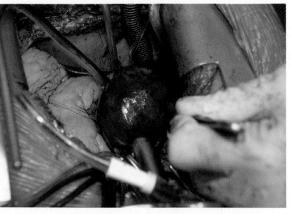

**Fig. 19.8a,b.** A 52-year-old woman with a right atrial mass. MDCT shows a large filling defect in the right atrium (**a**) that was confirmed to be a myxoma after surgical removal (**b**)

## 19.9
## Conclusion

In a routine clinical setting, MDCT provides invaluable structural and functional information on the heart and great vessels that is of particular interest for cardiac surgeons with regard to therapeutic decision-making, preoperative risk stratification, and definition of the surgical strategy, as well as postoperative evaluation.

## References

Abdulla J, Abildstrom SZ, Gotzsche O, Christensen E, Kober L, Torp-Pedersen C. (2007) Sixty-four-multi-detector-row detector computed tomography coronary angiography as potential alternative to conventional coronary angiography: a systematic review and meta-analysis. Eur Heart J; 28:3042–3050

Alkadhi H, Wildermuth S, Bettex DA, et al. (2006) Mitral regurgitation: quantification with 16-detector row CT—initial experience. Radiology; 238:454–463

Alkadhi H, Wildermuth S, Plass A, et al. (2006) Aortic stenosis: comparative evaluation of 16-detector row CT and echocardiography. Radiology; 240:47–55

Araoz PA, Mulvagh SL, Tazelaar HD, Julsrud PR, Breen JF. (2000) CT and MR imaging of benign primary cardiac neoplasms with echocardiographic correlation. Radiographics; 20:1303–1319

Baumert B, Plass A, Bettex D, et al. (2005) Dynamic cine mode imaging of the normal aortic valve using 16-channel multidetector row computed tomography. Invest Radiol; 40:637–647

Bogot NR, Durst R, Shaham D, Admon D. (2007) Cardiac CT of the transplanted heart: indications, technique, appearance, and complications. Radiographics; 27:1297–1309

Bonow RO, Carabello BA, Kanu C, et al. (2006) ACC/AHA guidelines for the management of patients with valvular heart disease: a report of the American College of Cardiology/American Heart Association Task Force on Practice Guidelines (writing committee to revise the 1998 Guidelines for the Management of Patients With Valvular Heart Disease): developed in collaboration with the Society of Cardiovascular Anesthesiologists: endorsed by the Society for Cardiovascular Angiography and Interventions and the Society of Thoracic Surgeons. Circulation; 114:e84–231

Debl K, Djavidani B, Seitz J, et al. (2005) Planimetry of aortic valve area in aortic stenosis by magnetic resonance imaging. Invest Radiol; 40:631–636

Dodd JD, Ferencik M, Liberthson RR, et al. (2007) Congenital anomalies of coronary artery origin in adults: 64-MDCT appearance. AJR Am J Roentgenol; 188:W138–146

Enzweiler CN, Wiese TH, Petersein J, et al. (2003) Diameter changes of occluded venous coronary artery bypass grafts in electron beam tomography: preliminary findings. Eur J Cardiothorac Surg; 23:347–353

Ferencik M, Gregory SA, Butler J, et al. (2007) Analysis of cardiac dimensions, mass and function in heart transplant recipients using 64-slice multi-detector computed tomography. J Heart Lung Transplant; 26:478–484

Fitzgibbon GM, Kafka HP, Leach AJ, Keon WJ, Hooper GD, Burton JR. (1996) Coronary bypass graft fate and patient outcome: angiographic follow-up of 5,065 grafts related to survival and reoperation in 1,388 patients during 25 years. J Am Coll Cardiol; 28:616–626

Gilard M, Cornily JC, Pennec PY, et al. (2006) Accuracy of multi-detector-row computed tomography in the preoperative assessment of coronary disease in patients with aortic valve stenosis. J Am Coll Cardiol; 47:2020–2024

Grebenc ML, Rosado de Christenson ML, Burke AP, Green CE, Galvin JR. (2000) Primary cardiac and pericardial neoplasms: radiologic-pathologic correlation. Radiographics; 20:1073–1103; quiz 1110–1071, 1112

Hamon M, Biondi-Zoccai GG, Malagutti P, et al. (2006) Diagnostic performance of multi-detector-row spiral computed tomography of coronary arteries as compared with conventional invasive coronary angiography: a meta-analysis. J Am Coll Cardiol; 48:1896–1910

Hamon M, Lepage O, Malagutti P, et al. (2008) Diagnostic performance of 16- and 64-section spiral CT for coronary artery bypass graft assessment: Meta-analysis. Radiology (Epub ahead of print)

Jacobs S, Grunert R, Mohr FW, Falk V. (2008) 3D-Imaging of cardiac structures using 3D heart models for planning in heart surgery: a preliminary study. Interact Cardiovasc Thorac Surg; 7:6–9

Jain VR, White CS, Pierson RN, 3rd, Griffith BP, Sorensen (2005) EN. Imaging of left ventricular assist devices. J Thorac Imaging; 20:32–40

Janne d'Othee B, Siebert U, Cury R, Jadvar H, Dunn EJ, Hoffmann (2008) U. A systematic review on diagnostic accuracy of CT-based detection of significant coronary artery disease. Eur J Radiol; 65:449–61

Jones CM, Athanasiou T, Dunne N, et al. (2007) Multi-detector computed tomography in coronary artery bypass graft assessment: a meta-analysis. Ann Thorac Surg; 83:341–348

Kim SY, Seo JB, Do KH, et al. (2006) Coronary artery anomalies: classification and ECG-gated multi-detector row CT findings with angiographic correlation. Radiographics; 26:317–333; discussion 333–314

Knisely BL, Collins J, Jahania SA, Kuhlman JE. (1997) Imaging of ventricular assist devices and their complications. AJR Am J Roentgenol; 169:385–391

Knisely BL, Mastey LA, Collins J, Kuhlman JE. (1999) Imaging of cardiac transplantation complications. Radiographics; 19:321–339; discussion 340–321

Knollmann FD, Bocksch W, Spiegelsberger S, Hetzer R, Felix R, Hummel M. (2000) Electron-beam computed tomography in the assessment of coronary artery disease after heart transplantation. Circulation; 101:2078–2082

Knollmann FD, Loebe M, Weng Y, et al. (1999) Radiologic anatomy of ventricular assist devices. J Thorac Imaging; 14:293–299

Laissy JP, Messika-Zeitoun D, Serfaty JM, et al. (2007) Comprehensive evaluation of preoperative patients with aortic valve stenosis: usefulness of cardiac multidetector computed tomography. Heart; 93:1121–1125

Ludman PF, Lazem F, Barbir M, Yacoub M. (1999) Incidence and clinical relevance of coronary calcification detected by electron beam computed tomography in heart transplant recipients. Eur Heart J; 20:303–308

Manghat NE, Morgan-Hughes GJ, Marshall AJ, Roobottom CA. (2005) Multidetector row computed tomography: imaging congenital coronary artery anomalies in adults. Heart; 91:1515–1522

Messika-Zeitoun D, Serfaty JM, Laissy JP, et al. (2006) Assessment of the mitral valve area in patients with mitral stenosis by multi-detector-row computed tomography. J Am Coll Cardiol; 48:411-413

Morino Y, Hara K, Tanabe K, et al. (2000) Retrospective analysis of cerebral complications after coronary artery bypass grafting in elderly patients. Jpn Circ J; 64:46–50

Omran H, Schmidt H, Hackenbroch M, et al. (2003) Silent and apparent cerebral embolism after retrograde catheterisation of the aortic valve in valvular stenosis: a prospective, randomised study. Lancet; 361:1241–1246

Pichler P, Loewe C, Roedler S, et al. (2008) Detection of high-grade stenoses with multi-detector-row computed tomography in heart transplant patients. J Heart Lung Transplant; 27:310–316

Pouleur AC, le Polain de Waroux JB, Pasquet A, Vanoverschelde JL, Gerber BL. (2007) Aortic valve area assessment: multidetector CT compared with cine MR imaging and transthoracic and transesophageal echocardiography. Radiology; 244:745–754

Ratliff NB, 3rd, Jorgensen CR, Gobel FL, Hodges M, Knickelbine T, Pritzker MR. (2004) Lack of usefulness of electron beam computed tomography for detecting coronary allograft vasculopathy. Am J Cardiol; 94:202–206

Romeo G, Houyel L, Angel CY, Brenot P, Riou JY, Paul JF. (2005) Coronary stenosis detection by 16-slice computed tomography in heart transplant patients: comparison with conventional angiography and impact on clinical management. J Am Coll Cardiol; 45:1826–1831

Salomon NW, Page US, Bigelow JC, Krause AH, Okies JE, Metzdorff MT. (1990) Reoperative coronary surgery. Comparative analysis of 6,591 patients undergoing primary bypass and 508 patients undergoing reoperative coronary artery bypass. J Thorac Cardiovasc Surg; 100:250–259; discussion 259–260

Scheffel H, Leschka S, Plass A, et al. (2007) Accuracy of 64-slice computed tomography for the preoperative detection of coronary artery disease in patients with chronic aortic regurgitation. Am J Cardiol; 100:701–706

Sigurdsson G, Carrascosa P, Yamani MH, et al. (2006) Detection of transplant coronary artery disease using multidetector computed tomography with adaptative multisegment reconstruction. J Am Coll Cardiol; 48:772–778

Simon AR, Baraki H, Weidemann J, Harringer W, Galanski M, Haverich A. (2007) High-resolution 64-slice helical-computer-assisted-tomographical-angiography as a diagnostic tool before CABG surgery: the dawn of a new era? Eur J Cardiothorac Surg; 32:896–901

Sun Z, Jiang W. (2006) Diagnostic value of multi-detector-row computed tomography angiography in coronary artery disease: a meta-analysis. Eur J Radiol; 60:279–286

Sun Z, Lin C, Davidson R, Dong C, Liao Y. (2007) Diagnostic value of 64-slice CT angiography in coronary artery disease: A systematic review. Eur J Radiol (Epub ahead of print)

Tanaka H, Shimada K, Yoshida K, Jissho S, Yoshikawa J, Yoshiyama M. (2007) The simultaneous assessment of aortic valve area and coronary artery stenosis using 16-slice multidetector-row computed tomography in patients with aortic stenosis comparison with echocardiography. Circ J; 71:1593–1598

Turi ZG. (2005) Whom do you trust? Misguided faith in the catheter- or Doppler-derived aortic valve gradient. Catheter Cardiovasc Interv; 65:180–182

van Beek EJ, Stolpen AH, Khanna G, Thompson BH. (2007) CT and MRI of pericardial and cardiac neoplastic disease. Cancer Imaging; 7:19–26

van der Linden J, Hadjinikolaou L, Bergman P, Lindblom D. (2001) Postoperative stroke in cardiac surgery is related to the location and extent of atherosclerotic disease in the ascending aorta. J Am Coll Cardiol; 38:131–135

## 20

# New Indications for Cardiac CT

Konstantin Nikolaou

## CONTENTS

### ABSTRACT

With recent technical advances in MDCT technology, such as DSCT or broad CT detectors with 256 or 320 slices, a number of new potential clinical indications for cardiac CT are being discussed, such as imaging of myocardial function, imaging of myocardial infarctions, imaging of patients with atrial fibrillation, or CT in the diagnosis of congenital heart disease. Although a number of other diagnostic modalities already exist for some of these clinical indications, and although cardiac CT will mostly and primarily be performed for noninvasive imaging of the coronary arteries, more and more information can be obtained from a single cardiac CT scan, and radiologists will increasingly have to deal with information and side findings present in the cardiac CT scan on which they should report. Thus, within this chapter, we hope to provide insight into a number of potential and new indications and techniques for noninvasive cardiac CT imaging, as well as technical implications, limitations and prerequisites.

## 20.1
## Introduction

CCA is considered the reference standard for the diagnosis of CAD and the grading of coronary artery stenoses. The established generation of 16- and 64-MDCT systems provides excellent results in terms of diagnostic accuracy, but certain limitations have hindered its full acceptance as a standard method in the clinical cascade for CAD patients. First, heavy calcium deposits in the coronary artery wall continue to negatively affect lu-

K. Nikolaou, MD
Department of Clinical Radiology, Ludwig-Maximilians-University of Munich, University of Munich Hospitals, Marchioninistrasse 15, 81377 Munich, Germany

men depiction due to partial volume effects, thereby impeding the detection and grading of significant CAD. Further limitations include the impaired assessibility of coronary artery branches smaller than 2 mm diameter and patients with high and/or arrhythmic heart rates (NIKOLAOU et al. 2006). Nevertheless, cardiac CT is increasingly used for a number of clinical indications, such as the noninvasive visualization of CABG (STEIN et al. 2005), the preoperative assessment of coronary anatomy before cardiac surgery and the depiction of coronary anomalies (GILKESON et al. 2003; RIST et al. 2004), or even stent assessment (RIST et al. 2006). Studies to date suggest that MDCT coronary angiography may become an important diagnostic modality in the routine workup of patients with suspected CAD and may prove particularly useful as a decision-maker in patients without a prior history of CAD to prove or exclude the presence of significant CAD and to decide on the need for invasive catheterization as a potentially therapy.

Recently, DSCT has been introduced into clinical routine. DSCT has been developed primarily to increase the temporal resolution (Fig. 20.1). The DSCT system is equipped with two X-ray tubes and two corresponding detectors, mounted onto the rotating gantry with an orthogonal orientation (FLOHR et al. 2006). Each detector acquires 64 overlapping 0.6-mm slices per rotation, and cross-sectional images are obtained with a very high temporal resolution of 82.5 ms, corresponding to one quarter of the gantry rotation time at a gantry rotation of 330 ms, using half-scan reconstruction algorithms (JOHNSON et al. 2006).

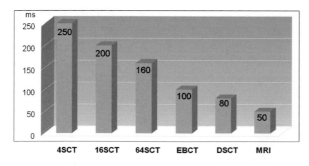

**Fig. 20.1.** Temporal resolution of different generations of CT scanners. With newest scanner technology like DSCT, a temporal resolution as low as 80 ms can be achieved. This should lead to increased robustness of the technique, with image quality more reliable even at higher or irregular heart rates, and to an improved capability for functional imaging, being close to the temporal resolution of the gold standard modality for functional imaging, i.e., MRI, with a temporal resolutions of about 50 ms. *4SCT* 4-slice CT, *16SCT* 16-slice CT, *64SCT* 64-slice CT, *EBCT* electron-beam CT

With these technical advances, a number of new potential clinical indications for cardiac CT are being discussed, such as imaging of myocardial function, imaging of myocardial infarctions, imaging of patients with atrial fibrillation, or CT in the diagnosis of congenital heart disease. Other diagnostic modalities already exist for some of these clinical indications, and though cardiac CT angiography is the most used for noninvasive imaging of coronary arteries, much information can be obtained from a single cardiac CT scan. Radiologists will be faced with this increase amount of information and present in the cardiac CT scan, and such findings should be reported.

## 20.2
## Coronary CT Angiography in Patients with Atrial Fibrillation

Motion artifacts have often constituted a diagnostic dilemma and continue to be the most important challenge in coronary CT angiography (CTA). Previous studies (WINTERSPERGER et al. 2003) have demonstrated a significant inverse correlation between image quality and heart rate. For 16-slice CT (-SCT) cardiac examinations, premedication with β-blockers (oral or intravenously administered) was routinely performed, typically in patients with heart rates of more than 65 bpm. Some authors still recommend the application of β-blockers, even for 64-SCT technology (RAF et al. 2005). Another report on 64-SCT shows that while good image quality can be obtained in patients with heart rates of more than 75 bpm, and in patients with heart rates below 65 bpm, intermediate heart rates of between 65 and 75 bpm may still be problematic; in a number of cases, neither systolic nor diastolic datasets yielded satisfactory image quality (WINTERSPERGER et al. 2006a). DSCT might overcome these limitations. Analysis of a larger number of DSCT datasets for image quality at different phases of the R–R interval, showed that diagnostic image quality could be obtained in both the systolic and diastolic phases over a wide range of heart rates (JOHNSON et al. 2006). However, a somewhat-limited diagnostic image quality was observed in diastolic reconstructions at heart rates of more than 75 bpm (LESCHKA et al. 2007). Similarly RIST et al. (2007) showed that diagnostic image quality can be obtained in nearly all patients, independent of the heart rate. In particular, the right coronary artery, which is particularly prone to motion artifacts due to its anatomical orientation and fast movement of up to 10 cm/s could be evaluated in all cases.

Apart from high heart rates, arrhythmia remained as a contraindication for CTA applications owing to between-beat variations, which led to inappropriate data sampling and resulted in severe motion artifacts (Sun and Jiang 2006). Atrial fibrillation (AF) is the most common type of arrhythmia, and the incidence increases markedly with advancing age (Fuster et al. 2007). AF is often associated with structural heart disease. Before initiating therapy, management of precipitating or re-versible causes of AF is recommended. Coronary artery disease is a cardiovascular condition associated with AF. Also, AF patients may manifest symptoms mimicking CAD. Therefore, the demonstration of CAD is an important issue in the management of AF patients (Sun and Jiang 2006). As motion artifacts, owing to high heart rates, particularly arrhythmia, impair image quality to a great extent, AF has remained as a contraindication for CTA applications. MDCT angiography was not

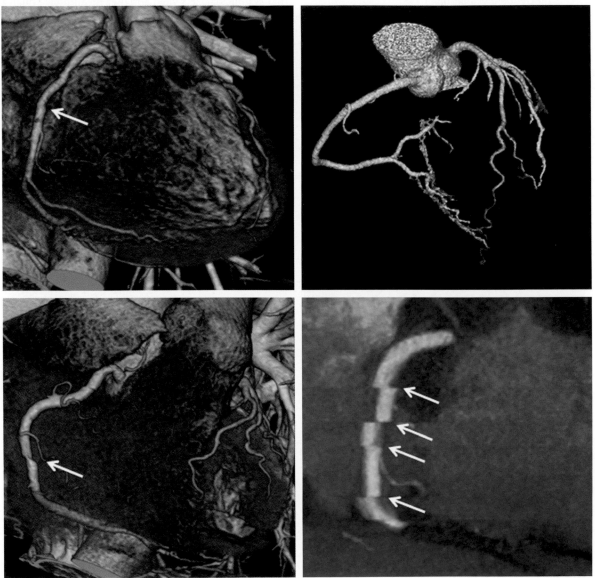

**Fig. 20.2a–d.** Dual-source coronary CTA performed in three patients with AF, causing an absolute arrhythmic heartbeat during the scan. In the first patient, image quality is optimal, and despite the absolute arrhythmia during scanning, no motion artifacts can be seen in the volume-rendered images (**a, b**). In the second patient with absolute arrhythmia, a minor step artifact can be seen in the midsegment of the RCA (**c** *arrow*), but this image quality can still be considered to be assessable. In the third patient, however, a number of step artifacts along the course of the RCA render this dataset uninterpretable (**d** *arrows*)

considered as a diagnostic tool in the clinical workflow of AF, but the improved temporal resolution achieved with DSCT may improve the visualization of coronary vessels in patients with AF. In a prospective study at our institution, 56 patients with AF have been enrolled, with the typical clinical indications for CTA:

1. Planning of radiofrequency ablations
   a. Anatomy of the pulmonary veins (mapping of radiofrequency points)
   b. Stenoses of pulmonary veins before or after radiofrequency ablations
2. Exclusion of CAD in patients with absolute arrhythmia
   a. To exclude CAD as a potential cause of the arrhythmia
   b. To exclude CAD before certain anti-arrhythmic medication (e.g., class 1c anti-arrhythmic drugs such as flecainide)
3. Exclusion of intracavitary thrombi if echocardiography is inconclusive

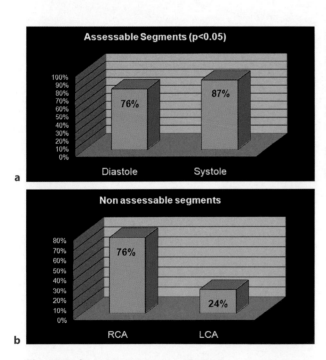
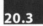

**Fig. 20.3a,b.** Fifty-six patients suffering from AF and chronic absolute arrhythmia were scanned with DSCT, and a systematic image quality assessment of all coronary artery segments was performed (our data). Comparing the number of assessable segments performing retrospective reconstructions during mid-diastole (i.e., at about 70–75% of the cardiac cycle), and during end systole (i.e., at about 30–40% of the cardiac cycle), it was shown that systolic reconstructions lead to a higher number of assessable segments (87% of segments assessable) RCA, as this vessel is moving faster than the LCA during the cardiac cycle (**b**)

In this patient cohort, the mean heart rate was 78±25 (range of 30–181), and all patients had irregular heart rates during the scan. Results were very promising: only two patients were considered as being nondiagnostic (4%), 39% did not show any artifacts, and in the remaining 57%, artifacts were present but not hindering diagnosis. Figure 20.2 shows a number of cases of patients with AF, with increasing levels of artifacts. Performing systolic and diastolic reconstructions of the datasets (at 300 ms and 70% of the R–R interval), it could be shown that systolic datasets yield a higher mean image quality than diastolic data do, and that most nondiagnostic vessel segments are found in the right coronary artery, as this vessel moves most (Fig. 20.3).

In conclusion, the recently introduced DSCT technology provides better temporal resolution and minimizes motion artifacts, which allows coronary angiography at higher heart rates, even in cases of arrhythmia. The high negative predictive value of CTA may be useful for obviating invasive coronary angiography in patients with AF, whose symptoms or abnormal stress test results make it necessary to rule out the presence of coronary artery stenosis to guide therapy. Therefore, DSCT has the potential to make noninvasive coronary angiography effective in a significantly increased number of patients and in a wider spectrum of clinical situations as compared with earlier scanners. Larger studies will be needed to determine if early results are reproducible.

## 20.3
## Imaging of Myocardial Function with CT

The evaluation of global left ventricular function with end-systolic and end-diastolic volumes and especially ejection fraction and myocardial mass is diagnostically important in multiple cardiac diseases. So far, parameters of cardiac function are routinely assessed with echocardiography or MRI with excellent temporal and spatial resolution. MRI is regarded as standard of reference in dynamic imaging and functional assessment of the myocardium (WINTERSPERGER et al. 2006b). But CT also is gaining increasing importance in cardiac imaging. Apart from the high clinical potential of noninvasive coronary CTA with its capability to reliably rule out significant coronary artery disease, the technique's inherent sharp depiction of the endocardial contours and the improving temporal resolutions of new scanner generations also make it possible to quantify ventricular function, adding to the value of the modality in a comprehensive cardiac assessment. The left ventricular functional parameters provide complementary information that can be derived from CTA datasets, using a standardized coronary CTA protocol, without additional contrast or radiation exposure to the patient. The evaluation of ventricular function has been facilitated by various fully and semiautomated reconstruction algorithms provided by several CT system vendors (Fig. 20.4). Early studies using 4-SCT and 16-SCT confirmed that evaluation of cardiac function is feasible by MDCT in patients with suspected or known CAD. However, a systematic underestimation of left ventricular ejection fraction (LV-EF) was characteristic for CT; the explanation for this is the limited temporal resolution of earlier CT scanners as compared with MRI. Interestingly, 64-SCT technology has already been reported to be able to identify wall motion abnormalities in a patient popu-

lation with a high prevalence of CAD, e.g., after myocardial infarction. Using DSCT, image reconstruction is possible in virtually any phase of the cardiac cycle, with a sufficiently high temporal resolution, clearly revealing global and regional functional abnormalities of the myocardium (Fig. 20.5) A recent report using DSCT confirmed these results: the image quality ratings for the coronary arteries, the myocardium and the heart valves at the optimal reconstruction interval were diagnostic even in patients with high heart rates (RIST et al. 2007).

Technically, functional CT data can be derived from the CTA dataset, without a second scan or adaptation of the contrast injection protocol. Even ECG pulsing (tube current modulation) can be used (with a reduction down to 25% of the nominal current value in sys-

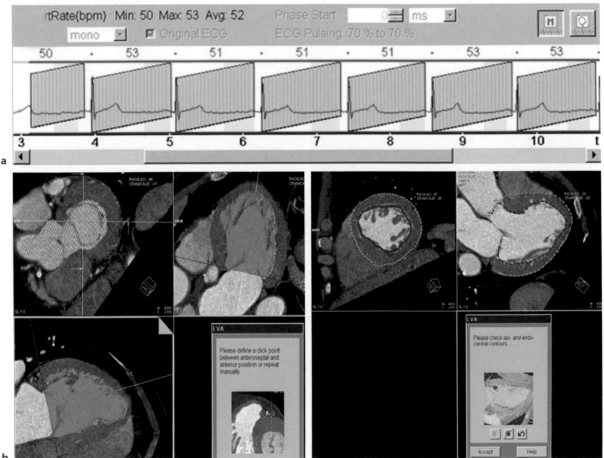

**Fig. 20.4a–c.** Retrospective reconstruction of a multiphasic dataset scanned with a DSCT scanner. Without exposing the patient to additional radiation exposure or contrast material application, a number of datasets can retrospectively be reconstructed from any coronary CT angiographic scan if a retrospective gating technique is used. For example, images can be reconstructed every 10% or every 50 ms throughout the cardiac cycle (**a**). This way, an analysis of functional parameters of the left ventricle is possible. New software tools will assist the physician by automatically performing a pixel-by-pixel segmentation of the left ventricular chamber (**b**), or, endo- and epicardial borders can be traced manually for functional analysis (**c**)

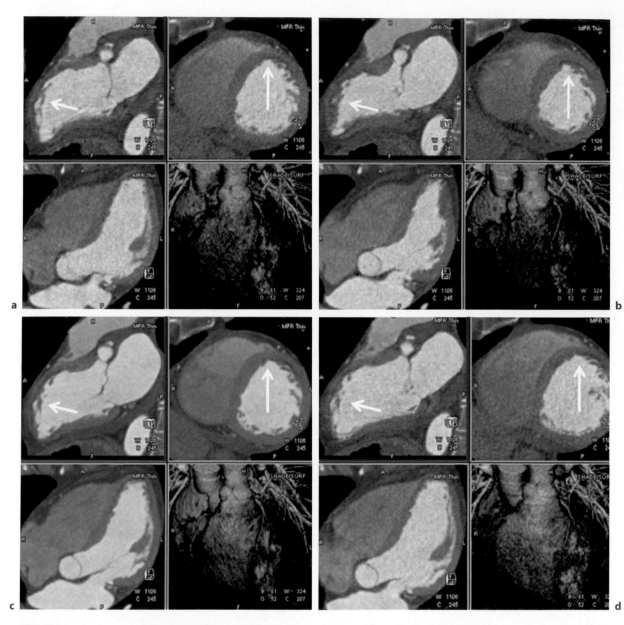

**Fig. 20.5a–d.** Contrast-enhanced DSCT of the heart performed in a 58-year-old male patient who had suffered a large myocardial infarction of the anterior and septal wall of the left ventricle (i.e., the vascular supply territory of the LAD). A se-lection of 4 out of 10 multiphasic datasets over the cardiac cycle clearly shows the wall motion abnormalities (akinesia and dys-kinesia) of the anterior and septal wall (*arrows*).

tole). To save data storing space, functional datasets can be reconstructed at 1-mm slice thickness (instead of 0.6 or 0.75 mm for CT coronary angiography) and with a reduced matrix size of 256 (instead of 512). This way, multiphase datasets can be reconstructed, e.g., every 5 or 10% throughout the cardiac cycle, resulting in 10–20 phases per R–R interval. For CT, functional evaluation software typically uses a region growing algorithm that quantifies the volume of voxels within certain density thresholds (e.g., between 150 and 300 HU). This procedure has to be done twice, for the end-systolic and for the end-diastolic phases of the R–R interval. The software then traces the left ventricular wall automatically in long-axis views, excluding papillary muscles and trabeculae, with the option to correct the contours manually, if necessary (Fig. 20.4).

Our results showed that DSCT data correlated well with functional MRI data, which served as the standard

**Table 20.1.** DSCT versus MRI in calculating cardiac function

| Function | DSCT (ml) | MRI (ml) |
|----------|-----------|----------|
| EF | 62±12 | 58±9 |
| EDV | 135±42 | 132±41 |
| ESV | 55±29 | 57±27 |
| SV | 80±21 | 75±18 |

Our results from 15 patients (modified from Busch et al. 2007). Values are means±standard deviations

of reference. EF, end systolic volume (ESV), end diastolic volume (EDV), and stroke volume (SV) were calculated for both modalities in 15 patients. Using DSCT, mean EDV was 135.8±41.9 ml versus 132.1± 40.8 ml EDV in MRI. Mean ESV was 54.9±29.6 ml in DSCT and 57.6±27.3 ml in MRI, and mean SV was 80.9± 20.9 ml in DSCT and 74.5±18.1 ml in MRI. LV-EF amounted to 61.6±12.4% in DSCT and 57.9±9.0% in MRI (Table 20.1). The observed nonsignificant differences between functional parameters acquired in CT and MRI may be caused by physiological effects due to rapid contrast material injection and the absence of β-blocker medication in CT, as well as differences in the software used for functional assessment.

In summary, a sufficient evaluation of the left ventricular function and wall motion is feasible with CTA datasets acquired for the examination of the coronary arteries, thus adding a comprehensive functional aspect to the static morphological assessment in CT and possibly rendering the modality a first choice for cardiac imaging in a wider range of indications.

## 20.4
## Imaging of Myocardial Infarctions with CT

Performing a standard coronary CTA, CT density values within the myocardium can give insight into pathologic ischemia of the myocardium, i.e., hypoperfusion or myocardial infarction, both reflected by a reduced CT density or hypoattenuation. Ischemic changes in the myocardium after coronary arterial occlusion consist of disruption of cell membrane function and integrity and increased permeability of small vessel walls. In contrast-enhanced CT, the initial area of low attenuation primarily reflects myocardial edema, i.e., a pronounced water content of the myocardium, which is followed by infiltration of inflammatory cells. Subsequently, necrotic myocardium is replaced by fibrous and/or fatty

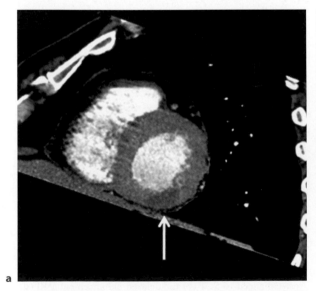
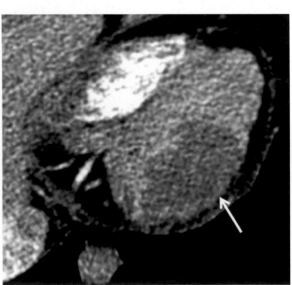

a            b

**Fig. 20.6a,b.** A 52-year-old male patient. The multiplanar reformation (MPR) in a short-axis view clearly depicts the extent of an inferior myocardial infarction and shows mild wall thinning in a (*arrow*). In the same patient, the original axial image of the inferior left ventricular wall reveals a recent infarction (<30 days), depicted as a moderately circumscribed area with CT densities of 60–80 HU (**b** *arrow*)

tissue, which is also characterized by a reduction of attenuation in CT as compared with normal myocardium (Fig. 20.6). In the early phase after contrast infusion, the infarct area is detectable as a perfusion defect. Such a myocardial perfusion defect in a standard contrast enhanced coronary CTA, however, is not specific for infarctions, since similar findings can occur in cases with severe local ischemia (but no infarction) or other cardiac diseases causing perfusion in-homogeneities, such as hypertrophic cardiomyopathy. Also, myocardial

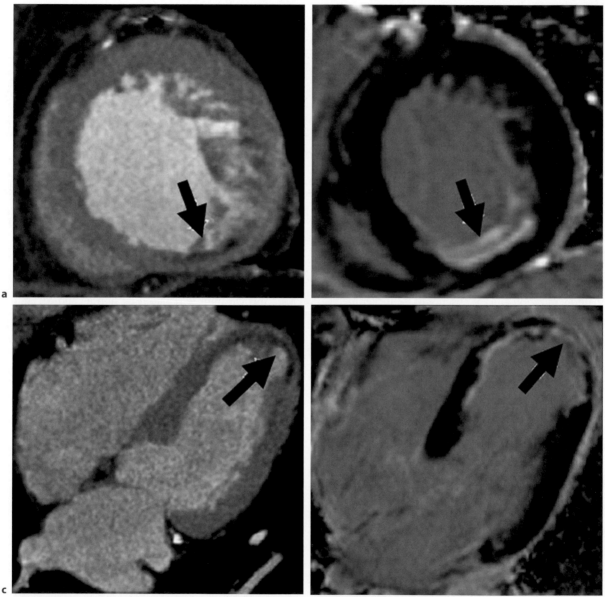

**Fig. 20.7a–d.** Cross-sectional (short axis) reconstruction of a first-pass, contrast-enhanced 16-slice coronary CT angiographic dataset (**a**) compared with delayed-enhancement MRI (**b**) of an 85-year-old male patient. In the contrast-enhanced CT images, an extensive area of decreased attenuation is seen in the free lateral and parts of the basal wall of the left ventricle (**a** arrow). In this area of myocardium, a large myocardial infarction is present, as proven my delayed-enhancement MRI imaging (**b** arrow). In another patient (68-year-old, male), contrast-enhanced 16-SCT (**c**) and delayed-enhancement MRI (**d**) depict an area of decreased attenuation in the CT data, seen in the apical and anterior region of the left ventricular wall (**c** arrow). In the same area of myocardium, a myocardial infarction is present, as proven by delayed-enhancement MRI (**d** arrow)

contrast enhancement depends on a number of independent variables, e.g., the contrast injection protocol or the cardiac output. That is why a significant variance of measured CT attenuation (Hounsfield units) can been observed in normal and infarcted myocardium, indicating that no absolute Hounsfield unit values can be defined, but the relative measurement of normal and infarcted tissue is the decisive factor (Nikolaou et al. 2004). Wall thinning in the left ventricle is one of the indirect findings associated with the healing process after myocardial infarction. In a longitudinal CT study on patients with myocardial infarction, the wall thickness at the site of infarction decreased significantly over time (Nikolaou et al. 2005).

Various imaging modalities have been tested for the detection and the exact assessment of myocardial infarctions. MRI and nuclear medicine procedures seem to be favorable, as these modalities can combine the assessment of myocardial perfusion and function, and are able to assess myocardial viability (Kim et al. 1999; Kitagawa et al. 2003). A number of reports on the application of CT in patients with myocardial infarction have been promising, including early animal studies (Huber et al. 1981; Slutsky et al. 1983) and experiences with EBCT (Georgiou et al. 1992, 1994; Schmermund et al. 1998), however, the clinical application of CT in the diagnosis of myocardial infarctions has not become popular thus far.

As described above, even from a standard MDCT coronary angiography protocol, i.e., without additional scans for the detection of late enhancement effects, and without additional radiation dose being applied to the patient, a variety of myocardial changes or pathologies can be detected. Infarctions can be seen on first-pass, contrast-enhanced datasets, evaluating CT attenuation (Hounsfield units) and wall thickness. Abnormal focal decrease of myocardial CT attenuation and abnormally reduced regional myocardial wall thickness can be indicative of myocardial infarction. It could be shown that recent infarctions are more difficult to detect using MDCT, as the decrease in Hounsfield units in the early arterial phase or the presence of wall thinning is not as pronounced as observed in chronic infarctions. Possible reasons for false-positive findings with MDCT for infarct detection might be a variety of causes other than infarctions that lead to perfusion defects or perfusion irregularities, as described above. False-positive results are typically more often detected in the posterior or inferior ventricular wall. Several studies have reported that CT underestimates the true extent of a myocardial infarction (Sanz et al. 2006). Figure 20.7 shows an example of infarctions being depicted on first-pass CTA versus late-enhancement MRI. This might be related to patchy and subendocardial infarctions, as collateral perfusion in the area of infarcted myocardium can obscure foci of necrosis surrounded by normal myocardium. In conclusion, one should interpret infarct size as assessed by contrast-enhanced, arterial-phase MDCT as an approximation to the true infarct size rather than as an absolute measurement.

In several CT studies, a "delayed contrast enhancement" was observed in the area of infarction (10 min to several hours after contrast administration), primarily found in recent infarctions, but also reported to be detectable in chronic infarctions (Adams et al. 1976; Mahnken et al. 2005, 2007; Fig. 20.8). However, detection of such delayed enhancement requires additional scans with an increased application of the radiation dose to the patient and prolonged examination times; therefore, it has hardly been used in clinical routine. It should therefore be the focus of future studies, to assess the diagnostic power of contrast-enhanced CT for the detection of myocardial infarctions, using the standard protocol that is being used widely for CTA of the coronary arteries. Any additional diagnostic information that can be derived from these standard CTA examinations is of considerable interest.

MDCT provides information on cardiac morphology in great detail, including findings or complications related to myocardial infarctions, such as left ventricular aneurysms, intramural calcifications, intracavitary thrombi, or infarct involvement of the papillary muscles (Fig. 20.9). Diagnostic criteria for the detection of aneurysms on CT scans are based on the anatomic definition, i.e., wall thinning and wall protrusion, which differs from the traditional angiographic criteria (Becker et al. 2000). CT does not include wall movement disturbance, while contrast ventriculography includes both anatomic protrusion of the left ventricle and functional disturbance of the wall movement but does not consider localized wall thinning of the aneurysm. Left ventricular thrombosis is one of the most significant complications of myocardial infarction. Two-dimensional echocardiography as well as MRI has been validated as reliable methods for the detection of thrombi. Using contrast ventriculography, the opacification of the left ventricular cavity precisely determines the surface area of thrombi, but the border between thrombi and the endocardium cannot always be identified sufficiently. MDCT allows for identification of subtle differences in attenuation of cardiac structures and can clearly distinguish mural from free-floating thrombi. Additionally, other possibly significant complications after myocardial infarction, like calcification of the myocardium and pericardial effusion, are easily detected on CT images.

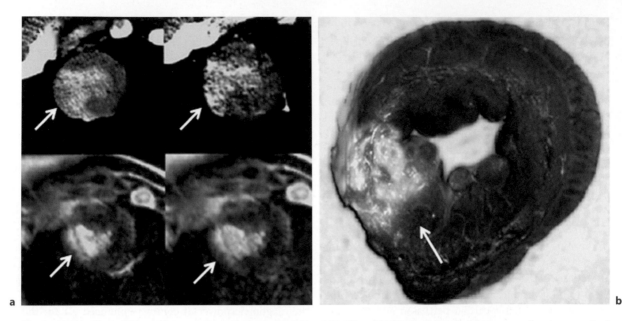

a                                                                    b

**Fig. 20.8a,b.** If an additional late scan is performed with CT after first-pass CTA of the heart, e.g., 15–20 min after initial contrast administration, then late enhancement effects can also be observed in CT, depicting infarcted myocardium. In these pictures from an animal model, a direct face-to-face comparison of delayed-enhancement CT (**a** *two upper row images*) versus delayed-enhancement MRI (**a** *two lower row images*) shows the different stages of early and chronic MI as visualized by MDCT and MRI. The *left* and *right* images of **a** were acquired on days 7 and 28, after artificial provocation of a left ventricular infarction. CT and MR images correlate well with the result of the triphenyl tetrazolium chloride (TTC) staining, displaying the exact extent of the myocardial infarction (**b**). (Images courtesy of Andreas Mahnken, University of Aachen, Aachen, Germany, modified from MAHNKEN et al. 2007, with permission)

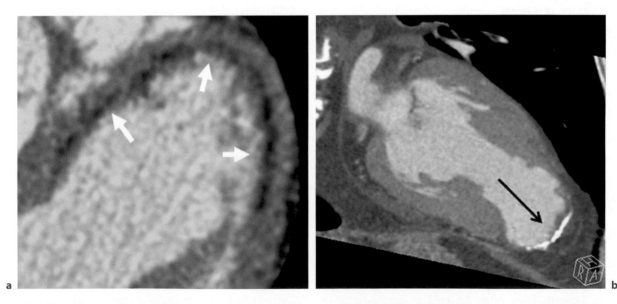

a                                                                    b

**Fig. 20.9a–d.** Typical morphologic aspects and potential sequelae of chronic myocardial infarctions. In a 47-year-old male patient scanned with 16-SCT, a sharply demarcated area with noticeable lower attenuation compared with the surrounding myocardium as well as a significant wall thinning is seen in the anterior left ventricular wall on the original axial CT source image, which is the typical appearance of a chronic myocardial infarction (**a**). Infarct sequelae and complications can also be depicted by contrast-enhanced CT, such as a circumscribed and partially calcified apical aneurysm in a 60-year-old male patient after myocardial infarction (**b** MPR, *arrow*).

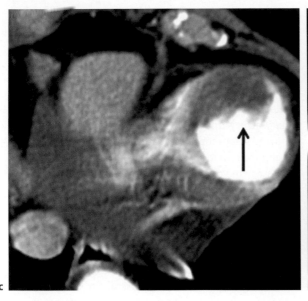

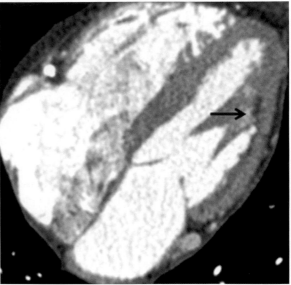

c

d

**Fig. 20.9a–d.** (*continued*) The axial source image in the basal part of the heart shows formation of a thrombus in an apical aneurysm in a 64-year-old female patient, with low CT attenuation (~25 HU) and an irregular surface (**c** *arrow*). Finally, an MPR in a four-chamber view shows a hypodense area in the lateral wall in a 65-year-old male patient, reflecting a myocardial infarction below the papillary muscle (**d** *arrow*)

## 20.5
## CT in the Diagnosis of Congenital Heart Disease

New-generation MDCT technology has changed the approach to noninvasive assessment of congenital heart disease, in both pediatric and adult patients. This is mainly because of rapid advances in spatial and temporal resolution and in postprocessing capability. In an increasing number of institutions, CT with multiplanar and 3D reconstruction has become a routine examination in the evaluation of congenital heart disease planning surgery, complex interventional catheterizations, and for follow-up. It has proved to be an invaluable diagnostic and decision-aiding methodology in these situations, as a complement to echocardiography or MRI, and as a potential substitute for diagnostic angiography. Currently, cardiac ultrasound is the most important diagnostic modality for the examination of cardiac structures in children. However, ultrasound is usually insufficient for the study of certain structures such as the coronary arteries, the aorta, and branches of the pulmonary artery, or for systemic and pulmonary venous structures. For visualizing these structures, both MRI and CT provide a better diagnostic capability, as a result of high-spatial resolution 3D imaging (Goo et al. 2005, 2007). While MRI has the advantage of applying no radiation to the patient and enabling protocols more comprehensive including functional information such as flow gradients, CT is much faster and easier to apply, especially in critical patients, or emergency situations, or where a lengthy MRI including full anesthesia cannot be performed.

In children younger than 5 years, they are unable to achieve a 5-s breath hold. Their heart rates are high, generally above 100 bpm. In this group of children, good image quality is difficult to obtain, owing to respiratory and cardiac movement artifacts, which are all the more marked when the child is anxious or agitated. The aim therefore is to acquire images as quickly as possible while the child is typically lightly sedated. This is one major advantage of MDCT over MRI, as for MRI, examination times are typically long (e.g., 30 min,) and full anesthesia of the child is required, which can be a contraindication for MRI in certain patients who are unstable or where a timely and quick diagnosis is critical. Therefore, the primary goal is to exploit the maximal speed of the CT scan along with an optimal injection of contrast medium. ECG gating is avoided in most cases, as it lengthens acquisition time. Contrast medium injection and image acquisition are carefully calculated (typically about 1.5–2 ml per kilogram body weight of the child) to achieve optimal image quality, either by hand injection or with a care-bolus technique. However, even in this patient cohort with high heart rates, in special clinical indications, coronary artery imaging can be possible with fast CT technology such as DSCT, and with ECG gating applied (Fig. 20.10).

For children older of 5 years of age, breath holding with appropriate and sympathetic coaching is generally possible. Sedation should be avoided if good cooperation from the child is possible, to ensure breath holding during the acquisition period. Choice of acquisition protocol depends above all on the malformation to be explored. Study of the great vessels (aorta, pulmonary arteries, systemic, or pulmonary venous return) is relatively straightforward: it is carried out by fast acquisition times without ECG gating. Study of the coronary arteries, on the other hand, is more difficult. The best image quality is obtained with ECG-gated acquisition in a child whose heart rate is maintained stably and slowly by administration of a β-blocker (<70 bpm). In all cases, the same precautions should be taken for contrast medium injection parameters and radiation dose as already described. Indications for CT coronary angiography in the diagnosis of congenital abnormalities of the coronary arteries are now well established in adults (Datta et al. 2005). In congenital heart disease, the coronary arteries are important if anomalous, or reimplanted after surgery in certain circumstances (Fig. 20.10). The main advantage of CT scanning is to provide a precise description of the 3D anatomy of the coronary arteries, in particular their origin and course. CT coronary angiography is especially useful in screening

for complications after coronary reimplantation in cases of anomalous LCA arising from the pulmonary artery or after the arterial switch operation for transposition of the great arteries (Fig. 20.11). Other nonradiation techniques—for example, MRI—are theoretically preferable for repeated screening examinations, particularly in children. Nevertheless, MRI is currently limited in coronary artery imaging by relatively poor spatial resolution and often-complex acquisition protocols, requiring a long examination so that general anesthesia is often necessary in young children (Taylor et al. 2005).

Currently, for imaging of the aortic arch, CT and MRI are the preferred modalities, for example, in the investigation of coarctation and congenital degenerative diseases of the aorta. Being complementary to echocardiography, CT and MRI allow precise pre- and postoperative assessment of the thoracic aorta (Lambert et al. 2005). CT is often extremely useful for neonates with isthmic coarctation associated with hypoplasia of the aortic arch. It precisely identifies the site of the coarctation, determines the degree of narrowing, and, above all, defines precisely the extent of hypoplasia of the aortic arch, thereby assisting the choice of surgical technique. CT is preferable to MRI for this group of children, owing to the simplicity of the examination and the rapidity of image acquisition, generally less than 5 days for neonates. For vascular rings, multiplanar and 3D reconstruction clearly demonstrates the origin and course of the great vessels and the relationship of the vessels to the adjacent airway (Fig. 20.12). Some authors have suggested that MRI is the gold standard for the evaluation of vascular rings (van Son et al. 1994). However, MRI examination of the aorta in children younger than

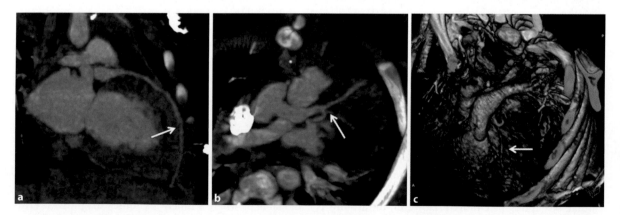

**Fig. 20.10a–c.** DSCT angiographic data from a 4-month-old baby suffering from a Bland-White-Garland syndrome and having undergone reimplantation of the LAD to the aorta. Despite the very small cardiac structures in such a young child and a very high heart rate of 144 bpm during the scan, the images show an excellent, motion-free visualization of the anastomosis between the LAD and the aorta, proving patency of the coronary artery and obviating the need for an invasive cardiac catheterization. **a, b** MPR of the LAD (*arrows*), **c** volume rendering of the thorax displaying the course of the LAD (*arrow*)

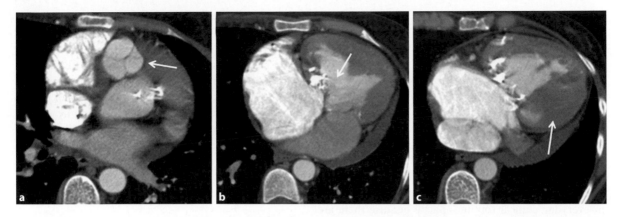

**Fig. 20.11a–c.** A 5-year-old male patient with a complex congenital heart disease. In patients in whom MRI is not feasible for a number of potential reasons, e.g., in unstable patients who cannot undergo a lengthy MRI scan lasting up to 60 min, MDCT offers a simple, fast, and noninvasive diagnostic approach, visualizing complex morphological features with a very high spatial resolution in a scan time of 5–10 s, however, done so by applying ionizing radiation and iodinated contrast. In this patient scanned with a 64-SCT scanner, a transposition of the great arteries can be seen, with the aorta arising ventrally to the pulmonary trunk (**a** *arrow*). Also, a large ventricular septum defect is depicted (**b**, *arrow*), as well as a hypo-plastic left cardiac chamber (**c** *arrow*)

7 years requires profound sedation or general anesthesia. Thus, for practical reasons, MRI is typically used to study older children, who can hold their breath repeatedly during an examination that takes about 30 min.

Concluding, MDCT undoubtedly represents a major advance in the imaging of congenital heart disease. Its application to small children, in particular, is promising, due to the ease and speed of acquisition and 3D imaging with high spatial resolution. However, it is equally true that for a large number of simple and common malformations, such as atrial septal defects or ventricular septal defects, echocardiography is sufficient for complete definition of the disease, and cardiac catheterization as well as MRI can provide essential hemodynamic data. Efforts should be made to minimize radiation dose, particularly in children for whom repeated examinations are necessary. CT examinations in children should generally be performed at low kilovoltage (80–100 kV). It is too early yet to regard MDCT as a substitute for invasive angiography or MRI, although this modality seems to be an important adjunct to current imaging techniques in CHD.

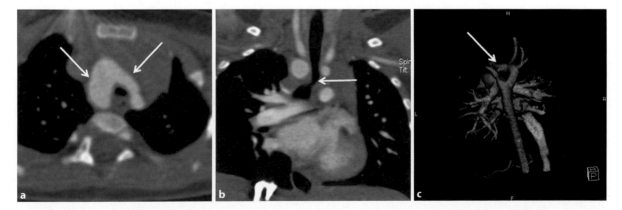

**Fig. 20.12a–c.** A 9-month-old boy with a double aortic arch, suffering from an increasing stridor and dyspnea, scanned with a 64-SCT scanner. On the axial source image, the two portions of the aortic arch embracing the trachea can clearly be seen (**a** *arrows*). The coronal MPR clearly shows the stenosing effect of this double aortic arch, compressing the trachea (**b** *arrow*). The 3D volume-rendered image gives a good overview of the complex cardiovascular anatomy in this patient (**c**)

## Conclusion

In conclusion, MDCT of the heart is a promising tool for cardiac imaging for a number of clinical indications. So far, it has mainly been used for morphological imaging, in particular for noninvasive angiography of the coronary arteries. However, a number of new indications are on the horizon, such as functional imaging, viability imaging, or imaging in congenital heart disease. While not all of these indications will be used in everyday clinical routine—partly because there are other imaging modalities of choice and partly because MDCT has some inherent drawbacks such as radiation exposure or application of iodinated contrast—the clinical value of these techniques might be significant and implementation in clinical routine will be tested in futures studies (Table 20.2). Today, even in patients with AF, new scanner technologies such as DSCT enable noninvasive imaging of the coronary arteries with a sufficiently robust image quality. Furthermore, performing standard, arterial-phase CTA of the coronary arteries can provide important additional information on the myocardium, including the possibility of detecting myocardial infarctions, with information on infarct size and age. The simultaneous depiction of the coronary arteries in considerable detail provides the opportunity to allocate the infarct area to the specific vascular supply territory. Future developments in postprocessing software will enable the assessment of global and regional myocardial function from MDCT datasets. These findings underscore the clinical value of contrast-enhanced cardiac MDCT, delivering noninvasive angiographic images of the coronary arteries and considerable information on the myocardium at the same time. Finally, 3D imaging obtained with the latest generation of CT scanners represents a real advance in the morphological study of cardiovascular malformations in children. In the near future and for dedicated indications and clinical requirements, CT could be established as an important new modality—besides echocardiography, cardiac catheterization and cardiac MRI—in the assessment of congenital heart disease.

## References

Adams DF, Hessel SJ, Judy PF, Stein JA, Abrams HL (1976) Computed tomography of the normal and infarcted myocardium. AJR Am J Roentgenol 126:786–791

Becker CR, Ohnesorge BM, Schoepf UJ, Reiser MF (2000) Current development of cardiac imaging with multidetector-row CT. Eur J Radiol 36:97–103

Busch S, Johnson TR, Wintersperger BJ, Minaifar N, Bhargava A, Rist C et al. (2007) Quantitative assessment of left ventricular function with dual-source CT in comparison to cardiac magnetic resonance imaging: initial findings. Eur Radiol 18:570–575

Datta J, White CS, Gilkeson RC, Meyer CA, Kansal S, Jani ML et al. (2005) Anomalous coronary arteries in adults: depiction at multi-detector row CT angiography. Radiology 235:812–818

Flohr TG, McCollough CH, Bruder H, Petersilka M, Gruber K, Subeta C et al. (2006) First performance evaluation of a dual-source CT (DSCT) system. Eur Radiol 16:256–268

Fuster V, Ryden LE, Cannom DS, Crijns HJ, Curtis AB, Ellenbogen KA et al. (2007) [ACC/AHA/ESC 2006 guidelines for the management of patients with atrial fibrillation—executive summary]. Rev Port Cardiol 26:383–446 (In Portuguese.)

**Table 20.2.** Synopsis: new indications for cardiac CT

| Indication | Feasible | Reasonable | Alternative | Discussion |
|---|---|---|---|---|
| CTA in patients with absolute arrhythmia | Yes | Yes | None | ECG pulsing is off or wide range, resulting in an increased radiation exposure |
| Myocardial function | Yes | Yes/no | MRI, echocardiography | Not the first line indication for CT  Interesting adjunct information to CTA  No flow values |
| Imaging of myocardial infarction | Yes | ? | MRI, nuclear medicine | CTA datasets: no viability information  CT late enhancement: additional scan  MRI: method of choice |
| Cardiac CT in congenital heart disease | Yes | Yes | MRI | Contra-CT: radiation exposure  Pro-CT: fast, no/very short anesthesia |

Georgiou D, Bleiweis M, Brundage BH (1992) Conventional and ultrafast computed tomography in the detection of viable versus infarcted myocardium. Am J Card Imaging 6:228–236

Georgiou D, Wolfkiel C, Brundage BH (1994) Ultrafast computed tomography for the physiological evaluation of myocardial perfusion. Am J Card Imaging 8:151–158

Gilkeson RC, Markowitz AH, Ciancibello L (2003) Multisection CT evaluation of the reoperative cardiac surgery patient. Radiographics 23 Spec No:S3–S17

Goo HW, Park IS, Ko JK, Kim YH, Seo DM, Park JJ (2005) Computed tomography for the diagnosis of congenital heart disease in pediatric and adult patients. Int J Cardiovasc Imaging 21:347–365

Goo HW, Yang DH, Park IS, Ko JK, Kim YH, Seo DM et al. (2007) Time-resolved three-dimensional contrast-enhanced magnetic resonance angiography in patients who have undergone a Fontan operation or bidirectional cavopulmonary connection: initial experience. J Magn Reson Imaging 25:727–736

Huber DJ, Lapray JF, Hessel SJ (1981) In vivo evaluation of experimental myocardial infarcts by ungated computed tomography. AJR Am J Roentgenol 136:469–473

Johnson TR, Nikolaou K, Wintersperger BJ, Leber AW, von Ziegler F, Rist C et al. (2006) Dual-source CT cardiac imaging: initial experience. Eur Radiol 16:1409–1415

Kim RJ, Fieno DS, Parrish TB, Harris K, Chen EL, Simonetti O et al. (1999) Relationship of MRI delayed contrast enhancement to irreversible injury, infarct age, and contractile function. Circulation 100:1992–2002

Kitagawa K, Sakuma H, Hirano T, Okamoto S, Makino K, Takeda K (2003) Acute myocardial infarction: myocardial viability assessment in patients early thereafter comparison of contrast-enhanced MR imaging with resting [201]Tl SPECT. Single photon emission computed tomography. Radiology 226:138–144

Lambert V, Sigal-Cinqualbre A, Belli E, Planche C, Roussin R, Serraf A et al. (2005) Preoperative and postoperative evaluation of airways compression in pediatric patients with 3-dimensional multi-detector-row computed tomographic scanning: effect on surgical management. J Thorac Cardiovasc Surg 129:1111–1118

Leschka S, Scheffel H, Desbiolles L, Plass A, Gaemperli O, Valenta I et al. (2007) Image quality and reconstruction intervals of dual-source CT coronary angiography: recommendations for ECG-pulsing windowing. Invest Radiol 42:543–549

Mahnken AH, Koos R, Katoh M, Wildberger JE, Spuentrup E, Buecker A et al. (2005) Assessment of myocardial viability in reperfused acute myocardial infarction using 16-slice computed tomography in comparison to magnetic resonance imaging. J Am Coll Cardiol 45:2042–2047

Mahnken AH, Bruners P, Kinzel S, Katoh M, Muhlenbruch G, Gunther RW et al. (2007) Late-phase MDCT in the different stages of myocardial infarction: animal experiments. Eur Radiol 17:2310–2317

Nikolaou K, Knez A, Sagmeister S, Wintersperger BJ, Reiser MF, Becker CR (2004) Assessment of myocardial infarctions using multirow-detector computed tomography. J Comput Assist Tomogr 28:286–292

Nikolaou K, Sanz J, Poon M, Wintersperger BJ, Ohnesorge B, Rius T et al. (2005) Assessment of myocardial perfusion and viability from routine contrast-enhanced 16-detector-row computed tomography of the heart: preliminary results. Eur Radiol 15:864–871

Nikolaou K, Knez A, Rist C, Wintersperger BJ, Leber A, Johnson T et al. (2006) Accuracy of 64-MDCT in the diagnosis of ischemic heart disease. AJR Am J Roentgenol 187:111–117

Raff GL, Gallagher MJ, O'Neill WW, Goldstein JA (2005) Diagnostic accuracy of noninvasive coronary angiography using 64-slice spiral computed tomography. J Am Coll Cardiol 46:552–557

Rist C, Nikolaou K, Wintersperger BJ, Bastarrika G, Reiser MF, Becker CR (2004) Indications for multi-detector-row CT angiography of coronary arteries. Radiologe 44:121–129

Rist C, von Ziegler F, Nikolaou K, Kirchin MA, Wintersperger BJ, Johnson TR et al. (2006) Assessment of coronary artery stent patency and restenosis using 64-slice computed tomography. Acad Radiol 13:1465–1473

Rist C, Johnson TR, Becker A, Leber AW, Huber A, Busch S et al. (2007) [Dual-source cardiac CT imaging with improved temporal resolution: Impact on image quality and analysis of left ventricular function]. Radiologe 47:287–284 (In German)

Sanz J, Weeks D, Nikolaou K, Sirol M, Rius T, Rajagopalan S et al. (2006) Detection of healed myocardial infarction with multidetector-row computed tomography and comparison with cardiac magnetic resonance delayed hyperenhancement. Am J Cardiol 98:149–155

Schmermund A, Gerber T, Behrenbeck T, Reed JE, Sheedy PF, Christian TF et al. (1998) Measurement of myocardial infarct size by electron beam computed tomography: a comparison with [99m]Tc sestamibi. Invest Radiol 33:313–321

Slutsky RA, Mattrey RF, Long SA, Higgins CB (1983) In vivo estimation of myocardial infarct size and left ventricular function by prospectively gated computerized transmission tomography. Circulation 67:759–765

Son JA van, Julsrud PR, Hagler DJ, Sim EK, Puga FJ, Schaff HV et al. (1994) Imaging strategies for vascular rings. Ann Thorac Surg 57:604–610

Stein PD, Beemath A, Skaf E, Kayali F, Janjua M, Alesh I et al. (2005) Usefulness of 4-, 8-, and 16-slice computed tomography for detection of graft occlusion or patency after coronary artery bypass grafting. Am J Cardiol 96:1669–1673

Sun Z, Jiang W (2006) Diagnostic value of multi-detector-row computed tomography angiography in coronary artery disease: a meta-analysis. Eur J Radiol 60:279–286

Taylor AM, Dymarkowski S, Hamaekers P, Razavi R, Gewillig M, Mertens L et al. (2005) MR coronary angiography and late-enhancement myocardial MR in children who underwent arterial switch surgery for transposition of great arteries. Radiology 234:542–547

Wintersperger BJ, Nikolaou K, Jakobs TF, Reiser MF, Becker CR (2003) Cardiac multidetector-row computed tomography: initial experience using 16 detector-row systems. Crit Rev Comput Tomogr 44:27–45

Wintersperger BJ, Nikolaou K, von Ziegler F, Johnson T, Rist C, Leber A et al. (2006a) Image quality, motion artifacts, and reconstruction timing of 64-slice coronary computed tomography angiography with 0.33-second rotation speed. Invest Radiol 41:436–442

Wintersperger BJ, Reeder SB, Nikolaou K, Dietrich O, Huber A, Greiser A et al. (2006b) Cardiac CINE MR imaging with a 32-channel cardiac coil and parallel imaging: impact of acceleration factors on image quality and volumetric accuracy. J Magn Reson Imaging 23:222–227

## 21

# Complementary Role of Cardiac CT and MRI

BERND J. WINTERSPERGER

## CONTENTS

## ABSTRACT

Both modalities, CT and MRI, have competed with each other in recent years to get to the ultimate goal: a one-stop-shop for comprehensive information on one's heart status. This race led to sophisticated technical innovations on both sides but has not yet succeeded, and it unlikely will. At present, the patient's clinical history is the most important information and basis for choosing the appropriate modality. As shown by many recent studies, cardiac CT allows for a reliable exclusion of significant CAD in proper patient populations, based on its constantly high NPV. In addition to this application, the assessment of bypass patency and even the morphologic evaluation in congenital heart disease (CHD) may be clinically relevant. MR is the modality of choice in any functional aspect of cardiac imaging, whether focusing on cardiac and valvular function or perfusion. Based on its imaging toolbox, it may also be applied in patients with advanced CAD and even more importantly, in the differential diagnosis of the wide variety of nonischemic cardiac diseases. Cardiac MR covers a substantially wider range of diseases than CT; suspicion of CAD though, a key indication for cardiac CT makes the largest share of all cardiac patients.

## 21.1
## Introduction

Noninvasive cardiac imaging has substantially emerged within recent years and is being included in clinical routine assessment of various cardiac diseases. In particular, the fast technical innovations of MDCT and MRI have pushed the envelope for noninvasive diagnosis of

B. J. WINTERSPERGER, MD
Department of Clinical Radiology, Ludwig-Maximilians-University of Munich, Munich University Hospitals, Marchioninistrasse 15, 81377 Munich, Germany

a wide variety of cardiac diseases. At present though, neither modality by itself can perform a one-stop-shop exam to provide the entire range of morphologic and functional information that can potentially be gathered by a combination of both exams. There are also aspects and information that can exclusively be shown and evaluated by only one of both modalities. The following chapter focuses on the strength and limitations of both noninvasive modalities, based on a variety of applications as well as on clinical situations.

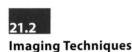

## Imaging Techniques

### 21.2.1
### Basics of Cardiac CT

Techniques of cardiac imaging based on CT are focused on in more detail in other chapters of this book, dedicated to cardiac CT only. However, with respect to some sections of this chapter, a few aspects need to be addressed.

The technique of cardiac CT based on MDCT scanners evolved in 1998, based on four-slice imaging technology. This new technique was soon picked up in order to focus on coronary CT imaging. The use in other applications followed later. Detailed imaging of the coronary arteries and other subtle intracardiac structures has long been limited to heart rates of ~70–80 or less. Heart rates in newborns and infants though are well beyond that range, and therefore the application of MDCT to assess cardiac structures has been limited. Only with the development of faster scanner techniques and thinner-slice collimation has this limit has been overcome. With regard to functional assessment, MDCT techniques were limited in accuracy before the advent of Dual-Source CT (DSCT), based on its mediocre temporal resolution in relationship to the speed of the beating heart. A major aspect of cardiac CT within recent years has been the discussion on its radiation dose issues. The most often-applied technique of cardiac MDCT is based on the use of retrospective ECG gating, and therefore the patient is exposed to a substantial amount of redundant radiation even when major dose-saving strategies are employed (JAKOBS et al. 2002). A new era may be initiated by the use of prospective ECG-triggered modes in contrast-enhanced cardiac CT imaging, a technique that has only recently become available with adequate image quality.

Imaging of the great vessels has been a standard application now for many years with MDCT scanners, and this technique typically is applied without ECG-related acquisitions and therefore applies substantially less radiation to the patient. In assessment of congenital heart disease (CHD), these techniques allow adequate morphologic information about the pulmonary circulation and the thoracic aorta. The application of dual-energy CT may even give information on blood-volume distribution, a valuable aspect in disease of the pulmonary vessels (JOHNSON et al. 2007).

### 21.2.2
### Basics of Cardiac MRI

Compared with CT techniques, MR methods have been in use for cardiac assessment since the 1980s. Technical development within recent years and the competition with MDCT though have further pushed the clinical use of cardiac MRI. Based on the fundamental technology properties, the spectrum of possible applications in cardiac MR has always been substantially wider than that of cardiac CT. While the various application of the latter technology is somewhat based on a general acquisition technique with variations in data reconstruction, MRI covers the various aspects of cardiac physiology and pathophysiology, based on substantially varying acquisition techniques.

While "morphologic" MRI with regard to mass assessment, detailed soft tissue differentiation, and cardiac morphology, is mainly carried out on T1-weighted or T2-weighted fast spin-echo (FSE) techniques, the majority of today's applications is covered with the use of gradient-recalled-echo (GRE) techniques.

While the high soft tissue contrast in MRI allows acquiring detailed information in many applications even without the application of Gd-chelate-based contrast agents, the assessment of mass vascularization and myocardial perfusion is linked to the use of Gd chelates. Also, the assessment of various myocardial diseases and myocardial viability is increasingly performed with the use of contract enhancement (VOGEL-CLAUSSEN et al. 2006).

Although being generally based on GRE techniques, the various clinical applications differ substantially. The major applications of GRE techniques include analysis of cardiac function, using cine techniques, assessment of blood flow based on cine phase-contrast (PC) sequences and myocardial perfusion, as well as delayed contrast enhancement imaging. These different applications are discussed separately within the clinical aspects of cardiac CT and MRI.

The vast majority of currently used techniques is based on ECG gating with segmented data acquisition schemes and therefore requires a somewhat regular sinus rhythm. The ongoing developments in MR technology including the application of higher field strength (e.g., 3 T), the use of parallel imaging techniques, and new coil developments enable the use of real-time data acquisition. However, these techniques still exhibit some limitations with regard to temporal and spatial resolution, and therefore are to be considered alternatives in cases in which standard techniques are not applicable or fail for various reasons (e.g., arrhythmia, limited patient compliance).


## 21.3
### Spectrum of Examinations

Cardiac CT and MRI allow for a variety of applications that typically focus on different aspects of cardiac function and morphology. The major applications are:
- Cardiac and coronary morphology
- Global, regional, and valvular function
- Myocardial perfusion
- Delayed myocardial enhancement imaging for assessment of myocardial viability and other myocardial diseases
- Cardiac and vascular flow imaging

As mentioned earlier, not every single aspect may be covered by both modalities, and further details are discussed separately.

### 21.3.1
### Imaging of Cardiac Morphology

Reliable and accurate imaging of cardiac morphology is of outmost importance in patients with CHD as well as cardiac masses. In the majority of CHD patients, initial diagnosis is accurately based on echocardiography, potentially complemented by catheter-based pressure level measurements. However, in complex diseases, additional cross-sectional imaging may be of substantial benefit for further therapeutic planning and prediction of patient outcome. This additional information may focus on morphologic information such as detailed anatomy of, especially, extracardiac structures such as pulmonary vessels or aortic changes. In particular, catheter-based imaging of the pulmonary vasculature may be extremely complicated if not almost impossible. In cases in which only static imaging information is of interest, both techniques, cardiac CT or MRI, may be performed (PRAKASH et al. 2007). Imaging of blood-flow dynamics though can only be revealed by cardiac MRI (see below). Beside the application of flow-sensitive techniques (phase-contrast techniques) to quantitatively assess blood flow within dedicated preselected vasculature, recently improved dynamic MRA techniques obtain an overview on gross central circulation (Figs. 21.1, 21.2). This is especially of added value for further planning of dedicated MR examination techniques. While MRI enables assessment of CHD without radiation exposure, the examination is somewhat time-consuming and necessitates adequate sedation or even anesthesia. In unstable infants or children, therefore, cardiac CT is

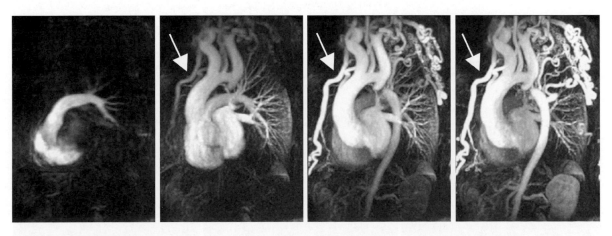

**Fig. 21.1.** Different frames (MIP reconstructions) of a dynamic MRA data set in a patient with suspicion of aortic coarctation. The frames demonstrate the consecutive contrast filling of the pulmonary vasculature, followed by the ascending aorta, the extensive collateral vessels, and the descending aorta (*arrow*: internal mammary artery)

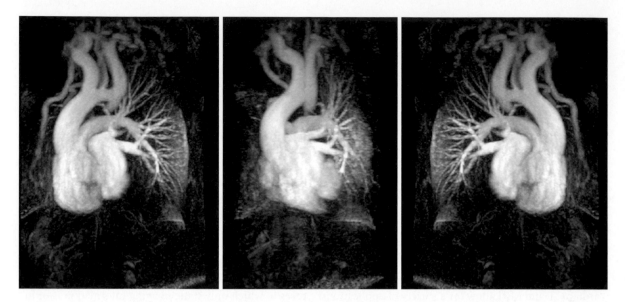

**Fig. 21.2.** Single-phase MIP reconstructions (different views) of the same dynamic MRA as shown in Fig. 21.1, demonstrating a total isthmic occlusion

more and more commonly performed to keep examination time as short as possible (Fig. 21.3).

Although being less commonly performed, assessment or exclusion of possible cardiac masses is a prime time indication for cardiac cross-imaging techniques. While screening for masses is typically performed using echocardiographic techniques, MR and CT techniques are commonly used for further workup of masses or inconclusive echocardiographic findings. While CT basically allows for higher spatial resolution with regard to

pixel size and slice thickness (~1–2 mm), MR shows its major benefits with its high soft tissue contrast, which potentially substantially narrows the differential diagnosis. In some masses such as cardiac lipomas or fibromas, MR may even allow a final diagnosis. The ability to evaluate contrast agent dynamics may aid in predicting tumor vascularization and differentiating cardiac masses and pseudolesions such as cardiac thrombi (Fig. 21.4). In the setting of disturbances of blood flow such as myocardial infarction with wall motion abnor-

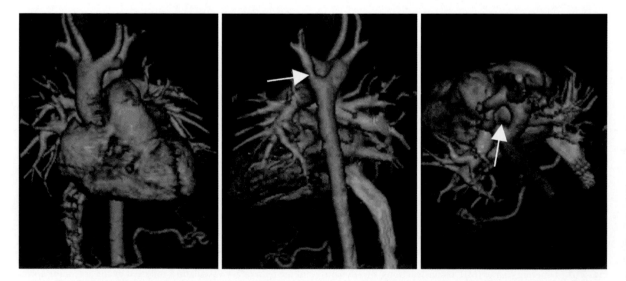

**Fig. 21.3.** MDCT angiography in a 9-month-old infant with sudden onset of dyspnea and unstable hemodynamic situation demonstrates a double aortic arch (*arrows*), which leads to intermittent tracheal constriction. CT imaging was performed using short sedation without breath holding

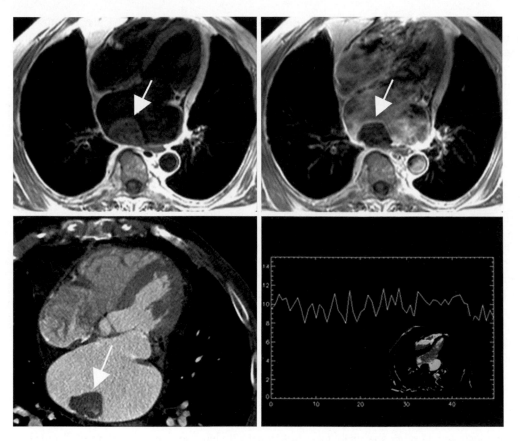

**Fig. 21.4.** Comparative CT and MR images in a patient after cardiac transplant, with suspicion of an atrial mass. Plain and postcontrast T1-weighted images demonstrate a mass (*arrow*) at the posterior wall, which is also shown by contrast-enhanced CT. Dynamic MR perfusion imaging prove the lack of contrast enhancement consistent with a partially calcified atrial thrombus

malities or cardiac rhythm distortion, when thrombotic clots are likely and differential diagnosis is somewhat less important, cardiac CT gives fast and reliable confirmation or exclusion of abnormalities (Fig. 21.5). In cases necessary, CT enables also an easy follow-up, and overall CT has proven to be almost as accurate as TEE while being less invasive (KIM et al. 2007).

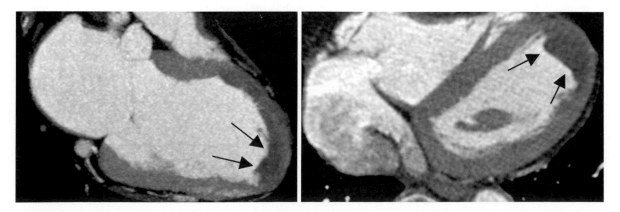

**Fig. 21.5.** Coronary CTA data sets of two different patients with apical clot formation (*arrows*) due to wall motion abnormalities after myocardial infarction

### 21.3.2
### Imaging of Coronary
### Anatomy and Morphology

Technical innovations of MDCT within recent years have almost exclusively been driven by coronary CT imaging, with the ultimate goal to reliably assess reliably coronary artery morphology. Based on several major studies, it has been proven that coronary CTA especially allows a reliable exclusion of significant coronary disease based on its constantly high NPV, ranging from 90 to 98%. With the constant improvement of spatial and especially temporal resolution, overall accuracy improved and the number of nonassessable coronary artery segments substantially decreased (MATT et al. 2007; SCHERTLER et al. 2007). With the advent of DSCT imaging, consistently high image quality can also be achieved at high heart rates, so pharmacologic (e.g., β-blockers) premedication to lower heart rates is therefore not longer necessary.

Although coronary imaging using MRA techniques has been developed and evaluated for many years, all techniques failed to compete with CT techniques after the advent of coronary MCDT angiography. Recent comparative studies of coronary MRA have mainly focused on patient populations with heavy calcified coronary arteries and demonstrated a higher specificity for MRA at comparative sensitivity (LIU et al. 2007; OZGUN et al. 2007). This aspect though represents only a niche indication. The assessment of coronary anomalies in children may also represent a niche indication, as MRA techniques are still not yet suitable to compete with coronary CTA in the vast majority of patients. Further aspects of coronary CT techniques, applications, and clinical indications will be elucidated more thoroughly in other chapters.

### 21.3.3
### Assessment of Cardiac
### and Valvular Function

As adequate cardiac function is of major importance in order to maintain proper hemodynamics, the non-invasive evaluation of functional parameters has long been a focus of imaging techniques. Based on its accuracy, reliability, and reproducibility, MR cine imaging is the current standard of reference in assessing global and regional cardiac function (SEMELKA et al. 1990a,b; ROMINGER et al. 2000). Reliable global functional parameters though necessitate adequate temporal resolution of imaging techniques. Based on the fast volumetric changes during the cardiac cycle and the short period of isovolumetric relaxation (least ventricular volume) and contraction (maximal ventricular volume), temporal resolution needs to be at least in the rage of 50 ms or better (SETSER et al. 2000). As segmented cine MR techniques can be adjusted for temporal resolution (number of lines/segment), these techniques can easily meet this criteria and potentially allow substantially better temporal resolution. Functional evaluation in cardiac CT imaging has been made available based on retrospective ECG-gated data acquisition. While for coronary CTA, retrospective gating is only been used for optimization of image quality at a single time point within the cardiac cycle, functional CT necessitates data reconstruction throughout the entire cardiac cycle. The temporal resolution of CT techniques has emerged within recent years. Based on the used data reconstruction techniques though, a stable and constant temporal resolution cannot exceed certain limits. With the use of single-detector CT scanner, the temporal resolution meets half the time necessary for a full 360° rotation. At a maximum possible rotation speed of 300 ms, this technique enables a temporal resolution of 150 ms. With dual-source scanners, the temporal resolution can be further reduced to a quarter of a full rotation, which reaches 83 ms at 330 ms/360° rotation speed. While earlier comparative studies of CT and MR demonstrated offsets of functional CT data especially regarding ESV and thus also affecting EF, initial results of dual-source CT scanners showed more accurate results when compared with MRI (BRODOEFEL et al. 2007).

Regarding initial data acquisition, CT and MRI are based on different strategies. While cine MR–based data sampling is based on acquisitions along the various cardiac axis, ECG-gated CT samples a 3D volume, with an original transverse slice orientation and possible secondary reconstruction along the cardiac axis. The latter is of major importance for evaluation of regional wall motion according to the AHA segmental classification (CERQUEIRA et al. 2002). The ability of cardiac CT to evaluate cardiac function though is opposed to the efforts of dose-saving strategies to reduce patients' radiation exposure (JAKOBS et al. 2002). The application of modern dose-modulation strategies may reduce the systolic tube current to a level as low as only ~4% of the nominal value. While this does not affect the quality of coronary artery reconstructions (mainly in diastole,) functional evaluation during systole may be substantially hampered or even impossible (Fig. 21.6). With the use of even prospective triggered cardiac CT imaging techniques, functional information cannot be processed anymore based on the same data acquisition, but requires an additional sampling with added radiation and the use of additional contrast agent.

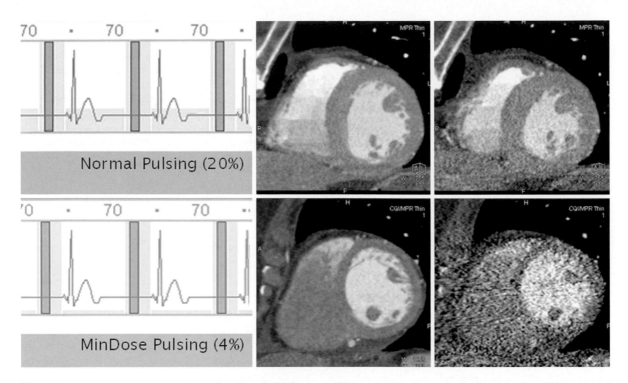

**Fig. 21.6.** MDCT cine imaging with ECG pulsing for reduction of radiation. The *upper row* demonstrate normal pulsing with 20% dose in systole, while image quality (*right*) still allows cardiac assessment. Images in the *lower row* have been acquired with MinDose protocol, lowering the radiation to only 4% within systole. Systolic image quality though is nondiagnostic

Acquired heart disease is often related to valvular pathologies, most often affecting the mitral and aortic valves. Deterioration of global functional parameters and possible subsequent heart failure may follow, based on constant pressure or volume overload. MRI has long been used in the assessment of stenotic and regurgitant valvular disease. Cine and PC flow imaging techniques are able to evaluate the relevant information to adequately assess and grade stenotic, regurgitant, or combined valvular disease (DJAVIDANI et al. 2005; GELFAND et al. 2006; POULEUR et al. 2007a). In evaluation of stenotic disease, two major approaches may be applied:

1. Measurement of the valve orifice area
2. Estimation of the maximum pressure gradient based on peak velocity measurements (or assessment of maximum acceleration)

The latter technique, unique to MRI, can easily be applied without the application of contrast agent (Fig. 21.7). The accuracy of PC-based velocity and flow assessment using through-plane PC imaging is related to the following factors:

• Perpendicular position of the slice in relation to the vessel of interest (proportional to the cosine of the angular offset)

• Correct velocity encoding gradient (VENC) adjusted to the estimated maximum velocity (possible detectable phase shift: $(-\pi)-\pi$)

The commonly used estimation of pressure gradients is based on the modified Bernoulli equation ($\Delta P = 4v^2$), while a more accurate technique would be the application of the Navier-Stokes equations. However, this would necessitate a higher temporal resolution of PC cine techniques, which would substantially prolong data acquisition (exceeding breath-hold periods). The application of PC cine techniques not only allows assessment of forward flow, but also enables the assessment of flow in the opposite direction and thus the quantification of regurgitant volumes.

The measurement of valve orifice area (most often applied for aortic valve disease) can be applied to both techniques, CT and MRI. Based on systolic images within the valvular plane, the outline of the valve orifice can be traced to evaluate the orifice area. The results of both methods show close correlation in comparison to echocardiography (FEUCHTNER et al. 2006b, 2007; POULEUR et al. 2007b). The measurement of the residual opening area in the setting of valve closure has also been used in CT imaging in order to assess and

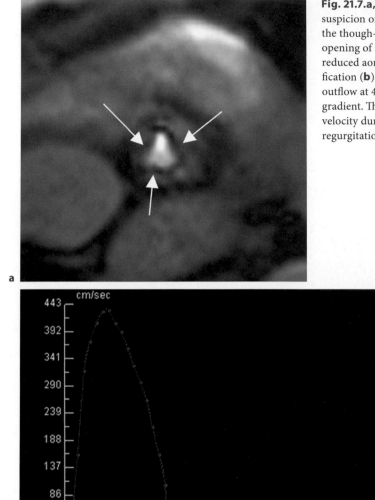

a

b

**Fig. 21.7.a,b** PC flow imaging in a 14-year-old girl with suspicion of aortic stenosis. The magnitude image (**a**) of the though-plane flow quantification shows an inadequate opening of the aortic valve at peak systole, with a markedly reduced aortic valve orifice (*arrows*). Peak velocity quantification (**b**) of the data set shows a substantially accelerated outflow at 435 cm/s, equivalent to a ~76-mmHg pressure gradient. The peak velocity curve also shows a negative velocity during diastole (*arrowheads*) consistent with aortic regurgitation

grade valvular insufficiency (ALKADHI et al. 2006, 2007; FEUCHTNER et al. 2006a). The regurgitant flow and volume though cannot be assessed with CT techniques.

Although both cross-sectional modalities can be used in valvular diagnosis, the direct visualization and assessment of the valvular leaflets or cusps is still a domain of echocardiography, based on its outstanding high temporal resolution and real-time capabilities. As already mentioned above, valvular diagnosis in CT may be hampered by dose-saving strategies, and with the advent of prospectively ECG-triggered data acquisition, it is unlikely that it will play a clinical role in the future. The assessment of valvular calcification may be of significant benefit in the setting of valve repair planning.

## 21.3.4
## Myocardial Perfusion Imaging

CAD is mainly based on atherosclerotic wall disease. Significant narrowing of the coronary vessel lumen reduces the coronary blood flow and may cause myocardial ischemia with its pathophysiologic changes and its potential symptoms. The morphologic degree of stenosis though not necessarily shows a strong correlation with its hemodynamic significance, its affects on coronary blood flow, and myocardial perfusion. In complex and eccentric coronary stenosis, these parameters might diverge. Thus, the most accurate way to adequately prove the potential relevance of coronary stenosis is not its morphologic assessment but the assessment of coronary blood flow and myocardial perfusion (WILSON 1996).

SPECT and PET imaging of myocardial perfusion have been used now for many years to assess myocardial perfusion and hemodynamic significance of coronary lesions. Although these techniques are still in use for clinical routine assessment, they also suffer from limitations:

- Application of radiation (radiotracers)
- Limited spatial resolution
- Time-consuming examinations
- Limited availability and costs of especially PET imaging

MRI allows the dynamic imaging of a contrast agent bolus through the cardiac chambers and the myocardium. In order to simulate physiologic stress levels, MR perfusion imaging is commonly performed at rest and during pharmacologic stress testing (e.g., adenosine infusion). Myocardial ischemia as a proof of significant coronary stenosis or even occlusion can easily be differentiated from normal perfused regions, based on a delayed and reduced contrast agent arrival. The use of quantitative analysis may even allow for absolute assessment of myocardial perfusion with good correlation to reference standards (AL-SAADI et al. 2001; NAGEL et al. 2003). Many studies support the efficacy of MR perfusion imaging in comparison to invasive coronary cathcterization or nuclear medicine studies in clinical scenarios, with sensitivities and specificities ranging from 85 to 90% compared with coronary angiography (SCHWITTER et al. 2001; NAGEL et al. 2003). Data from most recent studies suggest that the use of higher field strength (e.g., 3 T) further meliorates and improve results of MR myocardial perfusion imaging, mainly based on the improved signal-to-noise and contrast-to-noise levels (CHENG et al. 2007; THEISEN et al. 2007). With the further development of straightforward postprocessing algorithms that may even allow absolute quantification, MR perfusion imaging may replace SPECT and PET in daily routine application of myocardial perfusion assessment. This is not only based on the MR perfusion application, but also on the overall detailed insight into various pathologies.

CT perfusion techniques have been established in the assessment of brain perfusion for early detection of ischemic stroke. However, in the setting of a periodically fast-moving structure with overlaying additional respiratory motion, CT techniques have also been used for dynamic contrast agent studies of the heart to evaluate myocardial perfusion. These early studies though have been based on EBCT, with the lack of rotating gantry parts and thus enabling a fast-rotating X-ray beam.

MDCT techniques are currently under investigation with respect to myocardial perfusion imaging and show close correlation to microsphere data (GEORGE et al. 2006, 2007). With respect to real CT perfusion imaging with dynamic contrast agent tracing, the following facts may currently restrict the use to scientific evaluation only:

- Currently insufficient myocardial coverage, depending on the scanner configuration (may be solved with upcoming generations)
- Noncardiac axis-oriented acquisition with hindered assignment to coronary territories
- Necessity of prolonged contrast agent tracing with a substantial cumulating radiation dose

The principle of today's myocardial perfusion imaging techniques, no matter what modality actually being used, is based on the comparison of stress and rest studies. This strategy actually reliably differentiates persistent from reversible myocardial perfusion deficits. Application of this principle to CT techniques would in addition double the radiation dose. Overall, these current limitations prohibit CT dynamic perfusion imaging being used in clinical applications.

However, several clinical studies have reported the ability of CT to delineate myocardial hypoperfusion (NIKOLAOU et al. 2004). These data though are mostly gathered based on CT coronary angiography data sets, with constant contrast agent supply. The given information resembles myocardial blood distribution but does not give detailed information on myocardial perfusion. In nonacutely injured and ischemic myocardium, myocardial blood-volume parameters may be normal while myocardial blood flow is impaired, with the consequence of a prolonged myocardial mean transit time.

### 21.3.5
### Delayed-Enhancement Imaging

Delayed-enhancement (DE) imaging refers to assessment of the myocardium and other structures several minutes after the intravenous application of contrast agents. The technique was first described by HIGGINS et al. (1979) almost 30 years ago and surprisingly not for MRI, but with the use of CT techniques. The overwhelming success and today's widespread use of this technique though is based on its application to MRI techniques. Based on its systematic evaluation and clinical correlation, together with the development of new imaging techniques, DE imaging has rapidly emerged as standard of reference with regard to the assessment of myocardial viability (KIM et al. 1999; 2000; SIMON-

ETTI et al. 2001). This technique has further pushed the envelope for cardiac MRI in a routine setting and based on the high spatial resolution of DE imaging, results have been shown to be even superior SPECT and FDG-PET with respect to subtle, nontransmural infarctions (HUNOLD et al. 2002; WAGNER et al. 2003).

With the advent of multidetector row techniques, CT has picked up DE again. Several studies have focused on comparison to DE-MRI and on the optimization of imaging techniques. Based on animal studies, it has been shown that DE-CT imaging basically has the same potential in delineation of myocardial viability (AMADO et al. 2006; et al. GERBER 2006; LARDO et al. 2006). The clinical application of this technique though is hampered by the following factors:

- Additional radiation exposure with the use of a delayed scan after coronary CTA
- Necessity of high-contrast agent amounts to enable reasonable CNR

In order to improve contrast-to-noise ratio (CNR) of infarcted myocardium and to simultaneously reduce the radiation exposure, the use of lower tube voltage has been proposed (MAHNKEN et al. 2007). The clinical usefulness though is still questionable.

In recent years, the application of DE-MRI has been substantially broadened by its application to nonischemic myocardial diseases. The high CNR of DE-MR techniques even enables depiction of subtle intramyocardial foci and therefore has been given further insight in the differential diagnosis of myocarditis and various cardiomyopathies (HUNOLD et al. 2005; VOGEL-CLAUSSEN et al. 2006). In some entities, specific features of DE imaging have been described, substantially narrowing the range of differential diagnosis and thus enabling fast-track therapeutic decisions or even possible prediction of patient risk and outcome (MOON et al. 2003; VOGELSBERG et al. 2008). The application of DE-CT imaging to this detailed insight into these nonischemic diseases is mainly hampered by its ability to depict subtle changes in contract enhancement.

## 21.4
## Clinical Scenarios and Decisions

### 21.4.1
### How to Choose the Appropriate Modality?

The above-mentioned discussion on the various techniques of each modality is somewhat theoretical and needs to be applied to real clinical patient scenar-

ios. The clinical presentation and history of patients is extremely variable, and in many cases does not match the typical ones. However, the clinical information is of outmost importance with regard to further patient workup, with the ultimate aim to come to an accurate and fast diagnosis at reasonable costs. As both CT and MRI are two powerful tools in noninvasive cardiac imaging, which both also show limitations, the correct choice is of major importance. In some cases, even the use of both modalities may add valuable information and allow a more precise triage of disease.

In general, cardiac MRI shows a wide variety of clinically applicable techniques, while CT techniques are somewhat limited in their application. As the majority of symptoms and patients though are related to CAD, cardiac CT imaging still may cover a large patient population.

The following discussion is given to offer further insight into major clinical applications, with a dedicated focus to ischemic heart diseases.

### 21.4.1.1
### Imaging of CAD

As discussed above, coronary CTA is the tool to be used in patients presenting with a low to intermediate pretest probability of CAD. The exclusion of coronary changes reliably rules out CAD as the underlying cause of symptoms (high NPV). The technique may even replace coronary angiography in the setting of pretherapeutically planning of surgery in noncardiac diseases or add on information in other diseases. Cardiac MRI has attempted to improve further coronary MRA, but the best possible techniques today are still inferior to coronary CTA.

With the advent of prospectively triggered high-resolution coronary CTA that substantially reduces radiation exposure, even its application in assessment of coronary anomalies in a young patient population is justified.

In cases of positive findings (e.g., atherosclerotic wall changes, stenosis) in coronary CTA, further workup of patients is inevitable, as clinical cardiac CT is limited exclusively to image morphologic changes. Cardiac MRI may be suitable for further workup to identify the hemodynamic significance of CT detected coronary stenosis or even myocardial changes (e.g., silent infarctions).

Imaging of patients in the setting of known coronary disease substantially differs from the initial CT-based CAD diagnosis. Patients may have undergone surgical procedures (CABG) or interventional revasculariza-

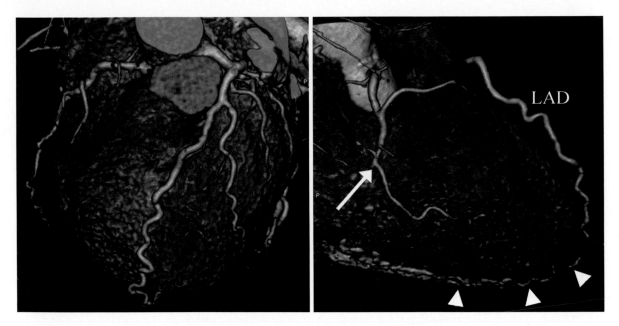

**Fig. 21.8.** High-resolution coronary CTA demonstrates an occluded (*arrow*) RCA and a tortuous LAD with collateral vessels (*arrowheads*) to the distal right coronary artery territory and inferior wall

tion (percutaneous transluminal coronary angioplasty [PTCA], stents), and thus the assessment is somewhat more complex. Patients may also have developed collateral vessels in order to provide blood supply to territories distal to severe stenosis or even occlusion. While CT may be able to demonstrate those collateralized territories, it cannot provide further information on the quality of collateral blood flow (Fig. 21.8). MR perfusion imaging can prove whether collateral blood flow is sufficient or insufficient (Fig. 21.9). In cases of recurrence of chest pain in patients post-CABG, CT bypass CTA is perfectly suited to assess bypass graft patency (Fig. 21.10); the judgment of the native vessels though is substantially hampered by the fact that coronary vessels may exhibit an accelerated atherosclerosis and calcification. In addition, CTA is limited in its accuracy in small distal coronary segments. Early after CABG, CT assessment of bypass patency may be of clinical value.

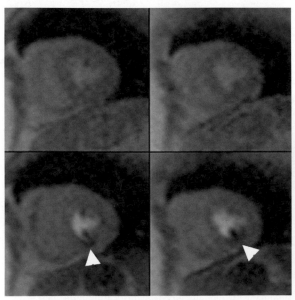

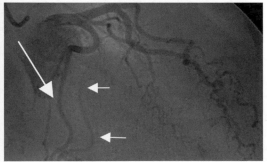

**Fig. 21.9a,b.** MR perfusion data (**a**) and conventional coronary angiography (**b**) of a 63-year-old female patient who presented with angina. While MR perfusion at rest (*upper row*) showed homogeneous contract enhancement, during adenosine stress, a hypoperfused area in the inferior wall is evident (*arrowheads*). The corresponding catheter examination shows a left main contrast injection with a late opacification of the RCA (*short arrows*) parallel to the left circumflex artery ([LCA] *long arrow*), which is filled via collaterals in the setting of ostial RCA occlusion

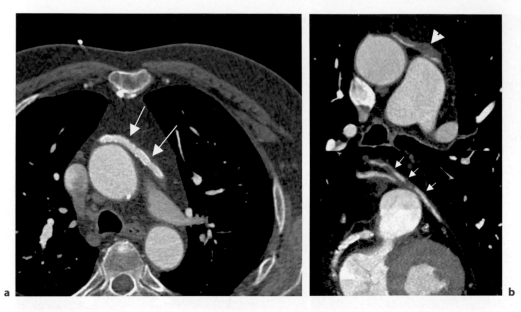

**Fig. 21.10a,b.** CTA of coronary bypass grafts. **a** Cross-sectional image of a patent saphenous vein graft (*arrows*) exhibiting severe calcified wall changes. Data of another patient (**b**) who presented with acute chest pain shows two venous grafts, with thrombus formation (*small arrows*) and total occlusion of one graft (*arrowhead*)

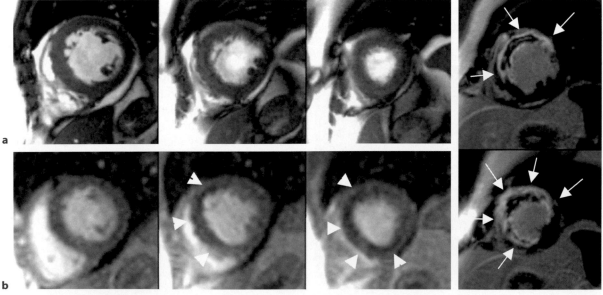

**Fig. 21.11a–c.** Comprehensive MR assessment of the cardiac status in a patient after myocardial infarction. **a** Cine imaging demonstrates normal end-diastolic thickness of the LV wall, while (**b**) myocardial perfusion (at rest) shows an extensive hypoperfusion within the anterior and anteroseptal LV wall (*arrowheads*). **c** Delayed enhancement imaging confirms a large transmural infarction, which also shows large areas with microvascular obstruction that do not show enhancement surrounded by enhancing nonviable myocardium (*arrows*)

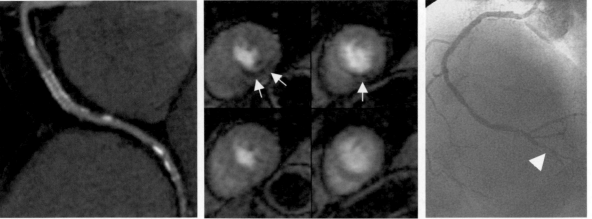

a,b                                                                                                        c

**Fig. 21.12a–c.** CTA (**a**) data set in a patient after stent placement and recurrence of chest pain. MPR of the RCA shows a patient stent within segment 2 and multiple lesions with unknown hemodynamic significance in the distal RCA. MR perfusion (**b**) demonstrates inferior wall hypoperfusion (*short arrows*) at stress (*upper row*) caused by a significant stenosis (*arrowhead*) proven in the cath lab examination (**c**)

In long-term follow-up when also changes of native vessels may have occurred (de novo stenosis), CT cannot perform an accurate triage of the patient.

The primary goal of noninvasive imaging tools in this patient population is the assessment of myocardial blood supply, which can be readily assessed by application of MR perfusion imaging. In combination with DE imaging and cine MRI, a comprehensive assessment of patient status is feasible including the extent of reversible perfusion deficits, the extent of infarcted myocardium, and the overall functional status (Fig. 21.11).

In patients after stent placement and recurrence of symptoms, the use of CTA also may be only of limited value. Assessment of overall stent patency can reliably be performed; the detailed insight into the stent though is heavily dependent on the stent type and design (RIST et al. 2006; DAS et al. 2007; HECHT et al. 2008). Applying MRI in these cases may allow insight into the functional status including possible de novo stenosis and collateral coronary flow (Fig. 21.12).

### 21.4.1.2
### Imaging of Nonischemic Cardiac Disease

Although ischemic disease makes up a large proportion of the overall patient population, there is a stunning variety of other cardiac diseases that also need to be addressed in noninvasive diagnostic procedures. This variety include diseases such as the entire range of CHD, the widespread range of cardiomyopathies and inflammatory diseases, and cardiac tumors.

As mentioned above, cardiac CT is somewhat limited as it "only" allows the clinical application of CTA techniques, possibly in combination with plain scans for identification of calcifications or delayed scanning to assess mass contrast agent uptake. MRI provides a much more sophisticated range of applications that may rule out or confirm clinical suspected pathologies or may narrow the list of differential diagnosis; in some cases, MRI may even be able to demonstrate features specific for a certain pathology and therefore yield a final diagnosis.

### Cardiomyopathies and Inflammatory Disease

As already pointed out earlier, DE imaging techniques assess differences in the myocardial texture and composition based on differences in contract agent wash-in, distribution, and wash-out mechanisms compared with normal myocardium. The technique though theoretically also works for MDCT imaging, but the CNR between normal and delayed enhancing myocardium is in the order of a magnitude higher in MRI and therefore eases depiction of even subtle pathologic changes (SIMONETTI et al. 2001). The easy combination of functional cine imaging and contract-enhanced tissue differentiation allows for a rapid and comprehensive diagnosis. The most important feature in the differential diagnosis, especially of cardiomyopathies and inflammatory diseases, is the pattern of delayed enhancement (HUNOLD et al. 2005; VOGEL-CLAUSSEN et al. 2006). The combination of the above-mentioned techniques with PC flow imaging gives even further insight into the functional status, as it allows for the assessment of diastolic dysfunction, parameters that already demonstrate changes while global systolic function remains normal. Thus, early diagnosis of disease is possible warranting early treatment options, with a possible effect on the patient's prognosis.

### Cardiac Masses and Pseudolesions

Imaging of cardiac mass in daily routine in mainly dedicated to the assessment of cardiac thrombi rather than primary cardiac neoplasms. Although not being superior to cardiac MR in terms of reliability and accuracy, cardiac CT allows for a substantially faster clot imaging and therefore eases the workflow in noninvasive clot assessment.

Assessment of real cardiac masses, no matter whether primary or secondary, may necessitate imaging techniques more sophisticated in order to narrow the final diagnosis and to be able to assess the true extent of a primary cardiac mass or the cardiac involvement of a primary extracardiac lesion (e.g., bronchiogenic carcinoma).

While based on typical mass features or characteristic imaging findings, cardiac CT may allow a substantial narrowing of the differential diagnosis (e.g., myxoma, calcified fibroma); especially masses that do not exhibit specific imaging features or typical tumor locations necessitate further MR workup for extensive soft tissue differentiation.

## 21.5
## Conclusion

As demonstrated within this chapter, cardiac MRI provides a substantially larger toolbox for the assessment of cardiac diseases. Using these techniques, MR can cover the majority of cardiac diseases. Cardiac CT though is, in comparison to MRI, substantially limited in techniques, and can only be reliably applied in a very narrow and specific range of cardiac diseases. This range includes CAD detection and exclusion, and thus the majority of patients being referred for cross-sectional diagnosis of cardiac pathology. Consensus statements and guidelines regarding the appropriate use of cardiac CT and MR have been published and provide further information on the clinical use of both modalities (HENDEL et al. 2006).

## References

al-Saadi N et al. (2001) Comparison of various parameters for determining an index of myocardial perfusion reserve in detecting coronary stenosis with cardiovascular magnetic resonance tomography. Z Kardiol 90:824–834 (In German)

Alkadhi H et al. (2006) Mitral regurgitation: quantification with 16-detector row CTinitial experience. Radiology 238:454–463

Alkadhi H et al. (2007) Aortic regurgitation: assessment with 64-section CT. Radiology 245:111–121

Amado LC et al. (2006) Multimodality noninvasive imaging demonstrates in vivo cardiac regeneration after mesenchymal stem cell therapy. J Am Coll Cardiol 48:2116–2124

Brodoefel H et al. (2007) Dual-source CT with improved temporal resolution in assessment of left ventricular function: a pilot study. AJR Am J Roentgenol 189:1064–1070

Cerqueira MD et al. (2002) Standardized myocardial segmentation and nomenclature for tomographic imaging of the heart: a statement for healthcare professionals from the Cardiac Imaging Committee of the Council on Clinical Cardiology of the American Heart Association. Circulation 105:539–542

Cheng AS et al. (2007) Cardiovascular magnetic resonance perfusion imaging at 3-tesla for the detection of coronary artery disease: a comparison with 1.5-tesla. J Am Coll Cardiol 49:2440–2449

Das KM et al. (2007) Contrast-enhanced 64-section coronary multidetector CT angiography versus conventional coronary angiography for stent assessment. Radiology 245:424–432

Djavidani B et al. (2005) Planimetry of mitral valve stenosis by magnetic resonance imaging. J Am Coll Cardiol 45:2048–2053

Feuchtner GM et al. (2006a) Multislice computed tomography for detection of patients with aortic valve stenosis and quantification of severity. J Am Coll Cardiol 47:1410–1417

Feuchtner GM et al. (2006a) Diagnostic performance of MDCT for detecting aortic valve regurgitation. AJR Am J Roentgenol 186:1676–1681

Feuchtner GM et al. (2007) Sixty-four slice CT evaluation of aortic stenosis using planimetry of the aortic valve area. AJR Am J Roentgenol 189:197–203

Gelfand EV et al. (2006) Severity of mitral and aortic regurgitation as assessed by cardiovascular magnetic resonance: optimizing correlation with Doppler echocardiography. J Cardiovasc Magn Reson 8:503–507

George RT et al. (2006) Multidetector computed tomography myocardial perfusion imaging during adenosine stress. J Am Coll Cardiol 48:153–160

George RT et al. (2007) Quantification of myocardial perfusion using dynamic 64-detector computed tomography. Invest Radiol 42:815–822

Gerber BL et al. (2006) Characterization of acute and chronic myocardial infarcts by multidetector computed tomography: comparison with contrast-enhanced magnetic resonance. Circulation 113:823–833

Hecht HS et al. (2008) Usefulness of 64-detector computed tomographic angiography for diagnosing in-stent restenosis in native coronary arteries. Am J Cardiol 101:820–824

Hendel RC et al. (2006) ACCF/ACR/SCCT/SCMR/ASNC/NASCI/SCAI/SIR 2006 appropriateness criteria for cardiac computed tomography and cardiac magnetic resonance imaging. J Am Coll Cardiol 48:1475–1497

Higgins CB et al. (1979) Evaluation of myocardial ischemic damage of various ages by computerized transmission tomography. Time-dependent effects of contrast material. Circulation 60:284–291

Hunold P et al. (2002) [Evaluation of myocardial viability with contrast-enhanced magnetic resonance imaging-comparison of the late enhancement technique with positron emission tomography]. Rofo Fortschr Geb Rontgenstr Neuen Bildgeb Verfahr 174:867–873 (In German)

Hunold P et al. (2005) Myocardial late enhancement in contrast-enhanced cardiac MRI: distinction between infarction scar and non-infarction-related disease. AJR Am J Roentgenol 184:1420–1426

Jakobs TF et al. (2002) Multislice helical CT of the heart with retrospective ECG gating: reduction of radiation exposure by ECG-controlled tube current modulation. Eur Radiol 12:1081–1086

Johnson TR et al. (2007) Material differentiation by dual energy CT: initial experience. Eur Radiol 17:1510–1517

Kim RJ et al. (1999) Relationship of MRI delayed contrast enhancement to irreversible injury, infarct age, and contractile function. Circulation 100:1992–2002

Kim RJ et al. (2000) The use of contrast-enhanced magnetic resonance imaging to identify reversible myocardial dysfunction. N Engl J Med 343:1445–1453

Kim YY et al. (2007) Left atrial appendage filling defects identified by multidetector computed tomography in patients undergoing radiofrequency pulmonary vein antral isolation: a comparison with transesophageal echocardiography. Am Heart J 154:1199–205

Lardo AC et al. (2006) Contrast-enhanced multidetector computed tomography viability imaging after myocardial infarction: characterization of myocyte death, microvascular obstruction, and chronic scar. Circulation 113:394–404

Liu X et al. (2007) Comparison of 3D free-breathing coronary MR angiography and 64-MDCT angiography for detection of coronary stenosis in patients with high calcium scores. AJR Am J Roentgenol 189:1326–1332

Mahnken AH et al. (2007) Low tube voltage improves computed tomography imaging of delayed myocardial contrast enhancement in an experimental acute myocardial infarction model. Invest Radiol 42:123–129

Matt D et al. (2007) Dual-source CT coronary angiography: image quality, mean heart rate, and heart rate variability. AJR Am J Roentgenol 189:567–573

Moon JC et al. (2003) Toward clinical risk assessment in hypertrophic cardiomyopathy with gadolinium cardiovascular magnetic resonance. J Am Coll Cardiol 41:1561–1567

Nagel E et al. (2003) Magnetic resonance perfusion measurements for the noninvasive detection of coronary artery disease. Circulation 108:432–437

Nikolaou K et al. (2004) Assessment of myocardial infarctions using multidetector-row computed tomography. J Comput Assist Tomogr 28:286–292

Ozgun M et al. (2007) Intraindividual comparison of 3D coronary MR angiography and coronary CT angiography. Acad Radiol 14:910–916

Pouleur AC et al. (2007a) Planimetric and continuity equation assessment of aortic valve area: Head to head comparison between cardiac magnetic resonance and echocardiography. J Magn Reson Imaging 26:1436–1443

Pouleur AC et al. (2007b) Aortic valve area assessment: multidetector CT compared with cine MR imaging and transthoracic and transesophageal echocardiography. Radiology 244:745–754

Prakash A et al. (2007) Usefulness of magnetic resonance angiography in the evaluation of complex congenital heart disease in newborns and infants. Am J Cardiol 100:715–721

Rist C et al. (2006) Assessment of coronary artery stent patency and restenosis using 64-slice computed tomography. Acad Radiol 13:1465–1473

Rominger MB et al. (2000) Left ventricular heart volume determination with fast MRI in breath holding technique: how different are quantitative heart catheter, quantitative MRI and visual echocardiography? Fortschr Roentgenstr 172:23–32

Schertler T et al. (2007) Dual-source computed tomography in patients with acute chest pain: feasibility and image quality. Eur Radiol 17:3179–3188

Schwitter J et al. (2001) Assessment of myocardial perfusion in coronary artery disease by magnetic resonance: a comparison with positron emission tomography and coronary angiography. Circulation 103:2230–2235

Semelka RC et al. (1990a) Interstudy reproducibility of dimensional and functional measurements between cine magnetic resonance studies in the morphologically abnormal left ventricle. Am Heart J 119:1367–1373

Semelka RC et al. (1990b) Normal left ventricular dimensions and function: interstudy reproducibility of measurements with cine MR imaging. Radiology 174:763–768

Setser RM et al. (2000) Quantification of left ventricular function with magnetic resonance images acquired in real time. J Magn Reson Imaging 12:430–438

Simonetti OP et al. (2001) An improved MR imaging technique for the visualization of myocardial infarction. Radiology 218:215–223

Theisen D et al. (2007) Myocardial perfusion imaging with gadobutrol: a comparison between 3 and 1.5 tesla with an identical sequence design. Invest Radiol 42:499–506

Vogel-Claussen, J et al. (2006) Delayed enhancement MR imaging: utility in myocardial assessment. Radiographics 26:795–810

Vogelsberg H et al. (2008) Cardiovascular magnetic resonance in clinically suspected cardiac amyloidosis: noninvasive imaging compared to endomyocardial biopsy. J Am Coll Cardiol 51:1022–1030

Wagner A et al. (2003) Contrast-enhanced MRI and routine single photon emission computed tomography (SPECT) perfusion imaging for detection of subendocardial myocardial infarcts: an imaging study. Lancet 361:374–379

Wilson RF (1996) Assessing the severity of coronary-artery stenoses. N Engl J Med 334:1735–1737

# Complementary Roles of Coronary CT and Myocardial Perfusion SPECT

Marcus Hacker

## CONTENTS

## ABSTRACT

Appropriate diagnosis and therapy of CAD frequently requires information about both the morphological and functional status of the coronary artery tree. Thus, combined imaging consisting of invasive coronary angiography (ICA) and myocardial perfusion imaging (MPI) has been practiced in clinical routine diagnostics of patients with stable angina for many years, and can therefore be accepted as the reference standard in the diagnosis of hemodynamically relevant coronary artery stenoses. Both morphological and functional information are mandatory for the decision of performing an interventional therapy or initiating/ maintaining medical treatment in numerous symptomatic patients. The hemodynamic relevance of coronary artery lesions is a major condition in deciding whether an interventional therapy should be performed. A noninvasive concept providing both morphological and functional information could provide accurate allocation of perfusion defects to their determining coronary lesion, and specific morphological and functional classification of patients with CAD. Complementary effects were observed for the combination of CTA and MPI in patients with suspected or known CAD, particularly when 3D image fusion was performed. Additionally, in the setting of patient screening, CT calcium scoring is accepted for exclusion of present CAD. Otherwise, in cases of coronary calcium burden >400, the probability of present ischemia increases to 25%, so that these patients require further functional diagnostic-like MPI.

M. Hacker, MD
Department of Nuclear Medicine, Munich University Hospitals, Ludwig-Maximilians-University of Munich, Marchioninistrasse 15, 81377 Munich, Germany

## 22.1
### Anatomic–Functional Imaging: Basic Principles

Appropriate diagnosis and therapy of CAD frequently require information about both the morphological and functional status of the coronary artery tree. Thus, combined morphological and functional imaging consisting of invasive coronary angiography and myocardial perfusion imaging (MPI) has been practiced in clinical routine diagnostic of patients with stable angina for many years, and is accepted as the reference standard in the diagnosis of hemodynamically relevant coronary artery stenoses.

Invasive coronary angiography (ICA) as the widely accepted gold standard in morphological imaging of the coronary artery tree has shown limited potential in predicting future cardiac events. This is due to the facts that atherosclerotic lesions cannot be detected in case of absent coronary artery stenoses, and that the functional relevance of coronary artery stenoses cannot be evaluated (WHITE et al. 1984; TOPOL and NISSEN 1995; LIBBY 2001). Consequently, the necessity of performing revascularization cannot be provided for many patients, using morphological criteria alone, particularly when multiple, profound stenoses are present.

Whenever intermediate stenoses are detected in ICA, MPI is performed to verify or rule out ischemia and, vice versa, when MPI shows reversible perfusion defects suggesting myocardial ischemia, ICA is required to allocate the respective coronary lesion. This information is mandatory in making the decision to performing an interventional therapy or initiating/maintaining medical treatment in numerous symptomatic patients (SMITH et al. 2001; KLOCKE et al. 2003). The hemodynamic relevance of coronary artery lesions is a major condition in determining whether an interventional therapy should be performed (GIBBONS 1996; SMITH et al. 2001; KLOCKE et al. 2003).

A noninvasive concept providing both morphological and functional information about coronary arteries could provide accurate allocation of perfusion defects to their determining coronary lesion, and specific morphological and functional classification of patients with CAD.

## 22.2
### Imaging Atherosclerosis, Coronary Stenoses, and Myocardial Perfusion

### 22.2.1
### Coronary CT

#### 22.2.1.1
#### CT for Calcium Scoring

Coronary artery calcification is highly specific for the presence of coronary atherosclerosis and is directly related to the total atherosclerotic plaque burden present in the epicardial coronary arteries (RUMBERGER et al. 1995). Significant CAD (>50% stenosis) is almost universally associated with the presence of coronary calcification. Conversely, in the largest published report to date, only 5/940 (0.5%) symptomatic patients referred for ICA had significant CAD if the coronary artery calcium score (CACS) was 0 (HABERL et al. 2001). A normal CT study is therefore reassuring for excluding significant CAD. The accuracy for identifying significant CAD increases with the CACS and may be further improved by incorporating age, gender, and traditional risk factor information (GUERCI et al. 1998; BUDOFF et al. 2002).

Since there is a strong relationship between CACS severity and the extent of atherosclerotic plaque, it is not surprising that the CACS predicts risk for subsequent cardiovascular events among otherwise heterogeneous patient populations with cardiac risk factors (RAGGI et al. 2000; WONG et al. 2000; WAYHS et al. 2002; KONDOS et al. 2003; SHAW et al. 2003; ARAD et al. 2005; TAYLOR et al. 2005). In the largest published series to date, in which 25,253 patients were followed for 6.8 years (BUDOFF et al. 2007), the mortality rate ranged from 0.6 to 23.1% for patients with a CACS of 0 to >1,000. The CACS predicts cardiac events independently of other standard risk predictors such as the Framingham risk score (ARAD et al. 2005; BUDOFF et al. 2007) and C-reactive protein (PARK et al. 2002), and irrespective of gender (WONG et al. 2000; SHAW et al. 2003). Although patients with diabetes have a higher mortality rate at every level of CACS as compared with nondiabetics, a CACS of 0 still confers a similar 99% 5-year survival in both groups (RAGGI et al. 2004). Finally, recent data indicate that serial CT imaging can assess the effects of intensive lipid-lowering therapy on CACS progression (ACHENBACH et al. 2002) and the risk for subsequent events (RAGGI et al. 2004).

## 22.2.1.2
## CTA

Recent developments in MDCT technology, with faster rotation times and higher spatial resolution created a good, noninvasive alternative to ICA. Latest publications reported high overall sensitivities ranging from 94 to 99% for 64-slice CTA compared with ICA in detecting coronary artery stenoses ≥50%. Also, the specificity with values between 95 and 97% was high, with a minimal fraction of nondiagnostic segments (ACHENBACH et al. 2000, 2001; KNEZ et al. 2001; KOPP et al. 2002; NIEMAN et al. 2002; ROPERS et al. 2003; HOFFMANN et al. 2004; KUETTNER et al. 2004; MOLLET et al. 2004; HOFFMANN et al. 2005; LEBER et al. 2005; LESCHKA et al. 2005; MOLLET et al. 2005; PUGLIESE et al. 2005).

However, MDCT angiography images are still impaired by motion artifacts, even though β-blocker medication is administered, and images are acquired at heart rates <65 bpm (HONG et al. 2001). Furthermore, quantification of lumen narrowing is inhibited in the case of heavy vessel calcifications or intracoronary stenting, resulting in low sensitivity, particularly in patients with advanced CAD (KUETTNER et al. 2004).

Additionally, even 64-slice scanners are lacking in accuracy compared with ICA if a lumen quantification more exact is required (LEBER et al. 2005), and it remains unclear if CT techniques even with 128- or 256-slice scanners will be able to achieve the high temporal and spatial resolution of ICA, which is a precondition for competing with the accepted invasive morphological gold standard in clinical routine diagnostic of the coronary tree.

The most important limitation of morphological imaging with MDCT angiography is the fact that like ICA, MDCT angiography is not able to predict the functional relevance of coronary artery stenoses. The positive predictive value of MDCT angiography for detecting hemodynamically relevant coronary artery stenoses on a vessel- and a patient-based level was published as between 32 and 60% (DI CARLI and HACHAMOVITCH 2007).

On the other hand, high NPVs were found for MDCT angiography in the detection of vessels, leading to reversible perfusion defects in MPI, suggesting a potential role for this very fast technique as a screening method for the exclusion of hemodynamically relevant CAD. High NPVs between 96 and 100% were already published for MDCT angiography compared with ICA using 16- or 64-slice scanners in the detection of significant coronary artery stenoses ≥50% (HOFFMANN et al. 2004, 2005; LESCHKA et al. 2005; MOLLET et al. 2005; PUGLIESE et al. 005).

## 22.2.2
## MPI SPECT

MPI SPECT is an established method for the noninvasive assessment of functional significance of coronary stenoses and, based on a huge amount of data, delivers valuable information for risk stratification (Fig. 22.1). Patients with stable angina and normal stress sestamibi SPECT have a very low risk of death or fatal myocardial infarction; therefore no intervention is required for those patients (GIBBONS 1996; ISKANDER and ISKANDRIAN 1998). Additionally, MPI has shown a high sensitivity to detect CAD compared with conventional coronary angiography (CCA) (BELLER and ZARET 2000) and a high NPV in the prediction of future cardiac events. Thus, no further examinations are scheduled for patients with a normal MPI (ISKANDER and ISKANDRIAN 1998).

Otherwise, there is limited potential of MPI to specify abnormal results, despite the use of newer imaging techniques like ECG-gated MPI, additional attenuation correction or quantitative analysis (TAILLEFER et al. 1997). Perfusion defects are not always caused by hemodynamically relevant epicardial coronary artery stenoses. In addition, intramural microangiopathic or functional changes like left bundle branch block can lead to left ventricular perfusion abnormalities.

Furthermore, it has to be considered that a negative MPI does not exclude the presence of atherosclerosis. And the allocation of perfusion defects to their determining coronary lesion, which is a major precondition for therapy planning, is impossible using MPI without morphological correlation (FABER et al. 2004).

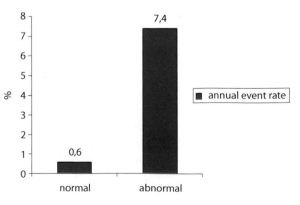

**Fig. 22.1.** Myocardial perfusion SPECT. A 12-fold increased annual event rate of an abnormal perfusion study as compared with a normal perfusion study. (Figure modified from ISKANDER and ISKANDRIAN 1998)

## 22.3
## Combining CT with SPECT

There are numerous possible advantages of a combined noninvasive imaging over each individual procedure.

First of all, accuracy of MPI in the diagnosis of CAD could be increased if morphological information is available, particularly in patients with three-vessel or left main disease and the presence of "balanced" ischemia (CHAMULEAU et al. 2002), even though combined assessment of perfusion and function with gated SPECT enhances the detection of defects in these patients (LIMA et al. 2003). Furthermore, false-positive findings could be reduced and particularly equivocal results in the case of inhomogeneous distribution of the radiotracer in the presence of small vessel disease or left ventricular hypertrophy, or of image artifacts in MPI (extracardial activity, attenuation artifacts), which could be minimized with the help of morphological information. Hybrid imaging modalities with systems such as SPECT–CT and PET–CT have been initially developed to overcome technical limitations by photon-attenuation correction, with the goal to improve further image quality, with subsequent enhancement of the diagnostic accuracy. For MPI SPECT, professional societies recommend incorporation of attenuation correction to improve diagnostic accuracy. On standalone SPECT scanners, the transmission scans necessary for determining tissue density maps for attenuation correction are obtained with an external radionuclide line or point source. With the advent of SPECT–CT hybrid systems, however, CT is now increasingly used for transmission scanning. Advantages of the CT method include higher-quality attenuation maps secondary to higher photon flux, lower noise, and improved resolution.

Second, morphological information could further increase the prognostic significance of MPI alone. In fact, MPI delivers high prognostic accuracy in the prediction of cardiac events, particularly in a short-term follow up period up to 12 months (GIBBONS 1996; IS-KANDER and ISKANDRIAN 1998). Otherwise, present artherosclerosis or significant coronary artery stenoses are missed if morphologic pathology does not lead to any perfusion defect in MPI. BERMAN et al. (2004) recently reported in a cohort of 1,195 patients with suspected CAD that normal MPI patients frequently had extensive atherosclerosis and followed a potential role for applying coronary artery calcification screening after MPI among patients manifesting normal MPI—information that could change the long-term prognoses of patients and consequently, their medical treatments.

Third, perfusion defects could better be allocated to their specific culprit lesion, which is not possible with MPI alone. Accordingly, in the presence of hemodynamically relevant coronary artery stenoses, accurate treatment stratification could be provided. Particularly in patients with known CAD and a more complex coronary anatomy with intracoronary stents or bypass grafts, exact morphological information has shown to be very useful.

Moreover, there are numerous advantages for MDCT angiography complementary to the functional information of MPI.

First, the presence of "nondiagnostic segments" including small coronary arteries or intracoronary stents could be outweighed in cases of absent perfusion abnormalities. Additionally, there is evidence that exact quantification of coronary artery stenoses is of minor priority for clinical decision making, if lesion location and functional status are known. In any case, functional information is indispensable for clinical decision making in MDCT angiography even if significant stenoses ≥50% are present. Our own group showed a low PPV for MDCT angiography to ascertain the hemodynamically relevance of coronary artery stenoses (HACKER et al. 2005, 2007) and, hence, to force revascularization therapy.

Second, previous myocardial infarction cannot always be identified by CTA alone, as the coronary and myocardial structure after infarction is heterogeneous, and not every patient shows vessel occlusions. In patients with intermediate or high-grade stenoses, revascularization could frequently be prevented if MPI shows a fixed perfusion defect, indicating prior myocardial infarction.

However, to date there is limited published experience combining MPI with various CT techniques in the diagnosis of CAD.

### 22.3.1
### Combination of CT Calcium Scoring and Myocardial Perfusion SPECT: Clinical Results

### 22.3.1.1
### Patient Screening

CT calcium scoring is mainly used for screening asymptomatic patients who are at least at intermediate risk for coronary atherosclerosis. Although myocardial perfusion SPECT can also predict outcome in asymptomatic subjects, CT is able to detect coronary atherosclerosis at earlier stages. Additionally, due to the simplicity and

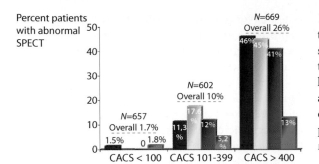

**Fig. 22.2.** Patients with a CACS <100 have a low likelihood of myocardial perfusion SPECT positivity with a dramatic increase when the CACS is >400. N = 1,928. *Red bar* HE et al. (2006) (*N* = 411); *yellow bar*, ANAND et al. (2006) (*N* = 220); *blue bar*, MOSER et al. (2003) (*N* = 102); *green bar*, BERMAN et al. (2004) (*N* = 1,195). (Figure reproduced with permission from MAHMARIAN 2007)

speed of image acquisition as well as the low radiation exposure, CT calcium scoring in this regard is a more robust technique (RUMBERGER et al. 1995) (Fig. 22.2).

There are four major studies (HE et al. 2000; MOSER et al. 2003; ANAND et al. 2004; BERMAN et al. 2004) that investigated the presence of myocardial ischemia as subject to patients' CACS, all in all some 2,000 asymptomatic subjects, which consistently reported very low incidence (1.7%) of an abnormal SPECT in patients with a CACS <100. Otherwise, a severe CACS >400 was associated with a 26% probability of present ischemia in MPI.

However, focusing on asymptomatic high-risk patients like diabetics, even patients with CACS 11–100 show abnormal SPECT results in 18.4%, which increases to 60% with a CACS of >400 (ANAND et al. 2006). The higher incidence of moderate and severe CACSs among asymptomatic diabetics, and their increased likelihood of an abnormal SPECT across all CACS ranges may explain their higher cardiac event rate as compared with nondiabetics at a given CACS threshold.

In a recent study by ANAND et al. (2006), multivariate analysis identified both the CT CACS severity and extent of ischemic myocardium as the only independent predictors of adverse cardiac events in a 2.2-year follow-up in 180 asymptomatic type 2 diabetic subjects, and the combination of the CT and SPECT results improved risk stratification.

A more recent study of 1,153 patients with a mean follow-up of 32±16 months reported no additional risk information from the CACS if SPECT was normal (ROZANSKI et al. 2007). However, most patients in this study had a low CACS of <400 (68%), and ischemia was present in only 64 patients. Larger patient series in more heterogeneous populations followed for longer periods will be needed to better clarify the interrelationship of these imaging modalities for defining risk (Fig. 22.3).

Current guidelines recommend that asymptomatic patients with a CACS of <100 not undergo MPI, since this group has a low likelihood of significant CAD, a very low incidence of stress-induced ischemia (<2%) and an exceedingly low cardiac event rate (BRINDIS et al. 2005). Notable exceptions may include asymptomatic high-risk patients, like diabetics. Conversely, patients with a CACS of ≥400 should routinely undergo

| CAC Score | Calcified Plaque Burden [*] | Likelihood of CAD[†] | CHD Risk[‡] | Recommended Clinical Action [*] | Additional Testing[§] |
|---|---|---|---|---|---|
| 0 | No identifiable atherosclerotic plaque | Very low | Very low | 1° prevention | 0 |
| 1-10 | Minimal plaque burden | Very low | Low | Optional | 0 |
| 11-100 | Mild plaque burden | Low | Moderate | Consider 2° prevention | 0 |
| 101-400 | Moderate plaque burden | Low-intermediate | Moderate-high | 2° prevention | Consider if >75th percentile, diabetes, or MetS |
| 401-1,000 | Extensive plaque burden | High-intermediate | High | 2° prevention | Yes |
| >1,000 | Very extensive plaque burden | High | Very high | 2° prevention | Yes |

CHD, coronary heart disease; MetS, metabolic syndrome.

[*] Sex, age and other issues: presence of chest pain, multiple risk factors, younger age subjects, or female sex should encourage a more aggressive approach to therapy/management.

[†] >50% stenosis.

[‡] 10 years CHD, death or MI.

[§] Most commonly, this recommendation is for stress imaging (MPS, echocardiography, MRI). In some patients and centers, coronary CTA is the recommended additional test.

**Fig. 22.3.** Classification of CAC Scores and Clinical Conditions/Recommendations Commonly Incorporated Into Clinical Reporting. (Figure reproduced with permission from BERMAN et al. 2007)

stress SPECT imaging—this group has a high likelihood of having an ischemic perfusion defect irrespective of symptom status, and particularly when diabetes mellitus is present.

The latter patients as well as patients with typical anginal symptoms, where a low CACS may not confer the same low risk as generally seen in heterogeneous groups, are best evaluated initially by SPECT rather than CT.

## 22.3.1.2
## Symptomatic Patients

A normal stress MPI confers a very low short-term risk for cardiac death and/or acute myocardial infarction (ROZANSKI et al. 2007). However, a normal MPI does not exclude the presence of underlying coronary atherosclerosis, which may be extensive although not yet flow limiting. BERMAN et al. (2004) recently reported 1,119 patients (45% symptomatic) with normal MPI, of whom 56% had a CACS greater than 100, 20% had a CACS of 400–999, and 11% had a CCS of 1,000 or greater. Another recent study of 200 symptomatic patients also showed high frequency of abnormal CT scans after an initial normal MPI, however, with 18% of patients having a CACS >100 (THOMPSON et al. 2005). This was particularly true in patients who were at intermediate or high risk by Framingham criteria. In this regard, CT will unmask a sizeable subgroup of patients with coronary atherosclerosis who should receive more intensive anti-atherosclerotic intervention than would have been indicated by MPI results alone. Knowledge regarding the presence and extent of subclinical coronary atherosclerosis in patients who do not have ischemia by MPI can be of importance in patient management. Recent statements from the American Society of Nuclear Cardiology have noted that patients with moderately high CACS >100 should be aggressively treated to meet secondary prevention goals. Additionally, current evidence now appears to indicate that if the likelihood of ischemia is high enough to warrant study by MPI, then the patients deserve consideration for assessment of subclinical atherosclerosis by CACS. Such assessment may provide a critical link in identifying those for whom targeted medical management may further improve outcome.

Furthermore, although a normal MPI study is generally associated with a low risk, an unacceptably large number of cardiac events occur in these patients. The current studies of the combination of MPI and CT coronary calcification scanning are providing the needed evidence on which recommendations for the broader use

of testing for subclinical atherosclerosis will be applied. Improved identification of at-risk patients through noninvasive imaging is likely to markedly improve the prevention of these unnecessary cardiac events.

CT may also play a significant role in clarifying equivocal MPI results when the latter images are compromised by soft tissue attenuation artifacts, high subdiaphragmatic count activity, or when the stress electrocardiogram and MPI results are disparate. A CACS of 0 associated with an equivocal MPI is reassuring due to the unlikely occurrence of obstructive CAD with a normal CT result.

## 22.3.2
## Combination of Coronary CTA and Myocardial Perfusion SPECT: Clinical Results

The combination of MPI and MDCT angiography was evaluated in three pioneer studies (Fig. 22.4).

In an initial proof-of-the-principle study, our own group focused on the allocation of MPI perfusion defects to their respective coronary artery lesion (HACKER et al. 2007). It was hypothesized that the combination of MDCT angiography and MPI provides accurate allocation of perfusion defects to their determining coronary lesions. Twenty patients with known CAD were studied with MPI, 16-detector CTA, and ICA. Reversible perfusion defects were subsequently allocated to their determining lesion separately for MDCT angiography and CCA. Interestingly, despite low accuracy of MDCT angiography compared with ICA in these patients with advanced stages of disease (sensitivity was 64 and 46% for detecting stenoses ≥50% and vessel- and lesion-based analyses, respectively), 5/5 reversible perfusion defects could be allocated to appropriate coronary artery stenoses for MDCT angiography compared with ICA. In a further study by our group, high sensitivity and specificity of 85 and 97%, respectively, were found for the combination of 64-detector CTA plus MPI compared with the combination of ICA plus MPI in the detection of hemodynamically significant coronary artery stenoses (HACKER et al. 2007). Additionally, high sensitivity and specificity of 93 and 87%, respectively, were shown on a patient-based level, suggesting high accuracy for combined noninvasive imaging in clinical decision making toward interventional or medical therapy. Only one of 15 patients requiring intervention due to a significant RCA stenosis in ICA and a resting perfusion defect in MPI without the history of myocardial infarction was missed with the noninvasive imaging concept. Consequently, we concluded that the combination of

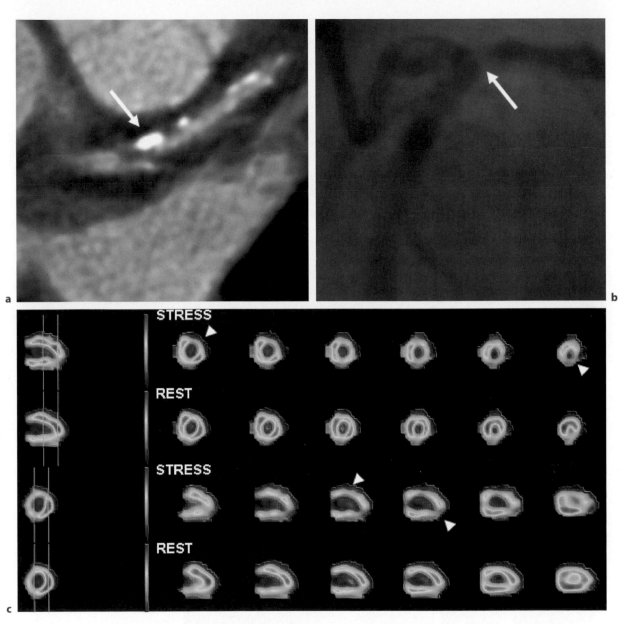

**Fig.22.4a–c.** A 69-year-old male patient with suspected CAD. MPI showed a reversible perfusion defect in the anterolateral wall. The defect was allocated to a significant stenosis located at the bifurcation of the left coronary artery in ICA. MDCT angiography showed a mixed plaque at the same location, also identified as the culprit lesion. The lesion was rated as a true-positive result for the combination of MDCT angiography and MPI. **a** Axial reconstruction of MDCT angiography showing a mixed plaque reaching from the bifurcation of the LM into the proximal LAD. Stenosis was classified ≥50% (*white arrow*). **b** ICA showed an extended stenosis located at the proximal LAD involving the bifurcation, classified as 60% lumen narrowing. The stenosis is partly overlapped by the LCX artery (*white arrows*). **c** Stress (*upper row*) and rest (*lower row*) perfusion images of MPI in axial and sagittal orientations showing a reversible perfusion defect in the anterolateral wall as well as a partly reversible perfusion defect inferoapical (*arrowheads*) (Figure reproduced with permission from HACKER et al. 2007)

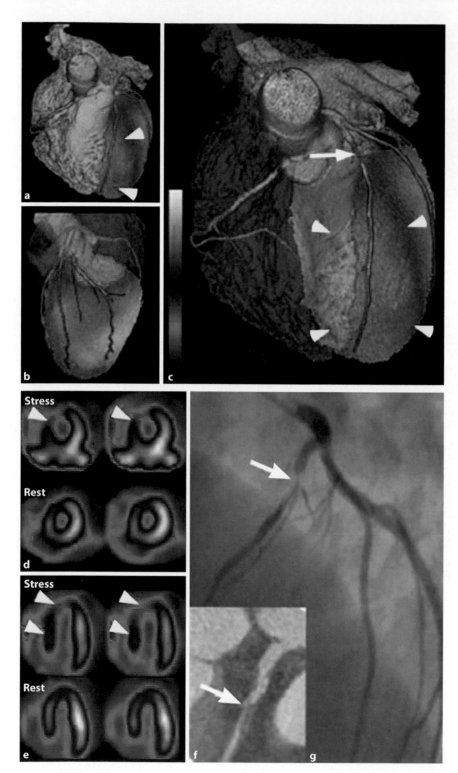

**Fig.22.5a–g.** A 50-year-old male patient (no. 9) referred for typical chest pain. Anterior (**a**) and lateral (**b**) views of the fused 3D SPECT–CT images show a large anterior perfusion defect (*arrowheads*) and preserved perfusion in the lateral and inferior wall. After fading away the right ventricle (**c**), the culprit lesion of the proximal LAD (*arrow*) and a corresponding large anteroseptal perfusion defect (*arrowheads*) can be seen. The short axis (**d**) and horizontal long axis (**e**) slices of the SPECT study confirm the partially reversible anteroseptal perfusion defect (*arrowheads*) The curved reformation of 64-slice CTA (**f**) shows a high-grade stenosis of the proximal LAD (*arrow*), which was confirmed by conventional CA (**g**) (Figure reproduced with permission from GAEMPERLI et al. 2007)

64-slice CTA and gated myocardial SPECT enables a comprehensive noninvasive view of the anatomical and functional status of the coronary artery tree.

These early results were recently confirmed by RISPLER et al. (2007) using an integrated SPECT–16-detector CT scanner for the assessment of hemodynamically significant coronary artery lesions in 56 symptomatic patients. The sensitivity, specificity, PPV, and NPV of MDCT angiography were 96, 63, 31, and 99%, respectively, as compared with 96, 95, 77, and 99%, respectively, for the combination of SPECT plus MDCT angiography. The authors concluded that hybrid SPECT–MDCT imaging results in improved specificity and PPV to detect hemodynamically significant coronary lesions in patients with chest pain.

SPECT–MDCT might play a potentially important role in the noninvasive diagnosis of CAD and introduce an objective decision-making tool for assessing the need for interventions in each occluded vessel.

### 22.3.3
### Image Fusion

Particularly in terms of planning not only interventional therapy, but also for clinical assessment and effective treatment of CAD the integration of sequential, near-simultaneous anatomic and physiologic information from CT and MPI might be of value. The combined SPECT–CT device provides noninvasive CT-based evaluation of coronary anatomy in the same setting with the MPI evaluation of its hemodynamic significance, and might therefore offer higher clinical efficacy than do current clinical diagnostic methods. Although this can be achieved by mental integration of the information from ICA and MPI, standard myocardial distribution territories correspond in only 50–60% to the real anatomic coronary tree (SCHINDLER et al. 1999). Several pioneering attempts of software-based image fusion from ICA and MPI have been paving the way, but are not implemented into clinical practice because its invasiveness precluded its use for noninvasive pre-interventional decision-making (SCHINDLER et al. 2000; FABER et al. 2004) (Fig. 22.5).

After several case repots (NAKAURA et al. 2005; GAEMPERLI et al. 2006, 2007), the recent publication by GAEMPERLI et al. (2007) for the first time investigated the potential clinical use of cardiac image fusion from stand-alone SPECT and CT in 38 consecutive patients with at least one perfusion defect on MPI. Most importantly, among 40 equivocal lesions on side-by-side analysis, the fused interpretation confirmed hemodynamic significance in 14 lesions and excluded functional rel-

evance in 10 lesions. Added diagnostic information by SPECT–CT was more commonly found in patients with stenoses of small vessels and involvement of diagonal branches. Consequently, in addition to being intuitively convincing, 3D SPECT–CT fusion images in CAD provides added diagnostic information on the functional relevance of coronary artery lesions.

## References

Achenbach S, Ulzheimer S et al. (2000) Noninvasive coronary angiography by retrospectively ECG-gated multislice spiral CT. Circulation 102:2823–2828

Achenbach S, Daniel WG et al. (2001) Noninvasive coronary angiography—an acceptable alternative? N Engl J Med 345:1909–1910

Achenbach S, Ropers D et al. (2002) Influence of lipid-lowering therapy on the progression of coronary artery calcification: a prospective evaluation. Circulation 106:1077–7782

Anand DV, Lim E et al. (2004) Prevalence of silent myocardial ischemia in asymptomatic individuals with subclinical atherosclerosis detected by electron beam tomography. J Nucl Cardiol 11:450–457

Anand DV, Lim E et al. (2006) Risk stratification in uncomplicated type 2 diabetes: prospective evaluation of the combined use of coronary artery calcium imaging and selective myocardial perfusion scintigraphy. Eur Heart J 27:713–721

Arad Y, Goodman KJ et al. (2005) Coronary calcification, coronary disease risk factors, C-reactive protein, and atherosclerotic cardiovascular disease events: the St. Francis Heart Study. J Am Coll Cardiol 46:158–165

Beller GA, Zaret BL (2000) Contributions of nuclear cardiology to diagnosis and prognosis of patients with coronary artery disease. Circulation 101:1465–1478

Berman DS, Wong ND et al. (2004) Relationship between stress-induced myocardial ischemia and atherosclerosis measured by coronary calcium tomography. J Am Coll Cardiol 44:923–930

Brindis RG, Douglas PS et al. (2005) ACCF/ASNC appropriateness criteria for single-photon emission computed tomography myocardial perfusion imaging (SPECT MPI): a report of the American College of Cardiology Foundation Quality Strategic Directions Committee Appropriateness Criteria Working Group and the American Society of Nuclear Cardiology endorsed by the American Heart Association. J Am Coll Cardiol 46:1587–1605

Budoff MJ, Diamond DA et al. (2002) Continuous probabilistic prediction of angiographically significant coronary artery disease using electron beam tomography. Circulation 105:1791–1796

Chamuleau SA, Meuwissen M et al. (2002) Usefulness of fractional flow reserve for risk stratification of patients with multivessel coronary artery disease and an intermediate stenosis. Am J Cardiol 89:377–380

Di Carli MF, Hachamovitch R (2007) New technology for non-invasive evaluation of coronary artery disease. Circulation 115:1464–1480

Faber TL, Santana CA et al. (2004) Three-dimensional fusion of coronary arteries with myocardial perfusion distributions: clinical validation. J Nucl Med 45:745–753

Gaemperli O, Schepis T et al. (2007) Validation of a new cardiac image fusion software for three-dimensional integration of myocardial perfusion SPECT and stand-alone 64-slice CT angiography. Eur J Nucl Med Mol Imaging 34:1097–1106

Gibbons RS (1996) American Society of Nuclear Cardiology project on myocardial perfusion imaging: measuring outcomes in response to emerging guidelines. J Nucl Cardiol 3:436–442

Guerci AD, Spadaro LA et al. (1998) Comparison of electron beam computed tomography scanning and conventional risk factor assessment for the prediction of angiographic coronary artery disease. J Am Coll Cardiol 32:673–679

Haberl R, Becker A et al. (2001) Correlation of coronary calcification and angiographically documented stenoses in patients with suspected coronary artery disease: results of 1,764 patients. J Am Coll Cardiol 37:451–457

Hacker M, Jakobs T et al. (2005) Comparison of spiral multidetector CT angiography and myocardial perfusion imaging in the noninvasive detection of functionally relevant coronary artery lesions: first clinical experiences. J Nucl Med 46:1294–1300

Hacker M, Jakobs T et al. (2007) Sixty-four slice spiral CT angiography does not predict the functional relevance of coronary artery stenoses in patients with stable angina. Eur J Nucl Med Mol Imaging 34:4–10

He ZX, Hedrick TD et al. (2000) Severity of coronary artery calcification by electron beam computed tomography predicts silent myocardial ischemia. Circulation 101:244–251

Hoffmann MH, Shi H et al. (2005) Noninvasive coronary angiography with multislice computed tomography. JAMA 293:2471–2478

Hoffmann U, Moselewski F et al. (2004) Predictive value of 16-slice multidetector spiral computed tomography to detect significant obstructive coronary artery disease in patients at high risk for coronary artery disease: patient-versus segment-based analysis. Circulation 110:2638–2643

Hong C, Becker CR et al. (2001) ECG-gated reconstructed multi-detector row CT coronary angiography: effect of varying trigger delay on image quality. Radiology 220:712–717

Iskander S, Iskandrian AE (1998) Risk assessment using single-photon emission computed tomographic technetium-99m sestamibi imaging. J Am Coll Cardiol 32:57–62

Klocke FJ, Baird MG et al. (2003) ACC/AHA/ASNC guidelines for the clinical use of cardiac radionuclide imaging—executive summary: a report of the American College of Cardiology/American Heart Association Task Force on Practice Guidelines (ACC/AHA/ASNC Committee to Revise the 1995 Guidelines for the Clinical Use of Cardiac Radionuclide Imaging) Circulation 108:1404–1418

Knez A, Becker CR et al. (2001) Usefulness of multislice spiral computed tomography angiography for determination of coronary artery stenoses. Am J Cardiol 88:1191–1194

Kondos GT, Hoff JA et al. (2003) Electron-beam tomography coronary artery calcium and cardiac events: a 37-month follow-up of 5,635 initially asymptomatic low- to intermediate-risk adults. Circulation 107:2571–2576

Kopp AF, Schroeder S et al. (2002) Noninvasive coronary angiography with high resolution multidetector-row computed tomography. Results in 102 patients. Eur Heart J 23:1714–1725

Kuettner A, Kopp AF et al. (2004) Diagnostic accuracy of multidetector computed tomography coronary angiography in patients with angiographically proven coronary artery disease. J Am Coll Cardiol 43:831–839

Kuettner A, Trabold T et al. (2004) Noninvasive detection of coronary lesions using 16-detector multislice spiral computed tomography technology: initial clinical results. J Am Coll Cardiol 44:1230–1237

Leber AW, Knez A et al. (2005) Quantification of obstructive and nonobstructive coronary lesions by 64-slice computed tomography: a comparative study with quantitative coronary angiography and intravascular ultrasound. J Am Coll Cardiol 46:147–154

Leschka S, Alkadhi H et al. (2005) Accuracy of MSCT coronary angiography with 64-slice technology: first experience. Eur Heart J 26:1482–1487

Libby P (2001) Current concepts of the pathogenesis of the acute coronary syndromes. Circulation 104:365–372

Lima RS, Watson DD et al. (2003) Incremental value of combined perfusion and function over perfusion alone by gated SPECT myocardial perfusion imaging for detection of severe three-vessel coronary artery disease. J Am Coll Cardiol 42:64–70

Mahmarian JJ (2007) Combining myocardial perfusion imaging with computed tomography for diagnosis of coronary artery disease. Curr Opin Cardiol 22:413–4121

Mollet NR, Cademartiri F et al. (2004) Multislice spiral computed tomography coronary angiography in patients with stable angina pectoris. J Am Coll Cardiol 43:2265–2270

Mollet NR, Cademartiri F et al. (2005) High-resolution spiral computed tomography coronary angiography in patients referred for diagnostic conventional coronary angiography. Circulation 112:2318–23

Mollet NR, Cademartiri F et al. (2005) High-resolution spiral computed tomography coronary angiography in patients referred for diagnostic conventional coronary angiography. Circulation 3:3

Moser KW, O'Keefe JH Jr et al. (2003) Coronary calcium screening in asymptomatic patients as a guide to risk factor modification and stress myocardial perfusion imaging. J Nucl Cardiol 10:590–598

Nieman K, Cademartiri F et al. (2002) Reliable noninvasive coronary angiography with fast submillimeter multislice spiral computed tomography. Circulation 106:2051–2054

Pugliese F, Mollet NR et al. (2005) Diagnostic accuracy of noninvasive 64-slice CT coronary angiography in patients with stable angina pectoris. Eur Radiol: 1–8

Raggi P, Callister TQ et al. (2000) Identification of patients at increased risk of first unheralded acute myocardial infarction by electron-beam computed tomography. Circulation 101:850–855

Raggi P, Callister TQ et al. (2004) Progression of coronary artery calcium and risk of first myocardial infarction in patients receiving cholesterol-lowering therapy. Arterioscler Thromb Vasc Biol 24:1272–1277

Ropers D, Baum U et al. (2003) Detection of coronary artery stenoses with thin-slice multi-detector row spiral computed tomography and multiplanar reconstruction. Circulation 107:664–6

Rozanski A, Gransar H et al. (2007) Clinical outcomes after both coronary calcium scanning and exercise myocardial perfusion scintigraphy. J Am Coll Cardiol 49:1352–1361

Rumberger JA, Simons DB et al. (1995) Coronary artery calcium area by electron-beam computed tomography and coronary atherosclerotic plaque area. A histopathologic correlative study. Circulation 92:2157–2162

Schindler TH, Magosaki N et al. (1999) Fusion imaging: combined visualization of 3D reconstructed coronary artery tree and 3D myocardial scintigraphic image in coronary artery disease. Int J Card Imaging 15:357–368; discussion 369–370

Shaw LJ, Raggi P et al. (2003) Prognostic value of cardiac risk factors and coronary artery calcium screening for all-cause mortality. Radiology 228:826–833

Smith SC Jr, Dove JT et al. (2001) ACC/AHA guidelines for percutaneous coronary intervention (revision of the 1993 PTCA guidelines)-executive summary: a report of the American College of Cardiology/American Heart Association task force on practice guidelines (Committee to revise the 1993 guidelines for percutaneous transluminal coronary angioplasty) endorsed by the Society for Cardiac Angiography and Interventions. Circulation 103:3019–3041

Taillefer R, DePuey EG et al. (1997) Comparative diagnostic accuracy of Tl-201 and Tc-99m sestamibi SPECT imaging (perfusion and ECG-gated SPECT) in detecting coronary artery disease in women. J Am Coll Cardiol 29:69–77

Taylor AJ, Bindeman J et al. (2005) Coronary calcium independently predicts incident premature coronary heart disease over measured cardiovascular risk factors: mean three-year outcomes in the Prospective Army Coronary Calcium (PACC) project. J Am Coll Cardiol 46:807–814

Topol EJ, Nissen SE (1995) Our preoccupation with coronary luminology. The dissociation between clinical and angiographic findings in ischemic heart disease. Circulation 92:2333–2342

Wayhs R, Zelinger A et al. (2002) High coronary artery calcium scores pose an extremely elevated risk for hard events. J Am Coll Cardiol 39:225–230

White CW, Wright CW et al. (1984) Does visual interpretation of the coronary arteriogram predict the physiologic importance of a coronary stenosis? N Engl J Med 310:819–824

Wong ND, Hsu JC et al. (2000) Coronary artery calcium evaluation by electron beam computed tomography and its relation to new cardiovascular events. Am J Cardiol 86:495–498

# CTA of the Aorta by MDCT

## 23

Wieland H. Sommer, Daniel Theisen and Bernd J. Wintersperger

W. H. Sommer, MD
Department of Clinical Radiology, Ludwig-Maximilians-University of Munich, Munich University Hospitals, Marchioninistrasse 15, 81377 Munich, Germany

D. Theisen, MD
Department of Clinical Radiology, Ludwig-Maximilians-University of Munich, Munich University Hospitals, Marchioninistrasse 15, 81377 Munich, Germany

B. J. Wintersperger, MD
Department of Clinical Radiology, Ludwig-Maximilians-University of Munich, Munich University Hospitals, Marchioninistrasse 15, 81377 Munich, Germany

### ABSTRACT

Since aortic pathologies are associated with high morbidity and mortality, they require an accurate and efficient diagnostic approach. The introduction of multidetector-row technology with option of high-resolution CTA has extensively improved and expanded the clinical applications and is the standard of reference in diagnosis and follow-up of patients with aortic pathologies. The aim of the present chapter is to provide technical details for CTA of the aorta and to overview the most common clinical pathologies of the aorta. These include different types of aortic aneurysms and dissections, penetrating aortic ulcers, intramural aortic hematomas, aortitis, and traumatic injuries of the aorta. Furthermore, this chapter outlines the role of CTA in endovascular aortic reconstruction.

## 23.1
## Technical Considerations

The technical advances of the last 10 years have given rise to a revolution in many domains of CTA. The most important advance for CTA consists in faster acquisition time of data; it is caused by the following three factors:

1. Development of MDCT
2. Increase of the width of the detector
3. Acceleration of rotation speed

### 23.1.1
### Data Acquisition

#### 23.1.1.1
#### Standard Algorithms (Not ECG Triggered)

Modern CT scanners are able to obtain collimations smaller than 1 mm over the complete range of the aorta. In many cases, the limiting factors of acquisition time are hemodynamic; therefore, the highest possible speed of acquisition (table movement, pitch) has to be reduced.

When CT scanners with less than 40 detector rings are used, the collimation may have to be adapted to values around 1.25–2 mm in order to reduce the acquisition time to less than 25–30 s. Since protocols of data acquisition are dependent on type and brand of the CT scanner, only some examples can be given here (Table 23.1). Further details are accessible on the Internet (e.g., http://www.CTisus.com, http://www.multidetector-row-ct.com).

Depending on the underlying pathology or clinical question, additional acquisitions beside arterial CTA are sometimes required, like unenhanced scans or late phases. To prevent unnecessary radiation exposure for the patient, these additional series should be limited to the relevant body region. Tube current and therefore radiation exposure can be significantly reduced by increasing the slice thickness in these scans.

#### 23.1.1.2
#### ECG-Gated Data Acquisition

Pulsation of the aorta causes artifacts, especially in the aortic root and ascending aorta. ECG-triggered data acquisition helps to significantly reduce these artifacts and therefore plays an important role in the examination of unclear chest pain or thoracic aortic dissection (Fig. 23.1). Furthermore, this technique enables the evaluation of coronary arteries and can replace invasive clinical diagnostics in some cases. However, detailed protocols of the thoracic aorta are normally based on protocols of coronary artery CT. Due to their specifications, they lead to longer acquisition times than those of standard protocols and do not properly visualize the abdominal aorta. This can be overcome by an ECG-gated acquisition of the thoracic aorta and a change to the standard protocol for the abdominal aorta. In order to achieve a sufficient contrast in the abdominal aorta, the time delay to modify the examination protocol should be minimized (Fig. 23.2).

### 23.1.2
### Administration of Contrast Agents

The vascular contrast in CTA is mainly dependent on the iodine flow (grams iodine per second), which de-

**Table 23.1.** Examples for protocols of CTA of the aorta with different generations of MDCT and vendors

|  | 16-SCT[a] | 40-SCT[b] | 64-SCT[c] | 64-SCT[d] | 64-SCT[e] | 64-SCT[f] | 64-DECT[g] |
|---|---|---|---|---|---|---|---|
| Collimation (mm) | 16 × 0.75 (16 × 1.5)[h] | 40 × 0.625 | 64 × 0.6 (z-sharp) | 64 × 0.625 | 64 × 0.625 | 64 × 0.5 | 24 × 1.2 |
| Rotation time (s) | 0.5 | 0.4 | 0.33 | 0.4 | 0.5 | 0.5 | 0.5 |
| Tube voltage (kV) | 100–120 | 120 | 100–120 | 120 | 120 | 120 | (80–140)[i] |
| Slice thickness (mm) | 0.5 | 0.9 | 0.75 | 0.9 | 0.625 | 0.5 | 1.5 |
| Increment (mm) | 1 | 0.45 | 0.5 | 0.45 | 0.4 | 0.3 | 0.75 |
| Table feed (mm/s) | ~25–30 | ~50 | ~60 | ~80 | ~110 | ~53 | ~42 |

Detailed protocols can be divergent from these presented here; further information is provided by the producers or via the following homepages: http://www.CTisus.com, http://www.multidetector-row-ct.com

*SCT* single-slice scanner, *DECT* dual-energy CT

[a]E.g., Sensation 16, Siemens AG, Forchheim, Germany

[b]E.g., Philips Brilliance 40, Philips Medical Systems, Best, The Netherlands

[c]E.g., Sensation 64, Siemens AG

[d]E.g., Philips Brilliance 64, Philips Medical Systems

[e]E.g., Lightspeed VCT, GE Healthcare, Milwaukee, Wis.

[f]E.g., Aquilion 64, Toshiba Medical Systems, Zoetermeer, Netherlands

[g]E.g., Sensation Definition, Siemens AG

[h]If the entire aorta is examined, then slice collimation is changed

[i]In dual-energy imaging, the tubes have different voltages

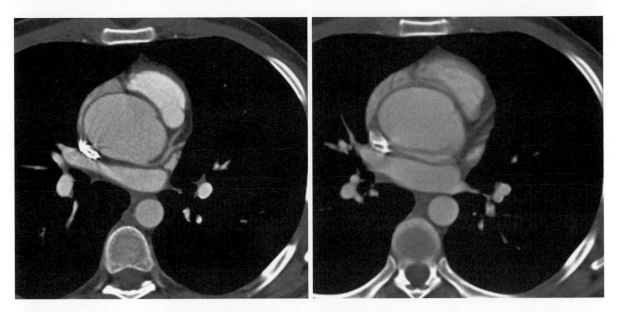

**Fig. 23.1.** Axial images of the aortic root and the left coronary ostium with (*left*) and without ECG gating (*right*). The images without ECG gating show pulsation artifacts, which could be misinterpreted as a dissection membrane

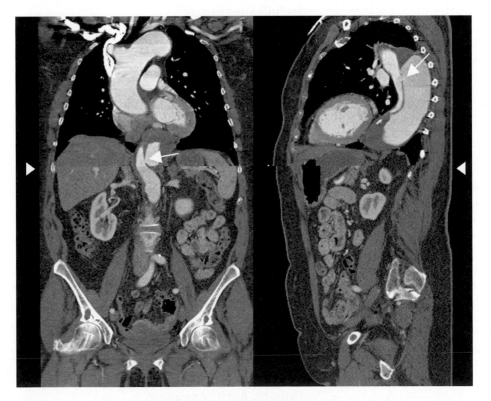

**Fig. 23.2.** Combination CTA of the thoracic and abdominal aorta with a single contrast application. *Left* coronary MPR, *right* sagittal MPR. The *white arrowheads* mark the change between the ECG-gated acquisition of the thoracic aorta and the standard acquisition of the abdominal aorta. There is a dissection Stanford type B in the descending aorta; the entry is distal of the left subclavian artery, the reentry is on a level with the diaphragm (*arrows*)

pends on the amount of iodine and the chosen flow rate (FLEISCHMANN 2003). This implies that a low iodine concentration of the contrast media can be partly balanced by a higher flow rate. For a sufficient vascular contrast in the aorta, an iodine flow rate of 1.5–2 g/s is adequate. With current iodine concentrations in contrast media (300–400 mg iodine per milliliter contrast agent), this can be achieved with flow rates around 4–5 ml/s. Two factors are decisive for the maximum flow rate, the diameter of the vein catheters used and the viscosity of the contrast agent (KNOLLMANN et al. 2004). In order to achieve high iodine flow at admissible flow rates, contrast agents with higher iodine concentration (≥350 mg/ml) should be used. Correct timing and homogenous contrast enhancement can be obtained using bolus tracking algorithms, which detect the arrival of contrast agent in the target vessel and trigger the acquisition of data. In the case of aortic wall dissection, the arrival is difficult to predict and sometimes requires manual activation of data acquisition.

### 23.1.3
### 3D Reconstruction

In order to better visualize certain aortic pathologies, 3D reconstructions of axial CT images can be helpful. There are ways to extract the relevant information for 3D reconstruction out of the primary data set:

- MIP: Voxels with the highest density are selected for 3D reconstruction. In MIPs, only these voxels are relevant and, in contrast to other reconstruction techniques, a summation of several voxels with lower densities does not come into account. MIPs extract structures with high contrast and they are especially helpful for an overview of contrast-enhanced vessels. They also can serve to evaluate and monitor endovascular aneurysm repair.
- Volume-rendering technique (VRT): Unlike MIPs, VRTs contain information about the complete depth of the volume. They result in a better 3D overview of anatomic structures by partially semitransparent visualization of structures with different densities. Thus, several anatomic structures can be examined at the same time (TENGG-KOBLIGK et al. 2007).

### 23.1.4
### Radiation Exposure

Modern CT scanners can modify the tube current in z-direction, as well as in anterior–posterior and lateral projections. This variation of tube current may partly be combined with ECG triggering. However, complete switching on and off according to different heart phases is not yet possible.

As BAHNER et al. (2005) showed, markedly reduced radiation exposure, as well as improved CNR in CTA can be achieved while using a reduced tube potential. The important issue of this method consists in getting closer to iodine's K-edge. Lowering the tube current moderately (e.g., from 120 to 100 kV) has two main effects, noise artifacts increase, but the vascular signal augments as well. Hence, these two effects cancel each other out to some extent (WINTERSPERGER et al. 2005). By reducing the tube potential from 120 to 100 kV, about 30% of radiation exposure can be prevented. A further reduction of the tube potential below 100 kV would lead to a disproportionately high disturbance of image quality. If narrow collimations and thin slices are chosen for image reconstruction, then a higher image noise must be accepted.

### 23.1.5
### Technical Advances

Dual-energy acquisitions greatly enlarge the possibilities of CTA. With one scan, data with two different voltages are acquired (e.g., 80 and 140 kV). Due to the different properties of iodine and calcium at changing tube voltages, a differentiation of those substances can be achieved. Among others, this facilitates an automatic bone removal (JOHNSON et al. 2007). Furthermore, it seems possible to reduce the number of scans, since "virtual nonenhanced scans" can be calculated from the combination of 80 and 140 kV images (Fig. 23.3). In the future, this may simplify examination protocols and even reduce radiation exposure of patients.

## 23.2
## Clinical Applications

### 23.2.1
### Aortic Aneurysm

#### 23.2.1.1
#### Thoracic Aortic Aneurysm

Thoracic aortic aneurysm (TAA) is defined as a persisting dilatation of the ascending aorta larger than 4 cm and of the descending aorta larger than 3 cm (ISSEL-

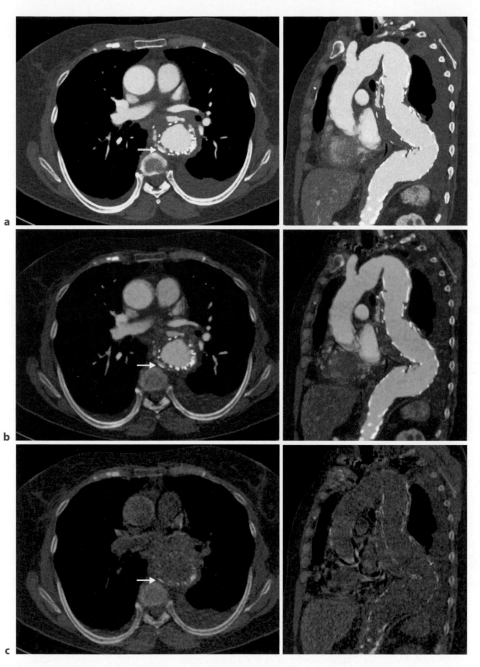

**Fig. 23.3a–c.** Dual-energy CTA of the thoracic aorta after endovascular aortic reconstruction. **a** Standard MPR, axial and sagittal. **b** Overlay of iodine content. **c** Virtual nonenhanced scan: structures containing iodine (contrast medium) are subtracted from these images. Therefore, endoleaks are no longer detectable, while calcifications in the aortic wall remain unchanged (*white arrows*)

BACHER 2005). The surgical classification of aortic aneurysms is graduated according to the Crawford classification (Fig. 23.4).

Morphologically, there are fusiform aneurysms (synonymous with *circumferential*) and sacciform aneurysms, which lead only to a partial dilatation of the aortic wall (ISSELBACHER 2005). The most common examinations for clinical diagnostics of TAA include echocardiography, MDCT, and MRI (RUBIN and KALRA 2006). CTA of the aorta provides a clear visualization of the diameter and allows an evaluation of the relative position of the aneurysm to the neighboring anatomic structures (Fig. 23.5). Dystrophic calcifications of thrombi adherent to the aortic wall can sometimes simulate a dissection of the aortic wall. In the case of a suspected leakage of the aneurysm, an additional nonenhanced scan is recommended in order to detect a periaortic hematoma.

To rule out a concomitant insufficiency of the aortic valve, echocardiography or MRI may be necessary. Be-

fore therapy of a TAA, imaging of the spinal vasculature is important due to the risk of damaging the spinal artery of Adamkiewicz with resulting paraplegia. In this domain, CT is less sensitive than MRI; it is, however, superior in examining the relevant collateral circulation via the internal mammary artery or to intercostal arteries, because of the larger coverage of volume.

### 23.2.1.2
### Abdominal Aortic Aneurysm

In the abdominal aorta, an aneurysm (AAA) is defined by a maximal diameter of ≥3 cm. CTA and MRA are appropriate examinations for diagnosis and clinical monitoring of abdominal aortic aneurysms. CTA or MRA can assess the form and extension of the aneurysm, as well as the relative position of originating arteries more exactly than with ultrasound. Additionally, CTA allows an exact and reproducible measurement of the aortic

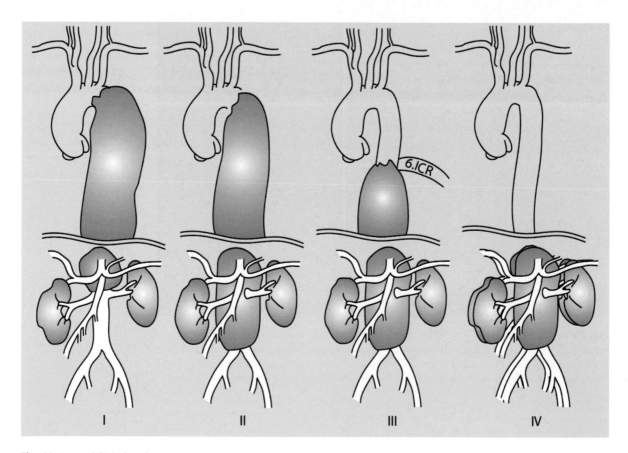

**Fig. 23.4.** Modified classification of thoracic and abdominal aortic aneurysms by Crawford. Type *I* distal of the left subclavian artery as far as the renal arteries; type *II* distal of the left subclavian artery, extending below the renal arteries; type *III* from the sixth thoracic vertebral body, extending below the re-

nal arteries; type *IV* from the twelfth thoracic vertebral body, extending below the renal arteries. (From LUTHER BLP (2007) Kompaktwissen, Gefäßchirurgie. Differenzierte Diagnostik und Therapie. Springer Berlin Heidelberg; Kapitel 8, Seite 127, Abbildung 8.1)

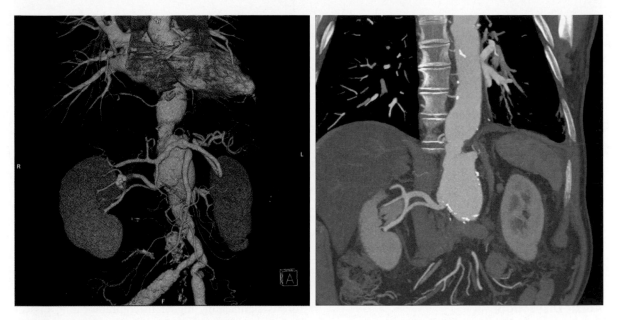

**Fig. 23.5.** Partially calcified thoracic and abdominal aortic aneurysm in a patient with Marfan syndrome. Coronary VR (*left*) and MPR (*right*)

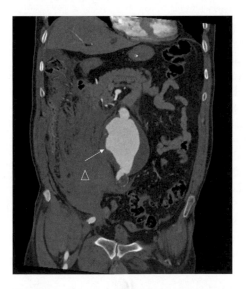

**Fig. 23.6.** Rupture of an infrarenal aortic aneurysm (*arrow*), with an extensive retroperitoneal hematoma (*arrowhead*). Coronary MPR of a CTA of the abdominal aorta

diameter, with low interobserver variability (Singh et al. 2003).

An early and specific sign of impendent aortic rupture can be observed in CT as a sickle-shaped hematoma within the thrombus of a large AAA (Rakita et al. 2007). Due to its high density, it can most clearly

be seen in nonenhanced scans. Further signs are the "draped aorta sign" which is made up of the unidentifiable posterior aortic wall, and an aspect of the posterior aortic wall that follows the vertebral contour. A periaortic, retroperitoneal hematoma with extension into the psoas muscle is the most frequent sign of acute rupture of an AAA. Periaortic blood may extend into the perirenal or pararenal space (Fig. 23.6) (Rakita et al. 2007).

Infected (mycotic) aneurysms can be identified by its lobulated contour, soft tissue infiltration, and periaortic abscesses or trapped air (Rakita et al. 2007). Primary aorto-enteric fistulas as a complication of an AAA are rare and can be identified by extraluminal periaortic trapped air or by the extravasation of the contrast agent into the gastrointestinal tract.

### 23.2.1.3
### Inflammatory Aortic Aneurysm

The inflammatory AAA is a variant of an AAA accompanied by a thickened aneurysm wall and a periaortic or retroperitoneal fibrosis. They are associated with increased morbidities. Some authors describe that they represent between 3 and 10% of AAAs (Tang et al. 2005), while others report between 10 and 30% (Theisen et al. 2007). The inflammatory components show increased enhancement of contrast agent in late phases, both in CT and MRI. Sensitivity and specificity of CT in the detection of inflammatory AAA were assessed by a retrospective survey of 355 patients in the year 2002. This gave a sensitivity rate of 83.3% for this imaging technique, with specificity and accuracy rates of 99.7 and 93.7%, respectively (IINO et al. 2002).

MRI shows advantages in the differentiation of pathologic contrast enhancement from retroperitoneal fat and in the estimation of infiltration of neighboring structures due to its frequency-selective fat saturation (WALLIS et al. 2000). In rare cases, the discrimination of a periaortic hemorrhage can cause problems. These can be overcome either by nonenhanced scans or by using MRI.

## 23.2.2
## Aortic Dissection

Most aortic dissections (ADs) occur in the thoracic aorta and extend into the abdominal aorta or even into the pelvis. An isolated dissection of the abdominal aorta is rare and should be distinguished from "classic" ADs. Penetrating atherosclerotic ulcers are considered as the origin of abdominal AD.

ADs occur due to a tear of the aortal intima and the inner layers of the media. This entry, which is most common in the lateral wall of the ascending aorta or in the aortic isthmus, leads to blood flow into the aortic wall and a consecutive separation of the media creating a "false" lumen. This lumen is separated from the "true" lumen by the dissection membrane.

The incidence of type I lesions of the aortic wall (TASK FORCE OF THE EUROPEAN SOCIETY OF CARDIOLOGY 2001) is about 5–15/100,000 inhabitants per year. In 60%, the origin is in the ascending aorta. The common Stanford classification distinguishes dissections according to the therapeutic approach. Dissections involving the ascending aorta are classified as Stanford A, whereas dissections without involvement of the ascending aorta are classified as Stanford B. The site of the intimal tear is irrelevant in this classification.

CT, MRI, and TEE yield equally reliable diagnostic values for confirming or ruling out thoracic AD (SHIGA et al. 2006). However, craniocaudal extension of the dissection is most easily detected by MDCT. Acute AD (≤2 weeks) is most commonly diagnosed by CTA, since it is an emergency indication. The appropriate imaging of the chronic type of dissection is by either CTA or contrast-enhanced MRA. If acute AD is suspected,

then CT examination should begin with a nonenhanced scan, in order to differentiate fresh thrombi of the false lumen and intramural hematomas by the higher density of old thrombi.

CTA enables the diagnosis of AD and its differentiation according to the Stanford classification, with a sensitivity and specificity of over 99% (HAYTER et al. 2006). Radiologically, the primary intimal tear (entry) and the extension of the AD should be located. Additionally, distal connections between the false and the true lumen (reentries) have to be located. In case of a circumferential dissection, there is an intimo-intimal intussusception and a floating true lumen in the center. A missing contrast enhancement of the lumen arises either from a significant reduction of the blood flow or from a thrombosis.

The differentiation of dissections with and without reentry is of clinical relevance, since the risk of rupture is significantly higher in communicating dissections with a flow in the false lumen than in noncommunicating dissections with a thrombosed false lumen (TAKAHASHI and STANFORD 2005). It can be achieved by an additional nonenhanced scan or by additional late phases (70–120 s).

In the evaluation of aortic side branches, it is essential to determine the origin. This can be in the true lumen, the false lumen or in both (Fig. 23.7). The reentry of a communicating dissection is generally located near the origin of a side branch and can occlude or dissect this branch. Sensitivity and specificity of MDCT for the involvement of side branches are between 95 and 100%. The detection of a dynamic obstruction by means of a prolapsing dissection membrane can be achieved by DSA or time-resolved MRA. This time-resolved acquisition could also be obtained in CT using ECG gating. However, this technique is associated with a relatively high radiation exposure.

The distinction between the true and false lumen is indispensable before endovascular aortic reconstruction (EVAR). Those lumens show the following characterizations:

- The true lumen is characterized by an early and strong contrast enhancement and by continuity into the aortic sections, which are not affected by the dissection. It often shows a smaller diameter than the false lumen.
- The false lumen is characterized by a mostly sickle-shaped configuration. Intimal flaps can be seen in some patients as small intraluminal lines looking like a cobweb, ("cobweb sign"). This sign is specific for the false lumen and can sometimes simplify the differentiation.

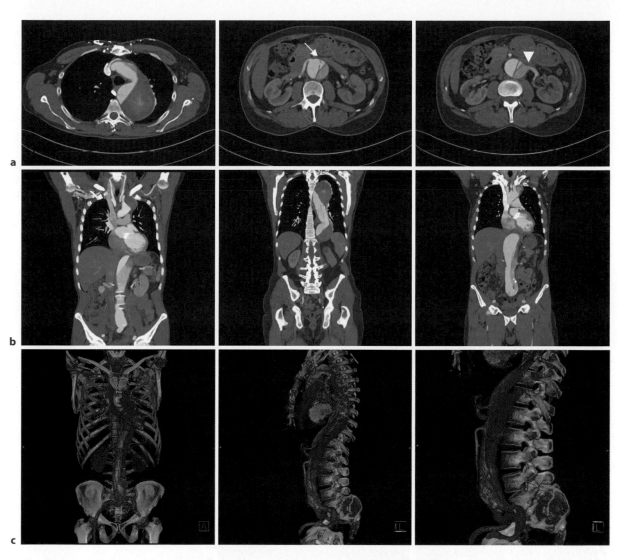

**Fig. 23.7a–c.** Stanford type A dissection with two separate false lumens. Axial (**a**) and coronary (**b**) standard MPR and a VR of the data in coronary and sagittal orientations (**c**). The lateral false lumen is partially thrombosed and shows a significant decrease of the blood flow. The medial false lumen shows a proper contrast enhancement and communicates with the true lumen at the level of the right renal artery (*arrow*). The left renal artery originates from the false lumen (*arrowhead*). Due to the decreased blood flow in the false lumen, the left kidney shows a decreased contrast enhancement due to the malperfusion

### 23.2.2.1
### Stanford A Dissection

An early diagnosis and operative treatment before hemodynamic aggravation or instability are most important for the prognosis of the patient (NIENABER and EAGLE 2003). In CTA, pulsation artifacts of the ascending aorta can imitate or mask an intimal tear. An exact evaluation of the aortic root and of the coronary arteries should therefore be achieved by CT scanners with a fast acquisition and ECG-gated algorithms (see Fig. 23.1).

Dangerous complications like aortic rupture, pericardial tamponade, or hemothorax can be identified easily by CT. However, echocardiography or MRI is required in order to determine the function of the valves.

### 23.2.2.2
### Stanford B Dissection

In Stanford B dissections (Fig. 23.8), conservative therapy is possible. Clinically asymptomatic cases without complications of the aortic side branches are generally treated conservatively. The underlying high blood pressure is reduced in order to minimize the risk of rupture of the false lumen. Regular morphological controls of the dissection are necessary in order to recognize a secondary expansion. This is the case in up to 30% of the cases and highly increases the risk of rupture. In this case, an invasive treatment becomes necessary (RICHTER et al. 2001).

### 23.2.3
### Penetrating Aortic Ulcer

The penetrating aortic ulcer (PAU) is defined as a type IV lesion of the aortic wall (TASK FORCE OF THE EUROPEAN SOCIETY OF CARDIOLOGY 2001). By definition, it is an ulcerating atherosclerotic lesion, which breaks through the inner elastic membrane of the media and may lead to an intramural hematoma (IMH). In many cases, there are multiple ulcers of diameters up to 25 mm and an expansion up to 30 mm deep into the aortic wall (SUNDT 2002). They are often accompanied by atherosclerotic aneurysms of the abdominal aorta. The PAU can be seen in CTA as a contrast-enhanced bulge of the aortic wall (spurious aneurysm). Additionally,

the aortic wall may show contrast enhancement itself (HAYTER et al. 2006).

Accompanying IMHs can be detected in nonenhanced scans and verify the penetrating character of the lesion. Furthermore, nonenhanced scans facilitate the therapeutically relevant differentiation between pseudoaneurysms as a complication of a PAU and a sacciform aortic aneurysm. Mural calcifications suggest an aneurysm. In the case of a spacious IMH or para-aortic hematoma, the differentiation between a ruptured aneurysm and a complicated PAU can be impossible. However, in both cases, an immediate therapeutic intervention is indicated. Complications of a PAU, like AD, formation of a pseudoaneurysm, or aortic rupture can all be detected or excluded in the same scan.

### 23.2.4
### IMH

Originally, IMH was defined as a dissection of the aortic wall without intimal tear. The pathogenesis includes rupture of the vasa vasorum, structural aortic wall fatigue, and loss of residual strain, leading to mechanical failure. Other clinicians doubted the missing intimal tear. Rather, they postulated that an intimal tear exists,

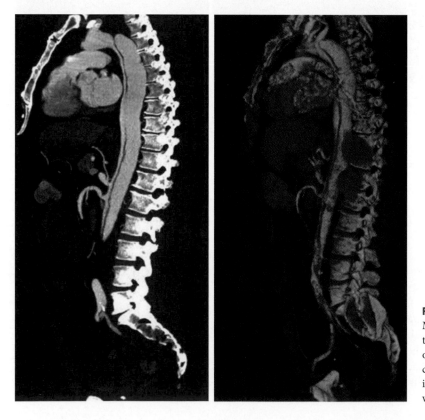

**Fig. 23.8.** Stanford type B dissection, MPR, and VR in the sagittal orientation. The dissection starts distal of the origin of the left subclavian artery. The celiac artery and the superior mesenteric artery originate from the true lumen, which is located ventrally

but cannot be visualized by imaging techniques. This view is supported by the pathological entity of PAU with IMH (SUNDT 2002).

Beside the lack of an intimal tear, there are several other differences between IMH and AD. The risk of malperfusion is lower in patients with IMH. Furthermore, the mean patient age in IMH is more advanced than it is in AD (67.7 vs. 61.7 years).

IMH is classified according to ADs in A and B types. Type A IMHs tend to have higher rates of progression and mortality than do type B IMHs (ROBBINS et al. 1993; NIENABER et al. 1995; MOHR-KAHALY et al. 1994). Both types require intensive follow-up examinations in order to monitor possible progress to an AD or aneurysm. In the vast majority of cases, IMH of the descending thoracic aorta can be treated noninvasively, and there is little indication for stent grafting in the absence of rupture. However, they normally have to be treated operatively when they involve the ascending aorta (SUNDT 2002).

## 23.2.5
## Aortitis

Aortitis often leads to a dilatation of the aortic root and a secondary aortic insufficiency. This dilatation is independent of the etiology of the aortitis. According to etiology, aortitis can be classified into infectious and noninfectious aortitis.

Rare *syphilitic aortitis* is specified by an unspecific thickening of the aortic wall, with increased contrast enhancement in early stages of the disease. This is subsequently replaced by a thinning and calcification of the aortic wall. The periaortic inflammation can better be visualized by fat-saturated techniques in MRI than in MDCT. A bark-like aspect of the aortic surface is characteristic for this subtype, but can also occur in other types of aortitis. The weakening of the aortic wall favors the development of luetic aneurysms with a high risk of rupture.

*Takayasu's arteritis* can affect the whole aorta and its side branches. In the acute stage of the disease, CT and MRI show an inflammatory thickening of the aortic wall, with increased contrast enhancement. This enables the differentiation from atherosclerotic transformations of the aortic wall. In MRI, edema of the wall can additionally be detectable (YAMADA et al. 1998). In chronic stages of the disease (weeks to months), long-segment stenosis of occlusion with the formation of collateral circulation, intraluminal thrombi, and calcifications of the aortic wall can be seen. The incidence of aortic aneurysms in Takayasu's arteritis lies between 30 and 50%

(TAVORA and BURKE 2006). Unlike the syphilitic aortitis, the risk of rupture is relatively low because of the reactive fibrosis of the intima and adventitia. Sensitivity and specificity of CT for characterizing chronic lesions of Takayasu's arteritis are reported already over 90% in single-slice CT scanners (YAMADA et al. 1998). The larger coverage of volume and higher spatial resolution of MDCT allow a more detailed evaluation of the aorta, its branches, and eventually of its collateral circulations. MRI is also suited to visualize the chronic changes and stenoses; however, the extent of aortic stenoses is partially overestimated.

*Giant cell arteritis* cannot be differentiated from Takayasu's arteritis in morphological terms. Only the distribution of the lesions with predominance in supra-aortic vessels is indicative for this type of arteritis.

## 23.2.6
## Injury of the Aorta

Nearly 90% of traumatic tears of the aorta are located between the left subclavian artery and the insertion of the ligamentum arteriosum. In the case of a trauma, this part of the aorta is affected by strong shearing forces because of the passage of an immobile to a mobile segment. The ascending aorta and the aortic passage through the diaphragm are other possible sites of injury, however less frequent. Additional accompanying injuries of the thorax or abdomen can be revealed by MDCT. Direct signs of a traumatic aortic injury include the detection of tear of the aortic wall, an IMH, or a dissection (TAKAHASHI and STANFORD 2005). The most important indirect sign is the periaortic hematoma. Its sensitivity and negative predictive value for the existence of an aortic injury are around 100% (TAKAHASHI and STANFORD 2005).

Hematomas of the anterior mediastinum should not be confounded in young patients with remaining thymus tissue. They are signs of a severe traumatism of the mediastinum, but not specific for an injury of the aorta. In a large survey including more than 1,500 patients, single-slice CT with reconstruction of thin layers led to a sensitivity of nearly 100% for the presence of an aortic injury; its specificity was around 82% (RUBIN 2003). New MDCT scanners with an isotropic resolution of 1 mm surely have the potential to further improve the detection (ALKADHI et al. 2004). Especially discrete irregularities of the aortic wall can be detected faster and more reliably by means of MPRs. In particular, nontransmural aortic ruptures favor the development of pseudoaneurysms, which appear in CT as fusiform or sacciform dilatations of the aortic wall.

### 23.2.7
### CTA in Endovascular Aortic Reconstruction

EVAR is an alternative to open surgery in selected patients. Since the outcome of the procedure and the rate of complications depend on anatomic factors, and poor patient selection is associated with a higher risk for complications, CTA plays an important role in patient selection, planning of the EVAR, and in follow-up examinations in order to monitor possible complications (Iezzi and Cotroneo 2006).

For reasons of planning an EVAR, especially the orthogonal diameter of the vessel, the length of the pathology and the relationship to aortic side branches should be determined before intervention using. Collimations and reconstructed slice thickness should be less than 1 mm.

After EVAR, follow-up examinations are essential in order to monitor possible complications. The most frequent complications include endoleaks, aneurysm expansion or rupture, graft migration, and graft deformation. Generally, the aneurysm size decreases if there is no perigraft blood flow. However, a significant number of aneurysms enlarge without apparent endoleak, and ruptures can occur in this situation. Also, stent deformation has been frequently noted, leading to graft thrombosis, endoleaks, or aneurysm rupture (Fillinger 1999).

Sandmann and Pfeiffer (2002) carried out a survey of 2,030 patients after EVAR due to abdominal aortic aneurysm. Within the first 4 years, 38% of patients had to undergo reintervention due to complications of the stent graft. The most common complications are endoleaks (Fig. 23.9), with a rate of 10% after 18 months. Endoleaks are generally classified into five types:
1. Type I: perigraft endoleak, leading to a persistent blood flow either at the proximal (type Ia) or distal attachment sites (type Ib)
2. Type II: retrograde blood flow into the aortic lesion from collateral branches (e.g. lumbar arteries)
3. Type III: midgraft leak, with blood flow through the graft due to inadequate or ineffective sealing of overlapping joints or rupture of the graft fabric
4. Type IV: graft wall porosity, leading to a blood flow into the aneurysm sac
5. Type V/endotension: persistent elevation of the pressure (>60 mmHg), leading to a risk of rupture without blood flow into the lesion. This can lead to graft thrombosis, endoleaks or aneurysm rupture (Fillinger 1999).

While type III endoleaks generally occur early after EVAR, types I and II can still develop years after the intervention. In order to detect endoleaks, both nonenhanced and enhanced scans are used in order to differentiate between calcifications in the aneurysm wall

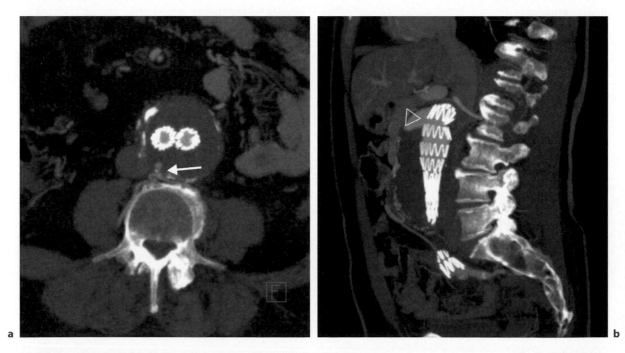

a       b

**Fig. 23.9. a** Type II endoleak after EVAR of an abdominal aortic aneurysm, with a bifurcation graft. The endoleak is filled from a retrograde flow out of a lumbar artery (*arrow*). **b** Type III endoleak after EVAR of an abdominal aneurysm. The graft is ruptured (*arrowhead*), leading to this type of endoleak

and an endoleak. Due to its ability in differentiating these substances, dual-source CTA seems to be a future perspective that might lead to a significant decrease of scans, since virtual nonenhanced scans can be calculated out of the contrast-enhanced scan.

While frequent follow-up scans are certainly required in the first years after EVAR, it is still under discussion, if lifelong, annual CTA scans are necessary in patients who have undergone EVAR.

## 23.3
## Conclusion

MDCT with high-resolution CTA is an excellent technique for the diagnosis, therapy, and follow-up of aortic pathologies. The examination protocol must be adapted to the clinical question in order to avoid excessive radiation exposure. Modern techniques like modulation of the tube current along the $x$-, $y$-, and $z$-axes can routinely reduce radiation exposure. In specific cases, it can even be further reduced by the reduction of the tube voltage. Depending on the clinical question, nonenhanced scans and venous contrast-enhanced phases can contribute important information for diagnosis.

## References

Alkadhi H, Wildermuth S, Desbiolles L, Schertler T, Crook D, Marincek B, Boehm T (2004) Vascular emergencies of the thorax after blunt and iatrogenic trauma: multi-detector row CT and three-dimensional imaging. Radiographics 24:1239–1255

Bahner ML, Bengel A, Brix G, Zuna I, Kauczor HU, Delorme S (2005) Improved vascular opacification in cerebral computed tomography angiography with 80 kVp. Invest Radiol 40:229–234

Fillinger MF (1999) Postoperative imaging after endovascular AAA repair. Semin Vasc Surg 12:327–338

Fleischmann D (2003) Use of high-concentration contrast media in multiple-detector-row CT: principles and rationale. Eur Radiol 13(Suppl):M14–M20

Hayter RG, Rhea JT, Small A, Tafazoli FS, Novelline RA (2006) Suspected aortic dissection and other aortic disorders: multi-detector row CT in 373 cases in the emergency setting. Radiology 238:841–852

Iezzi R, Cotroneo AR (2006) Endovascular repair of abdominal aortic aneurysms: CTA evaluation of contraindications. Abdom Imaging 31:722–731

Iino M, Kuribayashi S, Imakita S, Takamiya M, Matsuo H, Ookita Y, Ando M, Ueda H (2002) Sensitivity and specificity of CT in the diagnosis of inflammatory abdominal aortic aneurysms. J Comput Assist Tomogr 26:1006–1012

Isselbacher EM (2005) Thoracic and abdominal aortic aneurysms. Circulation 111:816–828

Johnson TR, Krauss B, Sedlmair M, Grasruck M, Bruder H, Morhard D, Fink C, Weckbach S, Lenhard M, Schmidt B, Flohr T, Reiser MF, Becker CR (2007) Material differentiation by dual energy CT: initial experience. Eur Radiol 17:1510–1517

Knollmann F, Schimpf K, Felix R (2004) [Iodine delivery rate of different concentrations of iodine-containing contrast agents with rapid injection]. Rofo 176:880–884

Luther BLP (2007) Kompaktwissen, Gefäßchirurgie. Differenzierte Diagnostik und Therapie. Springer, Berlin Heidelberg New York (In German)

Mohr-Kahaly S, Erbel R, Kearney P, Puth M, Meyer J (1994) Aortic intramural hemorrhage visualized by transesophageal echocardiography: findings and prognostic implications. J Am Coll Cardiol 23:658–664

Nienaber CA, Eagle KA (2003) Aortic dissection: new frontiers in diagnosis and management: Part II: therapeutic management and follow-up. Circulation 108:772–778

Nienaber CA, von Kodolitsch Y, Petersen B, Loose R, Helmchen U, Haverich A, Spielmann RP (1995) Intramural hemorrhage of the thoracic aorta. Diagnostic and therapeutic implications. Circulation 92:1465–1472

Rakita D, Newatiaa A, Hines JJ, Siegel DN, Friedman B (2007) Spectrum of CT findings in rupture and impending rupture of abdominal aortic aneurysms. Radiographics 27:497–507

Richter GM, Allenberg JR, Schumacher H, Hansmann J, Vahl C, Hagl S (2001) [Aortic dissection–when operative treatment, when endoluminal therapy?]. Radiologe 41:660–667 (In German)

Robbins RC, McManus RP, Mitchell RS, Latter DR, Moon MR, Olinger GN, Miller DC (1993) Management of patients with intramural hematoma of the thoracic aorta. Circulation 88:II1–10

Rubin GD (2003) CT angiography of the thoracic aorta. Semin Roentgenol 38:115–134

Rubin GD, Kalra MK (2006) MDCT angiography of the thoracic aorta. In: Saini S, Rubin GS, Kalra MK (eds) MDCT: a practical approach. Springer, Berlin Heidelberg New York, p 111

Sandmann W, Pfeiffer T (2002) Die endovaskuläre Therapie des abdominalen Aortenaneurysmas: Aus der Sicht des Gefäßchirurgen. Dtsch Arztebl 17:A1160–A1167 (In German)

Shiga T, Wajima Z, Apfel CC, Inoue T, Ohe Y (2006) Diagnostic accuracy of transesophageal echocardiography, helical computed tomography, and magnetic resonance imaging for suspected thoracic aortic dissection: systematic review and meta-analysis. Arch Intern Med 166:1350–1356

Singh K, Jacobsen BK, Solberg S, Bonaa KH, Kumar S, Bajic R, Arnesen E (2003) Intra- and interobserver variability in the measurements of abdominal aortic and common iliac artery diameter with computed tomography. The Tromso study. Eur J Vasc Endovasc Surg 25:399–407

Sundt TM (2002) Management of intramural hematoma of the ascending aorta: still room for debate. J Thorac Cardiovasc Surg 124:894–895

Takahashi K, Stanford W (2005) Multidetector CT of the thoracic aorta. Int J Cardiovasc Imaging 21:141–153

Tang T, Boyle JR, Dixon AK, Varty K (2005) Inflammatory abdominal aortic aneurysms. Eur J Vasc Endovasc Surg 29:353–362

Tavora F, Burke A (2006) Review of isolated ascending aortitis: differential diagnosis, including syphilitic, Takayasu's and giant cell aortitis. Pathology 38:302–308

Tengg-Kobligk H, Weber TF, Rengier F, Bockler D, Schumacher H, Kauczor HU (2007) [Image postprocessing of aortic CTA and MRA.]. Radiologe 47:1003–1011 (in German)

Wallis F, Roditi GH, Redpath TW, Weir J, Cross KS, Smith FW (2000) Inflammatory abdominal aortic aneurysms: diagnosis with gadolinium enhanced T1-weighted imaging. Clin Radiol 55:136–139

Wintersperger B, Jakobs T, Herzog P, Schaller S, Nikolaou K, Suess C, Weber C, Reiser M, Becker C (2005) Aorto-iliac multidetector-row CT angiography with low kV settings: improved vessel enhancement and simultaneous reduction of radiation dose. Eur Radiol 15:334–341

Yamada I, Nakagawa T, Himeno Y, Numano F, Shibuya H (1998) Takayasu arteritis: evaluation of the thoracic aorta with CT angiography. Radiology 209:103–109

# CTA of the Spinal Arteries

## 24

Hendrik von Tengg-Kobligk, Tim F. Weber and Dittmar Böckler

## CONTENTS

### ABSTRACT

Since vascular and nonvascular interventions in the vicinity of the spinal cord are challenged by the risk of spinal ischemia, cross-sectional imaging of spinal blood supply is gaining clinical importance. By identifying significant spinal feeders, spinal artery imaging using MDCT angiography can act as a roadmap for selecting an adequate surgical or interventional procedure, possibly including a preceded reimplantation of relevant spinal arteries or customization of the applied technique. The main spinal feeding artery is, in general, the Adamkiewicz artery, which is an anterior radicular ramus arising from a segmental aortic branch at the thoracolumbar region and supplies the anterior two thirds of the spinal cord. Visualization of tenuous spinal arteries necessitates an adapted scanning protocol that combines high spatial resolution with optimized contrast enhancement. Using a thin collimation and low pitch value as well an increased iodine dosage, spinal feeding arteries can be depicted reliably. Additional image postprocessing with adjustment of MPRs and MIPs improves evaluation of spinal vasculature. Interestingly, even after aortic stenting for endovascular aneurysm treatment, depiction of related spinal arteries may still be demonstrated, suggesting sufficient circumventing pathways that maintain spinal perfusion in individual cases.

H. v. Tengg-Kobligk, MD
Department of Radiology, German Cancer Research Center, Im Neuenheimer Feld 280, 69120 Heidelberg, Germany

T. F. Weber, MD
Department of Radiology, German Cancer Research Center, Im Neuenheimer Feld 280, 69120 Heidelberg, Germany

D. Böckler, MD
Department of Vascular and Endovascular Surgery, Ruprecht-Karls University Heidelberg, Im Neuenheimer Feld 110, 69120 Heidelberg, Germany

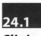

## 24.1
### Clinical Background

Paraparesis and paraplegia secondary to spinal cord ischemia are serious complications of surgical and interventional (e.g., endovascular aortic) procedures performed in the vicinity of the spinal cord or the feeding vasculature (HUNTOON and MARTIN 2004; SULLIVAN and SUNDT 2006). They result from a variety of mechanisms such as generalized ischemia, inadequate perfusion pressure (aortic clamping), reperfusion, and finally, the loss of critical spinal arteries. Operations in which spinal blood supply is at potential risk include interventions at the spine and posterior mediastinum as well as repair of thoracoabdominal aortic pathologies. In the latter, neurological injuries comprising paraplegia and milder forms of deficits have been reported to occur in up to 40% in earlier days of aortic surgery (CRAWFORD et al. 1986). Although neurological complication rates can nowadays be reduced to well below 10%, using either microinvasive EVAR or adjunctive techniques (e.g., monitoring of motor-evoked potentials [MEP], CSF, or reimplantation of intercostals) during a conventional operation, paraplegia is still a dreaded complication—elderly patients are particularly vulnerable (BÖCKLER et al. 2006, 2007b, STONE et al. 2006).

Reimplantation of feeding arteries is the surgical method of choice to maintain spinal perfusion (SAFI et al. 1998). This approach may be supported by test clamping of the aorta in the vicinity of the spinal suppliers (NIJENHUIS et al. 2007) or by intraoperative monitoring of neurophysiological parameters that help diagnosing ischemic injuries timely and refining the neurological outcome of patients (SVENSSON 2005; JACOBS et al. 2006). In addition, preoperative cross-sectional imaging of the spinal blood supply has become a feasible technique to identify relevant spinal feeders in the forefront of the procedure. Depicting these vessels, reimplantation of spinal arteries or a customization of the designated procedure can be considered, if necessary.

## 24.2
## Anatomy of Spinal Blood Supply

### 23.2.1
### Arterial Blood Supply

The arterial blood supply of the spinal cord is provided by the unpaired anterior spinal artery (ASA) and the paired posterior spinal arteries. These vessels constitute a longitudinally orientated arterial system that is interconnecting with numerous arteries entering transversely and resembling the segmental embryology of the spine (GILLILAN 1958; LASJAUNIAS and BERENSTEIN 1990).

The ASA is formed cranially at midmedullary level by side branches of each vertebral artery, descends on the ventral midline of the spinal cord along the anterior median sulcus, and reaches the filum terminale. It supplies the anterior two thirds of the spinal cord and inferiorly the cauda equina. The mean diameter varies between 0.5 mm in the cervical and usually not more than 1 mm in the lumbar region.

The ASA is transversely reinforced by branches of deep cervical arteries at the neck and by posterior intercostal (PIA) and upper lumbar arteries at the trunk. Both of the latter derive segmentally from the descending thoracic and abdominal aorta and range between 0.5 and 5 mm in diameter (BOLL et al. 2006). The PIA and lumbar arteries send rami dorsales, from which again the radicular arteries (synonymous with *radicomedullary artery* or *spinal branch*) as feeders of the spinal cord originate. The radicular arteries divide soon into anterior and posterior branches that support either the anterior or the posterior spinal arteries.

The posterior spinal arteries arise from the vertebral or posterior inferior cerebellar arteries and pass as two at each side along the dorsal aspect of the spinal cord. They are sustained to the lower spinal levels by being predominantly fed by the posterior branches of the radicular arteries. The posterior spinal arteries supply the dorsal third of the spinal cord and have a caliber of less than 0.5 mm.

### 24.2.1.1
### Arteria Radicularis Magna

While most anterior radicular arteries are small and end in the ventral nerve roots or the cord's pial plexus, only some are large enough to reach the anterior median sulcus to anastomose with the ASA. The largest of these is the arteria radicularis magna, or Adamkiewicz artery (AKA), and usually arises at variable sites between T5 and L2. If the AKA (synonymous with the *great anterior radiculomedullary artery*) arises in the region of T5 to T9, then a second anterior radicular artery of significant dimension may be found in the caudal area. In about 70% of the individuals, the AKA originates from the left and at the level of the 9th–12th thoracic vertebrae (BOLL et al. 2006; TAKASE et al. 2002).

After entering the spinal canal, it has a long course upward in company with the nerve root. When it finally reaches the anterior median sulcus, it turns downward in a characteristic acute, hairpin-like angle (Fig. 24.1). Typical average calibers of the AKA are between 0.8 and 1.2 mm. The AKA is of great importance, since it is con-

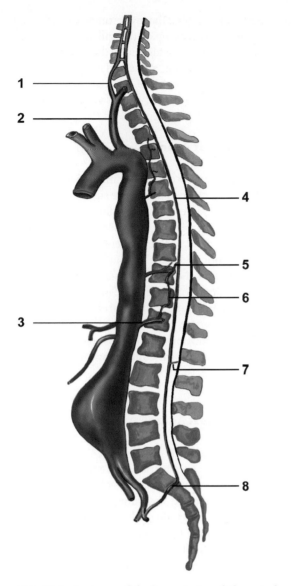

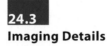

**Fig. 24.1.** Anatomy of feeding arteries of the spinal cord. *1* vertebral artery, *2* left subclavian artery, *3* posterior intercostal artery, *4* anterior spinal artery, *5* Adamkiewicz artery, *6* intersegmental anastomosis between radicular arteries, *7* anastomosis between anterior and posterior spinal artery, *8* iliolumbar artery. (Dirk Fischer; modified from Rogier Trompert and Robbert J. Nijenhuis)

sidered to be the main blood supplier to the lower two thirds of the spinal cord (GILLILAN 1958; LASJAUNIAS and BERENSTEIN 1990). In some individuals, a duplicate of the AKA may be found close to its origin (BOLL et al. 2006).

### 24.2.1.2
### Potential Arterial Collaterals

Several anastomoses between the cord supplying arteries give a complex picture of potential spinal collaterals. Although the AKA joins the ASA and is in general the dominant feeder to the thoracolumbar myelon, it usually sends a branch to anastomose with a sideline of the posterior spinal artery. Moreover, there may be a small ascending branch of the AKA joining the ASA at the superior segment. Other adjacent radicular arteries may be proximally interconnected by additional radicular twigs, forming further anastomoses within the spinal canal. The posterior spinal artery again is meant to form a series of communicating loops between intersegmental posterior arterial branches. The PIA gives off a collateral ramus that descends to and anastomoses with the subjacent intercostal vessel. Finally, the PIA—or the lumbar artery inferior to the thorax—merges during its course through the costal groove with the corresponding anterior branch (anterior intercostal artery), derived from the internal thoracic or superior epigastric artery, respectively (GILLILAN 1958; LASJAUNIAS and BERENSTEIN 1990).

### 24.2.2
### Venous Drainage

The venous drainage of the spinal cord is realized via the anterior medial vein and the great anterior radicomedullary veins (GARV) that drain into the radicular veins accompanying the corresponding arterial branches. A GARV may have a similar course as the AKA, and is known to be mixed up with the latter. The spinal veins drain as well into internal vertebral venous plexuses that are situated within the epidural space and connected to the sinuses of the brain, the external vertebral venous plexuses, and the segmental cervical, intercostal or lumbar veins.

### 24.3
### Imaging Details

### 24.3.1
### Imaging Modalities

In some centers, intra-arterial DSA is or has been used for identifying and visualizing spinal arteries, especially the AKA. However, this semi-invasive technique may lead to serious procedure related complications like spinal ischemia itself, dissections, and embolic infarcts in up to 5% (WILLIAMS et al. 1991; SAVADER et al. 1993). Furthermore, the success rate for AKA detection using DSA has been described to be only between 55 and 75% (HEINEMANN et al. 1998; WILLIAMS et al. 1991; SAVADER et al. 1993). Due to recent advancements in imaging techniques, cross-sectional imaging of the spinal blood supply has become feasible to identify relevant spinal feeders in the forefront of a procedure. CTA as well as contrast-enhanced MRA (CE-MRA) have both been described as capable methods for detecting the AKA in 56 to 90% of cases (NIJENHUIS et al. 2007; TAKASE et al. 2006; VON TENGG-KOBLIGK et al. 2007a). CTA is, however, the method of choice for surgeons who usually prefer CT to MR images for preprocedural work-up and decision making (BÖCKLER et al. 2007a, VON TENGG-KOBLIGK et al. 2007b). If the therapeutic approach requires use of DSA, then cross-sectional imaging can be used as a road map to reduce radiation exposure, contrast agent volume, and intervention time during interventional DSA.

### 24.3.1.1
### CT Image Acquisition

Since vessel diameters of the described spinal arteries may be of submillimeter size, and the fact that these arteries go through (intervertebral foramen) or run adjacent to the vertebrae, CTA of the spinal arteries is one of the most challenging tasks within the field of CT applications. Furthermore, a bidirectional flow along the ASA may be present, causing unpredictable opacifica-

tion of the arterial system. Extensive venous anastomoses, resembling the anatomy of the spinal arteries add additional challenges. In addition to the requirements for high spatial resolution, successful visualization of the typical hairpin-like course of the AKA may be optimized if the following imaging aspects are considered.

### Choice of Contrast Agent

An iodine concentration of equal or more than 350 mg/ml is highly recommended to achieve sufficient intraluminal attenuation values within the fine vessels of the spinal vasculature. Especially if venous access does not allow higher flow rates, iodine concentration should be 370 mg/ml or more (see Table 24.2). If a contrast agent with higher iodine concentration is available, then its increased viscosity should be kept in mind. For example, for iomeprol with an iodine concentration of 400 mg/ml, warming up prior to injection to refine its applicability by reducing viscosity is recommended. Possible side effects of each contrast agent need to be considered in the decision process.

### Volume of Contrast Agent

A volume that is routinely used for CTA of the entire aorta is sufficient for spinal artery imaging. Depending on scan time and venous access, the volume of contrast agent should be adjusted accordingly. To account for an additional scan delay after table movement, an appropriate amount of supplementary volume should be added. In the end, the technologist and the radiologist

**Table 24.1.** Overview of duration of contrast media administration(s), depending on flow rate and contrast media volume

| Contrast agent (ml) | Flow rate (ml/s) | | | |
|---|---|---|---|---|
| | 2 | 3 | 4 | 5 |
| 80 | 40 | 26.7 | 20 | 16 |
| 90 | 45 | 30 | 22.5 | 18 |
| 100 | 50 | 33.3 | 25 | 20 |
| 110 | 55 | 36.7 | 27.5 | 22 |
| 10 | 5 | 3.3 | 2.5 | 2 |

The *bottom row* represents the injection time (scan time) for 10 ml. Note that the maximum is set 5 ml/s, due to increased patient discomfort, danger of venous rupture, and lack of relevant impact on arterial HU values

do not know precisely how the bolus profile of the contrast agent will be stretched during passage of the lung and heart. The faster the flow rate and the faster the scanner, the more difficult it becomes to acquire every rotation at the maximum peak of arterial attenuation (Table 24.1).

Volumes used described in the literature go as high as 2 ml per kilogram body weight, using a contrast agent at a concentration of 370 mg I/ml. For a 70-kg individual, this would result in 140 ml contrast agent or 51.8 g iodine, respectively. The volume of contrast medium finally depends also on the speed of table movement, simultaneously used detector rows (e.g., 16 × 0.5-mm collimation), and the pitch. If the pitch is very low, e.g., 0.68 and only an 8-mm detector width is used per rotation, then higher volume of contrast medium need to be applied. The danger of venous overlay increases, however, with reduced speed of table movement.

## Administration of Contrast Media

As mentioned before, high Hounsfield unit values of arterial blood in the aorta (equal or greater than 350 HU) are highly recommended to allow for continuous visualization of spinal arteries. Therefore, an 18-G venous access via the right antecubital vein is suggested for higher flow rates. A flow rate of 5 ml/s is advised to achieve sufficient iodine delivery per second (Table 24.2). Higher flow rates did not show advantages aiming to increase aortic Hounsfield unit values and may cause patient discomfort and injection related complications.

If iomeprol is used at an iodine concentration of 400 mg/ml, then the power injector should allow keeping the contrast agent at body temperature. With the patient lying in final position with elevated arms above the head, a saline test run with approximately 40 ml is recommended, using identical flow parameters to evaluate if the desired flow rate can be achieved. A saline flush of ca. 40 ml after the contrast medium is advised as well.

## Timing of Scan Start

The challenge for spinal artery CTA is to provide sufficient arterial enhancement but to scan before arrival of contrast medium in the venous system. An ROI of the bolus tracking system placed in the ascending aorta might be affected by inflow artifacts of the SVC and may result in a mistimed early scan. Therefore, placement of the ROI in the aortic arch or descending aorta is recommended. In the presence of aortic dissection, caution should be taken that the ROI is not too big or positioned in the false lumen or across the dissection membrane, respectively. In these cases, manual start of the scan should be considered. The Hounsfield unit threshold should be around 100 HU above baseline. Scan start is usually delayed by time for table movement (<3 s), which is usually right above the origin of the vertebral arteries. An additional scan delay of 3 s is recommended for scanners with equal to or more than 16 rows and rotation time equal or less than 0.4 s. Hounsfield unit values of attenuated blood in the thoracic aorta should never be lower than within the pulmonary trunk.

## FOV

Ideally, the vertebral spine should be in the center of the scan FOV for the entire acquisition, since spatial resolution is highest in the center. Some CT scanners allow

**Table 24.2.** Overview of how much iodine per second can be administered, depending on flow rate and contrast media concentration

| Iodine concentration (mg/ml) | Flow rate (ml/s) | | | |
|---|---|---|---|---|
| | 2 | 3 | 4 | 5 |
| 350 | 0.7 | 1.05 | 1.4 | 1.75 |
| 370 | 0.74 | 1.11 | 1.48 | 1.85 |
| 400 | 0.8 | 1.2 | 1.6 | 2.0 |

Note that the maximum is set 5 ml/s, due to increased patient discomfort, danger of venous rupture, and lack of relevant impact on arterial HU values

the scan FOV to be adjusted to the volume of interest, i.e., spatial resolution can be improved by applying the 512 × 512 matrix (or 1024 × 1024, if available) to a smaller FOV. Other scanners acquire data always with a FOV of 500 mm and reconstruct smaller FOV, e.g., 90 mm, that can be manually applied. To optimize spatial resolution, a dedicated FOV can be reconstructed, comprising only the aorta and spinal canal (TAKASE et al. 2002; BOLL et al. 2006).

### Collimation, Pitch, and Slice Thickness

The goal is to achieve isotropic data with voxels 1 mm or smaller in edge length. Due to submillimeter diameter lumen of some of the spinal arteries, a collimation of 0.75 mm or less is advised. The pitch should not be >1. A pitch <1, e.g., 0.68, has been used for dedicated studies requiring longer scan time and larger volume of contrast medium (YOSHIOKA et al. 2006). The AKA has also been successfully visualized using a collimation of 1 mm but with a lower detection rate (VON TENGG-KOBLIGK et al. 2007a). Depending on the detector width, a collimation of 1 mm may be successful in some cases, but 0.75 or even 0.5 mm is preferred, provided 32 rows or more are available for fast image acquisition. The reconstructed slice thickness should not be bigger than 1 mm. With an increment, e.g., of 0.3 for 0.5 mm and 0.5 for 0.75 mm, collimation spatial resolution can be optimized. Some imaging groups prefer even an overlap of 50% for primary image reconstruction.

### Kernel

A kernel usually used for vascular imaging as well as a bone kernel is advisable since spinal arteries may be adjacent to bone, causing beam-hardening effects that might affect delineation and/or segmentation of arteries (BOLL et al. 2006).

### kV and mA

Depending on the indication, not only spinal arteries need to be evaluated, but also the entire aorta including its major branches. Dedicated studies comparing different kV settings (80 vs. 120 kV) show increased CNR for spinal artery imaging using 80 kV, but also increased noise (NIJENHUIS et al. 2007). Comparisons of different mA settings have not been published so far. The standard protocol used in clinical routine defines 120 kV; mA is nowadays adjusted to patient geometry

and anatomy by dose modulation in the $x$-, $y$-, and $z$-direction.

As for any other CT acquisition, there are also trade-offs for CTA of spinal arteries. To avoid venous overlay, table movement should not be too slow. Settings for kV, mA, and pitch described in the literature go as high as 400 mA (200 mA) at 120 kV in combination with a pitch of 0.68 and a collimation of 0.5 mm, using a 16-row scanner (YOSHIOKA et al. 2006). In the context of optimizing radiation exposure and lowering contrast media, volume protocols need to be designed for clinical routine use.

### 24.4
### Image Postprocessing and Identification of AKA

Standard transverse images reconstructed from a 3D data set with overlapping thin slices may be sufficient for visualization of the posterior intercostal and lumbar arteries as well as of their proximal rami dorsales. The AKA or other anterior radicular arteries of significant dimension may be localized on transverse sections as well, if a second vessel with arterial contrast begins to accompany the usually solitary ASA in the thoracolumbar region (Fig. 24.2).

The typical anatomy of the AKA, however, necessitates supplementary image postprocessing for its reliable identification and segmental attribution (BOLL et al. 2006; VON TENGG-KOBLIGK et al. 2007a). By using coronal MPRs, the spinal column can be screened fast for the characteristic hairpin of the AKA. For providing a perpendicular view on the ventral aspect of the myelon, it is sometimes necessary to interactively adjust oblique coronal MPR parallel to the curvature of the spine (Fig. 24.2). After identification of the AKA, additional curved MPRs generated manually help to delineate the individual course of a specific vessel and its aortic origin reformatted at one single image and proof herewith continuity of the AKA. Sliding thin-slab MIPs (STS-MIP) are also useful to grasp the 3D anatomy of the AKA and facilitate the depiction of several vessel portions on a single image if vessel contrast and vertebral anatomy allow continuous visualization (Fig. 24.2). To overcome the impairment of this technique as a result of bony, high-contrast objects in the vessel proximity, bone-removal algorithms can be applied to the data set, and thin-slab MIP with a thickness of 2 to 3 mm are recommended to scroll through the source data in either the transverse or the coronal orientation (Fig. 24.3). Although angiographic volume renderings

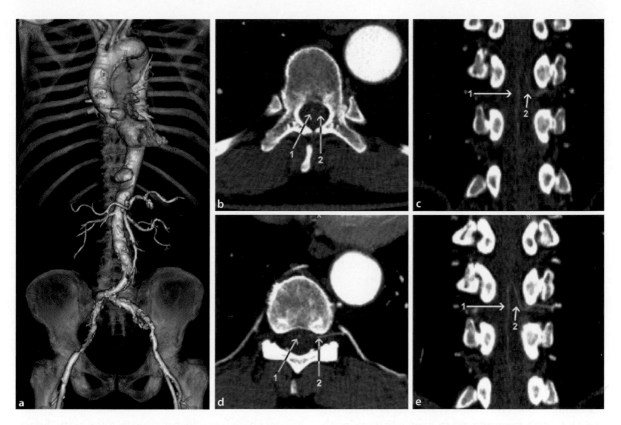

**Fig. 24.2.** **a** Patient with thoracoabdominal penetrating aortic ulcer. **b** Transverse section at T10, with evidence of anterior spinal artery, ASA (*1*) being accompanied by a second artery (Adamkiewicz artery [AKA]) (*2*). **c** Oblique coronal reforma-tion depicting more obvious ASA (*1*) and the pathognomonic hairpin of the distal segment of AKA (*2*). **d, e** Thin-slab MIP (3 mm) in corresponding orientations improve visualization of ASA (*1*) and AKA, including its intervertebral course (*2*)

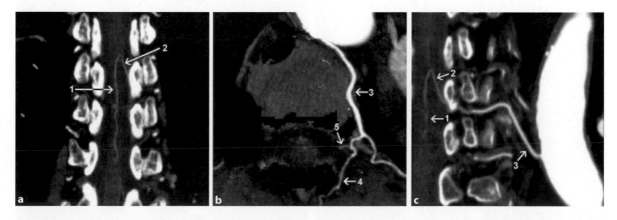

**Fig. 24.3.** **a** Oblique coronal MIP (3 mm) for excellent depiction of anterior spinal artery, ASA (*1*), and AKA (*2*). **b** MIP of a curved MPR with bone removal demonstrating a general view at the segmental arteries in one image and with depiction of PIA (*3*), muscular branch of ramus dorsalis (*4*), and radicular artery of ramus dorsalis (*5*). **c** Curved MPR proving continuity between ASA (*1*), AKA (*2*), PIA (*3*), and aorta

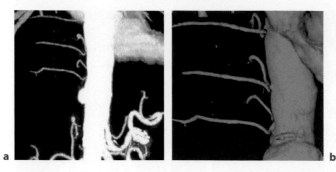

a

b

**Fig. 24.4a,b.** Oblique sagittal MIP and volume rendering after manual bone removal of the spine with continuous vessel delineation from aorta to anterior spinal artery, ASA

are made available automatically by several software vendors, this technique may not be sensitive enough to regularly depict the peripheral spinal arteries and is susceptible to unintentional elimination of fine structures (VON TENGG-KOBLIGK et al. 2007b) (Fig. 24.4).

## 24.5
## AKA Differentiation to Spinal Veins

Especially because GARV exhibit a comparable spatial configuration and course, challenges in identifying the AKA occur frequently when concomitant veins are already contrast enhanced at the time of data acquisition (JASPERS et al. 2007). To distinguish artery from vein, verification of continuity between the aorta, the suspected vessel, and the anterior spinal artery is certainly the most reliable criterion to aim at and is most notably documented on MIP and curved MPR. More-

over, corresponding veins are meant to be up to twice as thick compared with the AKA, which usually does not exceed a diameter of 1.2 mm. It has also been reported that the characteristic angle of the curvature of the anterior radicular vein is wider than that of the AKA and specifies a "coat hook" rather than a hairpin turn (LAS-JAUNIAS and BERENSTEIN 1990; YOSHIOKA et al. 2006).

## 24.6
## Postprocedural Observations

Placing an endovascular graft within the aortic lumen blocks the direct vascular supply of the spinal cord over the concluded segmental arteries and may induce spinal ischemia. In fact, besides covering the ostium of the LSA, the length of aortic coverage is being proposed as a major predictive factor for spinal ischemic complications after endovascular treatment of descending aortic

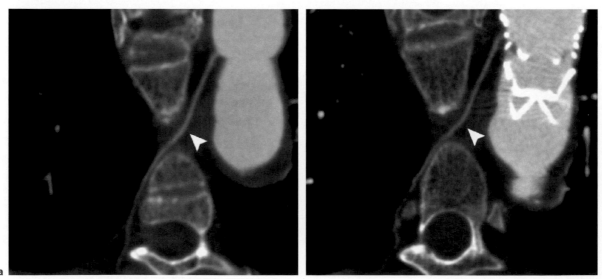

a

b

**Fig. 24.5a,b.** Curved MPR before and after endovascular repair. Although occluded by an endograft, the posterior intercostal artery, PIA (*arrowhead*) remains fully visible on the postoperative study

lesions (AMABILE et al. 2008). Some specialized clinical centers reimplant PIA prior to EVAR to preserve their antegrade perfusion and to reduce the danger of spinal ischemia in patients at high risk, as described above. However, occlusion of the aortic origins of some PIA may not be hazardous, if anterior spinal blood flow is maintained via the several potential collaterals described at the beginning of this chapter (Fig. 24.5).

If the internal thoracic arteries are still available (not redirected for coronary bypass surgery), then collateralization through the anterior intercostal branches may represent the most dominant flow compensatory at the thoracolumbar region. Consecutive flow reversal within the PIA may perpetuate blood supply to the spinal cord irrespective of lost aortic origin. Indeed, postoperative CTA of patients treated with thoracic EVAR have shown that the majority of PIA remains retrogradely perfused (VON TENGG-KOBLIGK et al. 2007a). In addition to the apparently retrograde perfusion of the PIA, it could be demonstrated in the same study that only 10% of the even more crucial dorsal branches of the PIA ($n = 203$, 18 patients) became occluded after EVAR, i.e., approximately one branch per patient. In individual cases, the capacity of collateral spinal pathways are shown to be sufficient for maintaining flow within the AKA overstented at the related aortic segment (Fig. 24.6).

## 24.7
## Imaging of Spinal Vascular Lesions

Spinal vascular lesions constitute a rare disease entity that includes spinal arteriovenous fistula and malformations, and is characterized by a shunt between dilated feeding arteries and usually engorged draining veins.

For classification, the anatomical relationship to associated extradural, intradural, or intramedullary vasculature has to be depicted. While extradural lesions are fed by arterial branches generally arising from extradural portions of the radicular arteries, intradural and intramedullary lesions show a supply from intradural radicular pedicles or from the ASA or posterior spinal arteries (KIM and SPETZLER 2006).

As a prerequisite for neurosurgical and endovascular management, exact identification of the level of origin is requested. Although conventional MRI of the spine may raise the suspicion of a spinal vascular lesion, standard modality for their localization providing both diagnostic imaging and therapeutic options is again selective DSA. Nevertheless, with current cross-sectional angiographic techniques, noninvasive preinterventional characterization of spinal vascular lesions has become possible and has shown to quicken a subsequent DSA by predicting the segmental origin of the vascular pathology (LAI et al. 2005; LUETMER et al. 2005; MULL et al. 2007).

In a few reports published so far, spinal CTA was feasible to detect and characterize the underlying vascular lesion and correlated well with corresponding conventional angiograms (BERTRAND et al. 2004; LAI et al. 2005, 2006; YAMAGUCHI et al. 2007). Since the arteriovenous transit time of these lesions is generally accelerated, an adaption of the imaging protocol is usually not necessary to covisualize their venous drainage. However, this implies that it may be impossible to distinguish between arterial and venous components or to identify the segmental origin of the lesions by CT imaging. Simultaneous identification of the AKA is of additional interest, because if the vascular lesion arises from the AKA or the related segment of the ASA endovascular treatment strategies may not be performed in these patients to assure spinal blood supply.

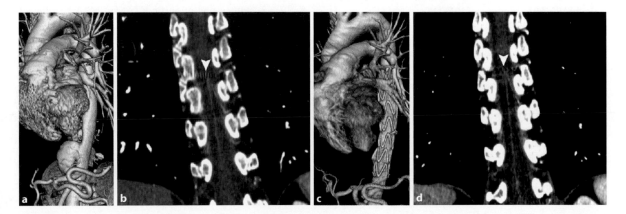

**Fig. 24.6a–d.** Adamkiewicz artery (AKA) (*arrowhead*) depicted on oblique coronal MPR before and after endovascular repair. The aortic origin of AKA was overstented for endograft implantation

# References

Amabile P, Grisoli D, Giorgi R et al. (2008) Incidence and determinants of spinal cord ischaemia in stent-graft repair of the thoracic aorta. Eur J Vasc Endovasc Surg 35:455–461

Bertrand D, Douvrin F, Gerardin E et al. (2004) Diagnosis of spinal dural arteriovenous fistula with multidetector row computed tomography: a case report. Neuroradiology 46:851–854

Böckler D, Schumacher H, Ganten M et al. (2006) Complications after endovascular repair of acute symptomatic and chronic expanding Stanford type B aortic dissections. J Thorac Cardiovasc Surg 132:361–368

Böckler D, Hylik-Durr A, von Tengg-Kobligk H et al. (2007a) Clinical requirements of aortic imaging. (In German) Radiologe 47:962–973

Böckler D, Schumacher H, Klemm K et al. (2007b) Hybrid procedures as a combined endovascular and open approach for pararenal and thoracoabdominal aortic pathologies. Langenbecks Arch Surg 392:715–723

Boll DT, Bulow H, Blackham KA et al. (2006) MDCT angiography of the spinal vasculature and the artery of Adamkiewicz. AJR Am J Roentgenol 187:1054–1060

Crawford ES, Crawford JL, Safi HJ et al. (1986) Thoracoabdominal aortic aneurysms: preoperative and intraoperative factors determining immediate and long-term results of operations in 605 patients. J Vasc Surg 3:389–404

Gillilan LA (1958) The arterial blood supply of the human spinal cord. J Comp Neurol 110:75–103

Stone DH, Brewster DC, Kwolek CJ et al. (2006) Stent-graft versus open-surgical repair of the thoracic aorta: midterm results. J Vasc Surg 44:1188–1197

Huntoon MA, Martin DP. (2004) Paralysis after transforaminal epidural injection and previous surgery. Reg Anesth Pain Med 29(5):494–5

Heinemann MK, Brassel F, Herzog T et al. (1998) The role of spinal angiography in operations on the thoracic aorta: myth or reality? Ann Thorac Surg 65:346–351

Kim LJ, Spetzler RF (2006) Classification and surgical management of spinal arteriovenous lesions: arteriovenous fistulae and arteriovenous malformations. Neurosurgery 59:S195–201; discussion S193–113

Jacobs MJ, Mess W, Mochtar B et al. (2006) The value of motor evoked potentials in reducing paraplegia during thoracoabdominal aneurysm repair. J Vasc Surg 43:239–246

Jaspers K, Nijenhuis RJ, Backes WH (2007) Differentiation of spinal cord arteries and veins by time-resolved MR angiography. J Magn Reson Imaging 26:31–40

Lai PH, Pan HB, Yang CF et al. (2005) Multi-detector row computed tomography angiography in diagnosing spinal dural arteriovenous fistula: initial experience. Stroke 36:1562–1564

Lai PH, Weng MJ, Lee KW et al. (2006) Multidetector CT angiography in diagnosing type I and type IVA spinal vascular malformations. AJNR Am J Neuroradiol 27:813–817

Luetmer PH, Lane JI, Gilbertson JR et al. (2005) Preangiographic evaluation of spinal dural arteriovenous fistulas with elliptic centric contrast-enhanced MR Angiography and effect on radiation dose and volume of iodinated contrast material. AJNR Am J Neuroradiol 26:711–718

Lasjaunias P, Berenstein A (1990) Functional vascular anatomy of brain, spinal cord and spine, 1st edn. Springer, Berlin Heidelberg, New York

Mull M, Nijenhuis RJ, Backes WH et al. (2007) Value and limitations of contrast-enhanced MR angiography in spinal arteriovenous malformations and dural arteriovenous fistulas. AJNR Am J Neuroradiol 28:1249–1258

Nijenhuis RJ, Jacobs MJ, Jaspers K et al. (2007) Comparison of magnetic resonance with computed tomography angiography for preoperative localization of the Adamkiewicz artery in thoracoabdominal aortic aneurysm patients. J Vasc Surg 45:677–685

Safi HJ, Miller CC III, Carr C et al. (1998) Importance of intercostal artery reattachment during thoracoabdominal aortic aneurysm repair. J Vasc Surg 27:58–66; discussion 66–8

Savader SJ, Williams GM, Trerotola SO et al. (1993) Preoperative spinal artery localization and its relationship to postoperative neurologic complications. Radiology 189:165–171

Sullivan TM, Sundt TM III (2006) Complications of thoracic aortic endografts: spinal cord ischemia and stroke. J Vasc Surg 43(Suppl):85A–88A

Svensson LG (2005) Paralysis after aortic surgery: in search of lost cord function. Surgeon 3:396–405

Takase K, Sawamura Y, Igarashi K et al. (2002) Demonstration of the artery of Adamkiewicz at multi-detector row helical CT. Radiology 223:39–45

Takase K, Akasaka J, Sawamura Y et al. (2006) Preoperative MDCT evaluation of the artery of Adamkiewicz and its origin. J Comput Assist Tomogr 30:716–722

Tengg-Kobligk H von, Böckler D, Jose TM et al. (2007a) Feeding arteries of the spinal cord at CT angiography before and after thoracic aortic endografting. J Endovasc Ther 14:639–649

Tengg-Kobligk H von, Weber TF, Rengier F et al. (2007b) [Image postprocessing of aortic CTA and MRA.] Radiologe 47:1003–1011 (In German)

Williams GM, Perler BA, Burdick JF et al. (1991) Angiographic localization of spinal cord blood supply and its relationship to postoperative paraplegia. J Vasc Surg 13:23–33; discussion 33–25

Yamaguchi S, Eguchi K, Kiura Y et al. (2007) Multi-detector-row CT angiography as a preoperative evaluation for spinal arteriovenous fistulae. Neurosurg Rev 30:321–326; discussion 327

Yoshioka K, Niinuma H, Ehara S et al. (2006) MR angiography and CT angiography of the artery of Adamkiewicz: state of the art. Radiographics 26(Suppl):S63–S73

# Lower-Extremity CTA

Dominik Fleischmann

CONTENTS

## ABSTRACT

Lower-extremity CTA has evolved into an accurate, robust, and widely available test for noninvasive vascular imaging of the lower extremities in patients with peripheral arterial occlusive disease (PAOD). This chapter reviews the acquisition and contrast medium administration techniques for peripheral CTA. Visualization of atherosclerotic disease with CTA in general requires "angiography-like" 3D images (such as VR or MIP images); however—notably in the presence of vessel wall calcifications and stents—cross-sectional views (such as CPRs) are also required to accurately assess the flow lumen of the aorta down to the pedal arteries. Adequate visualization and mapping of atherosclerotic lesions in patients with PAOD is not only a prerequisite for generating a dictated report, but more importantly, standardized postprocessed images serve as a treatment planning tool and are the key to communicating the findings to the treating physician. Treatment decisions (surgical versus transluminal revascularization, or conservative treatment), and percutaneous treatment planning (access site, antegrade versus retrograde puncture) can be made in the majority of patients with PAOD based on lower-extremity CTA.

D. Fleischmann, MD
Department of Radiology, Stanford University Medical Center, 300 Pasteur Drive, Room S-072, Stanford, CA 94305-5105, USA

## 25.1
## Introduction

Lower-extremity CTA has evolved into an accurate, robust, and widely available test for noninvasive imaging of the peripheral arterial tree, for a wide range of clinical indications: congenital abnormalities (e.g., popliteal entrapment syndrome), vascular (iatrogenic and non-iatrogenic) trauma, vasculitis, aneurysmal and thromboembolic disease, arterial mapping before fibula-graft procurement (Chow et al. 2005), follow-up, and surveillance of surgical and endovascular revascularization (Table 25.1). The main indication, for peripheral CTA, however, is treatment planning in patients with peripheral arterial occlusive disease (PAOD) (Kock et al. 2005; Ouwendijk et al. 2005; Fleischmann et al. 2006; Heijenbrok-Kal et al. 2007). Modern MDCT scanners provide high-resolution volumetric datasets of the entire peripheral arterial tree in less than 40 s of scan time, and the room time for mobile patients is in the range of only 10–20 min. Scanning and injection protocols can easily be standardized and individualized if certain physiologic constraints are taken into account. While data acquisition is thus straightforward, the practical bottleneck for routine lower-extremity CTA is often related to the problem of how to effectively visualize and communicate the complex multifocal manifestations of PAOD. Accurate mapping of the disease process—in terms of degree, number, length, and distribution of lesions—in the context of a patient's clinical symptoms is the basis for treatment planning. Comprehensive visualization is therefore highly desirable.

**Table 25.1.** Indications for lower-extremity CTA

| PAOD |
| --- |
| Trauma (accidental/iatrogenic) |
| Aneurysm/arteriomegaly |
| Anatomic mapping for fibula graft harvesting |
| Mass (vascular supply/anatomic relationship) |
| Acute ischemia (embolism) |
| Arteritis |
| Popliteal arterial entrapment syndrome |

The purpose of this chapter is to review the practical aspects of state-of-the-art lower-extremity CTA in its role as a treatment-planning tool for patients with PAOD. Taking full advantage of the capabilities of lower-extremity CTA in this role requires integration of acquisition and contrast medium injection parameters, with knowledge of therapeutic options and the ability to vi-

**Table 25.2.** Integrated 64-channel peripheral CTA acquisition and injection protocol

| Scanning range | First: T12 vertebra (level of superior mesenteric artery) through the toes |
| --- | --- |
| | Second (optional): above knee through the toes |
| Acquisition | $64 \times 0.6$ mm (number of channels × channel width) |
| | 120 kV, 250 quality reference mA (automated tube current modulation) |
| Pitch, table speed | Variable pitch (depends on volume coverage, usually <1) |
| | Variable table speed (usually ~30 mm/s) |
| Scan time | FIXED to 40 s (in all patients) |
| Injection duration | FIXED to 35 s (in all patients) |
| Scanning delay | $t_{CMT}$ + 2 s (minimum delay with automated bolus triggering, including breath-hold command) |
| Contrast medium | High concentration ($\geq 350$ mg I/ml) |
| Biphasic injections (body weight–adjusted) | Maximum flow rate for first 5 s of injection, continued with 80% of initial flow rate for 30 s |

| | Body weight (kg) | Biphasic injection |
| --- | --- | --- |
| | <55 | 20 ml (4 ml/s) + 96 ml (3.2 ml/s) |
| | <65 | 23 ml (4.5 ml/s) + 108 ml (3.6 ml/s) |
| | Average: 75 | 25 ml (5 ml/s) + 120 ml (4 ml/s) |
| | >85 | 28 ml (5.5 ml/s) + 132 ml (4.4 ml/s) |
| | >95 | 30 ml (6 ml/s) + 144 ml (4.8 ml/s) |

$t_{CMT}$ contrast medium transit time

sualize and convey the clinically relevant lesions to the treating physician.

## 25.2
### Imaging Strategy

Lower-extremity CTA can be performed with all currently available MDCT scanners. No special hardware is required. Because of the slightly thicker sections (2.5–3 mm) usually obtained with four-channel MDCT (4 × 2.5 mm), evaluation of crural and pedal arteries is slightly limited, notably if calcifications are present. The technical limitations of four-channel MDCT are only clinically problematic in a small subset of patients, such as individuals with critical limb ischemia who have no or mild inflow and femoropopliteal disease, and who have diseased and calcified infrapopliteal vessels. In the majority of patients—notably those with intermittent claudication where interventions are limited to above-knee arteries—even four-channel MDCT can provide all the therapeutically relevant information (HEIJEN-BROK-KAL et al. 2007; RUBIN et al. 2001; OFER et al. 2003; MARTIN et al. 2003; OTA et al. 2004 CATALANO et al. 2004).

The typical section thickness used with 8-, 16-, and 64-channel MDCT is between 1 and 2 mm. Even thinner, submillimeter sections can easily be obtained with 16- and 64-channel CT, and may have advantages for the depiction of very small vessels (e.g., pedal); however, the overall number of images and relatively more noise in the abdomen are the tradeoffs (WILLMANN et al. 2005). We routinely reconstruct 1-mm thick sections from scans acquired with a 64-channel scanner, which allows for reliable assessment of all therapeutically relevant arterial branches in the great majority of patients (Table 25.2).

The typical scanning range for a lower-extremity CTA extends from the celiac artery down through the feet. We also preprogram a second CT acquisition into our protocol, with a scanning range from above the knees through the feet (Fig. 25.1). This second acquisition is initiated when the technologist does not clearly see good arterial opacification below the knees in the first phase, which may ensue even when the CT data acquisition is deliberately slowed down. This can occur in patients with diffuse arteriomegaly, large aneurysms, and decreased cardiac output. As will be explained below, we generally use a long scan time of 40 s for lower-extremity CTA. This implies a small pitch, usually less than 1. The use of automated tube current modulation is therefore strongly recommended, not only to individ-

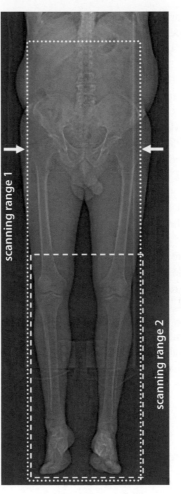

**Fig. 25.1.** Digital CT radiograph for prescribing a peripheral CTA. The patient's legs and feet are aligned with the long axis of the scanner. Scanning range (from the T12 vertebral body through feet) and reconstruction FOV (determined by the greater trochanters [*arrows*]) are indicated by the *dotted line*. A second, optional CTA acquisition is prescribed for the crural/pedal territory (*dashed line*) from above the knees through the feet

ualize radiation exposure, but also to achieve constant image–noise levels within a patient's dataset, and also across different patients.

## 25.3
### Integrated Scanning and Contrast Medium Injection Protocol for 64-Channel Lower-Extremity CTA

The technique of contrast medium injection always needs to be adapted to the scanner capabilities, but in the setting of lower-extremity CTA, also to the contrast medium flow dynamics. In patients with PAOD, the intravascular propagation of an intravenously injected contrast medium bolus may be substantially delayed within the dieseased lower extremity arterial tree. We have observed that the aortopopliteal bolus transit speed may be as slow as 30 mm/s (FLEISCHMANN and

RUBIN 2005). It is conceivable that if a CT scanner is operated at a table speed greater than the bolus transit speed, then the data acquisition can outrace the bolus down the peripheral arterial tree, resulting in inadequate opacification. The "risk" of outrunning the bolus is related to the table speed of the scanner, as illustrated in Fig. 25.2. While it is quite unlikely to outrace the bolus with a 4-channel MDCT scanner, where table speeds are in the range of 30 mm/s, the risk increases with faster table speeds: at 60 mm/s, approximately one third of patients with PAOD have slower bolus transit speeds, and at 90-mm/s table speed (which can be selected with 64-channel scanners), the data acquisition is faster than is the bolus in about half of the patients with PAOD.

The delayed flow dynamics in a diseased arterial tree therefore prohibit the use of the maximum scanning speed that is available with modern CT scanners. Our strategy for an integrated 64-channel lower-extremity CTA acquisition and injection protocol therefore uses an intentionally "slow" acquisition time of 40 s in all patients, which is combined with a 35-s injection duration in all patients (Table 25.2). Note, that the injection duration can be 5 s shorter than the scan time, because the scan "follows" the bolus down the peripheral arte-

rial tree. Also note that we use biphasic injections with high-concentration contrast medium (370 mg I/ml, which is the highest concentration agent available in the United States). The initially higher injection rates aim at achieving good proximal (i.e., aortic) enhancement (FLEISCHMANN et al. 2000, 2006; RUBIN et al. 2001).

The above example of an integrated 64-channel MDCT peripheral CTA protocol has several practical advantages: it is simple to execute (same scan time and same injection duration for all patients), it can be individualized to patient weight by using a simple look-up table, and it provides predictable image noise levels (by using automated tube current modulation), resulting in constant image quality for further image postprocessing.

## 25.4
### Visualization Techniques: 3D Overview (MIP and VR) and 2D Cross-Sections

Effective visualization of atherosclerotic changes within the peripheral arterial tree is challenging and generally requires the use of a 3D workstation to generate both 2D and 3D reformatted images. Three-dimensional VR or MIP images provide the most angiography-like views of the peripheral arterial tree displaying the conducting vessels as well as collaterals, if present. MIP and VR images are easy to interpret for everyone familiar with conventional angiography. One disadvantage of MIP is that it requires bone editing. VR is ideally suited to show vessels together with bones or soft tissues, such as in the setting of anatomic mapping for fibula graft harvesting, and popliteal arterial entrapment syndrome, and since VR does not require bone editing, it can be used to quickly interrogate a given dataset. Interactive VR is thus our preferred tool in the acute setting, such as trauma or acute lower-extremity ischemia. The most significant limitation of both MIP and VR is the fact that vessel wall calcifications or endoluminal stents obscure the vascular flow channels (Fig. 25.3). The majority of patients with PAOD have at least one arterial segment that is circumferentially calcified (ROOS et al. 2007). Therefore, 3D techniques need to be supplemented with 2D cross-sectional viewing for complete assessment of arterial flow channels in most patients with PAOD. Transverse CT source images (OFER et al. 2003; MARTIN et al. 2003; CATALANO et al. 2004; EDWARD et al. 2005; PORTUGALLER et al. 2004), coronal and sagittal MPRs (CATALANO et al. 2004), double-oblique MPRs perpendicular to the vessel centerline (OTA et al. 2004), and curved planar reformations (RUBIN et al.

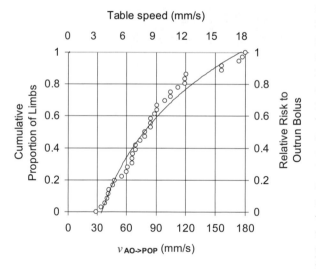

**Fig. 25.2.** Plot shows cumulative proportion of limbs as a function of aorto-popliteal bolus transit speed ($v_{AO \to POP}$), with a logarithmic trendline ($y = -0.6207\ln(x) + 3.203$) fitted to the data ($R^2 = 0.97$). The data can also be interpreted as the relative risk of outrunning the contrast medium bolus as a function of the table speed of the CT scanner, as indicated by the secondary $x$- and $y$-axes of the plot, respectively: an increase of the table speed (secondary $x$-axis) relates to an increased the risk of outrunning the contrast medium bolus (secondary $y$-axis). (From FLEISCHMANN et al. 2005, with permission)

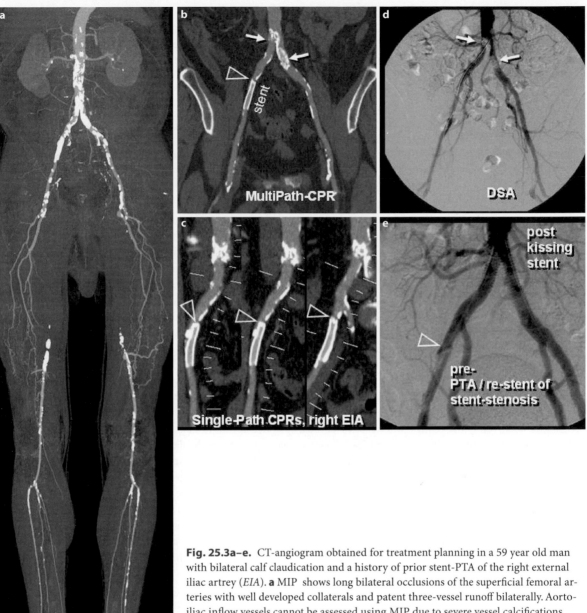

**Fig. 25.3a–e.** CT-angiogram obtained for treatment planning in a 59 year old man with bilateral calf claudication and a history of prior stent-PTA of the right external iliac artrey (*EIA*). **a** MIP  shows long bilateral occlusions of the superficial femoral arteries with well developed collaterals and patent three-vessel runoff bilaterally. Aorto-iliac inflow vessels cannot be assessed using MIP due to severe vessel calcifications (*arrows*). **b** MpCPR shows bulky calcifications with associated high-grade stenoses of the right common iliac artery (*CIA*) at the aortic bifurcation and a high-grade stenosis of the left CIA (*arrows*). A short stent is seen in the right EIA (*asterisk*). **c** Detailed analysis of the right EIA shows mild narrowing of the patent stent, however, a 'lid'-like calcification is seen obstructing the proximal end of the stent (*arrowheads*). **d** Diagnostic angiographic run confirms high-grade bilateral aorto-iliac stenois (*arrows*) which are subsequently treated with bilateral CIA 'kissing' stents. **e** Post-EIA-stent rerun clearly shows significant stenosis at the proximal end of the EIA stent (*arrowhead*), which was subsequently treatet with another stent (*not shown*)

2001; Ofer et al. 2003) all serve this purpose. Possibly the most efficient cross-sectional viewing modality is curved planar reformation (CPR), and its latest extension, the so-called multipath CPR (mpCPR) (Roos et al. 2007; Kanitsar et al. 2002) (Fig. 25.2). The advantage of mpCPR is that it simultaneously displays CPRs through all conducting vessels in a single image. The spatial arrangement of vessels is thus maintained, and anatomic identification of vessels is straightforward for anyone familiar with lower-extremity arterial anatomy. MpCPRs can be generated at arbitrary viewing angles. The disadvantage of mpCPR is that vessels may obscure each other from viewing angles, and certain artifacts may occur at vessel bifurcations (Roos et al. 2007). Standard single-path CPRs are also reconstructed routinely, and can be viewed if artifacts are present or if relevant regions of the arterial tree are incompletely visualized with mpCPR (Roos et al. 2007). All CPRs allow the assessment of the flow channels, the vessel wall, and the composition of clot or thrombus of an occluded segment. Display of plaque composition and vessel wall calcifications are helpful for both percutaneous and surgical treatment planning (Misare et al. 1996).

Both MIP and CPR generation requires labor-intensive postprocessing, such as bone editing for MIP and centerline extraction for CPR. Time-consuming postprocessing is currently the main bottleneck for clinical implementation of a routine lower-extremity CTA program. Automated or semiautomated bone editing and vessel-tracking algorithms are available on all modern workstations, and these tools have become faster and more efficient when tracking normal or minimally diseased vessels and for editing of large high-attenuation bone. All currently available techniques (commercial and academic), however, perform poorly when center-

lines need to be extracted from the clinically more relevant diseased arteries and when bone density is low. It is unreasonable to expect that postprocessing algorithms will provide accurate results without expert-user interaction in the near future.

## 25.5
## Workflow and Documentation

When peripheral CT angiograms are acquired on a routine, daily basis, it is important to establish an efficient and standardized workflow for image acquisition postprocessing, image interpretation, and for communication of imaging findings to the referring physician.

We have established a routine postprocessing protocol at our institution, which generates a standardized set of images—essentially a combination of 3D overview images (MIP) and cross-sectional images (e.g., CPR and mpCPR). These standardized set of images are produced by radiological technologists on a dedicated workstation, but all the resulting images can be viewed on any PACS viewing workstation. An example of such a protocol-driven set of images created at our institution for peripheral CTA using custom-built software is shown in Table 25.3. Figure 25.4 illustrates how these images can be displayed on a PACS viewing workstation. Our standard set of images includes the following images, which are grouped in separate DICOM series: 21 MIPs (after bone editing) of the entire peripheral arterial tree over a 180° viewing range. In the absence of stents or vessel wall calcifications, these MIP images may provide all the diagnostic information needed for image interpretation. The MIPs are supplemented by

**Table 25.3.** Standard set of postprocessed images for lower-extremity CTA (DICOM series)

| DICOM series name | Images (*n*) | Viewing range |
|---|---|---|
| MIP | 21 | 180° (9° increment) |
| MpCPR | 21 | 180° (9° increment) |
| CPR left | 3 × 11 | 180° (18° increment) |
| CPR right | 3 × 11 | 180° (18° increment) |
| Total | 108 | |

MIP images created after semiautomated bone editing; CPRs from the aorta through the bilateral plantar, dorsalis pedis, and distal peroneal arteries, respectively. Range of viewing angles is 180° in all series, from left lateral (–90°) through posteroanterior (0°) to (+90°)

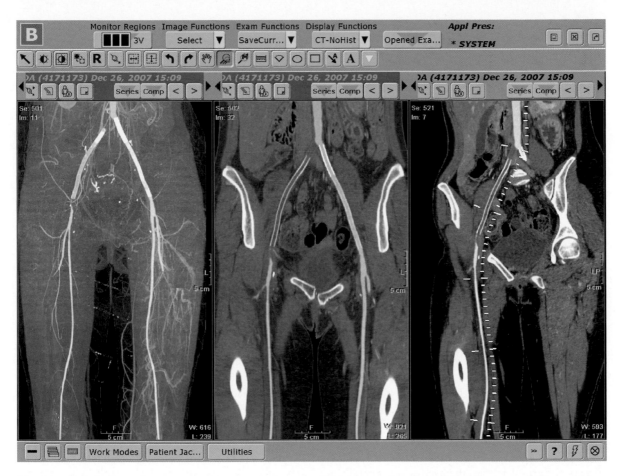

**Fig. 25.4.** Standard set of postprocessed images of a lower-extremity CT angiogram obtained in patient with bilateral iliac artery stents, as displayed on a standard PACS viewing station with side-by-side display of MIP, mpCPR, and single-path CPR. *Image on the left* MIP (anteroposterior view) shows bilateral stents in the common and external iliac arteries. Note, that the patency of the stents cannot be assessed on the MIP images. *Middle image* mpCPR allows simultaneous display of longitu-dinal cross-sections through the bilateral aorto-iliac and femoral arteries in a single image. Note the occlusion of the right iliac through common femoral artery and the occluded stent on the right side, whereas the stents in the left iliac territory are clearly patent. *Image on the right* standard single-path CPR with digital gauging ticks (right CPR) through the right iliac and femoral arteries displays the composition of thrombus and provides an estimate of the lesion length

21 mpCPRs, which show simultaneous cross-sections through all conducting vessels even in the presence of calcified plaque and stents. Side-by-side viewing of MIP and mpCPR images allows complete evaluation of the lower-extremity arterial tree in the majority of patients. Finally, we create standard single-path CPRs through all the conducting vessels. These images are reviewed if MIP and mpCPR images do not allow adequate assessment of certain vascular segments and for lesion length measurement (Figs. 25.3, 25.4).

Of course, there are many other ways how postprocessing of the data can be standardized using state-of-the-art commercial software as well. The importance of generating standardized, intuitive, and easily accessible images cannot be overemphasized in the setting of lower-extremity CTA because viewing of the transverse source images is not a practical option. One also cannot expect all treating physicians to be familiar with and have the time to operating a 3D postprocessing workstation.

## 25.6
### Clinical Interpretation

Knowledge of a patient's disease-specific clinical symptoms and the potential therapeutic consequences of imaging findings are a prerequisite for competent image interpretation. Detailed reviews of current clinical knowledge and therapeutic strategies in patients with PAOD can be found elsewhere (OURIEL 2001). The two major clinical categories of PAOD are *intermittent claudication* and *critical limb ischemia*. While therapeutic techniques are technically similar, their application is far more urgent in patients with critical limb ischemia because revascularization is required for limb salvage.

The therapeutic options in patients with *intermittent claudication* are conservative (exercise training), percutaneous intervention (PTA with or without stent), or surgical revascularization, with the goal to improve symptoms. Imaging is indicated if an invasive revascularization procedure is contemplated. Both percutaneous and surgical revascularization approaches are usually restricted to the aorto-iliac and femoropopliteal territories. The choice of treatment depends on the number, type, and length of lesions, and on local expertise and practice (TransAtlantic Inter-Society Consensus 2000). Although the status of crural arteries plays a role as a prognostic factor for treatment success, the crural arteries themselves are generally not the direct target of a revascularization attempt in this population. The implication for image interpretation is therefore that lesion detection and characterization in patients with intermittent claudication is primarily focused on aorto-iliac inflow and femoropopliteal arteries. It is not necessary to scrutinize crural or pedal arteries in this patient group. In this context, mpCPR is particularly helpful for percutaneous treatment planning because it reliably displays the entire aorto-iliac and bilateral femoropopliteal arterial flow channels in a single image, enabling very convenient planning of interventional procedures (Fig. 25.2) (SCHERNTHANER et al. 2007a,b). The interventional radiologist can select the best access site, decide on an antegrade or retrograde puncture, and visualize the length and character (calcified/noncalcified) of a lesion.

The therapeutic strategy in patients with *critical limb ischemia* is focused on revascularization for limb salvage, and is therefore urgent. If aorto-iliac and/or femoropopliteal lesions are identified, then these are the initial treatment targets, although direct crural artery intervention and/or infrapopliteal and pedal bypass grafts may also be necessary. In patients with critical limb ischemia, image interpretation also includes a detailed assessment of crural and pedal arteries as potential target vessels for peripheral bypass grafting. Although CPRs are the most helpful images for the assessment of conducting arteries, they are not well suited for assessment and evaluation of crural and pedal arteries or collateral vessels. Therefore, VRTs or even source image viewing may be necessary in order to answer the specific therapeutically relevant question. Even with the most advanced CT technology, accurate assessment of heavily calcified infrapopliteal arteries remains a challenge (OUWENDIJK et al. 2006).

## 25.7
### Pitfalls

Perhaps the most important pitfall related to the interpretation of peripheral CT angiograms is using viewing window settings too narrow in the presence of arterial wall calcifications or stents. Even at wider-than-normal "CT angiographic" window settings (window level/window width: 150HU/600 HU), high-attenuation objects (calcified plaque, stents) appear larger than they really are ("blooming" due to the point-spread function of the scanner), which may lead to an overestimation of a vascular stenosis or suggest a spurious occlusion. When scrutinizing a calcified lesion or a stented segment using any of the cross-sectional gray-scale images (transverse source images, MPR, or CPR), a viewing window width of 1,500 HU may be required. Interactive window adjustment on a PACS viewing station or on a 3D workstation is usually required during image interpretation. In the setting of extensive calcifications within small crural or pedal arteries, such as in diabetic patients and in patients with end-stage renal disease, the lumen may not be resolved regardless of the window width/level selection. In these circumstances, other imaging techniques, notably MRI, or selective intra-arterial DSA may be preferable to CTA.

The second pitfall in the interpretation of lower-extremity CTA is related to the lack of flow information, which may lead to the underestimation of high-grade stenoses or short occlusions. A typical case is shown in Fig. 25.5. The patient has an angiographically evident high-grade calcified stenosis of the proximal superficial femoral artery. The good opacification of the SFA distal to the lesion in the CT images makes the lesion appear less severe when compared with the corresponding DSA, which shows that there is no antegrade filling of the SFA. From the CT images, one cannot depict that the SFA is predominantly filled retrogradely via collaterals.

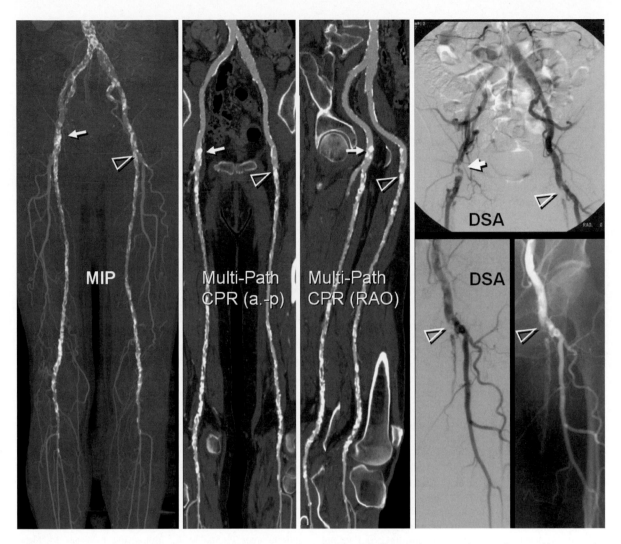

**Fig. 25.5.** Lower-extremity CTA in a 84-year-old woman with bilateral calf claudication, left greater than right. MIP shows significant calcifications in the right common femoral artery ([CFA] *arrow*) and in the proximal SFA (*arrowhead*), as well as in the bilateral distal SFA/popliteal arteries, respectively. Note, that the calcifications do not allow evaluation for the presence/degree of arterial stenoses. MpCPRs in anteroposterior and right anterior oblique views clearly demonstrate the extent of the CFA calcification that protrudes into the vessel lumen at the right CFA (*arrow*), and at the left SFA origin (*arrowhead*). Angiographic correlation confirms high-grade CFA/SFA stenoses. Note, that CTA "underestimates" the degree of stenosis; in this case, since it does not provide the flow information that is apparent during intra-arterial DSA

## 25.8
## Conclusion

Peripheral CTA has matured into an accurate, noninvasive vascular imaging technique in patients with PAOD. Peripheral CTA can safely replace intra-arterial angiography as a fist-line diagnostic test in patients with intermittent claudication (KOCK et al. 2005; OUWENDIJK et al. 2005; HEIJENBROK-KAL et al. 2007), and may also be helpful in patients with critical limb ischemia. While image acquisition is fairly straightforward with modern scanners, visualization remains a challenge. Standardized protocols for 2D and 3D image postprocessing play a central role in image interpretation and for communicating the findings to referring physicians, and are thus indispensable for therapeutic decision making and treatment planning in the increasing population of patients with PAOD.

# References

Catalano C, Fraioli F, Laghi A, Napoli A, Bezzi M, Pediconi F, Danti M, Nofroni I, Passarielloa R (2004) Infrarenal aortic and lower-extremity arterial disease: diagnostic performance of multi-detector row CT angiography. Radiology 231:555–563

Chow LC, Napoli A, Klein MB, Chang J, Rubin GD (2005) Vascular mapping of the leg with multi-detector row CT angiography prior to free-flap transplantation. Radiology 237:353–360

Edwards AJ, Wells IP, Roobottom CA (2005) Multidetector row CT angiography of the lower limb arteries: a prospective comparison of volume-rendered techniques and intra-arterial digital subtraction angiography. Clin Radiol 60:85–95

Fleischmann D, Rubin GD (2005) Quantification of intravenously administered contrast medium transit through the peripheral arteries: implications for CT angiography. Radiology 236:1076–1082

Fleischmann D, Rubin GD, Bankier AA, Hittmair K (2000) Improved uniformity of aortic enhancement with customized contrast medium injection protocols at CT angiography. Radiology 214:363–371

Fleischmann D, Hallett RL, Rubin GD (2006) CT angiography of peripheral arterial disease. J Vasc Interv Radiol 17:3–26

Heijenbrok-Kal MH, Kock MCJM, Hunink MGM (2007) Lower extremity arterial disease: multidetector CT angiography meta-analysis. Radiology 245:433–439

Kanitsar A, Fleischmann D, Wegenkittl R, Felkel P, Groeller E (2002) CPR—curved planar reformation. In: IEEE Visualization 2002. IEEE Computer Society, Boston, pp 37–44

Kock MCJM, Adriaensen MEAPM, Pattynama PMT, van Sambeek MRHM, van Urk H, Stijnen T, Hunink MGM (2005) DSA versus multi-detector row CT angiography in peripheral arterial disease: randomized controlled trial. Radiology 237:727–737

Martin ML, Tay KH, Flak B, Fry PD, Doyle DL, Taylor DC, Hsiang YN, Machan LS (2003) Multidetector CT angiography of the aortoiliac system and lower extremities: a prospective comparison with digital subtraction angiography. AJR Am J Roentgenol 180:1085–1091

Misare BD, Pomposelli FB, Jr., Gibbons GW, Campbell DR, Freeman DV, LoGerfo FW (1996) Infrapopliteal bypasses to severely calcified, unclampable outflow arteries: two-year results. J Vasc Surg 24:6–15; discussion 15–16

Ofer A, Nitecki SS, Linn S, Epelman M, Fischer D, Karram T, Litmanovich D, Schwartz H, Hoffman A, Engel A (2003) Multidetector CT angiography of peripheral vascular disease: a prospective comparison with intraarterial digital subtraction angiography. AJR Am J Roentgenol 180:719–724

Ota H, Takase K, Igarashi K, Chiba Y, Haga K, Saito H, Takahashi S (2004) MDCT compared with digital subtraction angiography for assessment of lower extremity arterial occlusive disease: importance of reviewing cross-sectional images. AJR Am J Roentgenol 182:201–209

Ouriel K (2001) Peripheral arterial disease. Lancet 358:1257–1264

Ouwendijk R, de Vries M, Pattynama PM, van Sambeek MR, de Haan MW, Stijnen T, van Engelshoven JM, Hunink MG (2005) Imaging peripheral arterial disease: a randomized controlled trial comparing contrast-enhanced MR angiography and multi-detector row CT angiography. Radiology 236:1094–1103

Ouwendijk R, Kock MC, van Dijk LC, van Sambeek MR, Stijnen T, Hunink MG (2006) Vessel wall calcifications at multi-detector row CT angiography in patients with peripheral arterial disease: effect on clinical utility and clinical predictors. Radiology 241:603–608

Portugaller HR, Schoellnast H, Hausegger KA, Tiesenhausen K, Amann W, Berghold A (2004) Multislice spiral CT angiography in peripheral arterial occlusive disease: a valuable tool in detecting significant arterial lumen narrowing? Eur Radiol 14:1681–1687

Roos JE, Fleischmann D, Koechl A, Rakshe T, Straka M, Napoli A, Kanitsar A, Sramek M, Groeller E (2007) Multipath curved planar reformation of the peripheral arterial tree in CT angiography. Radiology 244:281–290

Rubin GD, Schmidt AJ, Logan LJ, Sofilos MC (2001) Multidetector row CT angiography of lower extremity arterial inflow and runoff: initial experience. Radiology 221:146–158

Schernthaner R, Fleischmann D, Lomoschitz F, Stadler A, Lammer J, Loewe C (2007a) Effect of MDCT angiographic findings on the management of intermittent claudication. AJR Am J Roentgenol 189:1215–1222

Schernthaner R, Stadler A, Lomoschitz F, Weber M, Fleischmann D, Lammer J, Loewe C (2007b) Multidetector CT angiography in the assessment of peripheral arterial occlusive disease: accuracy in detecting the severity, number, and length of stenoses. Eur Radiol 18:665–671

TransAtlantic Inter-Society Consensus (2000) TransAtlantic Inter-Society Consensus: management of peripheral arterial disease. J Vasc Surg 1(Suppl):1–296

Willmann JK, Baumert B, Schertler T, Wildermuth S, Pfammatter T, Verdun FR, Seifert B, Marincek B, Bohm T (2005) Aortoiliac and lower extremity arteries assessed with 16-detector row CT angiography: prospective comparison with digital subtraction angiography. Radiology 236:1083–1093

# Lung

# Interstitial Lung Diseases

26

Christina Mueller-Mang, Christina Plank, Helmut Ringl, Albert Dirisamer and Christian Herold

## CONTENTS

## ABSTRACT

The term interstitial lung disease (ILD) comprises a diverse group of diseases that lead to *inflammation* and *fibrosis* of the alveoli, distal airways, and septal interstitium of the lungs. The ILDs consist of disorders of *known cause* (e.g., collagen vascular diseases, drug-related diseases) as well as disorders of unknown etiology. The latter include *idiopathic interstitial pneumonias* (IIPs), sarcoidosis and a group of miscellaneous, rare, but nonetheless interesting, diseases. In patients with ILD, MDCT enriches the diagnostic armamentarium by allowing volumetric high resolution scanning, i.e., continuous data acquisition with thin collimation and a high spatial frequency reconstruction algorithm. *CT* is a key method in the identification and man-

C. Mueller-Mang, MD
Department of Radiology, Medical University of Vienna, Waehringer Guertel 18–20, 1190 Vienna, Austria

C. Plank, MD
Department of Radiology, Medical University of Vienna, Waehringer Guertel 18–20, 1190 Vienna, Austria

H. Ringl, MD
Department of Radiology, Medical University of Vienna, Waehringer Guertel 18–20, 1190 Vienna, Austria

A. Dirisamer, MD
Department of Radiology, Medical University of Vienna, Waehringer Guertel 18–20, 1190 Vienna, Austria

C. Herold, MD
Department of Radiology, Medical University of Vienna, Waehringer Guertel 18–20, 1190 Vienna, Austria

agement of patients with ILD. It not only improves the detection and characterization of parenchymal abnormalities, but also increases the accuracy of diagnosis. The spectrum of morphologic characteristics that are indicative of interstitial lung disease is relatively limited and includes a reticular pattern (with or without traction bronchiectasis), thickening of interlobular septa, honeycombing, nodules, and ground-glass opacities. In the correct clinical context, some *patterns* or combination of patterns, together with the *anatomic distribution* of the abnormality, i.e., from the lung apex to the base, or peripheral subpleural versus central bronchovascular, can lead the interpreter to a specific diagnosis. However, due to an overlap of the CT morphology between the various entities, complementary *lung biopsy* is recommended in virtually all cases of ILDs.

## Introduction

The interstitial lung diseases (ILDs) are a heterogeneous group of lung disorders that result from damage to the lung by various forms of inflammation and fibrosis. By definition, ILDs involve the lung interstitium that forms a fibrous skeleton for the lungs. However, many of the conditions that have been traditionally included under the heading of ILDs are actually associated with extensive alterations of the alveolar and airway architecture. For this reason, the terms *diffuse infiltrative lung disease* or *diffuse parenchymal lung disease* are preferable. Still, the term ILDs remains in common clinical usage.

ILDs represent more than 200 different entities, and various and often-confusing classification systems are simultaneously used. One useful approach to classification is to separate the ILDs into diseases of known and

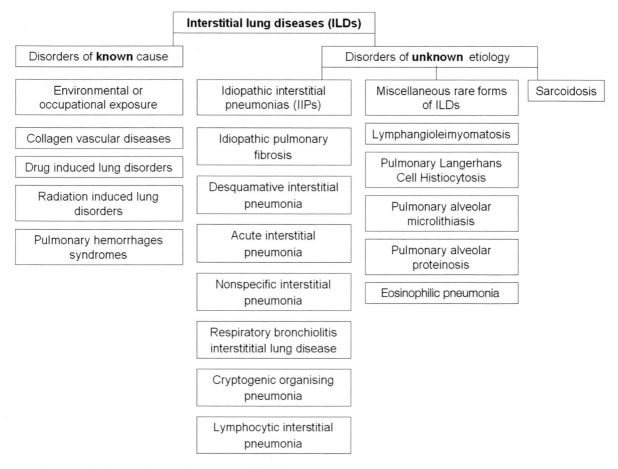

**Fig. 26.1** Classification of interstitial lung diseases (*ILDs*)

unknown etiology (Fig. 26.1). ILD of unknown etiology (65% of all ILDs) can be further subdivided into the group of idiopathic interstitial pneumonias (IIPs), and a group comprising several rare but interesting diseases with distinctive clinicopathologic features, such as lymphangioleiomyomatosis, Langerhans cell histiocytosis, pulmonary alveolar proteinosis, and pulmonary alveolar microlithiasis. Sarcoidosis has an exceptional position within the group of ILDs of unknown cause, as it is relatively common and can present as a systemic disease.

CT scanning is the most important noninvasive diagnostic key to the identification and characterization of ILD, and aids the radiologist and the clinician in the management of patients who carry this disorder. Among all noninvasive methods, it provides the highest sensitivity and specificity in the detection of ILD. Also, it has a higher accuracy in comparison to the clinical assessment, lung function tests, and chest radiography in diagnosing a specific disorder, and adds diagnostic accuracy and confidence when added to the clinical assessment and the chest radiogram. Finally, CT helps to identify the best location for lung biopsy, and provides an important basis for the follow-up of ILD patients.

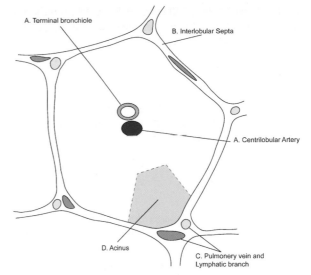

**Fig. 26.2.** Secondary pulmonary lobule (*A* centrilobular arteries and bronchioles with a diameter of approximately 1 mm, *B* interlobular septa with a thickness of approximately 0.1 mm, *C* pulmonary vein and lymphatic branch with diameters of 0.5 mm each, *D* acinus—never visible on CT scans)

## 26.2
## Anatomic and Technical Considerations

### 26.2.1
### Normal Lung Anatomy

The correct interpretation of CT and especially high-resolution CT (HRCT) requires a fundamental understanding of normal lung anatomy. In patients with ILD, the small anatomical structures of the lung parenchyma such as the secondary pulmonary lobule are involved in one way or another, and the identification of the patterns of infiltration and distribution is a key to the establishment of a correct list of differential diagnoses, and sometimes to the diagnosis itself. In this sense, HRCT provides an insight into lung morphology and architecture, comparable to or even beyond macroscopic pathology. The following anatomic structures and architectural components need to be considered:

#### The Secondary Pulmonary Lobule

The secondary pulmonary lobule is the smallest anatomical unit of the lungs that can be identified on high-resolution CT scans (Fig. 26.2). Whereas in normal

lungs, these polyhedral structures are only visible in the anterior and lateral portions of the pulmonary parenchyma, they may be identifiable in any region when ILD and other disorders such as lung edema are present.

Typical secondary pulmonary lobules are irregular polyhedral units that vary in size, measuring from approximately 1 to 2.5 cm in diameter and incorporating up to 24 acini (WEBB 2006). An average diameter for pulmonary lobules ranges from 11 to 17 mm in adults. The secondary pulmonary lobule is surrounded by a mantle of connective tissue septa. A central bronchovascular bundle, consisting of the lobular bronchiole and the accompanying pulmonary artery, enters the center of the secondary pulmonary lobule, where the bronchiole bifurcates into three to five terminal bronchioles. The region near the origin of the terminal bronchioles is termed the "centrilobular" region. Thus, on thin-section CT images, the secondary pulmonary lobule can be divided into three components: the interlobular septa, the centrilobular region, and the lobular parenchyma.

#### Interlobular Septa

The interlobular septa extend from the pleural surface of the lung inward, and surround the secondary lobule. They consist of connective tissue, house pulmonary veins, and lymphatics and belong to the peripheral interstitial fiber system (WEIBEL 1979). Interlobular septa are well developed in the periphery of the lungs, and in particular in the lung apex, and near the anterior, lower, mediastinal, and diaphragmatic surfaces. They are key structures to the identification of pulmonary involvement in ILD, because disorders such as interstitial pneumonia, sarcoidosis or lymphangitic carcinomatosis commonly lead to thickening and consequently, to better visibility of these structures.

### Centrilobular Region

The centrilobular region corresponds to the "axial fiber system" described by WEIBEL (1979). The central portion of the secondary pulmonary lobule contains the pulmonary artery and bronchiolar branches that supply the lobule. Because lobules do not arise at a specific branching generation of the bronchial or arterial tree, it is difficult to impossible to define exactly which specific bronchus or artery supplies that secondary lobule. However, lobular bronchioles are rarely seen in normal individuals since their lumen measures approximately 1 mm in diameter, and their wall 0.15 mm, respectively. Likewise, the more peripheral terminal and respiratory bronchioles cannot be resolved at CT (MURATA et al. 1986). It is only in diseases of the small airways that abnormal bronchi can be visualized through thickened walls, peribronchiolar inflammation, and/or intrabronchiolar fluid and mucus accumulations. Centrilobular arteries can be depicted on CT scans of normal and diseased individuals. Because of the anatomic properties of the lungs, centrilobular abnormalities are best seen in the lung periphery and near the hila.

### Lobular Parenchyma

The lung (lobular) parenchyma consists of alveoli, connective tissue, and the associated pulmonary capillary bed. These structures are too small to be directly visualized on thin-section CT, but may be indirectly assessed, as they are responsible for the background density of the lung on CT scans. Parenchymal background density reflects the proportions of fluid (blood and extravascular fluid), gas, and tissue. When ILD causes an increase of fluid or cells within the alveoli, or thickening of the alveolar septa through cellular infiltration or fibrosis, then parenchymal background density will change in turn and ground glass opacities may be identified at CT. Conversely, a decrease in fluid, cells, and tissue (in relation to air), as seen in emphysema, causes a reduction of the parenchymal density, in comparison to the normal state.

## 26.2.2
## CT Technique

For patients with ILD, the identification of the smallest possible structures of the lung parenchyma and the depiction of their abnormalities is of paramount importance for any imaging approach. Therefore, CT protocols have to utilize thin collimation and high-spatial-frequency reconstruction algorithms to achieve an optimal spatial resolution and consequently, facilitate an optimal assessment of interstitial and airspace disease. For decades, patients with ILD have traditionally been investigated with HRCT (MAYO et al. 1987). This technique consists of a "step-and-shoot" approach, in which 0.5- to 1-mm collimation scans are obtained at 10- to 20-mm intervals, a small FOV, and a high radiation dose per section. It provides excellent image quality, free of partial volume and projection artifacts, and combines high sensitivity in the detection of ILD with high accuracy in establishing the correct diagnosis. This "classic" HRCT technique still plays a decisive role in the noninvasive investigation of patients with pulmonary disease of a diffuse distribution pattern (HANSELL 2001).

With the advent of MDCT, volumetric high-resolution imaging has enriched the diagnostic armamentarium of the radiologist. New-generation MDCT scanners allow fast single-breath-hold scanning, volumetric data acquisition with thinly collimated scans, and high-spatial-frequency reconstruction when scanning the entire lung. They thus combine the advantages of "traditional" HRCT and modern spiral scanning techniques. Volumetric protocols enable the radiologist to detect those abnormalities that might have been missed during the classic HRCT step-and-shoot approach. Moreover, volumetric isotropic data sets permit the reconstruction of high-quality multiplanar images, which help to appreciate better the distribution of disease, for example, to identify a cephalocaudal gradient of disease severity in certain disorders. Finally, continuous data acquisition allows the generation of MIP images, which in our experience, are helpful in the detection of micronodular disease and centrilobular abnormalities.

There are also some trade-offs with volumetric HRCT scanning. The radiation dose is 5 to 10 times higher, and the image quality is discretely lower in comparison to classic sequential HRCT. This image quality reduction is most apparent in the depiction of small septa and of ground-glass opacities (STUDLER et al. 2005) (Fig. 26.3a,b), and its clinical significance has yet to be determined. In order to achieve the best possible balance between diagnostic accuracy, exploitation of the advantages of volumetric CT and radiation dose, the following options exist (Table 26.1):

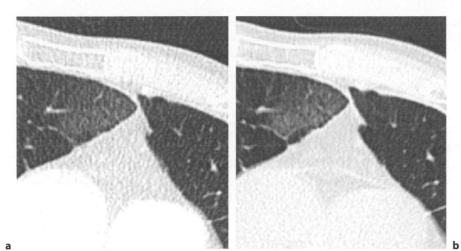

**Fig. 26.3a,b.** Difference in ground-glass depiction between sequential HRCT (**a**) and standard helical CT with 1-mm section thickness (**b**)

a                                                    b

1. Sequential HRCT protocol

   This protocol utilizes high milliampere-second and kilovolt peak values to obtain the best possible image quality. Thin collimation (1 mm) scans are obtained at 10- or 20-mm intervals. Therefore, the overall radiation dose is a 5th to a 10th in comparison to standard or high-resolution volumetric protocols. This protocol may be regarded as "imaging biopsy" in diffuse lung disease, as it detects disease, allows the specification of disease distribution, and helps in establishing a differential diagnosis with high accuracy and confidence levels. It is our protocol of choice in patients with proven ILD, and in those cases that require imaging follow-up during or after therapy. Because the classic HRCT leaves 9- to 19-mm broad gaps between the scanned sections unexamined, it should not be utilized as sole protocol in patients with suspicion of focal lung disease, in diffuse interstitial disorders where there is an increased risk associated with focal or even malignant abnormalities (such as dermatomyositis/polymyositis), or in entities with a distinct propensity to involve extrapulmonary sites in the mediastinum, the chest wall, the diaphragm, and the abdomen. In such instances, a combination with a standard volumetric protocol (Table 26.1) is highly

**Table 26.1.** Various MDCT protocols of the lung, valid for the Siemens Somatom Sensation 64 Cardiac scanner

| Protocol | Kilovolt peak | Current reference mAs/actual mAs | Dose modulation | Collimation (mm × slice no.) | Section thickness/reconstruction slice interval (mm/mm) | Dose length product (mGy × cm) | Effective dose (mSv) |
|---|---|---|---|---|---|---|---|
| HRCT sequential | 140 | 200/200 | Off | 1 × 2 | 1/20 | 60 | 1 |
| HRCT volumetric | 140 | 240/240 | Off | 0.6 × 64 | 1/0.8 | 800 | 13 |
| Standard volumetric | 120 | 200/80–120 | On | 0.6 × 64 | 1/0.8 | 300 | 5.1 |
| Low-dose volumetric | 80 | 30/30 | Off | 0.6 × 64 | 3/5 | 40 | 0.68 |

The reference mAs is the current preset of the protocol; the scanner controls the actual mAs within certain limits of this reference according its dose-modulation program

recommended. Another caveat is the assessment of patients with suspected air trapping at supine scans. In these cases, it is advisable to perform single slice step-and-shoot scans in prone positions instead of a continuous volumetric examination in order to reduce radiation burden.

2. Volumetric HRCT protocol
This protocol combines thin collimation with volumetric scanning and high milliampere-second and kilovolt peak values. During scanning, the dose modulation is off. The result is a high quality contiguous data set, which allows for high-resolution multiplanar and three-dimensional reconstructions with superb image quality. The latter is similar to that of sequential HRCT scanning, although it does not match it in every detail. The major disadvantage of this protocol is the radiation dose, which is approximately 10 times higher than that of conventional HRCT. We recommend using this protocol in ILD patients only when high-quality three-dimensional reconstructions are necessary, for example, for generating a data set for CT bronchoscopy.

3. Volumetric standard CT protocol
Here, the milliampere-second and kilovolt peak values are reduced in comparison to the sequential or volumetric high-resolution protocol, and dose modulation is switched on. The result is a substantial reduction in dose in comparison to the volumetric high-resolution protocol. Nevertheless, thin collimation and high-spatial-resolution reconstruction guarantee very good image quality, and volumetric data acquisition a continuous morphologic assessment of the lung investigated, respectively. In our view, this protocol is best used in combination with the classic sequential HRCT protocol in ILD patients. It provides a volumetric data set and the best high-resolution images, with a reasonable radiation dose that reaches roughly 50% of the dose resulting from the volumetric high-resolution protocol. It is advisable to utilize this combination protocol in all patients with ILD who are imaged for their first time, in cases where the chest radiogram indicates diffuse and focal disease, and in those who are at risk to develop focal disorders on top of a diffuse lung disease process.

4. Volumetric low-dose CT protocol
In patients with ILD, the low-dose high-resolution CT technique with a reduction of the milliampere-second values to approximately 40 mAs is in our view a valuable alternative to the standard volumetric protocol when combined with the sequential HRCT technique. It allows for the assessment of the pulmonary parenchyma in slim individuals, visualization of focal abnormalities in the lung parenchyma, and analysis of major airways disorders. The combination with the classic HRCT approach fosters almost the same advantages as those described for the combination of the standard volumetric protocol with classic HRCT. When using this protocol, one has to keep in mind that the somewhat reduced image quality may limit the diagnostic accuracy when scanning the parenchyma, the mediastinum, chest wall, and upper abdomen in obese patients.

## 26.3
## Interstitial Lung Diseases That Have No Known Cause

In the majority of ILDs, the etiology remains either largely or wholly unknown. Most are uncommon, and some, such as alveolar microlithiasis, are exceedingly rare, but others, such as idiopathic pulmonary fibrosis and sarcoidosis, are quite common.

### 26.3.1
### Idiopathic Interstitial Pneumonias

The term *idiopathic interstitial pneumonias* refers to a group of seven entities with distinct histologic patterns: idiopathic pulmonary fibrosis (IPF), characterized by the pattern of usual interstitial pneumonia (UIP); nonspecific interstitial pneumonia (NSIP); cryptogenic organizing pneumonia (COP); respiratory bronchiolitis-associated interstitial lung disease (RB-ILD); desquamative interstitial pneumonia (DIP); lymphoid interstitial pneumonia (LIP); and acute interstitial pneumonia (AIP).

In their idiopathic form, IIPs are rare diseases. They are, nevertheless, considered prototypes of more common secondary interstitial lung disorders, such as sarcoidosis, vasculitis, and connective tissue diseases, although they appear to follow a different and often less aggressive clinical course. The advent of HRCT has had a profound impact on the imaging of IIPs, because the detailed delineation of the lung anatomy allows a close correlation between the histologic patterns of IIPs and the CT features. On the basis of CT morphology and in the correct clinical context, the radiologist can achieve an accurate diagnosis in many cases. However, due to overlap between the various entities, complementary lung biopsy is recommended in virtually all cases.

### 26.3.1.1
### Idiopathic Pulmonary Fibrosis

IPF is by far the most common IIP, and has a substantially poorer long-term survival rate than do the other IIPs (median survival rate is 2.5–3.5 years) (KATZENSTEIN and MYERS 1998). IPF shares nonspecific clinical symptoms, such as gradual onset of progressive dyspnea and cough, with other IIPs. There is a slight male predominance, and patients are usually over the age of 50. Typically, patients do not respond to corticosteroid treatment, and currently, the only life-prolonging therapy consists of lung transplantation (THABUT et al. 2003). While the term IPF characterizes the clinical entity, the term *usual interstitial pneumonia* is used to describe the histologic and radiologic patterns associated with IPF. The histologic and radiologic features of UIP are characterized by heterogeneity with areas of normal lung alternating with patchy fibrosis. The typical CT findings in UIP are predominantly basal and

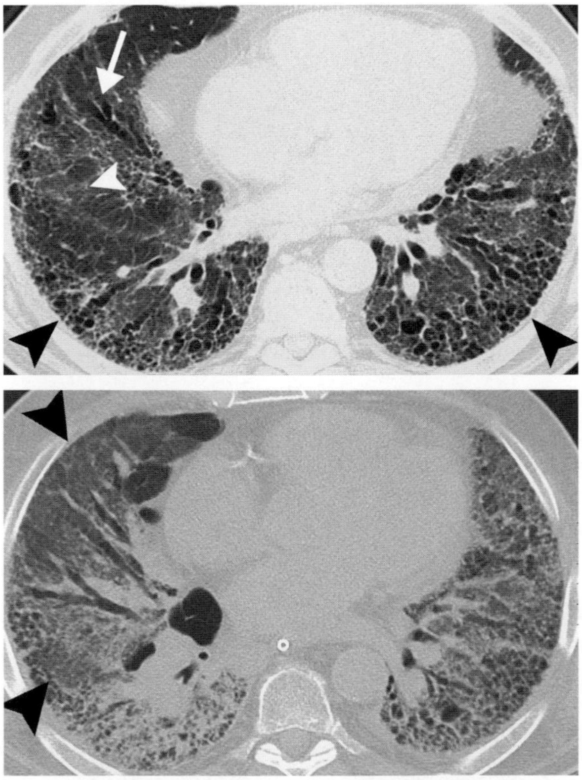

**Fig. 26.4a,b.** Axial CT image in a 63-year-old man with usual interstitial pneumonia (UIP)/idiopathic pulmonary fibrosis (IPF) shows bilateral reticular opacities, honeycombing (*black arrowheads*), and traction bronchiectasis (*arrow*). In addition, patchy, ground-glass opacities are present (*white arrowhead*) (**a**). Acute exacerbation in the same patient shows marked progression of ground-glass opacities (*arrowheads*) (**b**)

peripheral reticular opacities with honeycombing and traction bronchiectasis (Fig. 26.4a) (MUELLER-MANG et al. 2007). Ground-glass opacities are usually present, but limited in extent. However, in patients with rapid deterioration during the course of their illness, also referred to as acute exacerbation, widespread diffuse or patchy ground-glass opacities have been observed (Fig. 26.4b) (KIM et al. 2006). Other complications that should be noted in patients with IPF include opportunistic pulmonary infections (e.g., *Pneumocystis jiroveci*) and an increased risk of bronchial carcinoma (BOUROS et al. 2002). Therefore, CT scanning should involve a combination of standard volumetric CT with sequential HRCT at regular intervals.

### 26.3.1.2
### Nonspecific Interstitial Pneumonia

Given the clinical, radiologic, and pathologic variability of NSIP, the diagnostic approach to this entity is highly challenging, and the final diagnosis can be achieved only through interdisciplinary consensus. Patients with NSIP are usually between 40 and 50 years old, and men and women are equally affected. Compared with IPF, patients with NSIP have a variable, but overall more favorable, course of disease, and the majority of patients stabilizes or improves on corticosteroid therapy. According to the predominance of either inflammatory cells or fibrosis, NSIP is histologically subdivided into a cellular and a fibrotic subtype. Cellular NSIP is less common than is fibrotic NSIP and carries a substantially better prognosis (TRAVIS et al. 2000). On HRCT, NSIP is characterized by patchy ground-glass opacities combined with irregular linear or reticular opacities and scattered micronodules (JOHKOH et al. 2002) (Fig. 26.5a,b). In advanced disease, fibrotic changes, such as microcystic honeycombing and traction bronchiectasis, become more evident (DESAI et al. 2004). In contrast to the heterogeneous lung involvement and the typical apicobasal gradient in UIP, HRCT in NSIP reveals rather symmetric and homogeneous lung involvement without an obvious gradient (Fig. 26.6).

### 26.3.1.3
### Cryptogenic Organizing Pneumonia

COP was formerly referred to as *bronchiolitis obliterans organizing pneumonia (BOOP)* and is characterized by the histologic pattern of organizing pneumonia (OP). There is no gender predilection. Patients usually present between 50 and 60 years of age, and typically report

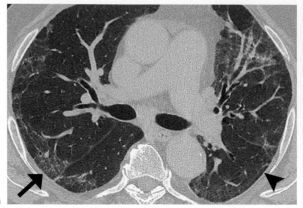
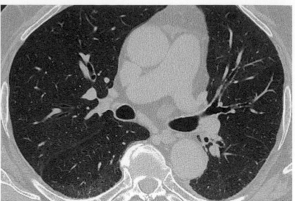

**Fig. 26.5a,b.** Axial CT image in a 61-year-old man with NSIP shows bilateral subpleural irregular linear opacities (*arrowhead*) and ground-glass opacities (*arrow*) (**a**). Follow-up CT image obtained after 6 months of corticosteroid therapy shows improvement, with partial resolution of the linear opacities and ground-glass opacities (**b**)

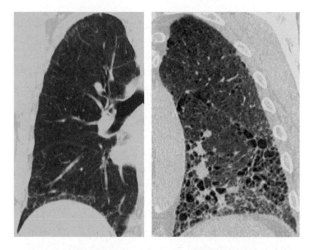

**Fig. 26.6.** Comparison of CT features between NSIP and UIP. NSIP (*left*) shows diffuse lung involvement with bilateral, peripherally located linear and reticular opacities. In UIP (*right*), the lung abnormalities show a typical apicobasal gradient with predominance of honeycombing

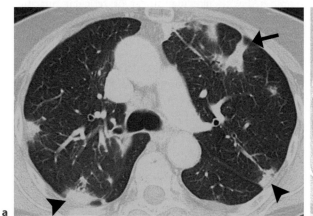

**Fig. 26.7a,b.** Axial CT image in a 75-year-old woman with COP shows bilateral, peripherally located patchy lung consolidation (*arrowheads*) In one of the lesions, the subpleural space is typically spared (*arrow*) (**a**). Follow-up CT image obtained after 4 weeks of corticosteroid therapy shows subtotal resolution of the lung abnormalities with residual ground-glass opacities (*arrowheads*) (**b**)

a respiratory tract infection preceding their symptoms. In its idiopathic form (as COP), OP is rare; however, it is frequently encountered in association with collagen vascular diseases, and in infectious and drug-induced lung diseases (CORDIER 2000). On corticosteroid therapy, patient usually experience complete recovery, but relapses are common. The histologic hallmark of COP is the development of granulation tissue polyps within the alveolar ducts and alveoli, with preservation of the lung architecture. On HRCT, COP is characterized by patchy peripheral or peribronchial consolidations that resemble pneumonic infiltrates and predominate in the lower lung lobes (LEE et al. 1994) (Fig. 26.7a,b). Frequently, air bronchograms and perifocal ground-glass opacities can be found. Other common findings include sparing of the outermost subpleural area and mild cylindrical bronchiectasis. In addition to these typical CT features, other less specific findings can be encountered, such as irregular linear opacities, solitary focal lesions, and multiple nodules (AKIRA et al. 1998), and diagnosis should be confirmed with surgical lung biopsy.

### 26.3.1.4
### Respiratory Bronchiolitis-Associated Interstitial Lung Disease

RB-ILD is exclusively encountered in smokers and is thought to represent a symptomatic variant of the his-tologically common and incidental finding of respiratory bronchiolitis (RB). Patients are usually 30–50 years old, and men are affected nearly twice as often as are women. After smoking cessation, prognosis is excellent. Histologically, RB-ILD is characterized by pigmented alveolar macrophages within the bronchioles. The typical HRCT features of RB-ILD are centrilobular nodules ("airspace nodules," small nodules with ground-glass opacity) that are randomly distributed or have upper lobe predominance (HEYNEMAN et al. 1999) (Fig. 26.8). Additional CT features are diffuse ground-glass opacities, bronchial wall thickening, and co-existing centrilobular emphysema (Fig. 26.9).

### 26.3.1.5
### Desquamative Interstitial Pneumonia

DIP is strongly associated with cigarette smoking and is considered to represent the end of a spectrum of RB-ILD. There is a male predominance, and patients usually present between 30 and 50 years of age. Most patients improve with smoking cessation and corticosteroid therapy. Histologically, DIP shows diffuse involvement, with filling of alveolar spaces with macrophages and desquamated alveolar cells, compared to the bronchiolocentric involvement in RB-ILD. On HRCT, DIP is characterized by extensive and diffuse ground-glass opacities with peripheral and lower lobe predominance (AKIRA et al. 1997) (Fig. 26.10). The presence of small cystic spaces and irregular linear opacities is indicative of fibrotic changes.

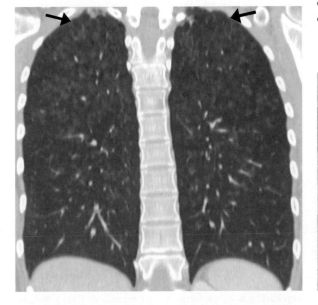

**Fig. 26.8.** RB-ILD in a 44-year-old female cigarette smoker. Coronal CT image shows scattered, poorly defined centrilobular nodules that are predominantly located in the upper lung lobes. Note mild coexisting centrilobular emphysema (*arrows*)

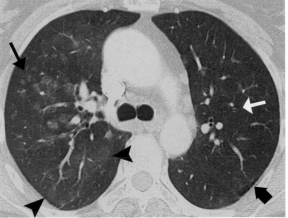

**Fig. 26.9.** RB-ILD. Axial CT image shows centrilobular nodules (*thin black arrow*), patchy ground-glass opacities (*arrowheads*), and mild bronchial wall thickening (*white arrow*). Note discrete paraseptal emphysema (*thick black arrow*)

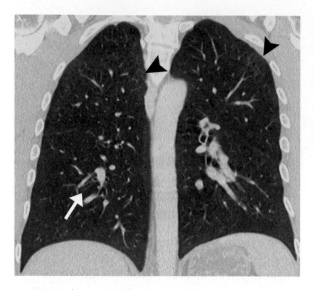

**Fig. 26.10.** Desquamative interstitial pneumonia (DIP). Coronal CT image shows bilateral, peripheral ground-glass opacities and coexisting moderate bronchial wall thickening (*arrow*). In some areas, small cystic spaces are present (*arrowheads*)

### 26.3.1.6
### Lymphoid Interstitial Pneumonia

LIP rarely occurs as an idiopathic disease. It is usually seen in conjunction with systemic disorders, most notably human immunodeficiency virus (HIV) infection, Sjögren's syndrome, and variable immunodeficiency syndromes (SWIGRIS et al. 2002). LIP is more common in women than in men, and typically, patients become symptomatic in the fifth decade of life. Histologically, LIP is characterized by diffuse interstitial cellular infiltrates that are composed of lymphocytes, plasma cells, and histiocytes. While the interstitium is expanded by these infiltrates, the alveolar airspaces are partially collapsed. The HRCT findings of LIP consist of bilateral, diffuse, or patchy ground-glass opacities, poorly defined centrilobular nodules, and cystic air spaces (Fig. 26.11). The mechanism of cyst formation has been postulated to be secondary to partial bronchiolar obstruction with air trapping due to peribronchiolar lymphocytic infiltration (DESAI et al. 1997).

### 26.3.1.7
### Acute Interstitial Pneumonia

AIP differs from the other IIPs in its acute course of disease, with rapid onset of dyspnea and cough, which is followed by respiratory failure and a high acute mortality rate of 50% or more (the AMERICAN THORACIC SOCIETY and the EUROPEAN RESPIRATORY SOCIETY 2002). AIP was formerly referred to as *Hamman-Rich syndrome*. The histological and radiological features of AIP are similar to those of acute respiratory distress syndrome (ARDS) and can be subdivided into an acute or exudative phase and a late or organizing phase. CT obtained in the early phase shows extensive ground-glass opacities, sometimes in a geographic distribution (Fig. 26.12a). In addition, areas of consolidation can be observed in the dependent areas of the lungs. In pa-

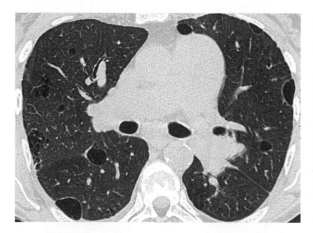

**Fig. 26.11.** Lymphoid interstitial pneumonia (LIP) in a 48-year-old woman. Axial CT image shows extensive ground-glass opacities and scattered thin-walled cysts

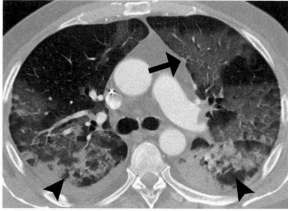

**Fig. 26.12a,b.** Acute interstitial pneumonia (AIP) in a 58-year-old patient. **a** Axial CT image shows bilateral ground-glass opacities in a geographic distribution (*arrow*). Consolidation is seen in the more dependent lung (*arrowheads*). Small, coexisting bilateral pleural effusions are present. **b** (*see next page*)

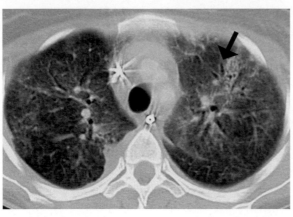

b

**Fig. 26.12a,b.** (*continued*) Acute interstitial pneumonia (AIP) in a 58-year-old patient. **b** Fibrotic changes with traction bronchiectasis (*arrow*) and architectural distortion in the late phase of acute interstitial pneumonia (AIP)

tients who survive the acute phase of disease, CT shows fibrotic changes with architectural distortion and traction bronchiectasis, predominantly in the nondependent areas of the lung (Fig. 26.12b).

## 26.3.2
## Sarcoidosis

Sarcoidosis is a common systemic disorder of unknown cause characterized by the presence of noncaseating granulomas, which either can dissolve or cause fibrosis. Almost any organ can be affected, but the lungs are most frequently involved.

The mean age of patients is between 20 and 40 years, and there is a slight female predominance (Costabel and Hunninghake 1999). In up to 50% of patients, sarcoidosis is incidentally discovered on radiographs. Common clinical symptoms include respiratory illness, skin lesions, fatigue, and weight loss. Lofgren's syndrome is a classic clinical presentation with fever, erythema nodosum, arthralgias, bihilar lymphadenopathy, and a usually benign course of disease.

The diagnosis is established on the basis of clinical and radiological findings, supported by histology from transbronchial biopsy. Spontaneous remissions occur in nearly two-thirds of patients, but the course is chronic or progressive in 10–30% (Costabel and Hunninghake 1999). The appropriate treatment depends on clinical and imaging findings and is based on corticosteroids. In patients with end-stage sarcoidosis, lung transplantation has been successfully performed,

but is associated with high recurrence rates of sarcoidosis (35%) (Collins et al. 2001).

For the staging of sarcoidosis, a system based on chest radiographs is in clinical use; stage I consists of bilateral hilar adenopathy; in stage II sarcoidosis, patients have bilateral hilar adenopathy and diffuse parenchymal infiltration; stage III describes parenchymal infiltration without hilar adenopathy. Some authorities use a stage IV classification to indicate irreversible fibrosis.

In patients with sarcoidosis, CT scans of the lung are now included routinely in the diagnostic workup at initial evaluation and at follow-up. Specifically, they are indicated in the setting of atypical clinical and/or chest radiograph findings, for the detection of complications of the lung disease (e.g., pulmonary fibrosis, superimposed infection, malignancy), and when chest radiographs are normal, despite clinical suspicion of the disease (Costabel and Hunninghake 1999). For these indications, the combination of the classic HRCT and a sequential MDCT protocol should be used.

The chest can be involved in sarcoidosis in many ways, and because of the multitude of potentially different findings, sarcoidosis can be regarded as one of the "great mimickers" in thoracic radiology. The most common intrathoracic manifestation of sarcoidosis is the presence of mediastinal lymphadenopathy with usually bilateral and rather symmetric involvement of hilar lymph nodes. They can calcify in chronic disease

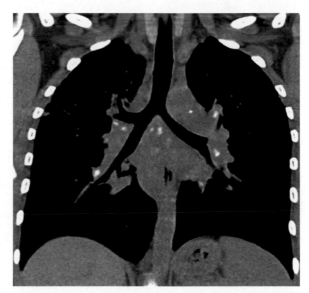

**Fig. 26.13.** A 27-year-old woman with chronic sarcoidosis. Coronal CT image displays extensive mediastinal lymphadenopathy. Lymph nodes show punctuate calcifications

and then show amorphous, punctate, or eggshell calcifications (Fig. 26.13). In patients with sarcoidosis and parenchymal involvement, nodular opacities are the predominant finding. These nodules typically range in size between 1 and 5 mm and are often ill defined. They have a perilymphatic distribution, and thus preferentially lie adjacent to the fissures, along pleural surfaces, and along central vascular structures (Fig. 26.14). There is a predilection for the upper lobes and the superior segments of the lower lobes of both lungs.

Sarcoid nodules sometimes tend to coalesce and form large parenchymal nodules with surrounding loosely aggregated small nodules. As the shape of these coalescent granulomas resembles a galaxy, it is referred to as the "sarcoid galaxy sign" (NAKATSU et al. 2002) (Fig. 26.15). Occasionally, a single, large nodule may be present in sarcoidosis and resemble bronchogenic carcinoma. Ground-glass opacities are common in sarcoidosis and have been postulated to represent alveolitis in early reports; however, according to pathologic correlation, ground-glass opacities in sarcoidosis are more likely to represent microgranulomas with or without perigranulomatous fibrosis (NISHIMURA et al. 1993). Patients with predominant ground-glass opacities on initial CT scan have a worse prognosis than have patients with a predominant nodular pattern (MURDOCH and MULLER 1992; AKIRA et al. 2005).

When sarcoidosis progresses to fibrosis, architectural distortion and traction bronchiectasis classically radiating from the hilum to the adjacent upper and lower lobes can be found. Other common CT abnormalities in fibrotic sarcoidosis include honeycombing, cysts, and bulla formation. Airway stenosis in sarcoidosis is usually due to extrinsic scarring, or to endobronchial granulomas, whereas lymphadenopathy alone is a rare cause of symptomatic airway narrowing.

Pneumoconiosis may simulate the appearance of sarcoidosis, but is usually easily diagnosed when correlated with clinical history. Primary tuberculosis, lymphoma, and mediastinal metastases from other tumors usually present with asymmetrical nodal enlargement as opposed to the bihilar, and often-symmetric hilar lymphadenopathy in stage I sarcoidosis.

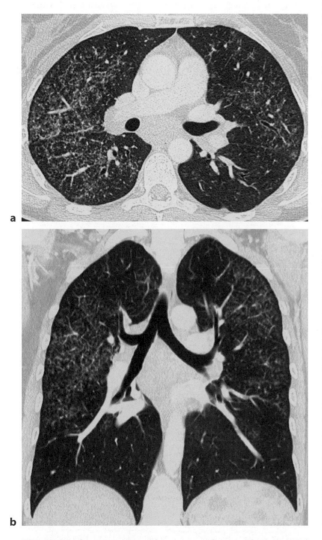

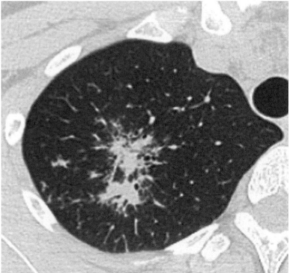

**Fig. 26.14a,b.** A 31-year-old woman with sarcoidosis. **a** Axial CT image shows multiple uniformly sized nodules as well as nodular thickening of the interlobar septa and the bronchial walls. **b** The upper lobe predominance of the nodules can be seen on the coronal CT image

**Fig. 26.15.** A 41-year-old man with sarcoidosis. The parenchymal nodules in the right upper lobe tend to coalesce and form a large parenchymal nodule surrounded by loosely aggregated small nodules. As this resembles a galaxy, it is referred to as the "sarcoid galaxy sign"

### 26.3.3
### Miscellaneous Rare Forms of Interstitial Lung Disease of Unknown Etiology

#### 26.3.3.1
#### Pulmonary Langerhans Cell Histiocytosis

Pulmonary Langerhans cell histiocytosis (PLCH) (formerly called *histiocytosis X*) is a rare interstitial lung disease of unknown cause that primarily affects cigarette smokers under 40 years of age. Most patients present with cough and dyspnea; sometimes additional systemic symptoms, such as fatigue, weight loss, and fever, are reported. Smoking cessation is the most important component in the therapeutic management of PLCH, with stabilization or regression of clinical and radiographic features in the majority of patients. CT is very sensitive for the detection of PLCH, and a correct diagnosis can be achieved in over 80% of cases (GRENIER et al. 1991). On CT, PLCH is characterized by a combination of small nodules (1–10 mm) and cysts. The cysts are thought to arise by cavitation of the nodules, have a variable wall thickness, and are often irregularly outlined (ABBOTT et al. 2004) (Fig. 26.16a). Usually, the lung abnormalities are most prominent in the upper lobes, with relative sparing of the lung bases near the costophrenic sulci (Fig. 26.16b). In later phases of the disease, nodules are less obvious, and cysts are the predominant feature. In this setting, PLCH may mimic lymphangioleiomyomatosis, but the latter occurs almost exclusively in women, affects the lung diffusely without sparing of the lung bases, and is characterized by uniformly sized cysts.

#### 26.3.3.2
#### Lymphangioleiomyomatosis

Lymphangioleiomyomatosis (LAM) is a rare interstitial lung disease that affects women of childbearing age exclusively. The tuberous sclerosis complex (TSC), an autosomal dominant inherited disorder, is associated with parenchymal lung changes identical to LAM (PALLISA et al. 2002).

Histologically, LAM is characterized by an abnormal proliferation of smooth muscle cells (LAM cells) in the lungs and in the thoracic and retroperitoneal lymphatics. The most common initial presenting symptoms are dyspnea, spontaneous pneumothorax, and cough (JOHNSON 1999). The clinical course of LAM is variable. Normally, the disease progresses slowly, with continuous deterioration of pulmonary function. Ultimately, it leads to respiratory failure. Because LAM deteriorates with pregnancy and the use of exogenous estrogen, several attempts at anti-estrogen therapies have been made, with controversial results (TAYLOR et al. 1990). Lung transplantation is indicated in patients with end-stage disease. Apart from the common postoperative complications of transplantation, recurrent disease in the donor lung can occur.

The key findings on CT are uniformly distributed, thin-walled cysts that tend to conflate (Fig. 26.17). The cysts can be up to 3 cm in diameter and are equally and symmetrically distributed throughout both lungs. Usu-

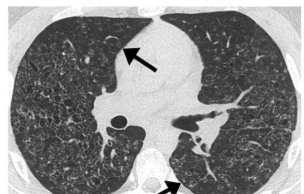

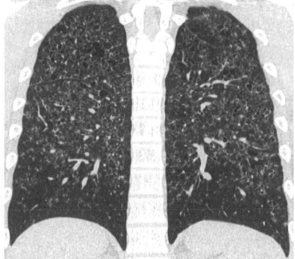

a          b

**Fig. 26.16a,b.** Pulmonary Langerhans cell histiocytosis in a 26-year-old man. **a** Axial CT image demonstrates bilateral, thin-walled cysts of variable size and multiple, ill-defined nodules (*arrows*). **b** Coronal CT image better demonstrates the upper and middle lung zone predominance, with relative sparing of the lung bases

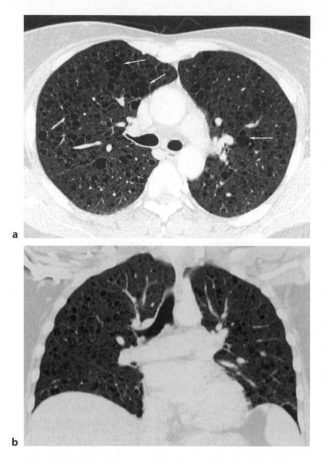

**Fig. 26.17a,b.** A 30-year-old woman with tuberous sclerosis complex. **a** Axial CT image shows multiple thin-walled cysts in a uniform distribution. The cysts adjacent to the upper right mediastinum tend to conflate (*white arrows*). **b** Coronal CT image displays the uniform and bilateral distribution of the cysts throughout both lungs. The lung parenchyma between the cysts is inconspicuous

ally, the cyst shape is round; however, in some cases, they can be of ovoid, polygonal, or irregular shape. Cyst wall thickness ranges from barely susceptible to up to 2 mm. On expiratory scans, cyst size decreases, suggesting a communication with the airway system. The lung parenchyma in between the cysts is usually inconspicuous, but, in the highly cellular forms of LAM, small nodules, reticular opacification, and ground-glass attenuation can be found (ABERLE et al. 1990). Pneumothorax is common in LAM, and occurs in about 80% of patients within the course of the disease. About 8–14% of patients develop pulmonary hemorrhage, which presents as ground-glass opacity on HRCT (LENOIR et al. 1990). Pleural chylous effusions can be found in up to 14% of patients, and are indistinguishable from protein-rich effusions of other origin on CT. In addition, dilatation

of the thoracic duct, as well as mediastinal, hilar, and retrocrural adenopathy, can be found in patients with LAM.

In more than 70% of patients with LAM, renal angiomyolipomas can be found, which show a characteristic appearance, with negative CT values due to their fat content. In some cases, retroperitoneal cystic hypoattenuating masses indicative of lymphangioleiomyomas can be found. Chylous ascites and lymphadenopathy are further extrathoracic findings in some patients (PALLISA et al. 2002).

The most important differential diagnoses for LAM are Langerhans cell histiocytosis, idiopathic pulmonary fibrosis, and panlobular emphysema. In contrast to LAM, in Langerhans cell histiocytosis, the costophrenic sulci are usually spared, the cysts can be thick-walled and irregularly outlined, and nodules are predominant in the early stage of disease. Idiopathic pulmonary fibrosis shows a volume loss in contrast to LAM, and the honeycomb cysts are predominantly located in the lower lobes and subpleural (BONELLI et al. 1998). Panlobular emphysema is associated with alpha-1-antiprotease deficiency. The most distinct feature of emphysema is the absence of defined walls in the areas of low attenuation, whereas cysts in LAM almost invariably present with walls (JOHNSON 1999).

### 26.3.3.3
### Eosinophilic Pneumonia

Eosinophilic pneumonia is divided into acute eosinophilic pneumonia (AEP) and chronic eosinophilic pneumonia (CEP). The pathogenesis of both forms is still unknown, but it is speculated to be a hypersensitivity reaction to an unknown antigen. However, AEP has been reported after cigarette smoking, dust exposure, and smoke from fireworks. The mean age of patients with CEP is 40; AEP occurs at all ages. AEP shows no gender predominance, whereas CEP occurs more often in women. Histologically, diffuse alveolar damage associated with interstitial and alveolar eosinophilia is found in AEP (TAZELAAR et al. 1997); in CEP, an accumulation of eosinophils and lymphocytes in the interstitium and alveoli, and sometimes, interstitial fibrosis, is found.

AEP clinically presents as an acute febrile illness with dyspnea, pleuritic chest pain, myalgias, and respiratory failure. In AEP, blood eosinophilia is often absent, but more than 25% eosinophils are found in the bronchial lavage fluid of these patients. CEP has an insidious onset with fever, malaise, weight loss, and dyspnea. About 90% of these patients suffer from asthmatic symptoms. In CEP, peripheral blood eosinophilia is present in more than 90% of cases, and there are an increased number of eosinophils in the bronchial lavage fluid as well (ALLEN and DAVIS 1994). Both AEP and CEP are often misdiagnosed as pneumonia, which can delay the correct diagnosis for months. Both AEP and CEP show a rapid response to corticosteroids, and there usually is rapid clearing of clinical and radiographic abnormalities within several days (ALLEN and DAVIS 1994).

At CT, AEP shows bilateral peripheral ground-glass opacities, with lower-lobe predominance (Fig. 26.18). In addition, interlobar septal thickening and thickening of the bronchovascular bundles, as well as localized areas of consolidation, can be seen. AEP is very commonly associated with pleural effusions, and band-like opacities paralleling the chest wall are nearly pathognomonic (ALLEN and DAVIS 1994; JOHKOH et al. 2000).

CEP shows upper lobe predominance and peripheral nonsegmental consolidations (Fig. 26.19). Consolidations can persist for some time, but, in the absence of treatment, they tend to migrate. Consolidations are often accompanied by ground-glass opacities, and a "crazy paving" appearance of the consolidations can also be appreciated in many cases. Pleural effusions are rare in CEP (MAYO et al. 1989; JOHKOH et al. 2000).

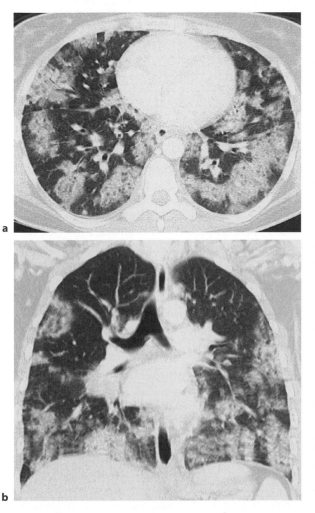

**Fig. 26.18a,b.** Acute eosinophilic pneumonia in a 37-year-old female with BAL fluid eosinophilia. **a** Axial CT image obtained 5 days after onset of dyspnea shows peripherally distributed patchy areas of consolidation and ground-glass opacities accompanied by interlobular septal thickening. **b** Coronal CT image displays the lower lobe predominance of the infiltrates

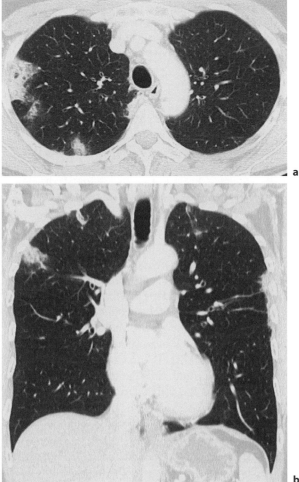

**Fig. 26.19a,b.** Chronic eosinophilic pneumonia in a 56-year-old man presenting with a 4-week history of cough and fever. Moderate blood eosinophilia is found in laboratory workup. **a** Axial CT image shows strikingly peripheral wedge-shaped airspace consolidations. **b** The upper lobe predominance of the consolidations is displayed on coronal CT image

The differential diagnoses include simple pulmonary eosinophilia (Löffler's syndrome), Churg–Strauss syndrome, cryptogenic organizing pneumonia (COP), pulmonary infarcts, aspiration pneumonia, and diffuse pulmonary hemorrhage. In Löffler's syndrome, patients are usually asymptomatic, and opacities are rather fleeting. Churg–Strauss syndrome is usually accompanied by a systemic disease, which is not present in CEP or AEP. In contrast to CEP, cryptogenic organizing pneumonia has lower lobe predominance, but the infiltrates can be similar to CEP. Pulmonary infarcts are more wedge-shaped than are infiltrates seen in CEP or AEP. Aspiration pneumonia is found in gravity-dependent lung regions and is commonly associated with small airways disease. Diffuse pulmonary hemorrhage presents with diffuse pulmonary consolidations, but these consolidations usually have a diffuse pattern, and a history of renal disease, anemia, and hemoptysis is common in such cases (Mayo et al. 1989; Allen and Davis 1994; Johkoh et al. 2000).

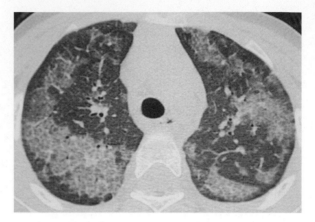

**Fig. 26.20.** Alveolar proteinosis in 40-year-old man with myelogenous leukemia presenting with cough and dyspnea. Axial CT image displays bilateral geographical areas of ground-glass opacity. Interlobular septa are thickened and within these areas, a fine reticular network of interlobular lines can be seen. These changes are referred to as the typical "crazy-paving" appearance of alveolar proteinosis

### 26.3.3.4
### Pulmonary Alveolar Proteinosis

Pulmonary alveolar proteinosis (PAP) is a rare interstitial lung disease, characterized by filling of the alveoli with a lipid-rich proteinaceous material (Rosen et al. 1958). Three different forms of PAP can be distinguished: an autosomal recessive congenital form (2%); a secondary form (10%) that is associated with various conditions, such as hematopoietic disorders (especially myelogenous leukemias), silicosis, immunodeficiency disorders, malignancies, and some infections; and an idiopathic form (90%). In idiopathic PAP, several mechanisms are responsible for phospholipid accumulation in the alveoli. Whether this accumulation is caused by reduced clearance or overproduction is not yet clear (Prakash et al. 1987). The median age of the patients is about 40 years, and most patients are men and have a history of smoking (Ben-Dov et al. 1999). Patients present with dyspnea or cough. The symptoms are usually out of proportion to the radiological findings (clinical–radiological discrepancy). In 13% of patients with PAP, secondary infections with nocardia, cryptococci, or mycobacteria are observed. The treatment for PAP is bronchoalveolar lavage with sterile saline, and prognosis is generally good with whole-lung lavage.

HRCT is characterized by bilateral, symmetrical, geometric areas of ground-glass attenuation (Fig. 26.20). The interlobular septa are thickened, and a fine network of interlobular lines can be seen. These changes

are responsible for the so-called "crazy-paving" pattern. The disease does not have any preferential zonal distribution (Holbert et al. 2001). Architectural distortion and bronchiectasis are absent normally; however, in a small percentage of patients, pulmonary fibrosis can be found. Although the crazy-paving pattern on HRCT is suggestive of PAP, this pattern can also be observed in a number of other interstitial and air-space diseases, such as pulmonary hemorrhage, pulmonary edema, hypersensitivity pneumonitis, and alveolar cell carcinoma. The diagnosis can be made by bronchoalveolar lavage and typical clinical findings. Nevertheless, the gold standard in diagnosis remains open lung biopsy.

### 26.3.3.5
### Pulmonary Microlithiasis

Pulmonary alveolar microlithiasis (PAM) is a rare condition characterized by the formation of intra-alveolar microliths (calcospherites). The pathogenesis of the micronodular calcifications is still unknown. In about 50% of cases, pulmonary alveolar microlithiasis occurs as an autosomal recessive hereditary lung disease (Sosman et al. 1957). Most cases of microlithiasis are found in Turkey (Ucan et al. 1993). The disease usually occurs between 30 and 50 years of age, and pediatric cases are rare. In hereditary cases, there is slight female predominance.

The disease is typically detected incidentally on chest films obtained for other reasons, and clinical symptoms are disproportional to the extent of radiologic findings. Occasionally, patients present with stress-induced dyspnea, malaise, or fatigue. As PAM progresses with the formation of tiny (0.01–3mm) microspheres in the alveoli, it can ultimately lead to respiratory failure and cor pulmonale.

In early stages, diffuse ground-glass opacifications are found throughout both lungs on CT. Still, the presence of calcified micronodules is most characteristic. The distribution of the micronodules is miliary, but there is a tendency toward greater involvement of the posterior segments of the lower lobes and the anterior segments of the upper lobes (Fig. 26.21). Due to the intra and periseptal accumulation of micronodules, interlobular septal thickening is found in almost all patients. In addition, subpleural septal thickening is frequently detected.

As the disease progresses, subpleural emphysema and the formation of thin-walled subpleural cysts are pathognomonic findings in PAM and might represent early lung fibrosis. The subpleural cysts are accountable for the black subpleural line on chest X-rays (KORN et al. 1992). The main differential diagnoses include miliary tuberculosis, sarcoidosis, metastatic pulmonary calcification associated with hemodialysis, silicosis, and pulmonary hemosiderosis.

Usually, the disease progresses very slowly, but can result in cardiac and pulmonary failure. There is no known treatment, except lung transplantation in end-stage disease.

# 26.4
## Interstitial Lung Diseases of Known Cause

### 26.4.1
### Occupational and Environmental Lung Disease

Occupational and environmental lung disease comprises a wide spectrum of lung disorders caused by the inhalation or ingestion of organic and inorganic particles and chemicals. CT is very sensitive in depicting the parenchymal, as well as airway and pleural abnormalities that are associated with these diseases.

#### 26.4.1.1
#### Hypersensitivity Pneumonitis

Hypersensitivity pneumonitis (HP), also known as *exogenous allergic alveolitis (EEA)*, is an immunologic lung disease caused by repeated exposure and sensitization to various organic and chemical antigens, which leads to diffuse inflammation of the lung parenchyma. The most common diseases are farmer's lung and bird fancier's lung due to *Aspergillus* antigens and avian proteins, respectively. Based on the length and intensity of exposure and subsequent duration of illness, clinical presentations of HP are categorized as acute, subacute, and chronic progressive. In acute HP, patients present 4–12 h after heavy exposure to an inciting agent with

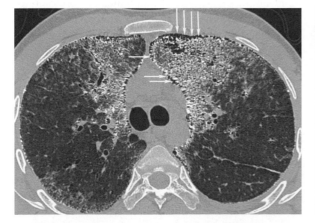

**Fig. 26.21.** A 37-year-old man with pulmonary alveolar microlithiasis. Axial CT image shows miliary distributed calcified micronodules predominantly located in the middle and lower zones of both lungs. Also note the formation of small subpleural cysts and subpleural emphysema and the formation of the pathognomonic black subpleural line (*white arrows*)

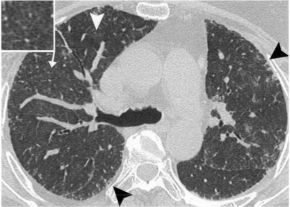

**Fig. 26.22.** Chronic hypersensitivity pneumonitis in a 52-year-old man, related to mold exposure. Axial CT image shows patchy ground-glass opacities with associated centrilobular nodules (*inset* magnified view of centrilobular nodules). Also note mild subpleural reticular opacities (*black arrowheads*) indicating fibrosis, and subtle mosaic attenuation (*white arrowhead*)

fever, chills, and myalgias. In subacute and chronic HP, patients have an insidious onset of cough, progressive dyspnea, fatigue, and weight loss. CT in acute HP typically shows diffuse ground-glass opacities and centrilobular nodules, most commonly in a random distribution (TOMIYAMA et al. 2000). In the subacute phase, centrilobular nodules become more prominent, and patchy ground-glass opacities can be found. In some patients, cystic lesions (3–25mm) have been observed (FRANQUET et al. 2003). Chronic HP is characterized by the presence of reticulation due to fibrosis superimposed on findings of subacute HP (Fig. 26.22). The abnormalities are usually predominantly located in the upper lobes, while the lung bases are relatively spared (SILVA et al. 2008). Other common findings in chronic HP include a mosaic attenuation pattern and air trapping on expiratory imaging (SMALL et al. 1996).

## 26.4.1.2
## Pneumoconiosis

Pneumoconiosis is a non-neoplastic reaction to the inhalation and accumulation of dust particles in the lung.

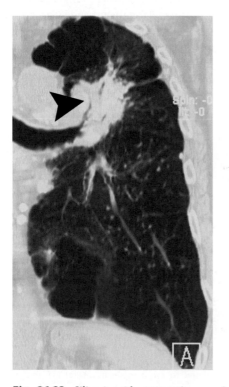

**Fig. 26.23.** Silicosis with progressive massive fibrosis in a 72-year-old man. Coronal CT image shows a large mass in the right medial upper lobe (*arrowhead*). There is retraction of the hilus and marked emphysema. In addition, some scattered small nodules are present

The particles are engulfed by alveolar macrophages that release inflammatory cytokines and induce fibrotic changes. The classification of pneumoconiosis is based on chest radiographs using the International Labor Organization (ILO) classification scheme. The CT features in patients with silicosis and coal worker pneumoconiosis consist of small, well-circumscribed nodules that are usually 2–5mm in diameter and predominantly affect the upper and posterior lung zones. The nodules in silicosis tend to be larger and better defined than those nodules in coal worker pneumoconiosis (KIM et al. 2001). Occasionally, eggshell calcifications in the hilar and mediastinal lymph nodes are seen. The presence of nodules larger than 1 cm is indicative of complicated pneumoconiosis, also known as *progressive massive fibrosis*. These nodules coalesce and form conglomerate masses that are typically located in the upper lobe of the lung. In large lesions, cavitation may occur, which is due to either ischemic necrosis or superinfection. In advanced disease, hilar retraction and compensatory emphysema, particularly in the lower lobes, is seen (Fig. 26.23).

The parenchymal lung manifestations related to asbestos exposure are referred to as *asbestosis* and differ from the previously described "classic" pneumoconiosis. Early asbestosis is characterized by subpleural linear and reticular opacities that are predominantly located in the posterior lung bases. To distinguish these abnormalities from gravity-related physiologic changes, prone scans should be included in cases of suspected asbestosis. Other typical findings in asbestosis include thickened interlobular septa and centrilobular nodules. In advanced disease, CT shows bands of fibrosis, traction bronchiectasis, and honeycombing. In addition, other asbestos-related lung abnormalities, such as pleural effusion, pleural plaques, and round atelectasis can be found.

## 26.4.1.3
## Drug-Induced Lung Injury

Drug-induced lung injury is a common cause of acute and chronic lung disease, and most commonly occurs with cytotoxic agents, such as bleomycin, busulfan, carmustine, and cyclophosphamide (ELLIS et al. 2000). Chemotherapeutic drugs can result in four main types of lung reaction: interstitial pneumonia (IP), diffuse alveolar damage (DAD)/ARDS, organizing pneumonia (OP) (formerly referred to as BOOP), and hypersensitivity reaction. The CT manifestations of IP are identical to the pattern of NSIP, and consist of scattered ground-glass opacities and irregular linear opacities

(Fig. 26.24). In early drug-induced DAD (first week after lung injury), CT shows diffuse ground-glass opacities and consolidations, whereas, in the late phase of disease (after 1 or 2 weeks), fibrotic changes occur, such as irregular linear opacities, architectural distortion, and traction bronchiectasis. Drug-induced OP is identical to COP, and manifests on CT with bilateral areas of ground-glass opacities or consolidations that are often peripheral in distribution. Hypersensitivity reactions usually become clinically apparent within hours or days after institution of drug therapy, and patients typically present with progressive dyspnea, cough, fever, and peripheral eosinophilia (ROSSI et al. 2000). Pulmonary involvement can result in either acute or chronic EP. CT in EP shows ground-glass opacities and consolidation that are typically distributed peripherally and in the upper lobe. EP usually responds well to cessation of the administered drug and is exceedingly sensitive to corticosteroid therapy. Within the group of noncytotoxic drugs, methotrexate and amiodarone frequently cause drug-induced lung diseases in 5–10% of patients. The most common lung injury associated with both drugs is interstitial pneumonia. Organizing pneumonia is less commonly associated with noncytotoxic drugs (Fig. 26.25).

## 26.4.2
## Radiation-Induced Lung Injury

Radiation-induced lung injury is subdivided clinically and radiologically into an early stage, characterized by acute radiation pneumonitis, and a late stage, charac-

terized by chronic radiation fibrosis. The degree of radiation damage to normal tissue depends particularly on total dose and the fraction of that dose, irradiated volume, individual susceptibility, preexisting lung disease, and previous or concomitant therapy. Early radiation pneumonitis usually develops 1 to 3 months after the therapy, and the radiographic findings are typically confined to the field of radiation, resulting in a geometric shape of pulmonary opacities with a sharp demarcation line at noninvolved lung areas and disregard of anatomic boundaries. The earliest CT findings consist of subtle ground-glass opacities (Fig. 26.26). These hazy abnormalities can progress to patchy consolidations that sometimes also involve lung areas outside the field of radiation (DAVIS et al. 1992). Chronic radiation fibrosis evolves within 6 to 24 months after radiation therapy and develops continuously from the phase of acute pneumonitis. At CT, it is characterized by the presence of reticular opacities, architectural distortion, traction bronchiectasis, and volume loss. The major differential diagnoses in radiation pneumonitis include infection, lymphangitic carcinomatosis, and recurrence of the original malignancy. Microbial infectious pneumonia is not usually confined to the field of irradiation and runs a clinical course more symptomatic than the course of radiation pneumonitis. In lymphangitic carcinomatosis, the rapid worsening of radiographic abnormalities, with development of irregular, often-nodular thickening of

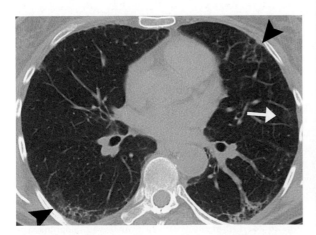

**Fig. 26.24.** A 50-year-old woman with interstitial pneumonia (IP)/nonspecific interstitial pneumonia (NSIP) after bleomycin chemotherapy for Hodgkin's lymphoma. Axial CT image shows irregular linear and reticular opacities (*arrowheads*) with subtle ground-glass opacities (*arrow*) in subpleural distribution

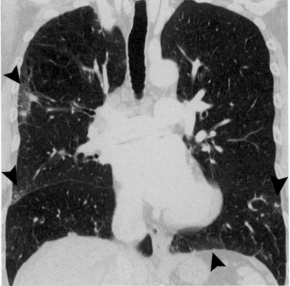

**Fig. 26.25.** A 63-year-old man with organizing pneumonia (OP). The patient was receiving amiodarone for cardiac arrhythmia. Coronal CT image shows bilateral areas of ground-glass opacities in subpleural distribution (*arrowheads*)

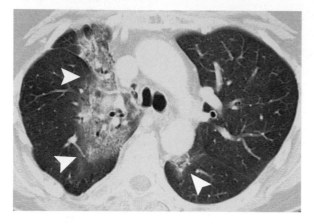

**Fig. 26.26.** Acute radiation pneumonitis after treatment of lung cancer. Axial CT image obtained at 4 months after completion of treatment shows paramediastinal ground-glass opacities with sharp lateral margins (*arrowheads*)

the interlobular septa and the bronchovascular bundles, pleural effusions, and diffuse spread to the lung, are the diagnostic clues. In patients with suspected radiation therapy, it is advisable to utilize a volumetric CT protocol in order to avoid missing focal disease representing tumor recurrence or metastases.

### 26.4.3
### Collagen Vascular Lung Disease

Lung involvement is common in patients with collagen vascular diseases and may be detected with CT before the disease has declared itself or been accurately characterized. Interstitial lung disease is probably most prevalent in systemic sclerosis, but is also a common problem in rheumatoid arthritis (RA), mixed connective tissue disease, dermatomyositis/polymyositis (DMPM), or Sjögren's syndrome. Lung involvement less frequently occurs with systemic lupus erythematosus (SLE). The parenchymal manifestations of collagen vascular diseases seen at CT closely resemble those found in IIPs and can be classified using the same system. Although the proportions of interstitial pneumonias vary, the NSIP is the most frequently encountered pattern in patients with collagen vascular lung disease, especially in progressive systemic sclerosis (Fig. 26.27). In keeping with the IIPs, the NSIP pattern is characterized by subpleural reticular opacities and varying proportions of ground-glass opacities, while in patients with UIP, honeycombing and traction bronchiectasis are the dominant abnormality. The predominance of the NSIP over the UIP pattern might explain the more favorable prognosis in patients with interstitial pneumonia associated with collagen vascular diseases than in those with IIPs (KIM et al. 2002). OP is more common in RA than in the other collagen vascular diseases and is characterized by patchy infiltrates in a peripheral distribution. LIP is a typical, but rare complication in Sjögren's syndrome in about 1% of patients during the course of their disease (SWIGRIS et al. 2002), and CT findings include diffuse or patchy ground-glass opacities and thin-walled perivascular cysts (Fig. 26.28). In addition to the patterns of interstitial pneumonias, other parenchymal manifestations in collagen vascular diseases include al-

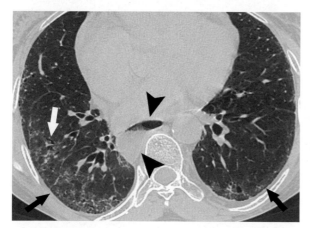

**Fig. 26.27.** Axial CT image in a patient with progressive systemic sclerosis shows a mixture of fine reticular and ground-glass opacities (*black arrows*), associated with mild traction bronchiectasis (*white arrow*), consistent with a nonspecific interstitial pneumonia pattern. Note esophageal dilatation (*arrowheads*)

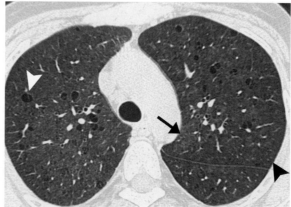

**Fig. 26.28.** LIP in a 44-year-old woman with Sjögren's syndrome. Axial CT image shows several thin-walled cysts (*white arrowhead*), bilateral patchy ground-glass opacities (*arrow*), and poorly defined centrilobular nodules (*black arrowhead*)

veolar hemorrhage, especially in patients with SLE, and necrobiotic nodules in patients with RA, which range in size from a few millimeters to a few centimeters (REMY-JARDIN et al. 1994), and are usually subpleural in distribution. The increased prevalence of malignant disorders complicating the course of some disorders such DMPM makes volumetric CT protocols mandatory in the follow-up of these patients.

## 26.4.4
## Diffuse Pulmonary Hemorrhage

Diffuse bleeding into the alveolar spaces most commonly occurs with immunological and hematological disorders and is clinically characterized by hemoptysis and anemia (ALBELDA et al. 1985); however, the absence of these symptoms does not rule out the diagnosis of diffuse pulmonary hemorrhage (DPH). DPH must be distinguished from localized pulmonary hemorrhage due to chronic bronchitis, bronchiectasis, tumor, and infection. DPH can occur in association with many collagen vascular diseases, notably SLE and Wegener's granulomatosis. Other rare causes of DPH include Goodpasture's syndrome and idiopathic pulmonary hemosiderosis. CT is more sensitive than is chest radiograph for the detection of pulmonary hemorrhage, and shows diffuse bilateral consolidation or ground-glass opacities in the acute phase (MARASCO et al. 1993). In the subacute phase of DPH, multiple small nodules associated with patchy ground-glass opacities and interlobular septal thickening have been observed (Fig. 26.29). In addition,

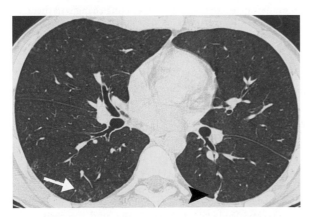

**Fig. 26.29.** Goodpasture's syndrome in a 21-year-old-man. CT scan shows multiple nodules, subtle ground-glass opacities (*arrow*), and mild interlobular thickening (*arrowhead*)

in patients with Wegener's granulomatosis, multiple, frequently cavitating nodules and masses, ranging from 5 mm to 10 cm, can be seen.

## References

Abbott GF, Rosado-de-Christenson ML et al. (2004) From the archives of the AFIP: pulmonary Langerhans cell histiocytosis. Radiographics 24:821–841

Aberle DR, Hansell DM et al. (1990) Lymphangiomyomatosis: CT, chest radiographic, and functional correlations. Radiology 176:381–387

Akira M, Kozuka T et al. (2005) Long-term follow-up CT scan evaluation in patients with pulmonary sarcoidosis. Chest 127:185–191

Akira M, Yamamoto S et al. (1997) Serial computed tomographic evaluation in desquamative interstitial pneumonia. Thorax 52:333–337

Akira M, Yamamoto S et al. (1998) Bronchiolitis obliterans organizing pneumonia manifesting as multiple large nodules or masses. AJR Am J Roentgenol 170:291–295

Albelda SM, Gefter WB et al. (1985) Diffuse pulmonary hemorrhage: a review and classification. Radiology 154:289–297

Allen JN, Davis WB (1994) Eosinophilic lung diseases. Am J Respir Crit Care Med 150:1423–1438

Anonymous (1999) Statement on sarcoidosis. Joint Statement of the American Thoracic Society (ATS), the European Respiratory Society (ERS) and the World Association of Sarcoidosis and Other Granulomatous Disorders (WASOG) adopted by the ATS Board of Directors and by the ERS Executive Committee, February 1999. Am J Respir Crit Care Med 160:736–755

Anonymous (2002) American Thoracic Society/European Respiratory Society International Multidisciplinary Consensus Classification of the Idiopathic Interstitial Pneumonias. This joint statement of the American Thoracic Society (ATS), and the European Respiratory Society (ERS) was adopted by the ATS board of directors, June 2001 and by the ERS Executive Committee, June 2001. Am J Respir Crit Care Med 165:277–304

Ben-Dov I, Kishinevski Y et al. (1999) Pulmonary alveolar proteinosis in Israel: ethnic clustering. Isr Med Assoc J 1:75–78

Bonelli FS, Hartman TE et al. (1998) Accuracy of high-resolution CT in diagnosing lung diseases. AJR Am J Roentgenol 170:1507–1512

Bouros D, Hatzakis K et al. (2002) Association of malignancy with diseases causing interstitial pulmonary changes. Chest 121:1278–1289

Collins J, Hartman MJ et al. (2001) Frequency and CT findings of recurrent disease after lung transplantation. Radiology 219:503–509

Cordier JF (2000) Organising pneumonia. Thorax 55:318–328

Costabel U, Hunninghake GW (1999) ATS/ERS/WASOG statement on sarcoidosis. Sarcoidosis Statement Committee. American Thoracic Society. European Respiratory Society. World Association for Sarcoidosis and Other Granulomatous Disorders. Eur Respir J 14:735–737

Davis SD, Yankelevitz DF et al. (1992) Radiation effects on the lung: clinical features, pathology, and imaging findings. AJR Am J Roentgenol 159:1157–1164

Desai SR, Nicholson AG et al. (1997) Benign pulmonary lymphocytic infiltration and amyloidosis: computed tomographic and pathologic features in three cases. J Thorac Imaging 12:215–220

Desai SR, Veeraraghavan S et al. (2004) CT features of lung disease in patients with systemic sclerosis: comparison with idiopathic pulmonary fibrosis and nonspecific interstitial pneumonia. Radiology 232:560–567

Ellis SJ, Cleverley JR et al. (2000) Drug-induced lung disease: high-resolution CT findings. AJR Am J Roentgenol 175:1019–1024

Franquet T, Hansell DM et al. (2003) Lung cysts in subacute hypersensitivity pneumonitis. J Comput Assist Tomogr 27:475–478

Grenier P, Valeyre D et al. (1991) Chronic diffuse interstitial lung disease: diagnostic value of chest radiography and high-resolution CT. Radiology 179:123–132

Hansell DM (2001) High-resolution CT of diffuse lung disease: value and limitations. Radiol Clin North Am 39:1091–1113

Heyneman LE, Ward S et al. (1999) Respiratory bronchiolitis, respiratory bronchiolitis-associated interstitial lung disease, and desquamative interstitial pneumonia: different entities or part of the spectrum of the same disease process? AJR Am J Roentgenol 173:1617–1622

Holbert JM, Costello P et al. (2001) CT features of pulmonary alveolar proteinosis. AJR Am J Roentgenol 176:1287–1294

Johkoh T, Muller NL et al. (2000) Eosinophilic lung diseases: diagnostic accuracy of thin-section CT in 111 patients. Radiology 216:773–780

Johkoh T, Muller NL et al. (2002) Nonspecific interstitial pneumonia: correlation between thin-section CT findings and pathologic subgroups in 55 patients. Radiology 225:199–204

Johnson S (1999) Rare diseases. 1. Lymphangioleiomyomatosis: clinical features, management and basic mechanisms. Thorax 54:254–264

Katzenstein AL, Myers JL (1998) Idiopathic pulmonary fibrosis: clinical relevance of pathologic classification. Am J Respir Crit Care Med 157:1301–1315

Kim DS, Park JH et al. (2006) Acute exacerbation of idiopathic pulmonary fibrosis: frequency and clinical features. Eur Respir J 27:143–150

Kim EA, Lee KS et al. (2002) Interstitial lung diseases associated with collagen vascular diseases: radiologic and histopathologic findings. Radiographics 22:S151–S165

Kim KI, Kim CW et al. (2001) Imaging of occupational lung disease. Radiographics 21:1371–1391

Korn MA, Schurawitzki H et al. (1992) Pulmonary alveolar microlithiasis: findings on high-resolution CT. AJR Am J Roentgenol 158:981–982

Lee KS, Kullnig P et al. (1994) Cryptogenic organizing pneumonia: CT findings in 43 patients. AJR Am J Roentgenol 162:543–546

Lenoir S, Grenier P et al. (1990) Pulmonary lymphangiomyomatosis and tuberous sclerosis: comparison of radiographic and thin-section CT findings. Radiology 175:329–334

Marasco WJ, Fishman EK et al. (1993) Acute pulmonary hemorrhage. CT evaluation. Clin Imaging 17:77–80

Mayo JR, Webb WR et al. (1987) High-resolution CT of the lungs: an optimal approach. Radiology 163:507–510

Mayo JR, Muller NL et al. (1989) Chronic eosinophilic pneumonia: CT findings in six cases. AJR Am J Roentgenol 153:727–730

Mueller-Mang C, Grosse C et al. (2007) What every radiologist should know about idiopathic interstitial pneumonias. Radiographics 27:595–615

Murata K, Itoh H et al. (1986) Centrilobular lesions of the lung: demonstration by high-resolution CT and pathologic correlation. Radiology 161:641–645

Murdoch J, Muller NL (1992) Pulmonary sarcoidosis: changes on follow-up CT examination. AJR Am J Roentgenol 159:473–477

Nakatsu M, Hatabu H et al. (2002) Large coalescent parenchymal nodules in pulmonary sarcoidosis: sarcoid galaxy sign. AJR Am J Roentgenol 178:1389–1393

Nishimura K, Itoh H et al. (1993) Pulmonary sarcoidosis: correlation of CT and histopathologic findings. Radiology 189:105–109

Pallisa E, Sanz P et al. (2002) Lymphangioleiomyomatosis: pulmonary and abdominal findings with pathologic correlation. Radiographics 22:S185–S198

Prakash UB, Barham SS et al. (1987) Pulmonary alveolar phospholipoproteinosis: experience with 34 cases and a review. Mayo Clin Proc 62:499–518

Remy-Jardin M, Remy J et al. (1994) Lung changes in rheumatoid arthritis: CT findings. Radiology 193:375–382

Rosen SH, Castleman B et al. (1958) Pulmonary alveolar proteinosis. N Engl J Med 258:1123–1142

Rossi SE, Erasmus JJ et al. (2000) Pulmonary drug toxicity: radiologic and pathologic manifestations. Radiographics 20:1245–1259

Silva CI, Muller NL et al. (2008) Chronic hypersensitivity pneumonitis: differentiation from idiopathic pulmonary fibrosis and nonspecific interstitial pneumonia by using thin-section CT. Radiology 246:288–297

Small JH, Flower CD et al. (1996) Air-trapping in extrinsic allergic alveolitis on computed tomography. Clin Radiol 51:684–688

Sosman MC, Dodd GD et al. (1957) The familial occurrence of pulmonary alveolar microlithiasis. Am J Roentgenol Radium Ther Nucl Med 77:947–1012

Studler U, Gluecker T et al. (2005) Image quality from high-resolution CT of the lung: comparison of axial scans and of sections reconstructed from volumetric data acquired using MDCT. AJR Am J Roentgenol 185:602–607

Swigris JJ, Berry GJ et al. (2002) Lymphoid interstitial pneumonia: a narrative review. Chest 122:2150–2164

Taylor JR, Ryu J et al. (1990) Lymphangioleiomyomatosis. Clinical course in 32 patients. N Engl J Med 323:1254–1260

Tazelaar HD, Linz LJ et al. (1997) Acute eosinophilic pneumonia: histopathologic findings in nine patients. Am J Respir Crit Care Med 155:296–302

Thabut G, Mal H et al. (2003) Survival benefit of lung transplantation for patients with idiopathic pulmonary fibrosis. J Thorac Cardiovasc Surg 126:469–475

Tomiyama N, Muller NL et al. (2000) Acute parenchymal lung disease in immunocompetent patients: diagnostic accuracy of high-resolution CT. AJR Am J Roentgenol 174:1745–1750

Travis WD, Matsui K et al. (2000) Idiopathic nonspecific interstitial pneumonia: prognostic significance of cellular and fibrosing patterns: survival comparison with usual interstitial pneumonia and desquamative interstitial pneumonia. Am J Surg Pathol 24:19–33

Ucan ES, Keyf AI et al. (1993) Pulmonary alveolar microlithiasis: review of Turkish reports. Thorax 48:171–173

Webb WR (2006) Thin-section CT of the secondary pulmonary lobule: anatomy and the image—the 2004 Fleischner lecture. Radiology 239:322–338

Weibel ER (1979) Fleischner lecture. Looking into the lung: what can it tell us? AJR Am J Roentgenol 133:1021–1031

# Pneumonia

Claus Peter Heussel

C. P. Heussel, PD Dr.
Department of Radiology, Chest-Clinic at University Hospital
Heidelberg, Amalienstrasse 5, 69126 Heidelberg, Germany

## ABSTRACT

Most patients suffering from community acquired pneumonia do not appear at a radiology department since diagnosis is made on a clinical basis. In severe or unclear situations, a chest X-ray is done and analysis is frequently done by interns. Radiologists frequently see those patients that suffer from recurrent, nosocomial pneumonia, or an additional predisposing disease. The appropriate investigational technique, frequently targeted differential diagnosis, and the special needs of these patients need to be understood by radiologists.

Early detection of a focus of infection is the major goal in immunocompromised patients. As pneumonia is the most common focus, chest imaging is to be done at the beginning. The sensitivity of chest X-rays, especially in the supine position, is known to be low. Therefore the very sensitive high-resolution CT (HRCT) became the gold standard in neutropenic hosts and is widely replaced by thin-section multi-detector-row-CT (MDCT). Underlying diseases such as pulmonary embolism or bronchial carcinoma might also be depicted. Furthermore, the costs of CT are low in comparison to antibiotics. The infiltrate needs to be localised, so that a physician can utilise this information as a guidance for invasive procedures for further microbiological work-up. The radiological characterisation of infiltrates gives a first and rapid hint to differentiate between different sorts of infectious (typical bacterial, atypical bacterial, fungal) and non-infectious aetiologies. Follow-up investigations need careful interpretation according to disease and concomitant treatment. Temporary exclusion of infectious involvement of the lung with high accuracy is, besides of pneumonia management, a hot topic for clinicians.

## 27.1
### Community Acquired Pneumonia

#### 27.1.1
#### Epidemiology

The community acquired pneumonia (CAP) is a frequently occurring disease. In Germany alone, approximately 800,000 people per year develop this disease. According to the Federal Statistical Office, nearly a third of them were hospitalize in 1998. The respective mortality rate is around 6%–8%.

#### 27.1.2
#### Radiological Procedure

Chest X-ray is recommended only in those patients with at least one of the following criteria:
- Regional auscultatory finding
- Clinical assessment
- Co-morbidity
- Differential-diagnostic consideration
- Severe disease with vital dysfunction
- Admission to a hospital.

If chest X-ray does not show an infiltrate, the symptoms may be a result of an acute bronchitis or exacerbation of COPD or influenza infection. If an infiltrate is evident, a community acquired pneumonia (CAP) is very probable. The type of infiltrate has to be described morphologically as typical (lobar or bronchial) or atypical (interstitial) pneumonia. This provides the first hint to an underlying spectrum of micro-organism.

## 27.2
### Forms of Pneumonia

#### 27.2.1
#### Aspiration Pneumonia

This involves acute or chronic aspiration of gastric contents with a typical history, frequently after ENT or oesophageal disease with typically bronchogenic spread in the dependent lung regions. Lung abscesses may be a result of aspiration depending on virulence of the micro-organism and the immuno-competence. A CT is recommended to localize and measure the abscess as well as to demonstrate the relationship to adjacent organs for a possible surgical treatment.

#### 27.2.2
#### Retention Pneumonia

The most frequent underlying disease for retention pneumonia is the endobronchial obstruction caused by a bronchial carcinoma. Further causes are metastases, cardiomegaly, pleural effusion, foreign-body aspiration, post lung surgery, pneumoconiosis, etc. These should be considered since imaging might be helpful in the differential diagnosis.

#### 27.2.3
#### Non-Infectious Disease

Several diseases may clinically appear like pneumonia and go along with infiltration. However, antibiotic treatment failure takes place. Some differential diagnosis should be considered, especially since imaging might provide characteristic information to point indicate the following:
- Crypogenic organizing pneumonia (COP, formerly BOOP)
- Non-specific idiopathic pneumonia (NSIP)
- Exogene allergic alveolitis (EAA)
- Eosinophilic pneumonia
- Sarcoid, M. Wegener
- Histiocytosis X
- Systemic Lupus eythematodes
- Rheumatoide arthritis
- Bronchiolo-alveolar carcinoma
- Lymphangiosis carcinomatosa
- Pulmonary congestion

etc.

## 27.3
### Pneumonia in Immuno-Compromized Patients

A variety of clinical situations go along with a certain kind of immuno-incompetence: acquired immuno-deficiency, immuno-suppression or temporal immuno-incompetence. Modern tumour therapy utilises a numerous of high-dose chemotherapy protocols. This induces an increasing number of long-term neutropenia (>10 days) with definitive immuno-deficiency (CHANOCK 1993; HÖFFKEN 1995). In long-term neutropenia, the risk for infections rises to more than 85% (HIDDEMANN et al. 1996). Furthermore, after initially successful empirical antibiotic treatment, an infectious relapse occurs in approximately 50% of the patients (Maschmeyer et al. 1994; Pizzo et al. 1982). Thus, physicians are confronted with an increasing number of immuno-compromised hosts showing non-specific clinical signs of infection. An empirical antibiotic strategy will be started initially, which covers the most frequent types of infections. This approach is very successful nowadays (Maschmeyer et al. 1994a, b; Maschmeyer 2001), but non-targeted. Because the underlying micro-organism remains unknown, empirical antibiotic strategy has several disadvantages:

- A de-escalation of a broad-spectrum to narrow antibiotic usage, at least at the end of the infectious course, remains troublesome. This enhances costs for antibiotics as well as the rates of adverse effects, possibly over utilised drugs, and bacterial resistance.
- Beside infections, non-infectious inflammatory diseases such as relapse of haematological disease, graft vs host disease etc. might mimic infection. Therefore non-infectious differential diagnoses remain underestimated.
- After an empirically treated episode of infection, the next chemotherapeutic course usually includes an antibiotic prophylaxis. The so-called "secondary prophylaxis" is again non-specific.
- The local epidemiology remains unknown without appropriate diagnostic procedures.

Thus, patients will profit from identification of the underlying disease, and are sent to a radiologist for iden-tification of the focus of infection. This early identifica-tion of the infection site is a major task for clinicians taking care for neutropenic patients. Frequently fever is the only sign for infection and different aetiologies have to be considered in this setting (Table 27.1).

The major role of the radiologist focuses on the detec-tion of the focus of infection or non-infectious disease. If an organ is affected, invasive diagnostic procedures can be undertaken for identification of the underlying micro-organism. The acquired information helps to lo-calise the most suspicious region within this organ. For example, the selection of a certain segment helps in guid-ing broncho-alveolar lavage or biopsy (Schaefer et al. 2001). Furthermore, characterisation of the detected fo-cus may give the clinician a clue for the underlying dis-ease (Table 27.3) (Tanaka et al. 2002a; Schaefer et al. 2001). The detected focus might additionally serve as a practicable follow-up parameter to document the course of the infection and therapeutical success.

Besides detecting infectious sites, the utilised tech-nique should also present a high negative predictive value to exclude the infectious involvement temporarily.

## 27.3.1
## Risk and Epidemiology

Bacterial infections are responsible for approximately 90% of infections in the early phase of neutropenia (Einsele et al. 2001) (Table 27.1, Fig. 27.1). In an allo-geneous transplantation setting, Gram-negative bacte-

**Table 27.1.** Overview of frequent infectious and infectious-like diagnoses in neutropenia and thereafter

| Causes | Description |
|---|---|
| Bacteria | Bacterial infections occur especially during the early phase of neutropenia. Approximately three-quar-ters of bacterial infections are caused by Gram positive bacteria (Kolbe et al. 1997) |
| Fungi | Invasive fungal infections (mycosis) occur especially during the late phase of neutropenia and espe-cially during broad spectrum antibacterial therapy (Maschmeyer et al. 1994b; Uzun and Anaissie 1995). In Europe, the most frequent fungal organisms are *Candida spp.* and *Aspergillus spp* (Figs. 27.3, 27.6, 27.8 and 27.10). The latter invades the lung parenchyma as well as the blood vessels. The mortality rate of invasive aspergillosis is high (50%–70%) |
| Viruses | These organisms lead to infection especially after allogeneous bone-marrow or stem-cell transplanta-tion (Figs. 21.1 and 21.12) |
| Atypical bacteria | These organisms lead to infection especially after allogeneous bone-marrow or stem-cell transplanta-tion (Fig. 21.11). They are frequently not covered sufficiently by the initial empirical antibiotic strategy |
| Non-infectious | Several aetiologies for fever or pulmonary infiltrates, particularly after allogeneous transplantation have to be considered (Fig. 21.13–21.17). Some of these infiltrates might appear very similar to those caused by infections |

**Table 27.2.** Risk factors for various infections in hosts suffering from different immunodeficiency

| Immuno-deficiency | Diagnosis | Microorganism |
|---|---|---|
| Neutropenia | Acute myeloid and lymphatic leukaemia | Extracellular Gram-positive and gram-negative bacteria, fungi |
| Hypogamma-globulinemia | Chronic lymphatic leukaemia, multiple myeloma | Encapsulated bacteria, *Streptococcus pneumoniae*, *Haemophilus influenzae*, *Neisseria meningitidis* |
| Steroids, lymphocyte dysfunction | Hairy-cell leukaemia, acute lymphatic leukaemia, lymphoma, conditioning therapy including T-cell depletion, AIDS | Intracellular bacteria, Listeria, Mycobacteria, Salmonella, *Cryptococcus neoformans*, *Pneumocystis jiroveci* |

ria are documented in 16%–31%, whereas in 65%–75% Gram-positive bacteria are found (EINSELE et al. 2001). On the other hand, the Gram-negative bacteria lead to a significantly higher morbidity (EINSELE et al. 2001).

Risk stratification and pharmacological improvements have enhanced the role of empirical antibiotic strategy (Table 27.2). Bacteria are covered sufficiently by antibiotic (antibacterial, i.e. neither antifungal nor antiviral) therapy (MASCHMEYER et al. 1994). If this approach fails or an infection breaks through, an antibacterial second-line treatment has limited success. The low cure rate of 30% in the second line demonstrates the limited role of antibiotic switching. Antifungal supplementation at this time point, however, reaches cure rates of up to 78% (Fig.27.1) (MASCHMEYER et al. 1999). This underlines the point, that the early detection of non-bacterial pneumonia is the major task. From a clinical point of view, the detection of an ongoing bacterial infection appears less important than detecting non-bacterial pneumonia, e.g. fungal pneumonia. Therefore, making a further characterisation of a bacterial pneumonia becomes less desirable for the clinician.

Besides prophylaxis and efficient initial broad-spectrum treatment, interventional therapy regimens for second- and third lines are formulated (EINSELE et al. 2001). In the treatment of pneumonia, prospective investigations demonstrate a major limitation of the empirical therapy due to fungal organisms (MASCHMEYER et al. 1999). Due to the recommendation of the European Organization for Research and Treatment of

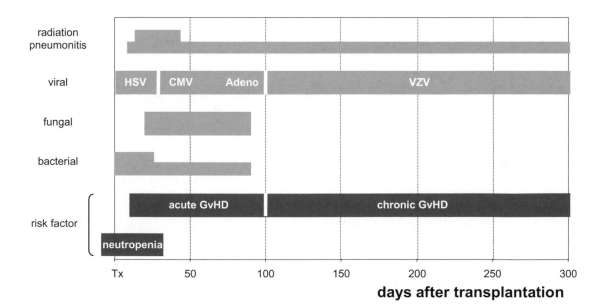

**Fig. 27.1.** Infectious and infectious-like syndromes as well as major risk factors at various times after bone marrow transplantation. Day 0 = day of transplantation. *HZV* = Herpes simplex virus, *CMV* = cytomegalo virus, *Adeno* = Adenovirus, *VZV* = Varicella zoster virus, *GvHd* = graft vs host disease (adapted to HEUSSEL et al. 2000a)

Cancer (EORTC)/Invasive Fungal Infections Cooperative Group and Bacterial and Mycosis Study Group (BAMSG), every new infiltrate is a minor criterion for fungal pneumonia and typical signs are a major criterion of fungal pneumonia (Ascioglu et al. 2002). This classification cannot be transferred to other immunodeficiencies such as AIDS (Edinburgh et al. 2000).

## 27.4
## Early Detection

The necessity for an early detection of the focus of infection bases upon high mortality of infections in immunocompromised hosts and high costs of prolonged hospitalisation. Newer antifungals as Voriconazole or Caspofungin alone result in daily therapy costs of 400–1000€. Combination with antibiotics result in even higher costs. This is a relevant amount of money in comparison to the costs of a non-enhanced CT scan of around 230€ (in Germany, in-patients, including report and comparison to previous scans). Thus, making expensive methods more cost-effective in early detection is important. Usually the search for the focus of infection consists of:

1. A physical examination and laboratory findings. Besides epidemiological knowledge, the results should be taken into account to identify the organ system which is most likely affected.
2. After identification of the most suspected organ system(s), select the appropriate imaging technique for investigation. A high sensitivity and useful negative predictive value are needed.

Exact frequencies of organ infections are difficult to determine and differ between clinical (i.e. patients alive) and pathological evaluation (i.e. patient deceased). Clinically, lungs are affected in 30% and paranasal sinuses in 3% of neutropenic patients, and 30% in an allogeneous transplantation setting (concomitant to pneumonia). Gastrointestinal tract, liver, spleen, central nervous system especially after allogeneous transplantation, and kidneys are rarely affected (Maschmeyer et al. 1994b). Due to the tremendously higher frequency of pneumonia in comparison to all other organ systems, this review focuses on early detection of pneumonia. A detailed discussion of the other organ systems and techniques is far beyond the scope of this review. The reader is referred to other publications in the literature (Heussel et al. 1998; Heussel et al. 2000b).

## 27.4.1
## Chest X-Ray

Chest X-ray (CXR) is widely performed when pneumonia is suspected or should be excluded (Azoulay et al. 2002; Navigante et al. 2002). CXR has several advantages such as: quick, widely available (even on the ward), inexpensive, low radiation dose. Some referrers prefer CXR in supine position done on the ward to keep the neutropenic patients isolated. However, supine CXR has the crucial disadvantage of superimposition and, therefore, a limited sensitivity for the detection of pneumonia (Figs. 27.2 and 27.3) (Azoulay et al. 2002; Barloon et al. 1991). In a study with 40 patients suffering from fever of unknown origin (FUO) after bone-marrow-transplantation (BMT), digital CXR in supine

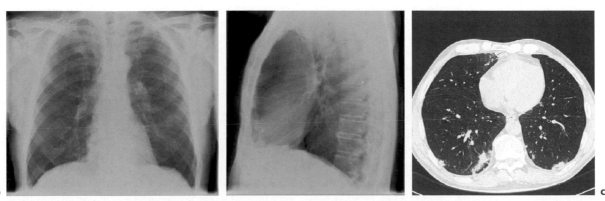

**Fig. 27.2a–c.** Neutropenic febrile patient receiving broad spectrum antibiotic therapy. CXR was normal at day 3 of fever (**a,b**). HRCT performed the same day demonstrates bilateral infiltrates, which were hidden behind the heart in posterior-anterior and the spine in lateral projection (**c**)

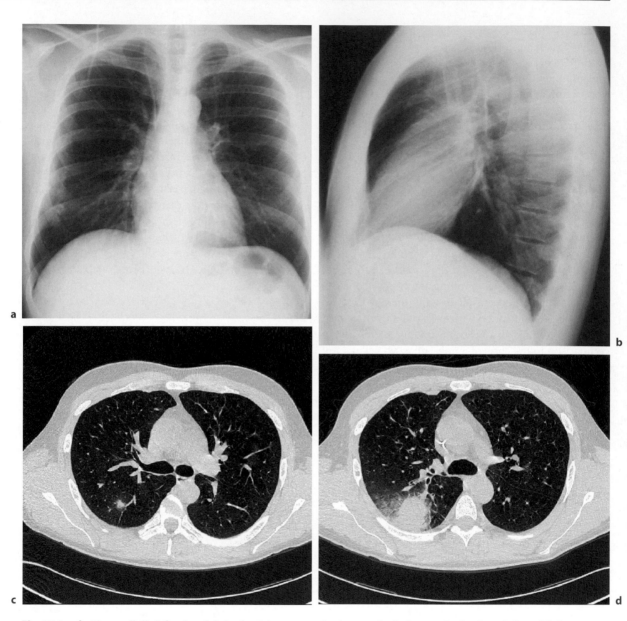

**Fig. 27.3a–d.** The small ill-defined nodule in the right upper lobe (**c**) of the 34 year-old neutropenic AML patient was even retrospectively not visible at chest X-ray done at the same day (**a,b**). Amphotericin B treatment was started due to suspicion of fungal pneumonia; however, the nodule size increased dur-ing haematological reconstitution 2 weeks later (**d**). In prepara-tion of bone marrow transplantation, the lesion was resected to prevent from septical spread. Aspergillus pneumonia was verified

position achieved a sensitivity for the early detection of pneumonia of only 46% (WEBER et al. 1999). Although CXR provides relevant clinical information concern-ing central venous catheters (CVC), pleural effusion, and pulmonary congestion (WEBER et al. 1999), it fails in the early detection or even exclusion of pneumonia, which is a major task in immuno-deficient patients. CXR in supine position alone is not recommended for the early detection of pneumonia in immuno-compro-mised hosts (MASCHMEYER 2001).

On the other hand, if an infiltrate is apparent at CXR, the options for pneumonia characterisation are very limited. Thus, if pneumonia is in question in these hosts, CT should be preferred at any time point if some-how available (MCLOUD and NAIDICH 1992).

## 27.4.2
## HRCT

The effective radiation dose of CXR is approximately 0.2 mSv but can be 10 times higher depending on the equipment used (CARDILLO et al. 1997). In low-dose multi-detector-row CT of the chest, an effective radiation dose of 1.1 mSv is reported, whereas the gap in single-slice HRCT can reduce the dose to approximately 10% of this value (SCHÖPF et al. 2001). Any low-dose technique goes along with a loss of low-contrast information. However, this information is essential for the determination of pneumonia (ground-glass opacification). Radiation dose is not a real limitation in the investigation of neutropenic patients because they frequently receive radiation for conditioning therapy for transplantation (total body irradiation, TBI) in more than 1000 times higher dosages than for diagnostic purposes. Furthermore, chemotherapy has similar cytotoxic effects on the patient. Thus, standard dose high-resolution or thin-section CT (HRCT) has been introduced as the standard technique in neutropenic patients.

After previous studies describing a limited use of CXR in these patients (BARLOON et al. 1991), a prospective study investigated the benefit of HRCT in comparison to CXR in the early detection of pneumonia: 188 febrile neutropenic patients who did not defer after 48 h on empirical antibiotic therapy (HEUSSEL et al. 1999)

were included. If CXR was normal at this time, HRCT was done. In approximately 60% of the patients with normal CXR, HRCT demonstrated infiltrates (Fig. 27.4). During the following days, in approximately 50% of the cases (total 30%) the pneumonia seen at HRCT was verified either by microbiology or an infiltrate became visible on CXR. Another 40% had a normal chest X-ray and a normal HRCT when entering the study. In these patients, pneumonia occurred in only 10% during follow-up (HEUSSEL et al. 1999). Methodological limitations are: (1) a mixed immune-status due to inclusion of patients after conventional chemotherapy or transplantation setting, and (2) the verification of underlying micro-organism, which is either uncertain, or when taking only certain identifications into account, a selection bias resulting (HEUSSEL et al. 1999). Also, the efforts in this trial (broncho–alveolar lavage, interdisciplinary clinical conference required) have limited effect. For the interpretation of microbiological results, super-infection, non-relevant isolates and contamination always have to be considered.

Besides the detection of pneumonia, the exclusion of pneumonia is a relevant information for the referring physician. Therefore the time point of pneumonia verification (by CXR or microbiology) has been evaluated in (HEUSSEL et al. 1999) to assess the negative predictive value of HRCT. In patients with normal HRCT pneumonia verification happened rarely, slowly, and con-

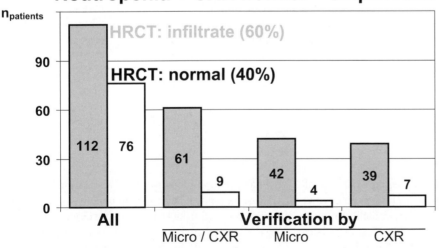

**Fig. 27.4.** Number of HRCT demonstrating an infiltrate (*shaded*) or no infiltrate (*white*) with normal CXR the same day in neutropenia and empirical antibiotic therapy (ABx). The verification of pneumonia was done either by detection of an infiltrate on CXR or evidence of a relevant micro-organism during follow-up after HRCT. Very few verifications occur after normal HRCT (*white*), whereas many verifications are done after HRCT demonstrating infiltrate (*shaded*)

## Probability of normal CXR & Micro    p < 0.0001, n_tot = 188

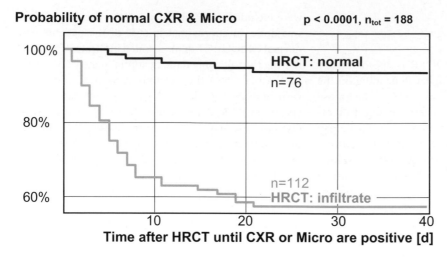

**Fig. 27.5.** Probability of verification of pneumonia by either detection of an infiltrate on a CXR or evidence of a relevant micro-organism during follow-up after HRCT. Kaplan–Meier analysis for patients with normal HRCT scans (*grey line*) and patients with pneumonia on HRCT scans (*black line*). The difference was highly significant (p<0.0001). Very few verifications occur very late after a normal HRCT, whereas most verifications after HRCT demonstrating infiltrate take place during the first 5–10 days

tinuously during the whole follow-up, but never during the first 5 days (Fig. 27.5). In patients with infiltrates at HRCT, pneumonia was verified during the next 5–10 days in most cases (Fig. 27.5) (HEUSSEL et al. 1999).

Thus, HRCT yielded very promising results to be used as a screening technique with good sensitivity (87%) and negative predictive value (88%). The gap to 100% was mainly caused by later occurring pneumonia leading to a false negative result, and minor infiltrates which were only detected at HRCT but, due to early detection and early treatment, did not progress to become visible on CXR. The additional and early use of HRCT achieved a time gain of approximately 5 days during which HRCT was able to exclude pneumonia (WEBER et al. 1999). This fact is essential in the management of immuno-deficient hosts (MASCHMEYER 2001).

in nodule detection and quantification. This topic is most relevant in follow-up scans and is solved by usage of contiguous thin-section multi-detector-row CT (MDCT) (GRENIER et al. 2002; FLOHR et al. 2002; EIBEL et al. 2003).

Contrast enhancement is generally unnecessary for detecting and characterising pneumonia (MCLOUD and NAIDICH 1992, SCHAEFER et al. 2001). Only in special situations, like pulmonary embolism or bleeding, e.g. due to vessel arosion by aspergillosis or mucormycosis, is CT-angiography beneficial (HEUSSEL et al. 1997). In an allogeneous setting, bronchiolitis obliterans has to be considered (CONCES 1999; GRENIER et al. 2002). Air-trapping is a relevant finding in this respect. Therefore, an additional expiratory CT scan is helpful (CONCES 1999; GRENIER et al. 2002).

### 27.4.3
### CT Technique

Besides HRCT, which is established as the technique of choice for detailed investigation of the lung parenchyma, multi-detector-row thin-section CT is available for lung imaging. Limitation of thick slices in CT is especially relevant in detection of inflammatory lung disease, especially ground-glass opacification (REMY-JARDIN et al. 1993). Therefore, thin-section CT should be performed as a standard (KAUCZOR et al. 1995). However, the non-contiguous scanning using HRCT involves limitations

### 27.4.4
### MRI

MRI has been evaluated for the investigation of pulmonary disease since it has a known benefit in lesion characterisation (LEUTNER et al. 2000; LEUTNER and SCHILD 2001). However, there are no studies that demonstrate the benefit of MRI in the early detection of pneumonia, where a high sensitivity is required (Fig.27.6). In advanced stages, CT and MRI are comparable in the visualisation of infiltrates (LEUTNER and SCHILD 2001). But CT is highly available, easier, and faster to perform

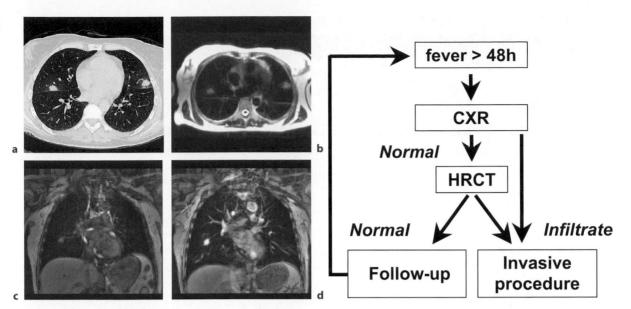

**Fig. 27.6a–d.** Fungal pneumonia in HRCT (**a**), T2w (**b**), non-enhanced T1w GE MRI (**c**) and after Gd application performed the same day (**d**). Lesion contrast is similar in CT and contrast enhanced MRI (Ullmann AU, personal communications)

**Fig. 27.7.** Recommendations of the Guidelines of the Infectious Diseases Working Party (AGIHO) of the German Society of Haematology and Oncology (DGHO) (Maschmeyer et al. 1999)

as well as less susceptible to breathing artifacts. MRI is superior to CT in the detection of abscesses due to a clearer detection of central necrosis in T2w images and rim enhancement after contrast application in T1w images (Leutner et al. 2000). However, this fact has limited clinical impact and duration of MRI and required compliance are substantially higher compared to CT.

## 27.4.5
## Standard Recommendation

In contrast to systemic infections, identification of the underlying organism in pneumonia is more difficult and complex. Trials to enforce this identification did not improve the therapeutical outcome significantly (Maschmeyer et al. 1999). Therefore, an empirical therapy in febrile immuno-deficient patients based on imaging results also is widely used.

The use of thin-section MDCT is recommended for early detection of pneumonia (Maschmeyer et al. 1999). The crucial fact is that CT allows for an optimisation for the indication and localisation of invasive diagnostic procedure, e.g. broncho-alveolar lavage (BAL). On the other hand, the exclusion of pneumonia can be obtained with a higher confidence compared to the exclusive use of CXR. The sequential cascade as shown in

Fig. 27.7 can be modified if the CT capacity allows for the skipping of CXR.

On the other hand, our own experience demonstrates the known limited success rate of invasive procedures. From 183 BAL specimens derived from 1/2002 until 11/2002, 71 had a positive bacterial/fungal result (39%). Only 9 of the 71 isolates were considered to be relevant for the suspected infection (8%), which results in an efficiency rate of 5% for the whole BAL and microbiological approach.

## 27.5
## Follow-up

The observation of growing infiltrates during haematological reconstitution has been quantified and documented recently (Caillot et al. 2001). Caillot et al. (2001) performed CT at a standard interval in 25 neutropenic patients with proven pulmonary Aspergillosis once a week. They documented the time point of different patterns and evaluated the size of the infiltrate. They frequently found the halo-sign (Fig. 27.8) in their first CT and report a low sensitivity of this well described pattern (68%). During follow-up this pattern disappeared. In contrast, the more specific air-crescent sign

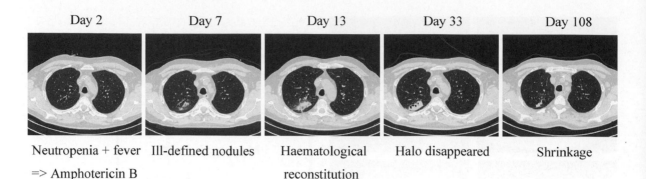

| Day 2 | Day 7 | Day 13 | Day 33 | Day 108 |

Neutropenia + fever   Ill-defined nodules   Haematological   Halo disappeared   Shrinkage
=> Amphotericin B                            reconstitution

**Fig. 27.8.** Neutropenic febrile patient who underwent autologous stem-cell transplantation due to non-Hodgkin lymphoma. At day 2 after transplantation, neutropenia and fever occurred. Therefore, antifungal treatment (Amphotericin B) was started. Ill-defined pulmonary nodules were diagnosed at day 7. Haematological reconstitution took place at day 13, simultaneously the nodule size reached its maximum during this course. Under continuously antifungal treatment and nearly normal leukocytes, the halo disappeared slowly, the lesions shrunk and a central cavitation occurred. Finally, the lesions almost disappeared

(Fig. 27.9) became more frequent during follow-up (from 8% to 63%). The size of the infiltrate increased four times despite of successful treatment and haematological reconstitution. In this approach, the mean first detection of pneumonia was at day 19 of neutropenia. This is late compared to day 11 in the study for early detection (HEUSSEL et al. 1999). The increasing infiltrate is an immunological phenomenon due to invasion of newly appearing neutrophile granulocytes at the beginning of haematological reconstitution. In critical ill patients, this is a known risk factor to develop ARDS (AZOULAY et al. 2002).

ciplinary co-operation between clinician and radiologist and the radiologists experience with these diseases. This requires an informational exchange concerning relevant patient data like standard neutropenia, allogeneous or autologous transplantation setting. Furthermore, the positivity for viral disease in graft and host is an essential information for correct interpretation of HRCT. Also the applied chemotherapeutical substances or the conditioning regimen need to be discussed (Table 27.3).

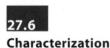

## Characterization

The radiologists' dream is to be capable to identify the underlying micro-organism in pneumonia of immunocompromised hosts with a sufficient specificity. In clinical routine, however, one has to wait for the results of microbiological and pathological analysis of samples. This requires several days to be obtained and it will only be feasible in some cases (DAVIES 1994). Furthermore, the isolated organism is not necessarily the underlying problem: Surface colonisation provides difficulties in the correct interpretation of microbiological results and super-infection with an additional organism takes place in approximately 20% (MASCHMEYER et al. 1999; SERRA et al. 1985).

In some cases, imaging can give more or less useful clues—instead of verifications—for the underlying disease. The quality of these clues depends on the interdis-

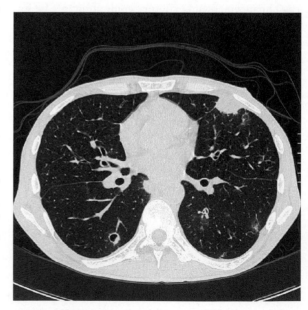

**Fig. 27.9.** The bilateral ill-defined nodules with cavitation appeared like fungal pneumonia. After taking the patients actual complaint into consideration, the patients suffered from port related infection with *Staphylococcus aureus*. The true disease septic emboli then became obvious

There are several differential diagnoses of FUO in immunocompromised hosts, which might appear clinically similar and where HRCT gives valuable hints for the differential diagnosis (Tanaka et al. 2002a, b; Schaefer et al. 2001; Reittner et al. 2003). The most useful clues are listed in Table 27.3.

## 27.6.1
## Bacterial Pneumonia

Since bacterial infections are responsible for approximately 90% of infections during the early phase of neutropenia (Einsele et al. 2001) (Tables 27.1 and 27.2, Fig. 27.1), their empirical treatment has been optimised during the last decades.

The radiological appearance of bacterial pneumonia includes consolidation, especially bronchopneumonia,

and positive pneumo-bronchogram (Fig. 27.2) (Conces 1998; Reittner et al. 2003). In contrast to immunocompetent patients, ground-glass opacification is found more often and remains non-specific.

## 27.6.2
## Fungal Pneumonia

Continuous febrile neutropenia is associated with invasive fungal infection (Pizzo et al. 1982). In Europe, *Aspergillus species* are the main underlying organism. Mucormycosis seems to increase, but besides the "bird's nest" sign, it is clinically and radiologically similar to aspergillosis. Ante mortem, *Candida species* are a rare pathogen entailing pneumonia (Fig. 27.10) (Maschmeyer 2001). Most isolates represent contamination due to surface colonisation. To describe typi-

**Table 27.3.** Clinical and radiological appearance for various infectious and non-infections lung diseases in neutropenic hosts and after bone-marrow or stem cell transplantation. *GGO* = ground-glass opacification

| Diagnosis | Clinical setting | Radiological appearance |
|---|---|---|
| Infection bacterial | Early phase neutropenia | Consolidation, bronchopneumonia pneumobronchogram, GGO |
| Fungal | Long-term neutropenia (>10 days) | Ill-defined nodules of each size cavitations (late phase) |
| Pneumocystis | Allogeneous transplantation | GGO left out subpleural space intralobular septa (late phase) |
| Mycoplasma pneumoniae | Outpatient | Angiotrophic micronodules, tree-in-bud |
| Mycobacterium tuberculosis | Each | Small ill-defined nodules/cavitations, tree-in-bud, homogeneous consolidation |
| Viral | Transplantation history in graft or host | GGO—mosaic pattern |
| Graft vs host | Allogeneous transplantation | GGO—mosaic pattern intralobular septa tree-in-bud air-trapping |
| Radiation toxicity | Total body irradiation | GGO—paramediastinal distribution intralobular septa |
| Drug toxicity | Bleomycine, Methotrexate, Cytarabine, Carmustine etc. | GGO—mosaic pattern intralobular septa |
| Pulmonary congestion | Extensive hydration, renal impairment, hypoproteinosis | GGO thickening interlobular septa |
| Leukemic infiltration | Chronic leukemic infiltration | Thickening bronchovascular bundles, thickening interlobular septa, GGO |
| Pulmonary hemorrhage | Thrombocytopenia, intervention | GGO—sedimentation phenomenon |

cal findings of fungal pneumonia caused by different pathogens, a dedicated review is necessary (HEUSSEL et al. 2000a). This manuscript focuses on the most relevant information for haematological patients. The appearance of pulmonary infiltrates with fungus typical patterns in the:

- Early phase:
    - Ill-defined nodules (Figs. 27.6, 27.8, and 27.10; REITTNER et al. 2003) in combination with the
    - Halo sign (Figs. 27.8 and 27.10; REITTNER et al. 2003), which is non-specific
- Late phase:
    - Air-crescent-sign (KIM MJ et al. 2001)
    - Cavitations (Fig. 27.10)

For use in the context of clinical and epidemiological research in neutropenic patients, the EORTC and BAMSO have defined standards for the interpretation of radiological findings in invasive fungal infections (AsCIOGLU et al. 2002): The new occurrence of these "typical" CT patterns (halo sign, air-crescent-sign, or cavity within area of consolidation) are classified as a major clinical criterion for fungal pneumonia. Furthermore, if a new infiltrate is observed even without a typical fungal pattern, it is classified as a minor clinical criterion for fungal pneumonia (ASCIOGLU et al. 2002).

Air-crescent-sign and cavitation occur simultaneously with haematological reconstitution during the late phase of infection (Fig. 27.10) (KIM MJ et al. 2001). Therefore air-crescent and cavitation signs are known

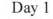
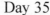
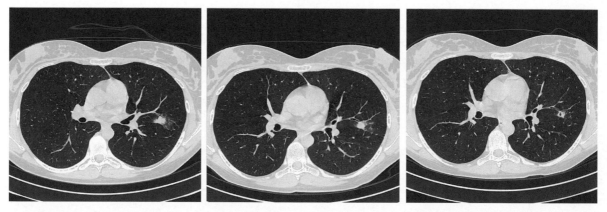

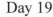
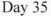
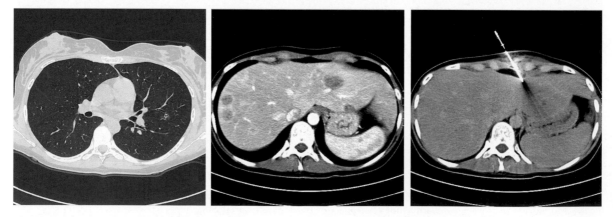

**Fig. 27.10.** Bilateral ill-defined nodules made the suspected diagnosis of a fungal infection which was treated accordingly. *Candida spp.* were identified from blood-culture and suspected to be involved with this pneumonia[1]. The small lesions developed into cavitations at haematological reconstitution and decreased. Due to increasing liver enzymes and because of known hepatospenic candidiasis after candidemia, contrast enhanced CT scan was done. Biopsy from the detected lesions revealed *Candida spp.* once again

---

[1] Candia pneumonia is a rare condition. Microbiological identification of Candida species in lavages or swabs usually have to be considered as colonization, not as infection.

to have a positive prognosis. However, the specificities of these findings are limited and relevant differential diagnoses have to be considered (Fig. 27.9) (Kim K et al. 2002). The histopathological work-up verified fungal pneumonia only in 56% (Kim K et al. 2002). Relevant differential diagnosis for the halo sign such as bronchiolitis obliterans organising pneumonia, pulmonary haemorrhage, and other infections (CMV, TBC, abscesses (Fig. 27.9), *Candida* (Fig. 27.10) etc.) have to be considered (Kim K et al. 2002).

There are other useful patterns in the identification of fungal pneumonia: distribution along the bronchovascular bundle resulting in the feeding vessel sign with an angiotropic location.

### 27.6.3
### Pneumocystis Jiroveci Pneumonia (PcP)

*Pneumocystis jiroveci* pneumonia (former: *P. carinii*, the abbreviation PcP continues for *Pneumocystis pneumonia*) (Stringer et al. 2002) is not a typical finding in haematological patients except in the late phase after allogeneous transplantation together with chronic GvHD (Einsele et al. 2001). Under the standard Trimethoprim/Sulfamethoxazol prophylaxis, 8% of the patients develop PcP, without prophylaxis even 29% (Einsele et al. 2001). Mortality is 4%–15% in these cases (Einsele et al. 2001).

CT provides a valuable characterisation for this micro-organism (Tanaka et al. 2002a; McLoud and Naidich 1992; Schaefer et al. 2001; Reittner et al.

2003) and is a reliable method for differentiating PcP from other infectious processes (Hidalgo et al. 2003; Reittner et al. 2003). A combination of ground-glass opacities and intralobular septa sparing out the subpleural space (i.e. perihilar distribution) are very typical for PcP (Fig. 27.11) (McGuinness and Gruden 1999; Reittner et al. 2003; Hidalgo et al. 2003; Reittner et al. 2003).

### 27.6.4
### Tuberculosis

Tuberculosis (TBC) has always to be considered as a rare but relevant differential diagnosis. In an immuno-compromised host, TBC appears different compared to immunocompetent hosts (e.g. gangliopulmonary (primary) forms) (Van Dyck et al. 2003). More widespread lymphogenic and hematogenous dissemination can occur and, therefore, the clinical course might be fulminant (Goo and Im 2002; Van Dyck et al. 2003). On the other hand, TBC might mimic or come along with other infections like pulmonary aspergillosis or systemic candidiasis (Goo and Im 2002).

In immuno-compromised hosts a peribronchial distribution (resulting in a "tree-in-bud" sign) of small, sometimes cavitated ill-defined nodules can be obtained due to miliar distribution (Goo and Im 2002; Van Dyck et al. 2003). Gangliopulmonary (primary) forms, however, present with In homogenous consolidation and necrotic mediastinal/hilar lymphadenopathy (Van Dyck et al. 2003).

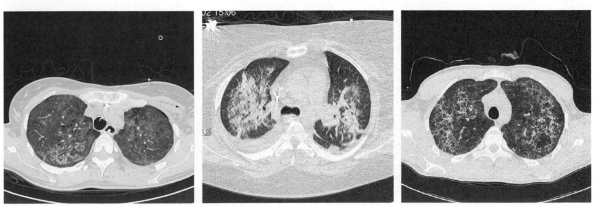

**a,b**                                                                                 **c**

**Fig. 27.11a–c.** Bilateral pneumonia caused by *Pneumocystis jiroveci* (PcP) at different stages of immunosuppression. The subpleural space is typically left out. Diffuse ground glass opacification appears typically in the early phase of infection (**a**), while consolidations appear at a fulminant course (**b**). The predominance of intralobular linear patterns takes place during a later and treated stage of PcP (**c**)

### 27.6.5
### Viral Pneumonia

Atypical pneumonia in neutropenic patients and especially after haematological reconstitution is frequently caused by virus infection. Viral pneumonia is associated with a mortality of approximately 50% in neutropenic hosts. The most frequent suspected microbe is cytomegalovirus (CMV); furthermore herpes, influenza, parainfluenza, adenovirus, respiratory syncytial (RSV) viruses have to be considered. There are no radiological patterns available to differentiate various forms of viral pneumonia. However, even the information that there is viral pneumonia is very valuable to the clinicians. Appropriate drug regimens are available for many of these viruses. The typical appearance of viral pneumonia in the early stage is ground-glass opacification (REITTNER et al. 2003) and mosaic pattern with affected and non-affected secondary lobules lying adjacent to one another (Fig. 27.12).

### 27.6.6
### Non-Infectious Disease

Certain non-infectious diseases have to be considered in hematological patients: graft vs host disease (GvHD),

radiation or drug toxicity, COP, pulmonary congestion, bleeding, or early tumour recurrence. Fever, dyspnoea or lab findings (C-reactive protein, transaminases) might be caused by some of these diseases and obscure the differentiation from infection. For instance, in GvHD the therapeutic approach to non-infectious caused infiltrates is in contrast to infection: further suppression of the immune system. This differential diagnosis is very helpful for clinicians. CT is able to assist in the detection and characterisation of these diseases (TANAKA et al. 2002a, b; McLOUD and NAIDICH 1992; SCHAEFER et al. 2001).

### 27.6.6.1
### Graft vs Host Disease

Pulmonary manifestation of chronic GvHD occurs in approximately 10% of patients usually 9 months after allogeneous transplantation (Fig. 27.13) (LEBLOND et al. 1994). Bronchiolitis obliterans is the pulmonary manifestation of this rejection (CONCES 1999). Unfortunately, the radiological appearance is similar to viral pneumonia, and to make things more complicated, clinical appearance and time point for both diseases are often similar (Fig. 27.1).

Ground-glass opacification and mosaic pattern, as

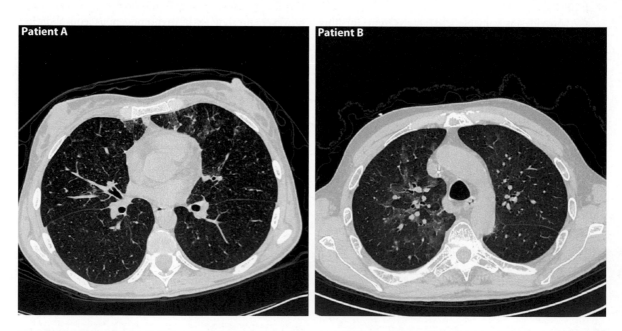

**Fig. 27.12.** Bilateral ground-glass opacification and mosaic pattern in both patients. However, pneumonia in patient A is caused by cytomegalo virus (CMV), patient B by respiratory syncytial virus (RSV). Note the mosaic pattern which results from affected and non-affected secondary lobules lying adjacent to one another

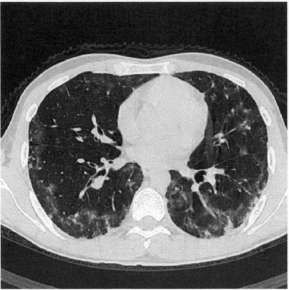

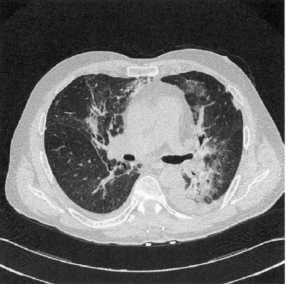

**Fig. 27.13.** A 28-year-old male after allogeneic re-transplantation due to CML. HRCT was performed due to fever, cough and dyspnoea. Peripheral intralobular septa (*arrow*) and ground-glass opacification was determined at HRCT at day 91 after transplantation. Tree-in-bud pattern (*arrowhead*) points to bronchiolitis obliterans. Acute GvHD was diagnosed from trans-bronchial biopsy. After increasing immunosuppression, the clinical symptoms and the radiological signs disappeared. Note the similarity to Fig. 27.15

**Fig. 27.14.** Three weeks after local radiation for a tumorous spine destruction, this patient suffered from fever and dyspnoea. Perihilar infiltrates appeared suddenly. Intralobular septa, consolidation, and ground-glass opacification were determined at HRCT. Especially the para-mediastinal distribution of the infiltrates led to the differential diagnosis of radiation pneumonitis. After failure of antibiotic escalation (chosen because of a concomitant abscess), steroids were applied additionally. This led to a quick improvement of the symptoms as well as reduction of infiltrates

well as signs of bronchiolitis obliterans such as air-trapping (CONCES 1999; GRENIER et al. 2002) and bronchus wall thickening occur during the early stage of pulmonary GvHD (Fig. 27.13), whereas intralobular septa and tree-in-bud follow in later stages (LEBLOND et al. 1994; TANAKA et al. 2002a; OIKONOMOU and HANSELL 2002).

et al. 1998; OIKONOMOU and HANSELL 2002). The key finding is the limitation of these patterns to the parenchyma within the radiation field. And even in TBI, lung parenchyma is blocked out, thus, para-mediastinal and apical lung parenchyma suffers mainly from radiation toxicity.

### 27.6.6.2
### Radiation Toxicity

An incidence of 5%–25% even after total body irradiation (TBI) is reported, which is applied for conditioning therapy prior to bone-marrow or stem cell transplantation (MONSON et al. 1998). One problem in detecting radiation toxicity is the time delay after radiation, which is approximately 3 weeks, but can also occur several months later (MONSON et al. 1998; OIKONOMOU and HANSELL 2002).

At CT, it is characterised by ground-glass opacities with transition to consolidations (Fig. 27.14) (MONSON

### 27.6.6.3
### Drug Toxicity

Especially high-dose chemotherapy protocols are used for conditioning therapy which results in pulmonary drug toxicity. Some of the frequently used agents are Bleomycin, Methotrexate (MTX), Cytarabine (Ara-C), Carmustine (BCNU), and many more (Fig. 27.15) (ERASMUS et al. 2002). Radiologists have to suspect treatment with these drugs and should ask for it. (www.pneumotox.com)

The term drug induced pneumonitis includes mainly diffuse alveolar damage, non-specific interstitial

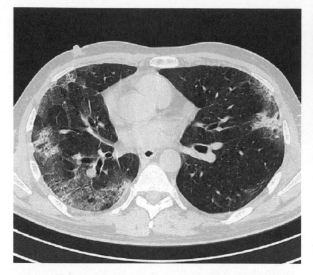

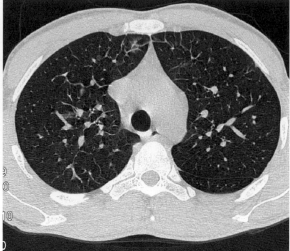

**Fig. 27.15.** A 40-year-old male received chemotherapy including Bleomycin (PEB protocol) for testicular cancer. HRCT was performed because of fever, cough and dyspnoea. HRCT revealed peripheral intralobular septa and ground-glass opacification. Due to the known pulmonary toxicity of the applied Bleomycin, a pulmonary drug toxicity was suspected and verified by open lung biopsy. Symptoms disappeared and findings decreased after application of steroids. Note the similarity to Fig. 27.13

**Fig. 27.16.** Thickening of the intralobular septa, which is a result of fluid overload in lymphatic vessels

pneumonia (NSIP) and cryptogenic organizing pneumonia (COP, former: bronchiolitis obliterans organizing pneumonia, BOOP) (ERASMUS et al. 2002). The CT appearance consists of ground-glass opacities with transition to consolidations, intralobular septa, air-trapping, and possibly the non-specific "crazy-paving" pattern (OIKONOMOU and HANSELL 2002; ERASMUS et al. 2002). This is quite similar to radiation toxicity but without being limited to the radiation field.

### 27.6.6.4
### Pulmonary Congestion

Dyspnea and infiltration are frequent in patients suffering from pulmonary congestion. Due to CVC, extensive hydration for renal protection during chemotherapy, frequent temporary renal impairment, hypo-proteinosis, or pulmonary congestion appear even in younger patients. It is one of the most frequent disorders in intensively treated patients.

At CXR, pulmonary congestion might be combined with infiltration. CT demonstrates a thickening of the lymphatic vessels, which corresponds to the well-known Kerley lines (Fig. 27.16).

### 27.6.6.5
### Leukemic Infiltration

Leukemic pulmonary infiltration is a less common clinical finding. Especially the peri-lymphatic pulmonary interstitium is involved (HEYNEMAN et al. 2000). This can be visualised at CT as thickening of the broncho-vascular bundles and interlobular septa. Besides this, non-lobular and non-segmental ground-glass opacifications can be seen (TANAKA et al. 2002b). This pattern arrangement might mimic pulmonary congestion (Fig. 27.16).

### 27.6.6.6
### Pulmonary Hemorrhage

In pancytopenia, pulmonary bleeding occurs spontaneously, after interventions (e.g. BAL), or during haematological reconstitution after fungal pneumonia (HEUSSEL et al. 1997).

Pulmonary bleeding might be a focal or diffuse pattern, and the phenomenon of sedimentation within the secondary lobules can sometimes be depicted (Fig. 27.17).

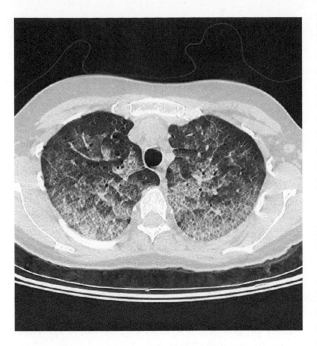

**Fig. 27.17.** The bilateral ground-glass opacification has an anterior-posterior gradient over the whole-lung and within certain secondary lobules. This gravity dependence sedimentation phenomenon may occur temporarily and localised, e.g. after BAL or in diffuse pulmonary bleeding

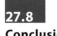
**27.7**

## Intervention

Radiological guided interventions in neutropenic patients suffer mainly from the coincidental thrombocytopenia. Interventions are limited to patients with at least 50,000 platelets/μL ideally with a running substitution during the biopsy.

### 27.7.1
### Biopsy

There is great interest in organ specimens for microbiological or pathological investigations. In most cases of fungal pneumonia, BAL fails to detect the fungi. Therefore, this frequent differential diagnosis is a special task for percutaneous intervention. There is no literature available, analysing risk and benefit in this population. Actually, neutropenic patients undergo biopsy rarely. On the other hand, the limited risk of radiological interventions in lungs or liver are known to radiologists:

Risk for pneumothorax requiring therapy is less than 3% (Froelich and Wagner 2001), for bleeding in liver lesions less than 2%. The probability to hit pulmonary nodules under CT guidance is approximately 95% (Froelich and Wagner 2001). Using CT fluoroscopy, investigation time and sensitivity are improved especially in small lesions. Non-culture detection tests on the other hand are becoming widely available (Galactomannan antigen test, Platelia©, Aspergillus-PCR) and reduce the necessity to perform invasive diagnostics procedures.

### 27.7.2
### Local Drug Instillation

As mentioned earlier, the response of fungal pneumonia to antifungal drugs is limited. Only when reconstitution of the leukocytes emerges can a substantial response be achieved. Dose escalation has been tested, but costs and adverse effects increase without significant improvement. Several groups have evaluated repeated local instillation of an Amphotericin B preparation into the fungal pneumonia under CT guidance. They had an improved outcome: eight lesions completely resolved, four greatly improved, and one was without change (Veltrei et al. 2000). Since a wide range of new antifungal drugs has become available, a local therapy appears not to be attractive any more.

**27.8**

## Conclusion

Imaging in pneumonia has to be indicated depending on the clinical status of the patient starting with no-imaging in simple respiratory infection, going over CXR in CAP and ending in early CT in immunocompromised patients.

Several chest complications occur in patients suffering from neutropenia after bone-marrow or stem-cell transplantation. Due to the clinical risk, CXR in the supine position is not recommended for early detection of pneumonia in these hosts. If pneumonia is suspected, HRCT or thin-section MDCT is suggested to identify the focus of fever or even to exclude pneumonia for some days.

In addition, characterisation of the infiltrate is a relevant topic in thoracic imaging. Therefore, close interdisciplinary co-operation as well as careful image interpretation may deliver rapidly a clear number of valid differential diagnoses.

# References

Ascioglu S, Rex JH, de Pauw B, Bennett JE, Bille J, Crokaert F, Denning DW, Donnelly JP, Edwards JE, Erjavec Z, Fiere D, Lortholary O, Maertens J, Meis JF, Patterson TF, Ritter J, Selleslag D, Shah PM, Stevens DA, Walsh TJ (2002) Defining opportunistic invasive fungal infections in immunocompromised patients with cancer and hematopoietic stem cell transplants: an international consensus. Clin Infect Dis 34:7–14

Azoulay E, Darmon M, Delclaux C, Fieux F, Bornstain C, Moreau D, Attalah H, Le Gall JR, Schlemmer B (2002) Deterioration of previous acute lung injury during neutropenia recovery. Crit Care Med 30:781–786

Barloon TJ, Galvin JR, Mori M, Stanford W, Gingrich RD (1991) High-resolution ultrafast chest CT in the clinical management of febrile bone marrow transplant patients with normal or nonspecific chest roentgenograms. Chest 99:928–933

Caillot D, Couaillier JF, Bernard A, Casasnovas O, Denning DW, Mannone L, Lopez J, Couillault G, Piard F, Vagner O, Guy H (2001) Increasing volume and changing characteristics of invasive pulmonary aspergillosis on sequential thoracic computed tomography scans in patients with neutropenia. J Clin Oncol 19:253–259

Cardillo I, Boal TJ, Einsiedel PF (1997) Patient doses from chest radiography in Victoria Australia. Phys Eng Sci Med 20:92–101

Chanock S (1993) Evolving risk factors for infectious complications of cancer. Hematol Oncol Clin North Am 7:771–793

Conces DJ (1998) Bacterial pneumonia in immunocompromised patients. J Thoracic Imaging 13:261–270

Conces DJ (1999) Noninfectious lung disease in immunocompromised patients. J Thoracic Imaging 14:9–24

Davies SF (1994) Fungal pneumonia. Med Clin North Am 78:1049–1065

Edinburgh KJ, Jasmer RM, Huang L, Reddy GP, Chung MH, Thompson A, Halvorsen RA Jr, Webb RA (2000) Multiple pulmonary nodules in AIDS: usefulness of CT in distinguishing among potential causes. Radiology 214:427–432

Eibel R, Ostermann H, Schiel X (2003) Thorakale Computertomographie von Lungeninfiltraten. http://www.dgho-infektionen.de/agiho/content/e134/e619/e657 (26.03.03)

Einsele H, Bertz H, Beyer J, Kiehl MG, Runde V, Kolb H-J, Holler E, Beck R, Schwertfeger R, Schumacher U, Hebart H, Martin H, Kienast J, Ullmann AJ, Maschmeyer G, Krüger W, Link H, Schmidt CA, Oettle H, Klingebiel T (2001) Epidemiologie und interventionelle Therapiestrategien infektiöser Komplikationen nach allogener Stammzelltransplantation. Dtsch Med Wochenschr 126:1278–1284

Erasmus JJ, McAdams HP, Rossi SE (2002) High-resolution CT of drug-induced lung disease. Radiol Clin North Am 40:61–72

Flohr T, Stierstorfer K, Bruder H, Simon J, Schaller S (2002) New technical developments in multi-detector-row CT—Part 1: Approaching isotropic resolution with sub-millimeter 16-slice scanning. Fortschr Röntgenstr 174:839–845

Froelich JJ, Wagner HJ (2001) CT-Fluoroscopy: tool or gimmick? Cardiovasc Intervent Radiol 24:297–305

Goo JM, Im JG (2002) CT of tuberculosis and nontuberculous mycobacterial infections. Radiol Clin North Am 40:73–87

Grenier PA, Beigelman-Aubry C, Fetita C, Preteux F, Brauner MW, Lenoir S (2002) New frontiers in CT imaging of airway disease. Eur Radiol 12:1022–1044

Heussel CP, Kauczor HU, Heussel G, Mildenberger P, Dueber C (1997) Aneurysms complicating inflammatory diseases in immunocompromised hosts: value of contrast-enhanced CT. Eur Radiol 7:316–319

Heussel CP, Kauczor H-U, Heussel G, Poguntke M, Schadmand-Fischer S, Mildenberger P, Thelen M (1998) Magnetic resonance imaging (MRI) of liver and brain in hematologic-oncologic patients with fever of unknown origin. Fortschr Roentgenstr 169:128–134

Heussel CP, Kauczor H-U, Heussel G, Fischer B, Begrich M, Mildenberger P, Thelen M (1999) Pneumonia in febrile neutropenic patients, bone-marrow and blood stem-cell recipients: use of high-resolution CT. J Clin Oncol 17:796–805

Heussel CP, Ullmann AJ, Kauczor H-U (2000a) Fungal pneumonia. Radiologe 40:518–529

Heussel CP, Kauczor H-U, Heussel G, Derigs HG, Thelen M (2000b) Looking for the cause in neutropenic fever. Imaging diagnostics. Radiologe 40:88–101

Heyneman LE, Johkoh T, Ward S, Honda O, Yoshida S, Muller NL (2000) Pulmonary leukemic infiltrates: high-resolution CT findings in 10 patients. AJR Am J Roentgenol 174:517–521

Hidalgo A, Falcó V, Mauleón S, Andreu J, Crespo M, Ribera E, Pahissa A, Cáceres J (2003) Accuracy of high-resolution CT in distinguishing between Pneumocystis carinii pneumonia and non-Pneumocystis carinii pneumonia in AIDS patients. Eur Radiol. DOI 10.1007/s00330-002-1641-6

Hiddemann W, Maschmeyer G, Runde V, Einsele H (1996) Prevention, diagnosis and therapy of infections in patients with malignant diseases. Internist 37:1212–1224

Höffken K (1995) Antibiotische Therapie bei neutropenischem Fieber. Onkologe 1:503–510

Kauczor HU, Schnuetgen M, Fischer B et al. (1995) Pulmonary manifestations in HIV patients: the role of chest films, CT and HRCT. Fortschr Roentgenstr 162:282–287

Kim K, Lee MH, Kim J, Lee KS, Kim SM, Jung MP, Han J, Sung KW, Kim WS, Jung CW, Yoon SS, Im YH, Kang WK, Park K, Park CH (2002) Importance of open lung biopsy in the diagnosis of invasive pulmonary aspergillosis in patients with hematologic malignancies. Am J Hematol 2002 71:75–79

Kim MJ, Lee KS, Kim J, Jung KJ, Lee HG, Kim TS (2001) Crescent sign in invasive pulmonary aspergillosis: frequency and related CT and clinical factors. J Comput Assist Tomogr 25:305–310

Kolbe K, Domkin D, Derigs HG, Bhakdi S, Huber C, Aulitzky WE (1997) Infectious complications during neutropenia subsequent to peripheral blood stern cell transplantation. BMT 19:143–147

Leblond V, Zouabi H, Sutton L, Guillon JM, Mayaud CM, Similowski T, Beigelman C, Autran B (1994) Late CD8+ lymphocytic alveolitis after allogeneic bone marrow transplantation and chronic graft-versus-host disease. Am J Respir Crit Care Med 150:1056–1061

Leutner C, Schild H (2001) MRI of the lung parenchyma Fortschr Röntgenstr 173:168–175

Leutner CC, Gieseke J, Lutterbey G, Kuhl CK, Glasmacher A, Wardelmann E, Theisen A, Schild HH (2000) MR imaging of pneumonia in immunocompromised patients: comparison with helical CT. AJR Am J Roentgenol 175:391–397

Maschmeyer G (2001) Pneumonia in febrile neutropenic patients: radiologic diagnosis. Curr Opin Oncol 13:229–235

Maschmeyer G, Link H, Hiddemann W, Meyer P, Helmerking M, Eisenmann E, Schmitt J, Adam D (1994a) Empirical antimicrobial therapy in neutropenic patients. Results of a multicenter study by the Infections in Hematology Study Group of the Paul Ehrlich Society. Med Klin 89:114–123

Maschmeyer G, Link H, Hiddemann W, Meyer P, Helmerking M, Eisenmann E, Schmitt J, Adam D (1994b) Pulmonary infiltrations in febrile neutropenic patients. Risk factors and outcome under empirical antimicrobial therapy in a randomized multicenter trial. Cancer 73:2296–2304

Maschmeyer G, Buchheidt D, Einsele H, Heussel CP, Holler E, Lorenz J, Schweigert M (1999) Diagnostik und Therapie von Lungeninfiltraten bei febrilen neutropenischen Patienten—Leitlinien der Arbeitsgemeinschaft Infektionen in der Hämatologie und Onkologie der Deutschen Gesellschaft für Hämatologie und Onkologie. Dtsch Med Wochenschr 9 124(Suppl 1):S18–23 Update: http://www.dgho-infektionen.de/agiho/content/e125/e670/lugeninfiltrate.pdf (26.03.03)

McGuinness G, Gruden JF (1999) Viral and Pneumocystis carinii infections of the lung in the immunocompromized host. J Thorac Imaging 14:25–36

McLoud TC, Naidich DP (1992) Thoracic disease in the immunocompromised patient. Radiol Clin North Am 1992 30:525–554

Monson JM, Stark P, Reilly JJ, Sugarbaker DJ, Strauss GM, Swanson SJ, Decamp MM, Mentzer SJ, Baldini EH (1998) Clinical radiation pneumonitis and radiographic changes after thoracic radiation therapy for lung carcinoma. Cancer 82:842–850

Navigante AH, Cerchietti LC, Costantini P, Salgado H, Castro MA, Lutteral MA, Cabalar ME (2002) Conventional chest radiography in the initial assessment of adult cancer patients with fever and neutropenia. Cancer Control 9:346–351

Oikonomou A, Hansell DM (2002) Organizing pneumonia: the many morphological faces. Eur Radiol 12:1486–1496

Pizzo PA, Robichaud KJ, Gill FA, Witebsky FG (1982) Empiric antibiotic and antifungal therapy for cancer patients with prolonged fever and granulocytopenia. Am J Med 72:101–111

Reittner P, Ward S, Heyneman L, Johkoh T, Müller NL (2003a) Pneumonia: high-resolution CT findings in 114 patients. Eur Radiol 13:515–521

Remy-Jardin M, Giraud F, Remy J, Copin MC, Gosselin B, Duhamel A (1993) Computed tomography assessment of ground-glass opacity: semiology and significance. J Thorac Imaging 8:249–264

Schaefer-Prokop C, Prokop M, Fleischmann D, Herold C (2001) High-resolution CT of diffuse interstitial lung disease: key findings in common disorders. Eur Radiol 11:373–392

Schöpf UJ, Becker CXR, Obuchowski NA, Rust G-F, Ohnesorge BM, Kohl G, Schaller S, Modic MT, Reiser MF (2001) Multi-slice computed tomography as a screening tool for colon cancer, lung cancer and coronary artery disease. Eur Radiol 11:1975–1985

Serra P, Santini C, Venditti M, Mandelli F, Martino P (1985) Superinfections during antimicrobial treatment with beta-lactam-aminoglycoside combinations in neutropenic patients with hematologic malignancies. Infection 13(Suppl 1):S115–122

Stringer JR, Beard CB, Miller RF, Wakefield AE (2002) A new name (Pneumocystis jiroveci) for Pneumocystis from humans. Emerg Infect Dis Sep 8 http://www.cdc.gov/ncidod/EID/vol8no9/02-0096.htm [26.03.03]

Tanaka N, Matsumoto T, Miura G, Emoto T, Matsunaga N (2002a) HRCT findings of chest complications in patients with leukemia. Eur Radiol 12:1512–1522

Tanaka N, Matsumoto T, Miura G, Emoto T, Matsunaga N, Satoh Y, Oka Y (2002b) CT findings of leukemic pulmonary infiltration with pathologic correlation. Eur Radiol 12:166–174

Uzun O, Anaissie EJ (1995) Antifungal prophylaxis in patients with hematologic malignancies: a reappraisal. Blood 86:2063–2072

Van Dyck P, Vanhoenacker FM, Van den Brande P, De Schepper AM (2003) Imaging of pulmonary tuberculosis. Eur Radiol DOI 10.1007/s00330-002-1612-y

Veltri A, Anselmetti GC, Bartoli G, Martina MC, Regge D, Galli J, Bertini M (2000) Percutaneus treatment with amphotericin B of mycotic lung lesions from invasive aspergillosis: results in 10 immunocompromised patients. Eur Radiol 10:1939–1944

Weber C, Maas R, Steiner P, Kramer J, Bumann D, Zander AR, Bucheler E (1999) Importance of digital thoracic radiography in the diagnosis of pulmonary infiltrates in patients with bone marrow transplantation during aplasia. Fortschr Röntgenstr 171:294–301

# CT of the Airways

Hans-Ulrich Kauczor, Michael Owsijewitsch and Julia Ley-Zaporozhan

## CONTENTS

H.-U. Kauczor, MD
Professor, Ärztlicher Direktor, Abt. Diagnostische und Interventionelle Radiologie, Universitätsklinikum Heidelberg, Im Neuenheimer Feld 110, 69120 Heidelberg, Germany

M. Owsijewitsch, MD
Department of Radiology, German Cancer Research Center (DKFZ), Im Neuenheimer Feld 280, 69120 Heidelberg, Germany

J. Ley-Zaporozhan, MD
Pädiatrische Radiologie, Universitätsklinikum Heidelberg, Im Neuenheimer Feld 153, 69120 Heidelberg, Germany

## ABSTRACT

Multislice CT is the method of choice for the morphological visualization of the airways and the associated diseases. High isotropic resolution and high contrast are the ideal prerequisites to generate MPRs in order to demonstrate the typical findings of airway disease, such as dilation, ectasis, wall thickening, increased collapsibility, and stenosis as well as visibility of small airways in bronchiolitis. The major diseases of the airways that can be adequately studied by multislice CT are tracheobronchomalacia, chronic obstructive pulmonary disease (COPD), and cystic fibrosis (CF).

## 28.1
### Introduction

### 28.1.1
### Anatomy

The airways denote the tubular and branching structures, which supply the lungs with air. They comprise the airways extending from the larynx downwards to the terminal bronchioles. In the context of CT, the airways can be subdivided in three major parts: (1) trachea and mainstem bronchi; (2) visible segmental and subsegmental bronchi; and (3) the small airways, which under normal conditions are not visible by CT.

The *trachea* begins at the larynx and extends for approximately 12 cm to the *carina*, where it bifurcates into the right and left mainstem *bronchi*. Since the trachea is rather mobile, it can change its length substantially. Thus, the carina can move from the level of the upper border of the fifth thoracic vertebra (position during tidal respiration) to the level of the sixth thoracic vertebra during deep inspiration (STANDRING 2004). The *an-*

*terior* and *lateral tracheal walls* are supported by 16–20 incomplete horseshoe-shaped cartilage rings. The *membranous posterior wall* (pars membranacea) connects the ends of the incomplete cartilaginous rings.

The right mainstem bronchus is wider, shorter, and has a course more vertical than the left one has. This is one of the reasons that aspirations, e.g., of foreign bodies, occur more frequently on the right side. The first branching of the right mainstem bronchus—into the upper lobe bronchus and the bronchus intermedius—is still localized within the mediastinum at a distance from the carina of approximately 2.5 cm. After this branching, the bronchus intermedius enters the *pulmonary hilum* and divides into the *middle lobe* and *lower lobe bronchus*. The left principal bronchus is narrower, less vertical than the right one is, and enters the lung before the branch-off of the upper lobe bronchus, which occurs at approximately 5 cm distal to the carina from where the lower lobe bronchi supply the lower lobe. As there is no middle lobe on the left side, the *lingula* is supported by the *lingular bronchus*, which originates from the left upper lobe bronchus.

The lobar bronchi subsequently divide into *segmental* and *subsegmental bronchi* and the subsequent generations. In each branching generation, the diameters and the wall thickness of the bronchi continuously decrease. This observation is also called *proximal-to-distal tapering*.

The cartilaginous support of the airways is continuously changing over the branching generations. The trachea and extrapulmonary bronchi contain incomplete rings of hyaline cartilage. The intrapulmonary bronchi only contain discontinuous plates or islands of cartilage, the irregularity of which increases with each further branching generation, and finally, the cartilaginous islands normally disappear when the airway diameter falls below 1 mm. Per definition, airways with diameters less than 1 mm are termed *bronchioles*, which do not contain cartilage within their walls. They represent about the 10th to the 20th generation of airways. They are the smallest and most peripheral, but still purely conducting airways, hence not containing any alveoli in their walls. Distal to the terminal bronchiole there are the *acini*, which consist of 3–4 generations of respiratory bronchioles, leading to 3–8 generations of *alveolar ducts*, finally leading to single *alveoli*.

The part of the lung distal to a single terminal bronchiole is defined as a *primary lobule* of the lung. The *secondary lobule* is the smallest subsection of the lung, surrounded by connective tissue septa and consists of approximately three to six primarily lobules. Secondary lobules have polygon shapes with each side ranging from 1 to 2.5 cm and are readily discernable on high resolution CT (Webb 2004; Weibel and Gomez 1962). The smallest airways discernable on high-resolution CT have a diameter of 2 mm.

## 28.1.2
## Anomalies and Diseases

The prevalence of tracheobronchial tree anomalies varies between 1 and 3%, which largely represents the fact that some of these anomalies do not cause symptoms such as recurrent episodes of pulmonary infections or airway obstruction. These anomalies include additional bronchi originating from the trachea (tracheal bronchus) (Bakir and Terzibasioglu 2007) or main bronchi (accessory cardiac bronchus), bronchopulmonary foregut malformations, and bronchial atresia.

The radiological key morphologies of airway diseases are dilation or stenosis of the lumen, wall thickening of the visible bronchi, and lack of tapering as well as the (pathologic) visibility of small airways. Morphological changes of the lung parenchyma such as hyperinflation, air trapping, and hypoxic vasoconstriction represent indirect signs of airway disease. Further, the increased collapsibility of the central airways can be depicted on dynamic examinations such as cine CT. As the morphologic changes of the airways in CT are limited to a small number of key morphologies imaging can—as often—be only one of the steps in a comprehensive clinical approach to a definitive diagnosis.

## 28.1.2.1
## Diseases with Airway Dilation

*Mounier-Kuhn syndrome* (tracheobronchomegaly) is a rare condition characterized by marked dilatation of the trachea and mainstem bronchi. It is associated with atrophy of cartilaginous, muscular, and elastic components of the tracheal wall, and may be seen in a variety of mostly congenital systemic diseases resulting in connective tissue abnormalities. CT findings include a thinning of the tracheal wall and a tracheal diameter of more than 3 cm at 2 cm above the aortic arch (Shin et al. 1988).

*Bronchiectasis* is defined pathologically as an abnormal permanent dilation of bronchi and bronchioles due to chronic necrotizing infection of these airways (Robbins et al. 1999). Based on gross morphologic appearance, Reid (1950) classified bronchiectasis into cylindrical, varicose, or cystic type. With the exception of infectious diseases, cystic fibrosis is probably the most common cause of clinically important bronchiectasis in the Caucasian population (Cartier et al. 1999). Bronchiectasis presents as local dilatation of the bronchi with or without bronchial wall thickening.

### 28.1.2.2
### Diseases with Airway Stenosis

Most tracheal stenoses are a complication of long-term tracheal intubation. Narrowing may occur at the stoma site after tracheostomy, at the level of the inflatable cuff, or, less commonly, where the tip of the tube has impinged on the tracheal mucosa (STARK 1995). Diffuse narrowing of the trachea or main bronchi may result from relapsing polychondritis, ulcerative colitis, amyloidosis, sarcoidosis, Wegener's granulomatosis, tracheopathia osteochondroplastica, and various infections including papillomatosis (MAROM et al. 2001). In the acute phase of these mostly diffuse inflammatory pathologies, the stenosis is due to wall thickening (mainly caused by edema). In the post-acute phase, the affected areas are likely to develop a stenosis without wall thickening due to fibrous scarring.

*Saber-Sheath trachea* is a fixed tracheal pathology in chronic obstructive pulmonary disease (COPD) patients, with a substantially decreased coronal diameter of the trachea, which is different from the excessive collapsibility of the trachea during expiration, which may also be encountered in COPD patients.

Further causes of airway narrowing are *neoplastic lesions*. They can exhibit a predilection for the one of the three compartments: lumen, wall, or surrounding soft tissue. For the trachea, 90% of the primary tumors in adults are malignant, mainly squamous cell carcinoma (55%) or adenoid cystic carcinoma (18–40%). Only 10% are benign neoplasms such as papilloma, true mucinous adenoma, hamartoma, fibroma, chondroma, leiomyoma, and granular cell myoblastoma. In the bronchi non-small cell lung cancer prevails (MAROM et al. 2001).

*External compression of the mediastinal airways* may occur due to enlarged lymph nodes or other mediastinal structures (most often thyroid goiter) or tumors (e.g., teratoma or thymoma). Intrapulmonary bronchial carcinoma or other tumors of more peripheral airways may also act as external compressors.

### 28.1.2.3
### Diseases with Wall Thickening of Visible Bronchi

Wall thickening of the bronchi is a consequence of acute or chronic inflammation and is a frequent abnormality

related to the severity of asthma (GRENIER et al. 1996). In addition, patients with chronic bronchitis or COPD may present with this airway abnormality. Since cystic fibrosis leads to a strong inflammatory response of the airways, bronchial wall thickening is also one of key features in this disease.

### 28.1.2.4
### Small Airways Disease

Pathologic visibility of air-filled airways within a 1.5-cm distance from the visceral pleura or presence of centrilobular nodular and V- or Y-shaped branching linear opacities (tree-in-bud pattern) are direct signs of small airways disease. The centrilobular opacities represent mucus-filled bronchioles with edematous, thickened walls. An indirect sign of bronchiolitis is air trapping, which leads to a mosaic attenuation pattern of the lung parenchyma, and represents the impaired ventilation of areas supplied by affected bronchioles (WAITCHES and STERN 2002). Small airways disease or bronchiolitis may be caused by a wide range of inflammatory and infectious processes including infection, cigarette smoking, connective tissue disease, toxic fume inhalation, drug reactions, graft-versus-host disease, and lung transplantation. Histopathologically, bronchiolitis can be subdivided into three main categories: cellular bronchiolitis, bronchiolitis obliterans with intraluminal polyps, and constrictive (obliterative) bronchiolitis.

### 28.1.2.5
### Diseases with Increased Collapsibility of the Central Airways

This feature is associated with the following diseases and conditions: COPD, relapsing polychondritis, history of prolonged intubation, or prior radiotherapy.

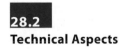

## 28.2
### Technical Aspects

### 28.2.1
### Basic Acquisition

Nowadays, a state-of-the-art MDCT of the thorax yields a volumetric dataset of images with an isotropic submillimeter resolution, which covers the complete thoracic cavity in a single breath hold. The combination of high spatial resolution and volumetric coverage of the lung is mandatory, as it results in 3D high-resolution CT (3D HRCT). For MPRs and other postprocessing tools, overlapping reconstruction is recommended. MDCT scanners with 16 or more detector rows routinely provide submillimeter collimation. The reconstructed slice thickness should match the collimation and the reconstruction increment and should be 80% of the slice thickness or less. Thin slices inherently carry a rather high level of image noise. Together with image reconstruction using a high-spatial-resolution kernel, noisy images might result. The trade-off between high-resolution images—what we are used to when looking at traditional HRCT—and noise represents a major challenge. The detailed assessment of small structures, such as peripheral airways in the lung parenchyma, normally requires a high-resolution kernel. At the same time, the performance of postprocessing, segmentation and quantification using dedicated software tools is often hampered by noisy, high-resolution images, and the use of images reconstructed with a regular soft tissue kernel might be more appropriate (MAYER et al. 2004). As the airways in the lung parenchyma are high-contrast structures, intermediate dose settings are appropriate. In general, a tube voltage of 120 kV together with a tube current between 50 and 150 mA is recommended (ZAPOROZHAN et al. 2006).

The isotropic datasets allow different postprocessing techniques to be used for evaluation and presentation purposes (GRENIER et al. 2003; FETITA et al. 2004). These techniques (which are described further on in more detail) encompass 2D MPRs, which allow to assess the central airways along their anatomical course and reduce the number of images to be analyzed (Fig. 28.1) as well as complex three dimensional segmentations and volume rendering (Fig. 28.2), which although a little more time-consuming, illustrate the important findings in a very intuitive way, e.g., a frontal view of the patient or a simulation of an intraoperative situs. Owing to this capability for continuous volumetric acquisitions during a single breath hold, MDCT has become the gold standard for visualization of intra- und extraluminal pathology of trachea and the bronchi. A presentation of overlapping thin slices in a cine mode allows identifying the bronchial divisions from the segmental origin down to the small airways. This viewing technique helps to identify intraluminal lesions, characterize the distribution pattern of any airway disease, and might also serve as a road map for the bronchoscopist. The perception of the anatomy of the tracheobronchial tree is further enhanced by MPRs as well as maximum (MIP) and especially minimum (minIP) intensity projections. Interactive viewing of MPRs and a workstation is the best

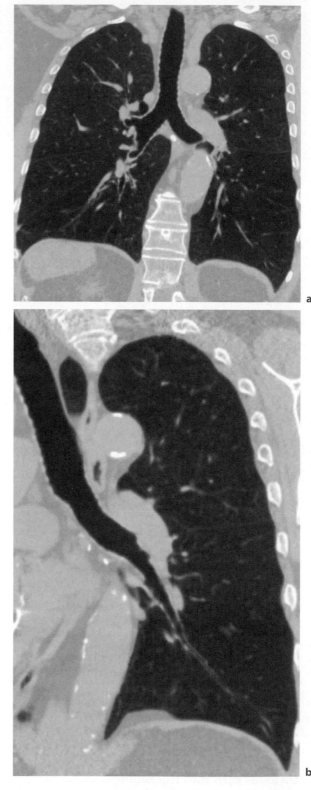

**Fig 28.1. a** Oblique MPR of central airways focused on the carina. **b** Curved MPR of the tracheobronchial tree following the course of the basal lateral segment bronchus (S9) on the left and one of its subsegmental branches

way to find the appropriate plan in which key features of the disease are displayed to confidently identify the main pattern of the disease, any associated findings, and the distribution of lesions relative to the airways. MPRs allow obviating the underestimation of the limits of the craniocaudal extension of a vertically oriented disease (such as tracheobronchial stenosis) from an axial slice only (GRENIER et al. 2002). Beyond the assessment of the extent of stenosis, they are of value in the treatment planning and follow-up as well as the quantification of pathological changes in obstructive lung disease.

The MIP technique may increase the detection and improve the visualization of the small centrilobular opacities in small airways disease (Fig. 28.3) (GRENIER et al. 2002; ZOMPATORI et al. 1997). This emphasizes the abnormal bronchioles and keeps the same high resolution as does a thin slice. Minimum intensity projections (minIP) are a simple form of volume rendering to visualize the tracheobronchial air column into a single viewing plane (Fig. 28.4). It is usually applied to a selected subvolume of the lung, which contains the airways under evaluation. The pixels encode the minimum voxel density encountered by each ray. Subsequently, an airway is visualized because the air contained within the tracheobronchial tree has a lower attenuation than has the surrounding pulmonary parenchyma. In clinical routine, minIPs are rarely used in the evaluation of the airways because numerous drawbacks have limited the technique's indications in the assessment of airway disease. In particular, the technique is susceptible to variable densities within the volume of interest and partial volume effects (GRENIER et al. 2002). 3D surface-rendering techniques as well as volume-rendering techniques are very helpful to enhance the visualization of the anatomy of the airway tree. CT bronchography consists in a volume-rendering technique applied at the level of the central airways after reconstruction of 3D images of the air column contained in the airways. Virtual bronchoscopy provides an internal analysis of the tracheobronchial walls and lumens, owing to a perspective-rendering algorithm that simulates an endoscopic view of the internal surface of the airways. In comparison to bronchoscopy, CT allows visualization beyond stenoses, which supports planning of endobronchial procedures (KAUCZOR et al. 1996). Thus, virtual bronchoscopy can be extremely helpful in a clinical setting, especially in planning transbronchial biopsies.

To assess the presence of expiratory obstruction, MDCT acquisitions in inspiration and expiration are recommended. For the acquisition, a low-mA protocol, 40–80 mA, is sufficient (ZHANG et al. 2003). Expiratory air trapping is the key finding to identify an obstruction of the small airways. At expiration, the cross-section of the lung will decrease, together with an increase of lung attenuation. Usually, gravity-dependent areas will show a greater increase in lung density during expiration than will non-gravity-dependent lung regions. At the same time, the cross-sectional area of the airways will also decrease. *Air trapping* is defined as the lack of an increase of lung attenuation as well as the decrease of the cross-sectional area of lung. Air trapping may be depicted in individual lobes in the dependent regions of the lung.

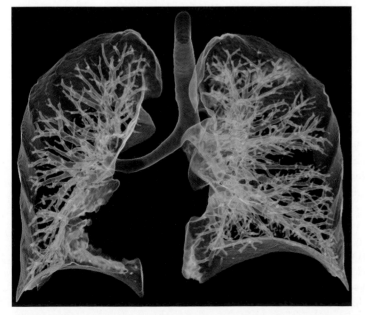

**Fig 28.2.** 3D volume rendering (VR) of the tracheobronchial tree based on a volumetric high-resolution MDCT acquisition (view from posterior to enhance the visibility of the left mainstem bronchus)

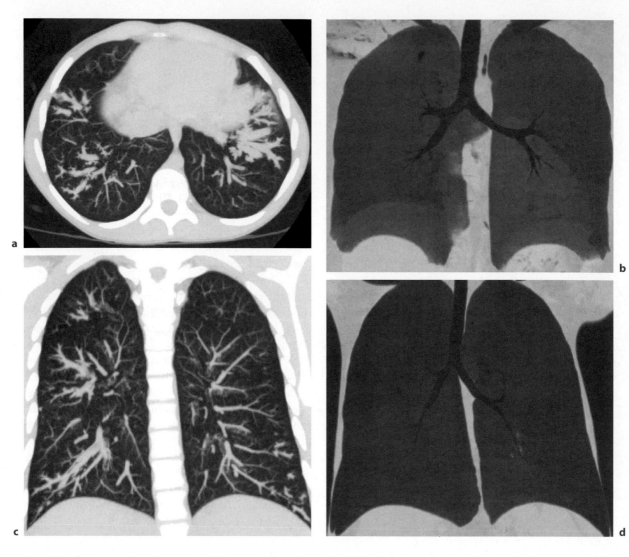

**Fig 28.3a,b.** Axial (**a**) and coronal (**b**) 1-cm thick MIPs showing widespread mucoid impaction, accentuated in the right lung as well as in the laterobasal aspect of the left lung

**Fig 28.4a,b.** minIP of the tracheobronchial tree in a healthy volunteer (**a**) and a CF patient (**b**). Due to bronchial wall thickening in CF, the depicted lumen caliber appears considerably reduced in all bronchi when compared with the healthy volunteer

In general, any air trapping involving less than 25% of the cross-sectional area of one lung at a single scan level can still be regarded as a physiological finding. Thus, physiological air trapping will be detected at an expiratory CT in up to 50% of asymptomatic subjects. The frequency of air trapping will increase with age and is associated with smoking. Some publications even suggest that the extent of air trapping is related to smoking history, independent from the current smoking habits. Air trapping has to be considered pathological when it affects a volume of lung equal or greater than a pulmonary segment and not limited to the superior segment of the lower lobe. Abnormal air trapping is a hallmark

of small airways disease, but it may also be seen in any other type of bronchial obstruction or in patients with asthma, COPD, or emphysema (KAUCZOR et al. 2000).

## 28.2.2
## Advanced Acquisition Techniques

Technically, the conventional assessment of air trapping is based on a CT acquired in a breath hold after deep expiration. Such post-expiratory scans are invariably obtained in conjunction with a routine examination obtained at end inspiration. Each post-expiratory scan is compared with its corresponding inspiratory scan to detect air trapping. In addition, significant work has been performed to elucidate the potential role of dynamic CT acquisitions during continuous expiration instead of collecting data at a fixed level during expiration only. Such acquisitions require high temporary resolution and are easily performed at a single axial level. CT scans acquired during continuous expiration are much more sensitive to diagnose bronchial collapse or air trapping (Fig. 28.5). The improvement by dynamic CT can be explained by the fact that patients have much less difficulty performing an active continuous exhalation instead of maintaining the residual volume after an exhalation for a breath hold period of up to 20 s.

However, modern MDCT scanners can also be used to generate volumetric 4D CT data, using a spirometric curve as a signal for retrospective gating. This technology is a recent translation from ECG-triggered CT scans of the heart to respiratory triggered scans of the lung parenchyma (Ley et al. 2006).

New techniques, such as DE CT, allow for a detailed assessment of the distribution of iodine as presented by the contrast agent. For CT of the lung, the dual-energy option will provide the chance to assess pulmonary perfusion from a single contrast-enhanced CT scan. From such a dataset, the virtual nonenhanced image as well as an iodine distribution image can be reconstructed. Color-coded superimposition of this information will then demonstrate the distribution of iodine given as an intravenous bolus of a contrast agent. This is a direct representation of the distribution of lung perfusion with a linear relationship between the concentration of iodine and the density measured by CT. Due to the reflex of hypoxic vasoconstriction, perfusion defects will match ventilation defects due to airway disease. As such, the functional impairment in airway disease can be assessed. The severity can be calculated as the lung volume affected by hypoxic vasoconstriction.

## Evaluation

### 28.3.1
### Visual Evaluation

Throughout the lung, the bronchi and pulmonary arteries run and branch together. The ratio of the size of the bronchus to its adjacent pulmonary artery is widely used as a criterion for detection of abnormal bronchial dilatation. In a healthy lung, it should be at the same at any

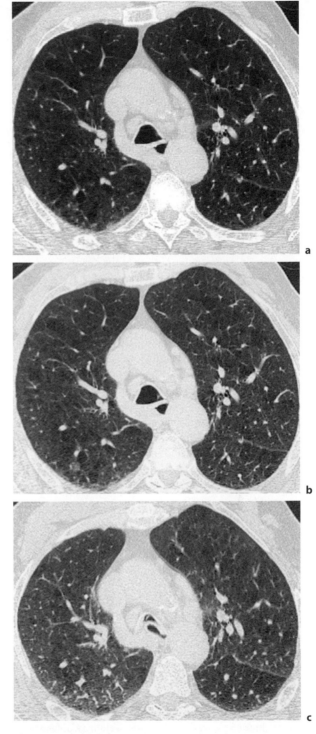

**Fig 28.5a–c.** Excessive expiratory collapse of the trachea in a patient with advanced COPD (**a** at suspended full inspiration, **b** at suspended full expiration, and **c** cine CT during shallow respiration, expiratory phase)

level with the mean ratio being 0.98±0.14 (with a wide range of 0.53 to 1.39) (Kim et al. 1995). The ratio of the internal luminal diameter of the bronchus to the diameter of its accompanying pulmonary artery has been estimated for the healthy subjects to be 0.62±0.13 (Kim et al. 1997). CT signs of bronchiectasis are nontapering or flaring of bronchi, dilatation of the bronchi with or without bronchial wall thickening (signet-ring sign), mucus-filled dilated bronchi (flame-and-blob sign), plugged and thickened centrilobular bronchioles (tree-in-bud sign), crowding of bronchi with associated volume loss, and areas of decreased attenuation reflecting small airways obliteration (Hansell et al. 2005). The bronchiectases are categorized in cylindrical (mild bronchial dilatation, regular outline of the airway), varicose (greater bronchial dilatation, accompanied by local constrictions resulting in an irregular outline of the airway), and cystic or saccular (ballooned appearance of the airways, reduced number of bronchial divisions) type.

Since normal centrilobular bronchioles are not visible at thin-section CT, the recognition of air-filled airways in the lung periphery usually means that the airways are both dilated and thick walled.

Small airways disease on CT can be categorized into visible and indirect patterns of the disease. The tree-in-bud sign reflects the presence of dilated centrilobular bronchioles with lumina that are impacted with mucus, fluid, or pus; it is often associated with peribronchiolar inflammation (Webb 2006). Cicatricial scarring of many bronchioles results in the indirect sign of patchy density differences of the lung parenchyma, reflecting areas of hypoventilation and air trapping, as well as subsequent hypoperfusion (mosaic perfusion).

## 28.3.2
## Quantitative Evaluation

The dramatically increased acquisition velocity, which reduces motion artifacts, as well as the increasing spatial resolution (especially $z$-axis resolution), open the door to quantitative evaluation of airway dimensions down to subsegmental bronchial level. Volumetric CT allows quantitative indices of bronchial airway morphology to be calculated, including lumen area, airway inner and outer diameters, wall thicknesses, wall area, airway segment lengths, airway taper indices, and airway branching patterns. The complexity and size of the bronchial tree render manual measurement methods impractical and inaccurate (Venkatraman et al. 2006). The use of curved MPR from 3D-CT datasets is a solution to accurately measure airway dimensions regardless of their course with respect to the transaxial CT scan. Airway tree segmentation can be performed manually, which, however, is tedious and extremely time-consuming (Aykac et al. 2003). Based on the volumetric data sets, sophisticated postprocessing tools will automatically segment the airways down to the sixth generation (Mayer et al. 2004). This allows for visualization of the tracheobronchial tree without any overlap by surrounding parenchyma, as well as for the reproducible and reliable measurements of the segmented airways.

The simplest segmentation method used a single threshold (cutoff) of pixel values in Hounsfield units. Pixels with Hounsfield unit values lower than the threshold were assigned to the lumen (air), while surrounding pixels with Hounsfield unit values higher than the threshold were assigned to the airway wall or other surrounding tissue. Based on this analysis, the 3D region–growing algorithm extracts all voxels that are definitely airway. However, using a simple global threshold often fails in detecting the wall of smaller airways; thereby such tools often require manual editing. To enhance this basic segmentation process some additional (add-on) algorithms were developed, i.e., based on fuzzy connectivity (Tschirren et al. 2005) or by wave propagation from the border voxels (Mayer et al. 2004). The luminal segmentation result is condensed to the centerline (or skeletization) running exactly in the center of the airway. These centerline points are the starting points for the airway wall detection and quantification. Approaches include methods based on the estimation of the full width at half-maximum (FWHM), brightness-area product and pixel-intensity gradient (Tschirren et al. 2005; Reinhardt et al. 1997; Saba et al. 2003; Nakano et al. 2005; Berger et al. 2005). The most frequently reported method is based on the FWHM approach (deJong et al. 2005a) that is explained in more detail: by identifying the lumen center, the scheme measures pixel values along radial rays casting from the lumen center outward beyond the airway wall in all directions. Along each ray, the boundary between the lumen and wall is determined by a pixel whose Hounsfield unit value is half the range between the local minimum in the lumen and the local maximum in the airway wall, whereas the boundary between the wall and lung parenchyma is determined by a pixel whose HU value is half the range between the local maximum in the wall and the local minimum in the parenchyma. Along each radial ray, these two FWHM pixels are used as the inner and outer (beginning and ending) pixels of the airway wall. All pixels inside the first FWHM pixel are assigned to a lumen, and all pixels outside the second FWHM pixel are assigned to the lung parenchyma.

## Diseases

### 28.4.1
### Tracheobronchomalacia

A common indication for imaging of the trachea is suspected *tracheobronchomalacia* (TBM). A definition used by many authors in the radiological as well as in the bronchoscopic field refers to TBM in case of a 50% decrease of the cross-sectional area (CSA) of the trachea during forced expiration (LORING et al. 2007). Excessive expiratory collapse of the trachea can be caused by two pathological mechanisms, either by weakness of the supporting airway cartilage or by an excessive invagination of the posterior membranous segment of the trachea. An in-depth review of this issue shows that these are distinct clinicopathological entities, which may or may not coincide. Following this review, only excessive collapsibility involving weakness of airway cartilage should be addressed as TBM, whereas the term excessive dynamic airway collapse (EDAC) should be used in case of excessive invagination of the posterior wall of the trachea without signs of cartilaginous involvement (MURGU and COLT 2006). However, most of the published work in the radiological literature does not separate these two mechanisms and mostly uses the term TBM for both mechanisms leading to expiratory collapse of the trachea. The definition mentioned above might be considered as a greatest common divisor of the two clinicopathological entities.

The acquired form of excessive expiratory collapse can be considered as one of common causes of chronic cough, expiratory dyspnea, and recurrent respiratory infections. Since these symptoms are highly unspecific and TBM/EDAC escapes detection on routine clinical and imaging investigations, it is considered a highly underdiagnosed condition. The prevalence varies from 23% in patients with chronic bronchitis (JOKINEN et al. 1976) over 10% in patients referred for evaluation of pulmonary embolism (HASEGAWA et al. 2003) to 4.5% in a large retrospectively reviewed bronchoscopic series (JOKINEN et al. 1977). Conditions leading to acquired TBM/EDAC include COPD, relapsing polychondritis, as well as a history of prolonged intubation or prior radiotherapy (CARDEN et al. 2005).

Since the pathology involves the dynamic process of expiration, TBM/EDAC cannot be sufficiently depicted by static end-inspiratory or end-expiratory CT scans alone. A paired inspiratory–expiratory investigation is the absolute minimum diagnostic approach. Dynamic examination protocols have been shown to be massively superior over breath-hold acquisitions for determination of TBM (HEUSSEL et al. 2001; BARONI et al. 2005). Dynamic imaging also resulted in a significant number of changes of therapy. At least two different protocols have been proposed.

The first one includes a dynamic expiratory spiral scan (40 mA, 0.5 s gantry rotation time, 120 kVp, 2.5-mm collimation, pitch equivalent of 1.5) during a forced expiration maneuver (BARONI et al. 2005). This scan covers the trachea and the main bronchi in the region between the low cervical region and the level 2 cm below the carina, and is acquired in the craniocaudal direction. Due to a naturally given high contrast between airway lumen and wall, low-dose techniques can be used without compromising the assessment of suspected TBM/EDAC (ZHANG et al. 2003). The examination protocol proposed by HEUSSEL et al. (2001) includes a temporally resolved scan (no table feed, cine CT; no interscan delay, reconstruction interval 100 ms.) over the region of suspected TBM/EDAC in shallow respiration. This work published in 2001 was performed on a four-detector-row CT with consecutively small spatial coverage. Modern 64-slice CT offer the possibility of simultaneous imaging a region with a craniocaudal extension of 3 cm with the same scan technique (BOISELLE et al. 2006).

The evaluation is two-fold, (1) evaluation of the degree of collapse, and (2) analysis of the shape change of the trachea. For this purpose, the dynamically acquired images are compared with those acquired at suspended end inspiration. The degree of collapse can be evaluated visually or better by calculating the change of the CSA with manual or semiautomatic segmentation tools for the tracheal lumen. Using the same diagnostic criterion for TBM/EDAC as bronchoscopy (greater than 50% reduction in CSA of the airway lumen at expiration), CT was shown to have similar accuracy when compared with invasive bronchoscopy (ZHANG et al. 2003; GILKESON et al. 2001; SUN and BOISELLE 2007). The reduction of the tracheal lumen is associated with an obvious change of the shape, which can be oval or crescentic. The crescentic form is due to the bowing of posterior membrane of the trachea (BOISELLE et al. 2006).

Concerning the therapeutic relevance of diagnosing TBM/EDAC, a short-term follow-up study of patients with severe TBM/EDAC undergoing central airway stabilization with silicone stents concluded that the intervention markedly improved dyspnea, health-related quality of life, and functional status in these patients (ERNST et al. 2007).

### 28.4.2
### COPD

COPD is characterized by airflow limitation that is not fully reversible. For diagnosis and severity assessment, pulmonary function testing (PFT) is the accepted and standardized workhorse, providing quantitative measures for forced expiration volume in 1 s ($FEV_1$), $FEV_1$/FVC (forced vital capacity), diffusing capacity for carbon monoxide ($DL_{CO}$) and others. As COPD is a broad disease entity with a functional definition, COPD obviously comprises several subtypes, which primarily can be related to the major site of involvement: the airways, mainly obstructive bronchiolitis, and the parenchyma, i.e., emphysema, and then further differentiated. PFT as a global measure is unable to categorize these subtypes. With the increasing number of therapeutic options in COPD, particularly when it is advanced, there is a high demand for a noninvasive imaging test to identify different phenotypes of the disease according to structural and functional changes and provide the regional information of such changes in order to target therapies accordingly. For phenotyping, a precise characterization of the different components of the disease, such as inflammation, hyperinflation, etc., is highly desirable for selecting the appropriate therapy. CT is a long-standing player in this field, with emphasis on structural imaging of lung parenchyma and airways. Several pathological studies have shown that a major site of airway obstruction in patients with COPD is in airways smaller than 2 mm in internal diameter (Hogg et al. 2004). The 2-mm airways are located between the 4th and the 14th generation of the tracheobronchial tree. Airflow limitation is closely associated with the severity of luminal occlusion by inflammatory exudates and thickening of the airway walls due to remodeling (Hogg 2006). Severe peripheral airflow obstruction can also affect the proximal airways from subsegmental bronchi to trachea. Cartilage abnormalities are also frequently present in COPD, associating atrophy and scarring. This deficiency of bronchial cartilage induces alternated narrowing and dilatation of the airways in advanced disease. This explains both loss of normal proximal to distal tapering of the airway lumen and the presence of bronchiectasis in COPD patients. In some COPD patients, the cartilage deficiency also involves the trachea and the main bronchi. The cartilage deficiency is also responsible for prominent collapse of airway lumen occurring at maximum forced expiratory maneuver (see Sect. 28.4.1, Fig. 28.5). On expiratory CT scans, also the lumen of segmental or subsegmental bronchi may collapse exaggeratedly, particularly in the lower lobes where the wall deficiency is the most apparent.

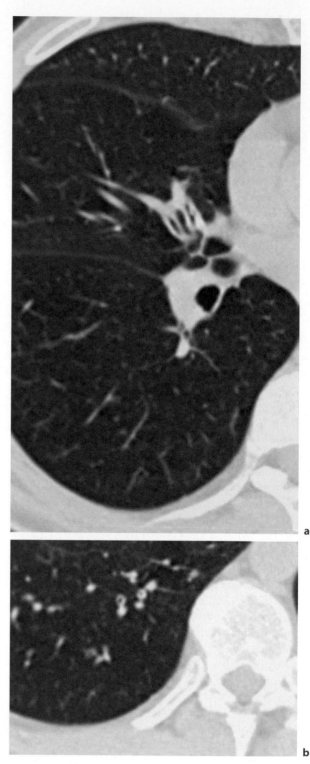

a

b

**Fig. 28.6a,b.** Bronchial wall thickening of subsegmental bronchi in the airway predominant phenotype of COPD

As a powerful adjunct to inspiratory scans, expiratory acquisitions reveal changes in lung attenuation related to air trapping and pulmonary blood volume. They also illustrate regional volumetric changes, providing deeper insights into local hyperinflation and expiratory obstruction (ZAPOROZHAN et al. 2005). Since the severity of emphysema, as evaluated by CT, does not necessarily show a very good correlation with $FEV_1$ (ZAPOROZHAN et al. 2005; BALDI et al. 2001), small airways disease appears to contribute more significantly to the airflow limitation in COPD. Regional air trapping reflects the retention of excess gas at any stage of respiration as an indirect sign of peripheral airway obstruction. It is best detected on expiratory CT as areas with abnormally low attenuation (BERGER et al. 2003). Air trapping is highly unspecific, as it occurs under physiological conditions as well as in a variety of lung diseases, including emphysema, bronchiectasis, bronchiolitis obliterans, and asthma (HANSELL 2001).

Using HRCT images visual assessment, bronchial wall thickness and the extent of emphysema were the strongest independent determinants of a decreased $FEV_1$ in patients with COPD and mild to extensive emphysema (AZIZ et al. 2005). However, visual assessment of bronchial wall thickening and bronchial dilatation is highly subjective and poorly reproducible (Figs. 28.6, 28.7) (PARK et al. 1997). The quantitative analysis can be performed by manual delineation of bronchial contours (ORLANDI et al. 2005). NAKANO et al. (2000) were the first to perform computer-assisted automated quantitative measurements of airway wall thickening in COPD patients, and reported a significant correlation between wall thickness of the apical right upper lobe bronchus and $FEV_1$% predicted. Due to technical limitations of HRCT, neither the generation of the bronchus measured could be determined nor could measurements be performed exactly perpendicular to the axis of the bronchus. Other groups demonstrated that the normalized airway wall thickness was larger in smokers with COPD than it was in smokers or nonsmokers without COPD (BERGER et al. 2005); however, the measurements were restricted to bronchi running almost perpendicular to the transverse CT section. Using dedicated software tools for 3D quantification of bronchial parameters, it is possible to measure airway dimensions accurately and reproducibly. Such measurements revealed high correlations between airway luminal area, and to a lesser extent for wall thickening, with $FEV_1$% predicted in patients with COPD. The correlation actually improved as airway size decreased from the third ($r = 0.6$ for airway luminal area and $r = 0.43$ for wall thickening) to sixth bronchial generation ($r = 0.73$ and $r = 0.55$, respectively) (HASEGAWA et al. 2006).

### 28.4.3
### Cystic Fibrosis

Cystic Fibrosis (CF) is an autosomal recessive disorder caused by mutations of a gene located on the long arm of chromosome 7. It codes for CFTR (CF transmembrane regulator protein), which functions as an anion channel. The impaired CFTR function causes aberrations of volume and ion composition of airway surface fluid, leading to viscous secretions, with the consequence of bacterial colonization, chronic lung infection, airway obstruction, and consecutive destruction of the lung parenchyma (PUDERBACH et al. 2007). Despite improved understanding of the underlying pathophysiology and introduction of new therapies, CF is still the most frequent life-shortening inherited disease in the Caucasian population. Advantages in knowledge and medical care resulted in a dramatic increase of the life span for these patients. The median of survival in CF patients in Germany is up to 36.8 years. CF affects most body systems, but the majority of morbidity and mortality in CF patients is due to lung disease.

As life expectancy is limited by pulmonary complications, repeated imaging of the chest is required. The standard radiological tools for imaging of the chest are chest X-ray and CT. CT has been shown to be more sensitive to early CF lung disease than PFT is, likely due to the regional nature of the information obtained. The

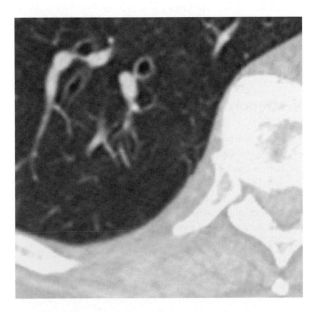

**Fig. 28.7.** Bronchial dilation of subsegmental bronchi without wall thickening, also typical for the airway predominant phenotype of COPD

structural changes of CF lung disease include bronchial wall thickening, mucus plugging, bronchiectasis, air fluid levels, consolidation, and segmental/lobar destruction (Fig. 28.8) (PUDERBACH et al. 2006). The better sensitivity of CT in the detection of lung damage beyond that of chest radiography has long been recognized (BHALLA et al. 1991; MAFFESSANTI et al. 1996). Thin-section CT scoring systems have frequently been used to quantify airway abnormalities (BHALLA et al. 1991; HELBICH et al. 1999; DEJONG et al. 2004). All of these scoring systems rely on composite scores to enable subjective estimation of features on CT scans. A strong correlation between the $FEV_1$ value and the CT scoring system has been reported (HELBICH et al. 1999; DEJONG et al. 2004). However, this approach was limited to patients with mild lung disease in whom the $FEV_1$ value usually is normal despite the presence of abnormal airways and an exaggerated inflammatory response (KAHN et al. 1995; TIDDENS 2002). This reflects that in case of mild disease, the maintenance of normal PFT results does not necessarily indicate a lack of lung damage (BRODY 2004). It was reported that thin-section CT scoring systems may be more sensitive than the PFT in the detection of disease progression (DEJONG et al. 2004).

Quantification of the structure of the lung includes evaluation of the parenchyma and the airway walls. Large airway wall abnormalities can be assessed by airway wall measurement, and small airway and parenchymal abnormalities can be assessed by changes in lung parenchymal attenuation or air trapping. (BRODY et al. 2005). The first quantitative airway analysis was performed on HRCT images. Thicker walls and dilated airways were reported for infants and young children with CF when compared with normal infants (LONG et al. 2004). The ratio between airway lumen area and the area of the accompanying pulmonary artery as well as between airway wall area and the area of the accompanying pulmonary artery was increased, and the airway walls were thickened (DEJONG et al. 2005b). Although lung function did not change significantly over a 2-year follow-up period, there were significant changes in quantitative airway wall thickening (DEJONG et al. 2005b). Due to technical limitations of HRCT as pointed out above, the acquisition of volumetric datasets with subsequent quantification in 3D obviously makes sense. MONTAUDON et al. (2007) compared bronchial measurements obtained with 3D quantitative thin-section CT with those obtained with thin-section CT scores in the assessment of the severity of CF. Wall area and wall thickness were assessed with dedicated software tools and were valuable indexes for determining the severity of airway disease in patients with CF.

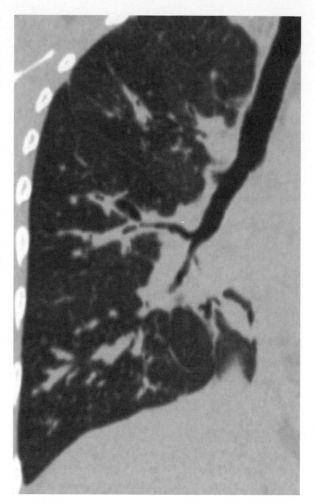

**Fig. 28.8.** Curved MPR of a segmental bronchus in CF showing bronchial wall thickening, mucoid impaction, and bronchiectasis

# References

Aykac D, Hoffman EA, McLennan G, Reinhardt JM (2003) Segmentation and analysis of the human airway tree from three-dimensional X-ray CT images. IEEE Trans Med Imaging 22:940–950

Aziz ZA, Wells AU, Desai SR et al. (2005) Functional impairment in emphysema: contribution of airway abnormalities and distribution of parenchymal disease. AJR Am J Roentgenol 185:1509–1515

Bakir B, Terzibasioglu E (2007) Images in clinical medicine. Tracheal bronchus. N Engl J Med 357:1744

Baldi S, Miniati M, Bellina CR et al. (2001) Relationship between extent of pulmonary emphysema by high-resolution computed tomography and lung elastic recoil in patients with chronic obstructive pulmonary disease. Am J Respir Crit Care Med 164:585–589

Baroni RH, Feller-Kopman D, Nishino M et al. (2005) Tracheobronchomalacia: comparison between end-expiratory and dynamic expiratory CT for evaluation of central airway collapse. Radiology 235:635–641

Berger P, Laurent F, Begueret H et al. (2003) Structure and function of small airways in smokers: relationship between air trapping at CT and airway inflammation. Radiology 228:85–94

Berger P, Perot V, Desbarats P, Tunon-de-Lara JM, Marthan R, Laurent F (2005) Airway wall thickness in cigarette smokers: quantitative thin-section CT assessment. Radiology 235:1055–1064

Bhalla M, Turcios N, Aponte V et al. (1991) Cystic fibrosis: scoring system with thin-section CT. Radiology 179:783–788

Boiselle PM, Lee KS, Lin S, Raptopoulos V (2006) Cine CT during coughing for assessment of tracheomalacia: preliminary experience with 64-MDCT. AJR Am J Roentgenol 187:175–177

Brody AS (2004) Scoring systems for CT in cystic fibrosis: who cares? Radiology 231:296–298

Brody AS, Tiddens HA, Castile RG et al. (2005) Computed tomography in the evaluation of cystic fibrosis lung disease. Am J Respir Crit Care Med 172:1246–1252

Carden KA, Boiselle PM, Waltz DA, Ernst A (2005) Tracheomalacia and tracheobronchomalacia in children and adults: an in-depth review. Chest 127:984–1005

Cartier Y, Kavanagh PV, Johkoh T, Mason AC, Muller NL (1999) Bronchiectasis: accuracy of high-resolution CT in the differentiation of specific diseases. AJR Am J Roentgenol 173:47–52

deJong PA, Ottink MD, Robben SG et al. (2004) Pulmonary disease assessment in cystic fibrosis: comparison of CT scoring systems and value of bronchial and arterial dimension measurements. Radiology 231:434–439

deJong PA, Muller NL, Pare PD, Coxson HO (2005a) Computed tomographic imaging of the airways: relationship to structure and function. Eur Respir J 26:140–152

deJong PA, Nakano Y, Hop WC et al. (2005b) Changes in airway dimensions on computed tomography scans of children with cystic fibrosis. Am J Respir Crit Care Med 172:218–224

Ernst A, Majid A, Feller-Kopman D et al. (2007) Airway stabilization with silicone stents for treating adult tracheobronchomalacia: a prospective observational study. Chest 132:609–616

Fetita CI, Preteux F, Beigelman-Aubry C, Grenier P (2004) Pulmonary airways: 3-D reconstruction from multi-detector-row CT and clinical investigation. IEEE Trans Med Imaging 23:1353–1364

Gilkeson RC, Ciancibello LM, Hejal RB, Montenegro HD, Lange P (2001) Tracheobronchomalacia: dynamic airway evaluation with multidetector CT. AJR Am J Roentgenol 176:205–210

Grenier P, Mourey-Gerosa I, Benali K et al. (1996) Abnormalities of the airways and lung parenchyma in asthmatics: CT observations in 50 patients and inter- and intraobserver variability. Eur Radiol 6:199–206

Grenier PA, Beigelman-Aubry C, Fetita C, Preteux F, Brauner MW, Lenoir S (2002) New frontiers in CT imaging of airway disease. Eur Radiol 12:1022–1044

Grenier PA, Beigelman-Aubry C, Fetita C, Martin-Bouyer Y (2003) Multidetector-row CT of the airways. Semin Roentgenol 38:146–157

Hansell DM (2001) Small airways diseases: detection and insights with computed tomography. Eur Respir J 17:1294–1313

Hansell DM, Armstrong P, Lynch DA, McAdams HP (eds) (2005) Imaging of disease of the chest, 4th edn. Elsevier, London

Hasegawa I, Boiselle PM, Raptopoulos V, Hatabu H (2003) Tracheomalacia incidentally detected on CT pulmonary angiography of patients with suspected pulmonary embolism. AJR Am J Roentgenol 181:1505–1509

Hasegawa M, Nasuhara Y, Onodera Y et al. (2006) Airflow limitation and airway dimensions in chronic obstructive pulmonary disease. Am J Respir Crit Care Med 173:1309–1315

Helbich TH, Heinz-Peer G, Eichler I et al. (1999) Cystic fibrosis: CT assessment of lung involvement in children and adults. Radiology 213:537–544

Heussel CP, Hafner B, Lill J, Schreiber W, Thelen M, Kauczor HU (2001) Paired inspiratory/expiratory spiral CT and continuous respiration cine CT in the diagnosis of tracheal instability. Eur Radiol 11:982–989

Hogg JC (2006) State of the art. Bronchiolitis in chronic obstructive pulmonary disease. Proc Am Thorac Soc 3:489–493

Hogg JC, Chu F, Utokaparch S et al. (2004) The nature of small-airway obstruction in chronic obstructive pulmonary disease. N Engl J Med 350:2645–2653

Jokinen K, Palva T, Nuutinen J (1976) Chronic bronchitis. A bronchologic evaluation. ORL J Otorhinolaryngol Relat Spec 38:178–186

Jokinen K, Palva T, Sutinen S, Nuutinen J (1977) Acquired tracheobronchomalacia. Ann Clin Res 9:52–57

Kauczor HU, Wolcke B, Fischer B, Mildenberger P, Lorenz J, Thelen M (1996) Three-dimensional helical CT of the tracheobronchial tree: evaluation of imaging protocols and assessment of suspected stenoses with bronchoscopic correlation. AJR Am J Roentgenol 167:419–424

Kauczor HU, Hast J, Heussel CP, Schlegel J, Mildenberger P, Thelen M (2000) Focal airtrapping at expiratory high-resolution CT: comparison with pulmonary function tests. Eur Radiol 10:1539–1546

Khan TZ, Wagener JS, Bost T, Martinez J, Accurso FJ, Riches DW (1995) Early pulmonary inflammation in infants with cystic fibrosis. Am J Respir Crit Care Med 151:1075–1082

Kim JS, Muller NL, Park CS et al. (1997) Bronchoarterial ratio on thin section CT: comparison between high altitude and sea level. J Comput Assist Tomogr 21:306–311

Kim SJ, Im JG, Kim IO et al. (1995) Normal bronchial and pulmonary arterial diameters measured by thin section CT. J Comput Assist Tomogr 19:365–369

Ley S, Ley-Zaporozhan J, Unterhinninghofen R et al. (2006) Investigation of retrospective respiratory gating techniques for acquisition of thin-slice 4D-multidetector-computed tomography (MDCT) of the lung: feasibility study in a large animal model. Exp Lung Res 32:395–412

Long FR, Williams RS, Castile RG (2004) Structural airway abnormalities in infants and young children with cystic fibrosis. J Pediatr 144:154–161

Loring SH, O'Donnell C R, Feller-Kopman DJ, Ernst A (2007) Central airway mechanics and flow limitation in acquired tracheobronchomalacia. Chest 131:1118–1124

Maffessanti M, Candusso M, Brizzi F, Piovesana F (1996) Cystic fibrosis in children: HRCT findings and distribution of disease. J Thorac Imaging 11:27–38

Marom EM, Goodman PC, McAdams HP (2001) Focal abnormalities of the trachea and main bronchi. AJR Am J Roentgenol 176:707–711

Mayer D, Bartz D, Fischer J et al. (2004) Hybrid segmentation and virtual bronchoscopy based on CT images. Acad Radiol 11:551–565

Montaudon M, Berger P, Cangini-Sacher A et al. (2007) Bronchial measurement with three-dimensional quantitative thin-section CT in patients with cystic fibrosis. Radiology 242:573–581

Murgu SD, Colt HG (2006) Tracheobronchomalacia and excessive dynamic airway collapse. Respirology 11:388–406

Nakano Y, Muro S, Sakai H, et al. (2000) Computed tomographic measurements of airway dimensions and emphysema in smokers. Correlation with lung function. Am J Respir Crit Care Med 162:1102–1108

Nakano Y, Wong JC, de Jong PA, et al. (2005) The prediction of small airway dimensions using computed tomography. Am J Respir Crit Care Med 171:142–146

Orlandi I, Moroni C, Camiciottoli G, et al. (2005) Chronic obstructive pulmonary disease: thin-section CT measurement of airway wall thickness and lung attenuation. Radiology 234:604–610

Park JW, Hong YK, Kim CW, Kim DK, Choe KO, Hong CS (1977) High-resolution computed tomography in patients with bronchial asthma: correlation with clinical features, pulmonary functions and bronchial hyperresponsiveness. J Investig Allergol Clin Immunol 7:186–192

Puderbach M, Eichinger M, Gahr J, et al. (2007) Proton MRI appearance of cystic fibrosis: Comparison to CT. Eur Radiol 17:716–724

Puderbach M, Eichinger M, Haeselbarth J et al. (2007) Assessment of morphological MRI for pulmonary changes in cystic fibrosis (CF) patients: comparison to thin-section CT and chest x-ray. Invest Radiol 42:715–725

Reid LM (1950) Reduction in bronchial subdivision in bronchiectasis. Thorax 5:233–247

Reinhardt JM, D'Souza ND, Hoffman EA (1997) Accurate measurement of intrathoracic airways. IEEE Trans Med Imaging 16:820–827

Robbins SL, Cotran RS, Kumar V, Collins T (eds) (1999) Pathologic basis of disease, 6th edn. Saunders, Philadelphia

Saba OI, Hoffman EA, Reinhardt JM (2003) Maximizing quantitative accuracy of lung airway lumen and wall measures obtained from X-ray CT imaging. J Appl Physiol 95:1063–1075

Shin MS, Jackson RM, Ho KJ (1988) Tracheobronchomegaly (Mounier-Kuhn syndrome): CT diagnosis. AJR Am J Roentgenol 150:777–779

Standring S (ed) (2004) Gray's anatomy: the anatomical basis of clinical practice, 39th edn. Elsevier, Edinburgh

Stark P (1995) Imaging of tracheobronchial injuries. J Thorac Imaging 10:206–219

Sun M, Ernst A, Boiselle PM (2007) MDCT of the central airways: comparison with bronchoscopy in the evaluation of complications of endotracheal and tracheostomy tubes. J Thorac Imaging 22:136–142

Tiddens HA (2002) Detecting early structural lung damage in cystic fibrosis. Pediatr Pulmonol 34:228–231

Tschirren J, Hoffman EA, McLennan G, Sonka M (2005) Segmentation and quantitative analysis of intrathoracic airway trees from computed tomography images. Proc Am Thorac Soc 2:484–487, 503–484

Venkatraman R, Raman R, Raman B et al. (2006) Fully automated system for three-dimensional bronchial morphology analysis using volumetric multidetector computed tomography of the chest. J Digit Imaging 19:132–139

Waitches GM, Stern EJ (2002) High-resolution CT of peripheral airways diseases. Radiol Clin North Am 40:21–29

Webb WR (2006) Thin-section CT of the secondary pulmonary lobule: anatomy and the image—the 2004 Fleischner lecture. Radiology 239:322–338

Weibel ER, Gomez DM (1962) Architecture of the human lung. Use of quantitative methods establishes fundamental relations between size and number of lung structures. Science 137:577–585

Zaporozhan J, Ley S, Eberhardt R et al. (2005) Paired inspiratory/expiratory volumetric thin-slice CT scan for emphysema analysis: comparison of different quantitative evaluations and pulmonary function test. Chest 128:3212–3220

Zaporozhan J, Ley S, Weinheimer O et al. (2006) Multi-detector CT of the chest: influence of dose onto quantitative evaluation of severe emphysema: a simulation study. J Comput Assist Tomogr 30:460–468

Zhang J, Hasegawa I, Feller-Kopman D, Boiselle PM (2003) 2003 AUR Memorial Award. Dynamic expiratory volumetric CT imaging of the central airways: comparison of standard-dose and low-dose techniques. Acad Radiol 10:719–724

Zompatori M, Poletti V, Rimondi MR, Battaglia M, Carvelli P, Maraldi F (1997) Imaging of small airways disease, with emphasis on high resolution computed tomography. Monaldi Arch Chest Dis 52:242–248

# Oncology

# Liver Tumors

CHRISTOPH J. ZECH

## ABSTRACT

With the introduction of multidetector CT (MDCT), *multiphasic examinations* of the liver can be performed without compromise with regard to spatial or temporal resolution. However, an adequate *examination technique* is still critical for sensitive detection and specific characterization of focal liver lesions. The limiting factor for *lesion detection* in CT is usually the *contrast* and not just the *geometrical resolution*. For good lesion detection results, a reasonable balance of both these parameters has to be chosen. The criteria for the *characterization of focal liver lesions* are derived from their behavior and degree of contrast agent enhancement in the different *vascular phases of liver CT*. For a valid characterization, usually at least two different phases are mandatory, so that changes of enhancement over time (e.g., wash-in and wash-out of contrast agent) can be appreciated. Although MR still has distinctive advantages for dedicated liver examinations, the fast and reliable approach of MDCT makes it an indispensable modality for imaging of liver pathologies.

## 29.1
## Introduction

Imaging of patients with liver tumors is an important and highly relevant field of diagnostic imaging, due to the large number of patients with diffuse or focal liver disease (e.g., the increasing number of patients with viral hepatitis) or with at least potential involvement of the liver (e.g., patients with extrahepatic malignancies such as breast cancer or colorectal cancer). The aim of

C. J. ZECH, MD
Department of Clinical Radiology, Ludwig-Maximilians-University of Munich, Munich University Hospitals, Marchioninistrasse 15, 81377 Munich, Germany

imaging has to be an accurate assessment of number, size, and localization of malignant liver lesions. Moreover, various benign liver lesions have to be differentiated from malignant lesions, since these benign entities seldom need treatment. For malignant lesions, therapeutic decisions usually depend strongly on the extent of liver involvement–a limited number of lesions can be surgically resected or treated with local ablative therapies, whereas multifocal lesions require a different approach including systemic chemotherapy, and various treatment options including Y-90 radioembolization.

Depending on the logistics within the hospital and the clinical background, several modalities can be selected for imaging patients with liver tumors. CT has gained high importance in this setting, since it combines wide availability and fast access with high diagnostic accuracy. Although in most cases sonography might be the first and easiest accessible imaging modality for the liver, and MR imaging–especially with liver-specific contrast agents–is appreciated in difficult cases due to the highest available noninvasive diagnostic accuracy, CT of the abdomen including a high-quality scan of liver represents a pragmatic imaging modality and cannot be excluded from today's radiological practice. This chapter aims to give practical aids for setting up a protocol for CT examinations of the liver on a multidetector row CT scanner and introduces the most important liver lesions, their appearance in CT, and the diagnostic capabilities of CT for the specific diagnosis.

For focal liver lesions in general, detection rates of biphasic spiral CT typically ranging from roughly 60 to 75%, and differentiation of benign and malignant lesions in around 70% have been reported in literature (KONDO et al. 1999; SEMELKA et al. 1999; REIMER et al. 2000; BARTOLOZZI et al. 2004; OUDKERK et al. 2002). CT (even with recent multidetector CT [MDCT] technology) has shown to be inferior with regard to lesion detection (and lesion characterization) in trials that compared it directly to gadolinium-enhanced MRI (SEMELKA et al. 2001) or liver-specific MRI (REIMER et al. 2000; BARTOLOZZI et al. 2004; OUDKERK et al. 2002). This was especially seen in the subgroup of lesions smaller than 1 cm in diameter. This limitation is presumably due to the limited contrast resolution of CT that is not compensated by the excellent geometric spatial resolution. Just how far latest technology or future innovations might further increase the potential of MDCT remains to be seen.

Recently developed PET–CT scanners, which combine the advantages of PET (functional imaging with high sensitivity) with the advantages of CT (morphological imaging with high spatial resolution) within one

examination and nearly perfect image co-registration, are with regard to imaging in oncological patients a real contribution.

## 29.2
## Protocols for MDCT of the Liver

CT has developed dramatically with the introduction of multidetector technology. This is especially true with regard to the abdomen, where disturbing motion artifacts due to respiratory motion and bowel peristalsis are lessened to a great degree because of this technique. While scanners with 64 or more detector rows are still most common in large community or university hospitals, scanners with 2–16 slices are widely available even in private practice or in small hospitals. Recent technical developments have gone in two directions. One the one hand, scanners with two x-ray tubes and detector systems (so-called dual-source CT) were introduced, needing only a quarter rotation to reconstruct an image and thereby increasing the temporal resolution to acquire an image to the value of 83 ms (Somatom Definition, Siemens Medical Solutions, Erlangen, Germany). On the other hand, scanners with more than 300 detector rows have been introduced, increasing the anatomical coverage up to 16 cm per rotation and thereby giving new possibilities to cover whole organs for functional and time-resolved applications (Aquilion One, Toshiba Medical Systems, Tustin, Calif.). Nevertheless, at present these innovations will only have impact on research applications.

With the introduction of MDCT bi-, tri-, or even quadruple-phasic examinations of the liver can be combined into a thoraco-abdominal CT examination, without compromise with regard to spatial or temporal resolution. The acquisition of the liver with a 64-slice scanner for example only requires a few seconds, despite a submillimeter collimation. Even patients with a compromised general state of health are able to tolerate these breath-hold times. However, even on single-slice spiral CT scanners adequate image quality of the liver can be obtained. However, combination with thoraco-abdominal examinations is not possible without compromises in temporal and spatial resolution.

Adequate examination technique is critical for sensitive detection and specific characterization of focal liver lesions. A biphasic examination of the liver with a late arterial (arterial dominant) and a portovenous phase can be regarded as standard today. For specific indications like follow-up of hepatocellular carcinoma

(HCC) after transarterial chemoembolization (TACE) or for the depiction of the arterial vessels prior to angiography, an early-arterial-phase scan, which can be postprocessed into a CT angiography, is helpful (Fig. 29.1). The value of delayed scans (e.g., 5 min after contrast agent injection) is controversial in the literature; mainly, centers with a focus on imaging in liver cirrhosis consider the use of late-phase images as necessary, whereas other authors see no benefit for it (HWANG et al. 1997; SCHIMA et al. 2006).

With the short acquisition times of MDCT, contrast agent timing has become critical, since the optimal enhancement phase has to be included within a very short acquisition window. Therefore, the use of modern contrast agent power injectors and bolus timing are mandatory (SCHIMA et al. 2005). For bolus timing, automatic bolus triggering is recommended, which is available from all CT vendors. Non-ionic, iodine-based contrast agents with a concentration of 300–400 mg iodine per milliliter have become standard. Depending on the iodine concentration, fast flow rates up to 5 or 6 ml s$^{-1}$ are recommended (SCHIMA et al. 2005). The dosing of the contrast agent should be related to body weight, with 1.5–2 ml per kilogram body weight (for a concentration of 300 mg iodine per milliliter) (BARON 1994). Whereas the enhancement in the arterial phases can be optimized with help of high-concentration (370–400 mg iodine per milliliter) contrast agents or increased injection speed, the enhancement in the portovenous phase is not dependent on the iodine delivery per time but rather on the total amount of iodine (BRINK 2003). Therefore, even with sophisticated injection protocols, the total iodine dose should not be significantly below the value of 38–45 g iodine or 1.5 ml per kilogram body weight for contrast agents containing 300 mg iodine per milliliter (BRINK 2003). However, with dual-head power injectors, a saline-chaser of 30–50 ml can be injected directly after contrast agent injection, allowing for a somewhat-reduced contrast agent dose, despite optimal contrast enhancement in the arterial phase (SCHOELLNAST et al. 2003).

Usually, liver protocols are set up with a tube voltage of 120 kV and a tube current of 140–180 mA, where the tube current is nowadays usually adapted to the patients' constitution with special algorithms. The bolus timing is achieved with the already-mentioned technique of bolus triggering. A single transversal slice in the level of the diaphragm is placed before the start of contrast agent application. The aorta in this slice has to be identified and a region-of-interest (ROI) is drawn. This transversal section is scanned in 1-s steps after contrast agent injection. In case the ROI exceeds 100 HU, the diagnostic scan is started with a certain delay, either automatically or by hand. The delay between reaching the triggering threshold and starting the scan is usually 5 s for the early arterial phase (or CT angiographic phase) and

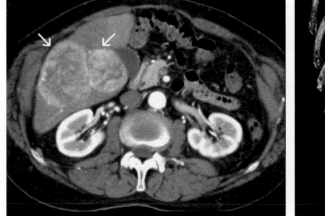

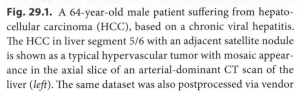

**Fig. 29.1.** A 64-year-old male patient suffering from hepatocellular carcinoma (HCC), based on a chronic viral hepatitis. The HCC in liver segment 5/6 with an adjacent satellite nodule is shown as a typical hypervascular tumor with mosaic appearance in the axial slice of an arterial-dominant CT scan of the liver (*left*). The same dataset was also postprocessed via vendor software (Siemens Syngo, Siemens Medical Solutions, Erlangen, Germany) as a CT angiography showing the vascular supply of the tumors via the right hepatic artery (*left*). This multimodal information of MDCT is useful especially for treatment planning in liver surgery or minimally invasive therapies like transarterial chemoembolization (TACE) or thermoablation

15 s for the late arterial (or arterial dominant) phase. In case only a portovenous phase of the liver is acquired, bolus triggering is usually not mandatory, since generally a sufficient result can be reached with a fixed delay of 65–75 s. In case timing is needed for the portovenous phase, a single transversal slice for bolus triggering can be placed in the upper level of the liver, so that the large liver veins can be delineated. For an optimal venous enhancement, the scan should be started with a delay of 5 s, after contrast enhancement in the main liver veins has been noticed. Figure 29.2 gives an overview of the different phases and delays of MDCT of the liver.

The optimal slice thickness of reconstructed CT images of the liver is still under debate. The effects of a submillimeter collimation versus a 2.5-mm collimation, for example, to achieve 3-mm reconstructed slices have not been determined. With regard to this point, at least the pragmatic view today is that the availability of high-resolution submillimeter raw data is an advantage, due to the possibilities for unlimited postprocessing, including standard or curved MPR reconstructions or MIPs, and CT angiographic images. There are only a few publications on this issue that showed that a general comment cannot be given, since different vendor-specific filtering and postprocessing steps do not allow evaluating the mere effect of low versus high collimation for all scanner types (VERDUN et al. 2004). In general, it is advised, therefore, to use the lowest possible collimation.

This is different when it comes to the parameter of reconstructed slice thickness. Past publications have been quite restricted here and have recommended that the slice thickness should not be lower than 5 mm for low-contrast organs like the liver (KAWATA et al. 2002; HAIDER et al. 2002). Recent publications discovered, however, advantages for a reconstructed slice thickness down to 3 mm (WEDEGÄRTNER et al. 2004). If the slice thickness is further decreased, then image noise and low contrast overwhelm the positive effect of geometrical resolution. This phenomenon can only be covered with inadequately high radiation doses.

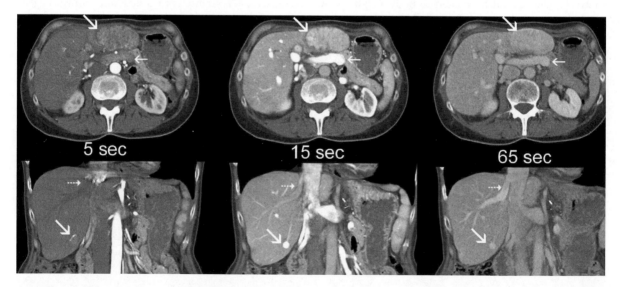

**Fig. 29.2.** Axial and coronal sections in the early arterial phase (*left*), late arterial phase (*middle*), and portovenous phase (*right*) in a female patient suffering from HCC under treatment with transarterial chemoembolization (TACE). In the early arterial phase, only the liver arteries are properly enhanced, the portal vein and the liver parenchyma are not yet opacified. The two HCC nodules in segment 2/3 and segment 6 (marked by *large arrows*) are also both not properly demarcated. The early arterial phase is, therefore, not suitable for detection of hypervascular tumors; it is rather a CT angiographic phase and can be omitted in most cases. The most important phase for detection of hypervascular tumors is the late arterial phase (also called arterial-dominant phase or phase of portovenous inflow). In this phase, there is already enhancement in the por-tal vein (*small arrow in the upper row*) and in the liver parenchyma. The liver veins are not yet opacified in this phase (*small arrow in the lower row*). Most hypervascular tumors reach their highest attenuation in this phase. In the portovenous phase, enhancement of the liver parenchyma is highest; the vascular enhancement in the portovenous system and in the hepatic vein is similar. Hypervascular tumors show decreased attenuation compared to the late arterial phase; depending on the degree of wash-out, they can be still hyperdense (as in this case), isodense (see Fig. 29.4) or even hypodense (figure reprinted with permission from Zech CJ, Reiser MF [2008] Radiological evaluation of patients with liver tumors. In: Bilbao JI, Reiser MF [eds] Liver radioembolization with Y90 microspheres. Springer, Berlin Heidelberg New York)

## Radiological Appearance of Different Focal Liver Lesions

The criteria for the characterization of focal liver lesions are derived from their behavior and degree of contrast agent enhancement in the different vascular phases of liver CT. For a valid characterization, usually at least two different phases are mandatory, so that changes of enhancement over time (e.g., wash-in and wash-out of contrast agent) can be appreciated. Nowadays, the necessity for an additional precontrast scan is usually denied; however, some centers still use it, depending on the clinical situation and referring diagnosis.

### 29.3.1
### Solid Benign Lesions

The group of solid benign lesions is mainly formed by focal nodular hyperplasia (FNH) and hepatocellular adenoma. (Regenerative nodules also belong to that group, but are listed in Chap. 29, Sect. 3.3, since they are usually found in the cirrhotic liver.) The current concept of FNH is that of a congenital arteriovenous malformation (seen as "central scar") with an area of surrounding hyperplasia (WANLESS et al. 1985). Thus, histologically, the cells found in FNH are normal, non-neoplastic polyclonal liver cells in an abnormal arrangement (REBOUISSOU et al. 2008). Hepatocellular adenomas on the other hand are true neoplastic lesions with monoclonal hepatocytes (REBOUISSOU et al. 2008). They are associated with a substantial risk of complications like bleeding or malignant transformation (WEIMANN et al. 1997). Benign solid liver lesions, such as FNH or liver cell adenoma, can be detected in CT by the characteristic tumor blush, seen in the late arterial phase, with following wash-out to iso- or slight hyperdensity (GRAZIOLI et al. 2001; CARLSON et al. 2000). In addition to the contrast agent behavior, morphological features like the hypodense central scar recognizable in FNHs (Fig. 29.3) or fatty or regressive changes and hemorrhage in adenomas contribute to establishing the correct diagnosis (WINTERER et al. 2006). The differential diagnosis between hepatocellular adenoma and FNH is, however, still a problematic point, especially if typical morphological features like, e.g., the central scar, are missing (Fig. 29.4). In these cases, MRI with liver-specific contrast agents can contribute to the differential diagnosis (GRAZIOLI et al. 2005). The differentiation of solid benign lesions from hypervascular malignant tumors can also be difficult. In case of HCC, the underlying cirrhosis and the wash-out to hypointensity are the most useful criteria for HCC. However, for lesions with only moderate wash-out like hypervascular metastases of, e.g., neuroendocrine tumors or for lesions mimicking the central scar of FNH like fibrolamellar HCC, this differentiation can be nearly impossible in CT sometimes.

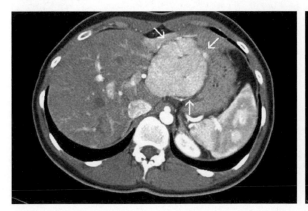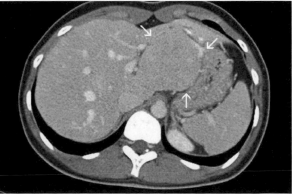

**Fig. 29.3.** Focal nodular hyperplasia of the liver in a young female patient in the late arterial (*left*) and portovenous phases (*right*). Note the strong, homogenous enhancement of the lesion in the arterial phase, with a spot of hypodensity in the central parts, representing the central scar. The adjacent liver parenchyma is compressed rather than infiltrated by the lesion. Together with additional features like the return to isointen-sity and the lobulated, well-defined margin, the diagnosis of an FNH can be made with confidence in this case (figure reprinted with permission from Zech CJ, Reiser MF [2008] Radiological evaluation of patients with liver tumors. In: Bilbao JI, Reiser MF [eds] Liver radioembolization with Y90 microspheres. Springer, Berlin Heidelberg New York)

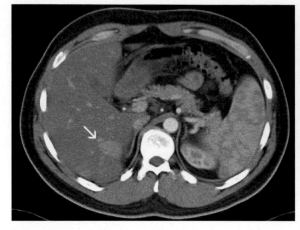
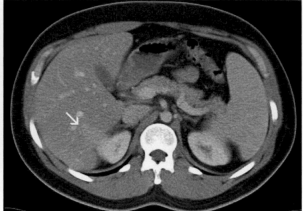

**Fig. 29.4.** A 36-year-old male patient with a hepatocellular adenoma in liver segment 5 (*arrow*). Note the homogenous hypervascularity of the lesion in the arterial-dominant phase (*left*); in the portovenous phase (*right*), the lesion is only just appreciable as a faintly hyperdense area. The comparison to FNH (Fig. 29.3) illustrates the difficulties in making a confident diagnosis noninvasively in a hypervascular tumor, with only faint wash-out in the venous phase if a central scar is missing

In the literature, values of about 70% correct characterization of FNH with help of dual-phase CT have been reported (VAN HOE et al. 1997). Other authors describe that characterization of a lesions is quite confident in case the above-mentioned typical morphological features like, e.g., a central scar, can be delineated without providing exact sensitivity/specificity data (WINTERER et al. 2006; KAMEL et al. 2006). A quite interesting approach seems the quantitative evaluation of attenuation values of triphasic CT of the liver and calculation of a relative enhancement ration as introduced by RUPPERT-KOHLMAYR and coworkers (2001), in which only minor overlap between FNH and adenoma was encountered; however, these results did not establish themselves in daily practice.

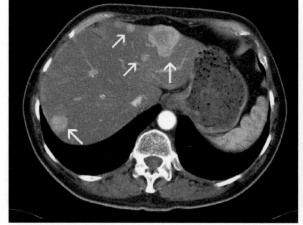
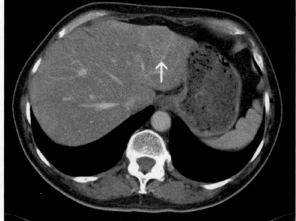

**Fig. 29.5.** MDCT in the late arterial (*left*) and portovenous phase (*right*) in a male patient suffering from a neuroendocrine carcinoma with liver metastases (*arrows*). Note the strong wash-out of the metastases to nearly isointensity, so that even the larger lesions can retrospectively not be properly detected in the portovenous phase in contrast to the excellent conspicuity of the lesions in the arterial phase. This example strikingly demonstrates the importance of a correctly timed late arterial phase (figure reprinted with permission from Zech CJ, Reiser MF [2008] Radiological evaluation of patients with liver tumors. In: Bilbao JI, Reiser MF [eds] Liver radioembolization with Y90 microspheres. Springer, Berlin Heidelberg New York)

## 29.3.2
## Metastatic Liver Lesions

Depending on the primary tumor, liver metastases can present with different morphological and enhancement characteristics, which mainly correspond to the consistency (cystic, mucinous, solid) and the vascularity (hypovascular or hypervascular). Some primary tumors usually have hypervascular liver metastases. These include thyroid carcinoma, carcinoid tumors, neuroendocrine tumors, and renal cell carcinoma (DANET et al. 2003). Metastases from pancreatic carcinoma, breast carcinoma, and colonic carcinoma may sometimes also be hypervascular (DANET et al. 2003). In liver metastases from a cancer of unknown primary (CUP), hypervascular lesions can be seen occasionally. The hypervascular nature of these lesions can be best appreciated in the arterial-dominant phase of the liver. The pronounced vascularity leads to a fast wash-out of the contrast agent in later phases (Fig. 29.5), which underlines the need for a proper timing of the arterial-dominant phase as described above (ZECH et al. 2007). Hypovascular metastases appear hypodense in both arterial and portovenous phases. One should be aware of the fact that this classification reflects only the degree of lesion enhancement compared with the normal liver parenchyma in the arterial and portovenous phases. It is known that even hypovascular lesions have a considerable amount of vascularization (which is a basic presumption for, e.g., the radioembolization treatment of hypovascular metastases) and show contrast uptake, but to a lesser degree compared with the surrounding liver parenchyma (DANET et al. 2003).

In case of hepatic steatosis, the contrast between metastatic lesions and the surrounding liver parenchyma can be alternated (Fig. 29.6). In some cases, this leads to isodensity of hypovascular liver metastases, which makes lesion detection virtually impossible. This problem can be regarded as one of the major reasons for false-negative findings of CT. The problem gets even more pronounced when taking into account that patients having been treated with chemotherapies often show variable degrees of hepatic steatosis, depending on the protocol used.

According to the literature, liver metastases can be detected with spiral CT with a sensitivity ranging from 58 to 85% (LENCIONI et al. 1998; WARD et al. 1999; VALLS et al. 2001; BARTOLOZZI et al. 2004). In case of hepatic steatosis, lower detection rates are described due to the missing contrast between typical hypovascular metastasis and the hypodense liver parenchyma in steatosis (KATO et al. 1997; LLAUGER et al. 1991).

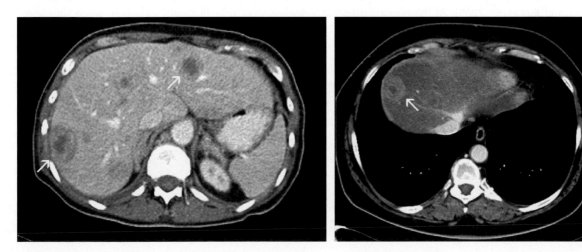

**Fig. 29.6.** CT images in the portovenous phase of two different patients suffering from extrahepatic malignancies with liver metastases. On the *left side*, typical hypovascular metastases from a breast cancer are depicted (*arrows*); the larger lesions show central regressive changes with the corresponding "bull's-eye appearance." On the right side, a metastasis from a colorectal carcinoma is shown (*arrow*). This lesion is also a typical hypovascular metastasis with the bull's-eye appearance; however, due to extensive steatosis hepatis (most likely as a consequence of the systemic chemotherapy), the contrast between the lesion and the adjacent liver is inverted, so that the metastasis appears hyperdense. In cases of intermediate steatosis hepatis, sometimes even liver metastasis with larger sizes can be masked as liver-isodense lesions

### 29.3.3
### Lesions in the Cirrhotic Liver

Imaging of the cirrhotic liver is a challenging task for every modality. The main diagnostic criterion for HCC is the presence of neoangiogenesis based on increased arterial supply. Therefore, typically HCC presents as a hyperdense lesion in the arterial-dominant phase, with following wash-out to iso- or mostly hypodensity in the portovenous phase. In addition to the intrahepatic staging with regard to number and size of lesions, complicating factors like liver cirrhosis and patency of the portal vein are of relevance for assigning patients to a proper treatment regimen (Fig. 29.7). Only a low percentage of mostly anaplastic hepatocellular tumors of mixed hepatocellular and cholangiocellular origin show no hypervascularity. Therefore, the presence of hypervascularity can be considered a specific finding for HCC in case underlying liver cirrhosis is present. The proof of hypervascularity with one or two imaging techniques in lesions ranging from 1–2 cm and larger than 2 cm, respectively, allows the definite diagnosis of a HCC noninvasively, according to the American Association for the Study of Liver Diseases (AASLD) practice guidelines (Bruix and Sherman 2005). For lesions smaller than 1 cm, characterization remains doubtful with any modality, so that follow-up is recommended. For lesions larger than 2 cm without the typical contrast agent dynamic (wash-in/wash-out), an elevated α-fetoprotein value is also diagnostic of HCC.

Although based on the AASLD practice guidelines (Bruix and Sherman 2005), all hypervascular lesions exceeding 1 and 2 cm, respectively, are considered to be HCC; from a radiological/pathological aspect, the differentiation between regenerative nodules, low-grade, and high-grade dysplastic nodules and early HCC would be desirable. This so-called gray zone of hepatocarcinogenesis remains unclear for imaging (either with CT or MRI) as well as sometimes for pathology (Bartolozzi et al. 2007). MDCT as a modality that works based on attenuation differences due to different vascular supply, as well as mere extracellular MRI, does not contribute to the differential diagnosis (Burrel et al. 2003). Although not recommended in the guidelines, many centers sucessfully apply MR imaging with liver-specific contrast agents (e.g., SPIO [superparamagnetic iron oxide] or hepatobiliary contrast agents) to characterize smaller hypervascular foci in patients with liver cirrhosis (Fig. 29.8) as either regenerative nodules or HCC (Yamamoto et al. 1996; Ward et al. 2000; Imai et al. 2000; Bartolozzi et al. 2007).

The detection rates of HCC reported in the literature are highly variable. One trial with a very stringent methodology showed a sensitivity of 61%, a specificity of 66%, and a negative predictive value of 30% for the detection of HCC (Burrel et al. 2003). A subgroup analysis in this trial revealed a strong influence of the lesion size. While lesions larger 2 cm were detected in 100%, lesions smaller than 1 cm were only detected in 10% (Burrel et al. 2003). Another trial with a four-row MDCT demonstrated an overall sensitivity of 73% for lesion detection, with also markedly reduced detection rates (33%) for lesions smaller than 1 cm (Kawata et al. 2002). Since CT can only depict the vascularity of lesions, it is difficult to distinguish between simple regenerative nodules, high-grade dysplastic nodules, and

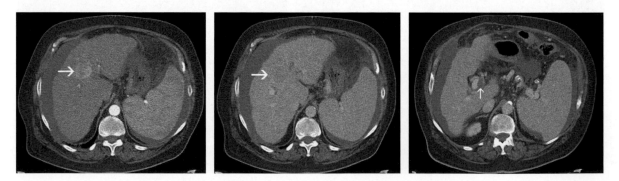

**Fig. 29.7.** A 75-year-old male patient with liver cirrhosis. An unclear lesion was depicted with ultrasound. The MDCT in arterial-dominant (*left*) and portovenous (*middle*) phases show a lesion with distinctive hypervascularity and strong wash-out 2.8 cm in size (*large arrows*). According to the AASLD practice guidelines (2005), this contrast agent behavior in a cirrhotic liver is diagnostic for HCC–in the presented lesions exceeding 2 cm in diameter, no further diagnostic tests have to be applied to establish the diagnosis. Consistent with the diagnosis of an HCC, the α-fetoprotein levels were highly elevated. Note the additional findings of perihepatic ascites, splenomegaly, and of a partial thrombosis of the main branch of the portal vein (*small arrow, right image*), which can be relevant for the indication of transarterial chemoembolization and/or surgery

early HCC in the cirrhotic liver (BURREL et al. 2003). The advantages of MRI in this respect are the possibility of tissue characterization based on different contrast weightings of the pulse sequences (T1, T2) and the availability of several liver specific contrast agents.

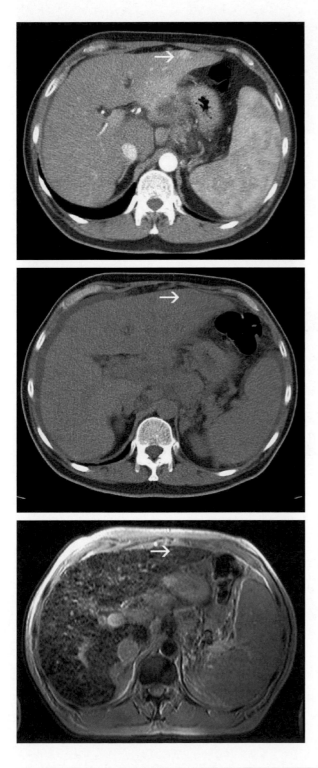

### 29.3.4
### Other Lesions

Congenital simple liver cysts are the most commonly encountered focal liver lesions. Cysts larger than 1 cm usually do not pose any differential diagnostic difficulties in cases in which the typical morphological features like sharp delineation, homogenous attenuation characteristic of fluid (0–15 HU), and absent contrast agent uptake can be seen. However, simple cysts have to be delineated from parasitic cysts (usually with inner septations and calcifications of the cyst wall) or cystic neoplasms like, e.g., cystic metastases, which can be differentiated usually by unclear margins and higher attenuation values (Fig. 29.9).

Hemangiomas are frequently encountered benign focal liver lesions histologically composed of large, cystic, blood-filled spaces with endothelial lining. These large, blood-filled spaces are responsible for the typical imaging features of hemangioma. In the arterial-dominant phase, usually a nodular, dot-like enhancement in the periphery is seen, which tends to progress centripetal in the portovenous phase (CASEIRO-ALVES et al. 2007). In later phases (5 min postinjection), the whole lesions is contrasted, since the slow flow in the enlarged vascular space of hemangiomas pools the extracellular contrast agent for a certain time. Deviations from this classical pattern are described mostly for small hemangioma, with usually homogenous enhancement already in the arterial phase and faster wash-out, and for large hemangioma with missing complete enhancement seen due to central thrombosis (CASEIRO-ALVES et al. 2007) (Fig. 29.10).

◄ **Fig. 29.8.** Patient with known hepatocellular carcinoma in liver segment 8 (not shown here). In a follow-up CT prior to transarterial chemoembolization, another hypervascular lesion in segment 2 was discovered (*arrow*). During the subsequent chemoembolization of the main tumor manifestation, no visible enhancement was noted in projection of segment 2. Even probationary lipiodol injection in the left liver artery did not result in depiction of a lesion in the suspected area in the following plain lipiodol CT (*middle*). The corresponding MR of the liver with a T2* gradient echo sequence 10 min after injection of the SPIO (super-paramagnetic iron oxide) contrast agent Ferucarbotran (Resovist, Bayer Schering Pharma AG, Berlin, Germany) confirms the finding of a regenerative nodule with uptake of the iron contrast agent. MRI with liver-specific contrast agents is, in this respect, a very powerful tool to distinguish between regenerative nodules and HCC because it helps to establish this differential diagnosis noninvasively

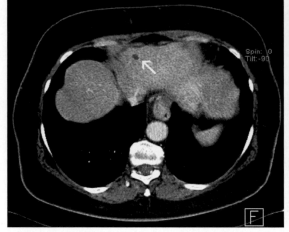

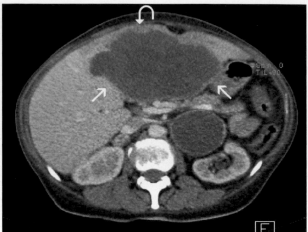

**Fig. 29.9.** CT images in the portovenous phase of two different patients suffering from extrahepatic malignancies. In the patient on the *left side*, a small, sharply delineated lesion without contrast uptake and CT values of 5–10 HU is depicted. This lesion can be characterized as a simple cyst despite the small size of only 0.8 cm in diameter. The large hypodense lesion on the *right side* shows CT values of 15–20 HU (*arrows*) and might on first glance be confused with a cyst; however, definite morphological signs like the unclear margins (*curved arrow*) in the ventral part, the inner inhomogeneity, and the shape of the lesion are signs of a "complicated" cystic lesion. A percutaneously core biopsy of the lesion revealed a cystic metastasis of a squamous cell carcinoma. The corresponding primary tumor was not discovered on further examinations; however, MDCT revealed additional tumor manifestations in the retroperitoneal space (not shown) as well as in the left adrenal gland with a similar cystic morphology as depicted

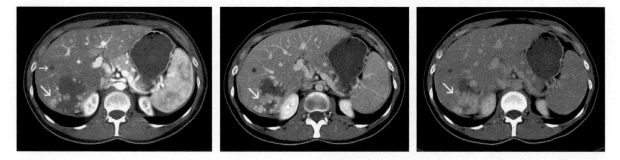

**Fig. 29.10.** Female patient with known colorectal carcinoma. In the arterial-dominant (*left*) and portovenous phases (*middle*) scans of a staging CT, a focal liver lesion in segment 6/7, with nodular peripheral contrast agent enhancement was depicted (*large arrow*). To increase the confidence of diagnosis an additional delayed scan after 5 min was added (*right*), where the ongoing centripetal enhancement and contrast agent pooling is documented. The lesion can be characterized as a hemangioma. Due to the large size of the lesion, even after 5 min not all parts have been contrasted properly. However, the remaining features of hemangioma can be depicted nicely in this case. Note the additional simple cyst nearby in liver segment 5/8 (*small arrow*)

## Role of MDCT for Follow-Up After Radiological Interventions

In emergency cases, such as acute hemorrhage within the liver (e.g., in a preexisting tumor, after liver biopsy, or after blunt abdominal trauma), acute vascular occlusion, or inflammatory lesions such as abscesses, MDCT is the modality of choice, since it is broadly available, allows for very fast scanning, and is based on well-established examination techniques. After surgical and interventional procedures, MDCT allows for reliable diagnosis of complications, such as hematomas, abscesses, or biliomas (ROMANO et al. 2005), which can be treated percutaneously with CT guidance, if required (Fig. 29.11). In the follow-up after TACE, the accumulation of lipiodol is readily visualized with CT,

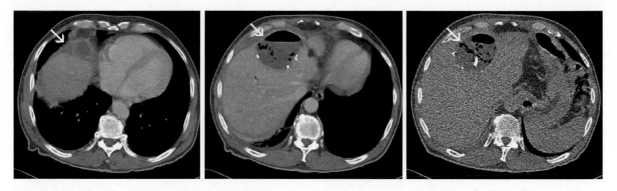

**Fig. 29.11.** Male patient with a history of liver surgery due to liver metastasis of a pancreatic adenocarcinoma. In the fourth week after surgery, the patient complained about increasing abdominal discomfort and underwent CT. The CT scan in the portovenous phase at two different axial levels (*left* and *middle*) shows a fluid collection with gas bubbles (*middle*) and strong enhancement in the rim (*left*) just at the area of liver resection, marked by surgical clips, highly suspicious of a liver abscess. The lesion was treated directly by a percutaneously CT-guided drainage insertion (CT fluoroscopic image on the right), which confirmed the diagnosis of an abscess

even on noncontrast scans without contrast enhancement, contributing to predict the success of the therapy (GUAN et al. 2004; TAKAYASU et al. 2000). Figure 29.12 shows a typical case of liver hemorrhage after a percutaneous biopsy.

In all cases of suspected inflammatory processes of the liver, a portovenous enhanced scan can be regarded as sufficient to answer diagnostic questions. In cases of acute hepatic hemorrhage, it is of clinical interest to determine the source of bleeding–whether from the hepatic veins or the portovenous system, or whether from liver arteries and/or arteries of the liver capsule arising from the phrenic artery. This differentiation as well as the degree of acute bleeding can be only addressed when an arterial-dominant or even an early-arterial-phase scan is added. In case of known calcifications, lipiodol deposition or in case of bleeding complications after, e.g., percutaneous transhepatic cholangiography (PTC), an additional plain CT scan can be helpful to distinguish between other hyperdense structures than extravasal contrast agent.

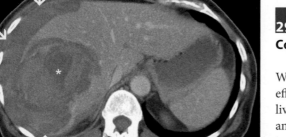

**Fig. 29.12.** CT images of a female patient 3 h after percutaneously biopsy of a focal liver lesion (*asterisk*). The patient complained about increasing pain in the right upper abdomen. CT in the portovenous phase confirms the clinical suspicion of acute liver hematomas subcapsular and in the area of the focal liver lesion postbiopsy (*arrows*). It is advisable to perform the CT in such a constellation as a biphasic examination to show potential contrast agent extravasation as a sign of an active arterial bleeding, which was not present in this patient

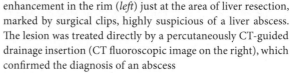
**29.5**
## Conclusion

With MDCT, radiology has a versatile, fast, and highly efficient modality available for the assessment of the liver and the upper abdomen. It is suitable for the examination of emergency patients as well as for elective treatment planning. The great advantages over other modalities are mainly the easy access, the possibility to examine the whole thorax and abdomen within seconds and, therefore, the time-efficient diagnosis, with usually excellent image quality, without motion artifacts. Disadvantages are the radiation exposure and the lower soft tissue contrast when compared with MRI. Although MRI of the liver (especially with liver-specific contrast agents) remains the noninvasive gold standard in liver imaging, MDCT has its benefits as above mentioned and has its definite place in the workup of liver disease.

# References

Baron RL (1994) Understanding and optimizing use of contrast material for CT of the liver. AJR Am J Roentgenol 163:323–331

Bartolozzi C, Lencioni R, Caramella D, Palla A, Bassi AM, Di Candio G (1996) Small hepatocellular carcinoma. Detection with US, CT, MR imaging, DSA, and lipiodol-CT. Acta Radiol 37:69–74

Bartolozzi C, Donati F, Cioni D et al. (2004) Detection of colorectal liver metastases: a prospective multicenter trial comparing unenhanced MRI, MnDPDP-enhanced MRI, and spiral CT. Eur Radiol 14:14–20

Bartolozzi C, Crocetti L, Lencioni R, Cioni D, Della Pina C, Campani D (2007) Biliary and reticuloendothelial impairment in hepatocarcinogenesis: the diagnostic role of tissue-specific MR contrast media. Eur Radiol 17:2519–2530

Brink JA (2003) Contrast optimization and scan timing for single and multidetector-row computed tomography. Eur J Radiol 27(Suppl.):S3–S8

Bruix J, Sherman M (2005) Practice Guidelines Committee, American Association for the Study of Liver Diseases. Management of hepatocellular carcinoma. Hepatology 42:1208–1236

Burrel M, Llovet JM, Ayuso C et al. (2003) MRI angiography is superior to helical CT for detection of HCC prior to liver transplantation: an explant correlation. Hepatology 38:1034–1042

Carlson SK, Johnson CD, Bender CE, Welch TJ (2000) CT of focal nodular hyperplasia of the liver. AJR Am J Roentgenol 174:705–712

Caseiro-Alves F, Brito J, Araujo AE et al. (2007) Liver haemangioma: common and uncommon findings and how to improve the differential diagnosis. Eur Radiol 17:1544–1554

Danet IM, Semelka RC, Leonardou P et al. (2003) Spectrum of MRI appearances of untreated metastases of the liver. AJR Am J Roentgenol 181:809–817

Grazioli L, Federle MP, Brancatelli G, Ichikawa T, Olivetti L, Blachar A (2001) Hepatic adenomas: imaging and pathologic findings. Radiographics 21:877–894

Grazioli L, Morana G, Kirchin MA, Schneider G (2005) Accurate differentiation of focal nodular hyperplasia from hepatic adenoma at gadobenate dimeglumine-enhanced MR imaging: prospective study. Radiology 236:166–177

Guan YS, Zheng XH, Zhou XP et al. (2004) Multidetector CT in evaluating blood supply of hepatocellular carcinoma after transcatheter arterial chemoembolization. World J Gastroenterol 10:2127–2129

Haider MA, Amitai MM, Rappaport DC et al. (2002) Multidetector row helical CT in preoperative assessment of small (< or = 1.5 cm) liver metastases: is thinner collimation better? Radiology 225:137–142

Hwang GJ, Kim M-J, Yoo HS, Lee JT (1997) Nodular hepatocellular carcinoma: detection with arterial-, portal- and delayed-phase images at spiral CT. Radiology 202:383–388

Imai Y, Murakami T, Yoshida S et al. (2000) Superparamagnetic iron oxide-enhanced magnetic resonance images of hepatocellular carcinoma: correlation with histological grading. Hepatology 32:205–212

Kamel IR, Liapi E, Fishman EK (2006) Focal nodular hyperplasia: lesion evaluation using 16-MDCT and 3D CT angiography. AJR Am J Roentgenol 186:1587–1596

Kato M, Saji S, Kanematsu M et al. (1997) A case of liver metastasis from colon cancer masquerading as focal sparing in a fatty liver. Jpn J Clin Oncol 27:189–192

Kawata S, Murakami T, Kim T et al. (2002) Multidetector CT: diagnostic impact of slice thickness on detection of hypervascular hepatocellular carcinoma. AJR Am J Roentgenol 179:61–66

Kondo H, Kanematsu M, Hashi H et al. (1999) Preoperative detection of malignant hepatic tumors: comparison of combined methods of MR imaging with combined methods of CT. AJR Am J Roentgenol 174:947–954

Lencioni R, Donati F, Cioni D, Paolicchi A, Cicorelli A, Bartolozzi C (1998) Detection of colorectal liver metastases: prospective comparison of unenhanced and ferumoxides-enhanced magnetic resonance imaging at 1.5 T, dual-phase spiral CT, and spiral CT during arterial portography. MAGMA 7:76–87

Llauger J, Pérez C, Coscojuela P, Sanchís E, Traid C (1991) Hepatic metastases: false-negative CT portography in cases of fatty infiltration. J Comput Assist Tomogr 15:320–322

Oudkerk M, Torres CG, Song B et al. (2002) Characterization of liver lesions with mangafodipir trisodium-enhanced MR imaging: multicenter study comparing MR and dual-phase spiral CT. Radiology 223:517–524

Rebouissou S, Bioulac-Sage P, Zucman-Rossi J (2008) Molecular pathogenesis of focal nodular hyperplasia and hepatocellular adenoma. J Hepatol 48:163–170

Reimer P, Jähnke N, Fiebich M et al. (2000) Hepatic lesion detection and characterization: value of nonenhanced MR imaging, superparamagnetic iron oxide-enhanced MR imaging, and spiral CT–ROC analysis. Radiology 217:152–158

Romano S, Tortora G, Scaglione M et al. (2005) MDCT imaging of post interventional liver: a pictorial essay. Eur J Radiol 53:425–432

Ruppert-Kohlmayr AJ, Uggowitzer MM, Kugler C, Zebedin D, Schaffler G, Ruppert GS (2001) Focal nodular hyperplasia and hepatocellular adenoma of the liver: differentiation with multiphasic helical CT. AJR Am J Roentgenol 176:1493–1498

Schima W, Kulinna C, Ba-Ssalamah A, Grunberger T (2005) Multidetector computed tomography of the liver. Radiologe 45:15–23

Schima W, Hammerstingl R, Catalano C et al. (2006) Quadruple-phase MDCT of the liver in patients with suspected hepatocellular carcinoma: effect of contrast material flow rate. AJR Am J Roentgenol 186:1571–1579

Schoellnast H, Tillich M, Deutschmann HA et al. (2003) Abdominal multidetector row computed tomography. Reduction of cost and contrast material dose using saline flush. J Comput Assist Tomogr 27:847–853

Semelka RC, Cance WG, Marcos HB, Mauro MA (1999) Liver metastases: comparison of current MR techniques and spiral CT during arterial portography for detection in 20 surgically staged cases. Radiology 213:86–91

Semelka RC, Martin DR, Balci C, Lance T (2001) Focal liver lesions: comparison of dual-phase CT and multisequence multiplanar MR imaging including dynamic gadolinium enhancement. J Magn Reson Imaging 13:397–401

Takayasu K, Arii S, Matsuo N et al. (2000) Comparison of CT findings with resected specimens after chemoembolization with iodized oil for hepatocellular carcinoma. AJR Am J Roentgenol 175:699–704

Valls C, Andia E, Sanchez A et al. (2001) Hepatic metastases from colorectal cancer: preoperative detection and assessment of resectability with helical CT. Radiology 218:55–60

Van Hoe L, Baert AL, Gryspeerdt S et al. (1997) Dual-phase helical CT of the liver: value of an early-phase acquisition in the differential diagnosis of noncystic focal lesions. AJR Am J Roentgenol 168:1185–1192

Verdun FR, Noel A, Meuli R et al. (2004) Influence of detector collimation on SNR in four different MDCT scanners using a reconstructed slice thickness of 5 mm. Eur Radiol 14:1866–1872

Wanless IR, Mawdsley C, Adams R (1985) On the pathogenesis of focal nodular hyperplasia of the liver. Hepatology 5:1194–1200

Ward J, Naik KS, Guthrie JA, Wilson D, Robinson PJ (1999) Hepatic lesion detection: comparison of MR imaging after the administration of superparamagnetic iron oxide with dual-phase CT by using alternative-free response receiver operating characteristic analysis. Radiology 210:459–466

Ward J, Guthrie JA, Scott DJ et al. (2000) Hepatocellular carcinoma in the cirrhotic liver: double-contrast MR imaging for diagnosis. Radiology 216:154–162

Wedegärtner U, Lorenzen M, Nagel HD et al. (2004) Image quality of thin- and thick-slice MDCT reconstructions in low-contrast objects (liver lesions) with equal doses. Rofo 176:1676–1682

Weimann A, Ringe B, Klempnauer J et al. (1997) Benign liver tumors: differential diagnosis and indications for surgery. World J Surg 21:983–990

Winterer JT, Kotter E, Ghanem N, Langer M (2006) Detection and characterization of benign focal liver lesions with multislice CT. Eur Radiol 16:2427–2443

Yamamoto H, Yamashita Y, Takahashi M (1996) Development of hepatomas in hyperplastic nodules induced in the rat liver: detection with superparamagnetic iron oxide-enhanced magnetic resonance imaging. Acad Radiol 3:330–335

Zech CJ, Reiser MF (2008) Radiological evaluation of patients with liver tumors. In: Bilbao JI, Reiser MF (eds) Liver radioembolization with Y90 microspheres. Springer, Berlin Heidelberg New York

Zech CJ, Herrmann KA, Reiser MF, Schoenberg SO (2007) MR imaging in patients with suspected liver metastases: value of liver-specific contrast agent Gd-EOB-DTPA. Magn Reson Med Sci 6:43–52

# MDCT of Pancreatic Tumors

**30**

Wolfgang Schima, Claus Kölblinger and Ahmed Ba-Ssalamah

W. Schima, MD, MSc
Abteilung für Radiologie und bildgebende Diagnostik, KH Göttlicher Heiland, Dornbacher Strasse 20–28, 1170 Vienna, Austria

C. Kölblinger, MD
Department of Radiology, Medical University of Vienna, Waehringer Guertel 18–20, 1090 Vienna, Austria

A. Ba-Ssalamah, MD
Department of Radiology, Medical University of Vienna, Waehringer Guertel 18–20, 1090 Vienna, Austria

**ABSTRACT**

Dual-phasic contrast-enhanced MDCT in the pancreatic parenchymal and the venous phase is the method of choice for detection and staging of pancreatic cancer. Three-dimensional reconstructions (CPR, MIP, or VRT) are of great value for demonstration of tumors and the anatomical relationship between tumor and peripancreatic for the surgeon. For cystic lesion characterization, MDCT is comparable to MRI with MRCP, although MRI will increase the diagnostic confidence. For detection of small, hypervascular neuroendocrine tumors, no single imaging method will reveal all tumors. In this respect, MDCT and MRI are complementary methods.

## 30.1
## Introduction

In most institutions, MDCT is the radiologic study of choice for the evaluation of patients with suspected pancreatic tumors. The technical advances of MDCT, which allow the acquisition of well-defined CT imaging protocols of the pancreas and 3D visualization techniques, has made CT the preferred tool, well accepted by surgeons. Fully exploiting the advantages of MDCT imaging of the pancreas, dedicated scan protocols, and newly defined imaging criteria should be used, which are summarized in this chapter.

## 30.2
## CT Scan Protocols

As for other abdominal CT protocols, several important points for pancreatic CT imaging have to be observed.
1. The number of CT acquisitions
2. Oral contrast material
3. Amount of intravenous contrast material
4. Contrast material flow rate
5. Scan delay
6. Slice thickness and reconstruction interval for 2D and 3D viewing

## 30.2.1
## Number of CT Scans

MDCT of the pancreas is performed using triphasic acquisition obtained prior to, and biphasic acquisition after, intravenous contrast material injection (FREENY 2005). It has been shown that an arterial-phase scan (similar in timing to the typical arterial-phase scan of the liver) is not of value for detection of pancreatic adenocarcinoma (FLETCHER et al. 2003; GRAF et al. 1997). Pancreatic adenocarcinoma, which is by far the most common pancreatic tumor, is hypovascular and shows only little to no contrast to the minimally enhancing pancreatic parenchyma in the early arterial phase. LU et al. (1996) implemented a two-phase CT protocol evalu-

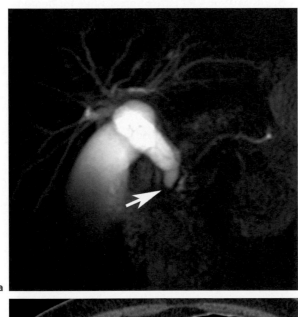

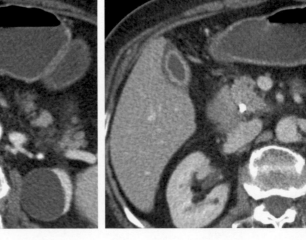

**Fig. 30.1a–c.** Pancreatic adenocarcinoma: superior tumor delineation in the pancreatic parenchymal phase. **a** MRCP reveals stenosis of the distal CBD (*arrow*) with massive biliary dilatation, suggestive of tumor. **b** Contrast-enhanced in the CT in the pancreatic phase revels a low-density mass in the uncinate process (*arrows*), adjacent to the biliary plastic stent in situ, indicative of pancreatic cancer. A hypodense mass is a direct sign of tumor at CT. **c** In the venous-phase CT image, the lesion is not discernible

ation of pancreatic tumors, which involves acquisition during maximum pancreatic enhancement (the so-called pancreatic parenchymal phase) and during the venous phase. They suggested using a fixed delay of 40 s after start of intravenous injection at a flow rate of 3 ml s$^{-1}$ for pancreatic parenchymal-phase imaging. Subsequently, it has been shown that the tumor-to-gland attenuation difference is greatest on images obtained in the pancreatic phase (mean: 57 HU) versus that on images obtained in the hepatic phase (mean: 35 HU) (Fig. 30.1) (Boland et al. 1999). In the pancreatic parenchymal phase, the contrast material filling of the superior mesenteric vein and the portal vein may still be insufficient, which renders the acquisition in the hepatic venous phase valuable for detection of vascular invasion (Fletcher et al. 2003). Moreover, the hepatic venous phase is crucial for detection of liver metastases. Therefore, there is consensus that a triphasic CT protocol including unenhanced scans and contrast-enhanced scans in the pancreatic parenchyma and the venous phases is essential for detection and staging of pancreatic cancer. Only for detection of neuroendocrine tumors (NET), which tend to be hypervascular, are biphasic, contrast-enhanced scans in the arterial phase and the venous phase recommended.

## 30.2.2
## Oral Contrast Material

The administration of oral contrast material is necessary to improve delineation of the pancreatic head against the duodenum. Administration of a positive oral contrast material may sometime impair the delineation of the pancreatic head if dilution of the ingested contrast material by retained fluid in the stomach yields the same CT density as the pancreatic head enhanced by intravenous contrast material. Thus, Richter et al. (1998) developed the concept of hydro-CT of the pancreas: Patients are to drink at least 1,000 ml of water prior to the examination. To impair peristaltic contractions of the stomach and duodenum during the helical CT acquisition, intravenous administration of Buscopan® is recommended. Filling of the stomach and duodenum with water, which acts as a negative contrast agent, allows excellent delineation of the pancreatic head and even the papilla, which improves detection of pancreatic tumors adjacent to the duodenum. With the evolution of MDCT and the dramatic shortening of acquisition times, the administration of scopolamine (e.g., Buscopan®) to paralyze the stomach is not necessary anymore.

## 30.2.3
## Amount of intravenous Contrast Material

The amount of contrast material administered may vary. In many institutions, a fixed amount of contrast material of 140–150 ml (at 300 mg ml$^{-1}$) has been shown to give good results (Fletcher et al. 2003; Lu et al. 1996; McNulty et al. 2001; Schima et al. 2007). This contrast material dosage amounts to a total iodine load of 42–45 g. If contrast material of higher concentration (350 to 400 mg ml$^{-1}$) is to be used, then the amount of contrast material, accordingly, should be reduced. Other studies have shown that for a weight-adjusted contrast material acquisition scheme, an amount of contrast material of 2 ml per kilogram body weight is superior to 1.5 ml per kilogram body weight. A weight-adjusted contrast material protocol will yield satisfactory pancreatic and liver enhancement, irrespective of patient weight (Yanaga et al. 2007).

## 30.2.4
## Contrast Material Flow Rate

Higher contrast material flow rates have been shown to be advantageous. Tublin et al. (1999) showed that a flow rate of 5 ml s$^{-1}$ is superior to 2.5 ml s$^{-1}$ regarding enhancement of the pancreas and the liver parenchyma. Many authors recommend using a flow rate of 4–5 ml s$^{-1}$ to optimize pancreatic enhancement and tumor-to-pancreas contrast. Schueller at el. (2006) demonstrated that an even higher flow rate of 8 ml s$^{-1}$ (compared with the standard flow rate of 4 ml s$^{-1}$) has its merits. They demonstrated that a flow rate of 8 ml s$^{-1}$ results in better enhancement of the pancreas, but not of the typically hypovascular adenocarcinomas, which resulted in a higher tumor-to-pancreas contrast.

## 30.2.5
## Scan Delay

In the helical CT era, a fixed scan delay for the pancreatic parenchymal phase of 40 s was recommended. With an acquisition time of approximately 20 s for a helical scan of the pancreas, good enhancement of the pancreas was guaranteed for most of the patients. However, with the evolution of MDCT scanners, which has considerably shorted the acquisition time of a pancreatic CT scan to not more than 3–5 s for modern scanners, a fixed scan delay may be suboptimal to catch the phase of maximum enhancement. Schueller et al. (2006) compared fixed scan delays of 40 s with an individual scan delay based on aortic transit time. They showed that an individualized scan delay is superior to a fixed delay of 40 s. Using a flow rate of 4 ml s$^{-1}$ (at 140 ml with 300 mg ml$^{-1}$), an individual scan delay of aortic transit time plus 28 s renders optimal enhancement of the pancreas and maximum contrast of adenocarcinomas. GOSHIMA et al. (2006) evaluated a different approach: they used a weight-based amount of contrast material (2 ml per kilogram body weight) with fixed injection duration of 3 s (thus, the flow rate is variable!). According to their results, peak enhancement of pancreatic parenchyma occurs quite consistently at 35–45 s post-start of contrast material injection. Thus, as an alternative to an individual scan delay with a fixed dose and fixed flow rate for pancreatic CT, with a weight-based contrast dose of 2 ml kg$^{-1}$ and a fixed injection duration of 30 s, a fixed scan delay will render good results.

## 30.2.6
### Slice Thickness and Reconstruction Interval for 2D and 3D Viewing

Similar to MDCT scanning of the liver, two different slice thicknesses are to be reconstructed. For viewing of axial images, a slice thickness of 3 mm with a reconstruction interval of 2 mm (i.e., an overlap of 1 mm) is a good compromise between spatial resolution in the z-axis and image noise. However, reconstruction of thin slices (e.g., 1 mm with a reconstruction interval of 0.7 mm) is necessary for 3D reconstructions. Multiplanar reconstructions (MPR) in the coronal plane, made with a few mouse clicks, are helpful for demonstration of pancreatic anatomy and tumor morphology. Other, slightly more advanced 3D reconstructions, such as stacked curved planar reconstructions (CPR) along the pancreatic duct, are helpful to reveal subtle indirect signs of tumor obstruction. Volume-rendered images are able to demonstrate vascular tumor encasement very convincingly for surgeons.

## 30.3
### Adenocarcinoma

Pancreatic cancer is the fourth to fifth leading cause of cancer-related deaths in the Western world. The prognosis for patients with pancreatic cancer is bleak, with an overall 5-year survival rate of <5%. According to the histopathologic classification, there are wide varieties of malignant tumors that arise from the exocrine pancreas, adenocarcinoma being by far the most common (approximately 80%). The incidence peaks in the sixth to seventh decades of life. The etiology of pancreatic adenocarcinoma is not exactly known. However, some risk factors have been identified. Cigarette smoking is the most important environmental risk factor. Chronic pancreatitis increases the risk to develop risk pancreatic cancer (up to 16 times) (LOWENFELS et al. 1993). In select cases, hereditary factors may play a role. In hereditary chronic pancreatitis, there is a cumulative risk of up to 40% for the development of pancreatic cancer until the age of 70 (LOWENFELS et al. 1997).

Adenocarcinomas are located in the pancreatic head in 60–70%. In surgical series, 80–90% of tumors are located in the head of the gland because they are the only ones amenable to surgery (ALEXAKIS et al. 1997; TREDE et al. 1990). In contrast to the pancreatic head tumors, which present with jaundice, tumors of the pancreatic body and tail lead only very late to clinical symptoms due to invasion into the stomach or spleen or due to liver metastases. Tumors located in the pancreatic body or tail are almost in an advanced stage at the time of diagnosis, and therefore not resectable (WARSHAW et al. 1992). Overall, potentially curative resection can be performed in only about 10–20% of patients. Although surgery offers a low cure rate, it is also the only chance for a cure.

## 30.3.1
### Direct and Indirect Tumor Signs and CT Detection Rates

A direct sign of tumor at contrast-enhanced CT is the presence of a hypoattenuating mass in the pancreas. The value of pancreatic phase CT lies in its superiority over venous-phase CT for detection of subtle attenuation difference suspicious for tumor (Fig. 30.1). However, even with dual-phase MDCT imaging, direct tumor signs are absent approximately 10% of cases because adenocarcinoma may be isoattenuating with contrast-enhanced CT (PROKESCH et al. 2002). There are other, indirect signs of pancreatic cancer of which the reader should be aware: the presence of a biliary dilatation due to a stenosis of the distal common bile duct, pancreatic duct dilatation due to a stenosis of the pancreatic duct, and the presence of a "double-duct sign" (dilatation of both pancreatic ducts and biliary ducts), even without demonstrable tumors are highly suspicious for cancer! Focal loss of lobulation of the pancreatic parenchyma and deformity of pancreatic contour are other indirect signs of pancreatic cancer (Fig. 30.2). CPR images along the pancreatic duct are superior to axial images alone

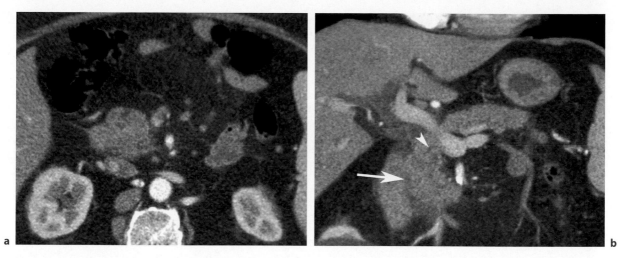

**Fig. 30.2a,b.** Pancreatic adenocarcinoma: indirect signs of tumor at CT. **a** Axial CT shows enlargement and loss of lobulation of pancreatic head, which (**b**) is much better seen on the CPR. This loss of lobulation of the pancreatic head, leading to pancreatic duct dilatation (*arrowhead*), is highly suspicious of tumor

regarding the detection of cancer (sensitivity: 91 vs. 79%) (FUKUSHIMA et al. 2006).

Several studies have assessed the sensitivity of helical CT for the detection of pancreatic cancer. Contrast-enhanced dual-phase helical CT yields a sensitivity for cancer detection of 76–92% (BLUEMKE et al. 1995; ICHIKAWA et al. 1997; LEGMANN et al. 1998; SCHIMA et al. 2002). The sensitivity of helical CT suffers when only small tumors (≤2 cm) are analyzed. In a study by IRIE et al. (1997), helical CT could detect only 6 of 8 (63%) of small tumors. A recent study by BRONSTEIN et al. (2004) demonstrated a sensitivity of 77% for helical CT for the detection of small tumors. The reconstruction of 3D reconstructions (MPR, CPR) of MDCT data sets improves the depiction of the main pancreatic duct and, thus, the detection of small tumors not appreciated on axial slices. Only a few studies have addressed the value of MDCT for the detection of pancreatic cancer. GRENACHER et al. (2004) found a sensitivity of 100% for four-row MDCT, which has to be corroborated in larger studies. DEWITT et al. (2004) noted that MDCT was inferior to endosonography (EUS) in detection overall (sensitivity: 86 vs. 98%) and in detection of small cancers. DEWITT et al.'s results confirm earlier studies, which showed that EUS is superior to CT in the detection of small cancers. Large series have shown that EUS has a very high negative predictive value to rule out pancreatic cancer of 100% in experienced hands (KLAPMAN et al. 2005). Thus, in patients with equivocal CT, a EUS (if available) or an MRI examination would be the next step in a patient with suspected cancer. A negative result then obviates the need for further studies.

### 30.3.2
### Staging of Adenocarcinoma

The *T stage* of pancreatic cancer is defined by tumor size and local spread (SCHIMA et al. 2007). Tumors stage T1 is defined by a tumor size of <2 cm in the largest. In stage T2, the tumor diameter exceeds 2 cm, the tumor being still confined to the pancreas. In stage T3, there is local invasion of the tumor into the peripancreatic fatty tissue and/or infiltration into the duodenum (Fig. 30.3) or the common bile duct or limited invasion of the portal or superior mesenteric vein. Because of the very close anatomic relationship between the pancreatic gland and the large peripancreatic vessels, a stage T4 infiltration of the tumor into the superior mesenteric artery or vein, portal vein, hepatic artery, or celiac trunk may occur quite early. Infiltration into surrounding organs, such as the stomach, spleen, or transverse colon is also defined as a stage T4. The *N stage* of pancreatic cancer is defined by the presence of peripancreatic lymph node metastasis. *Lymph node metastases*, apart from the peripancreatic nodes (such as para-aortic lymph node metastases), are defined as stage M1 (distant metastases). The most common causes of distant metastases (M1) are liver metastases (Fig. 30.3) and peritoneal carcinomatosis.

In pancreatic cancer staging, several questions are to be answered by the radiologist to define patients amenable to curative surgery. Absolute contraindications against surgical resection are as follows:

- Infiltration in adjacent organs: stomach, spleen, colon (T4)

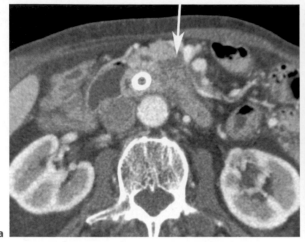
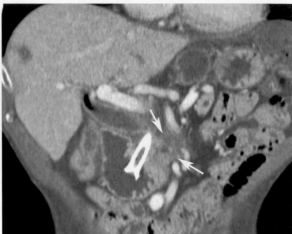

a

b

**Fig. 30.3a,b.** Adenocarcinoma with spread into duodenum and liver metastasis. **a** There is a large, low-density mass in the uncinate process (*arrow*), but the duodenum is not well seen. There is a metallic biliary stent in place. **b** Coronal MPR demonstrates tumor invasion into the ascending part of the duo-denum (*arrows*) with dilatation of the fluid-filled duodenum. Note that no oral contrast material was given due to symptoms of gastric outlet obstruction. There is a hypoattenuating metastases present in the liver

- Invasion into peripancreatic arteries: celiac trunk, hepatic artery, superior mesenteric artery (T4)
- Invasion into peripancreatic veins: portal vein, superior mesenteric vein (relative contraindication, T3)
- Distant metastases: liver, peritoneum, para-aortic lymph nodes, lung (M1)

When tumor–vessel contact was absent (grade 0, according to Lu et al. 1997), the likelihood of vessel invasion was 0%. With a tumor–vessel contact of less than 90° of the vessel circumference (grade 1, according to Lu et al. 1997), the probability of vessel infiltration is close to zero (Fig. 30.4). When the tumor–vessel contact is 90–180° of the vessel circumference (grade 2), the likelihood of vessel invasion is approximately 50%, and with a tumor–vessel contact of >180° of the vessel (grade 3), there is a very high likelihood of vessel invasion. With more than 270° tumor–vessel contact, vessel infiltration is almost certain (Figs. 30.5, 30.6) (Lu et al. 1997). Nakayama et al. (2001) modified the grading system for definition of vascular encasement: involvement of the venous system exceeding 180° of vessel circumference (grades 3 and 4) was suggestive of vascular invasion. However, for arterial encasement, the criteria are different: with CT grade 3 involvement resectability may still be found, because the circumferential soft tissue cuff may be due to perivascular fibrosis with tumor invasion.

For the superior mesenteric vein and the portal vein, the "teardrop sign" has been described, which is also a strong indicator for tumor vessel infiltration (Fig. 30.5). It means that a teardrop-like deformity of the su-perior mesenteric vein or portal vein (which are normally round in shape) by an adjacent tumor is indicative of vascular invasion (Hough et al. 1999). Likewise, the presence of dilated pancreaticoduodenal veins is indicative of obstructed venous outflow at the level of the superior mesenteric vein and, thus, of vessel invasion by tumor (Yamada et al. 2000). In general, 3D reconstructions techniques such as MIP, CPR, and volumerendered techniques (VRT) are superior to a stack of axial images for demonstration of vascular involvement (Fig. 6) (Prokesch et al. 2002; Vargas et al. 2004).

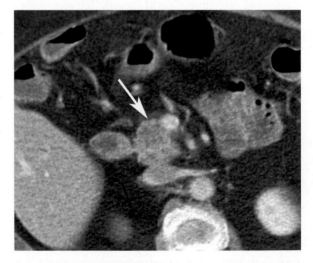

**Fig. 30.4.** Adenocarcinoma in the pancreatic head shows minimal contact to the SMV (grade 1, less than 90° of the vessel circumference). During surgery, no vessel infiltration was found and the tumor could be resected

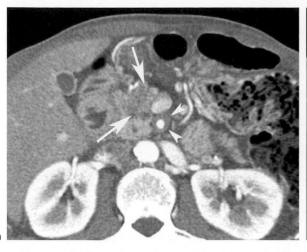

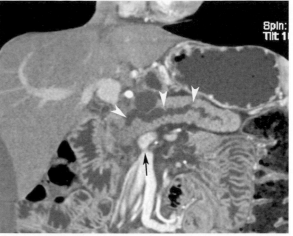

a

b

**Fig. 30.5a,b.** Adenocarcinoma with extensive vascular infiltration of SMA and SMV (teardrop sign). **a** Axial CT shows a low-density mass in the pancreatic head abutting the SMV, which is not round anymore. Deformation of the SMV is better seen on adjacent CT slices reviewed in cine mode (not shown). There is also circumferential tumor growth around the SMA (*arrowheads*). **b** The volume-rendered image in the coronal plane demonstrates in one image the deformation the superior mesenteric vein (teardrop deformity). There is massive dilatation of the pancreatic duct in the body and tail proximal to the stenosis (*arrowheads*)

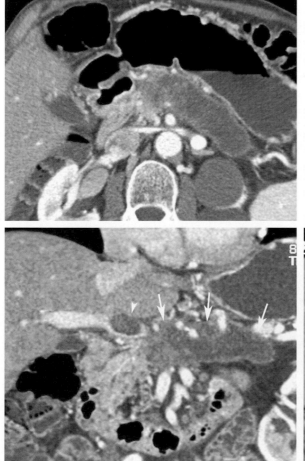

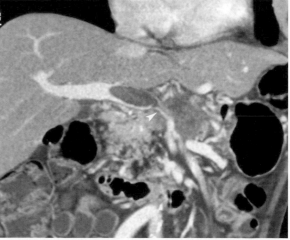

a

b

c

**Fig. 30.6a–c.** Extensive vascular involvement: superior demonstration by CPR and VRT. **a** The axial image demonstrates a large cancer in the body and tail, with compression of the venous confluence. **b** The CPR image demonstrates the whole tumor (*arrows*) involving the celiac trunk and a thrombus (*arrowhead*) in the portal vein. **c** The volume-rendered image delineates extensive compression of the venous confluence (*arrowhead*) with subsequent thrombosis of the portal vein

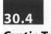

## 30.4
## Cystic Tumors

There is a variety of cystic lesions in the pancreas. The most common cystic mass in the pancreas is the pseudocyst, which has been estimated to compose up to 80% of cystic lesions of the pancreas. However, with the development of MDCT and contrast-enhanced MRI of the pancreas as well as EUS, an increasing prevalence of small- to medium-sized cystic lesions of the pancreas are found in patients without any history of pancreatitis. Many of these cystic masses are neoplasms, which pose an increasing challenge to radiologists in terms of lesion characterization and involvement in further management of these tumors (SAHANI et al. 2005). As contrast-enhanced CT is often the first imaging modality to detect these tumors, readers have to be aware of the typical features of cystic lesions in the pancreas, although definitive characterization is often left to MRI or EUS with guided aspiration biopsy.

## 30.4.1
## Serous Cystadenoma

The serous cystadenoma (formally known as "microcystic" cystadenoma) predominantly affects women in the sixth to seventh decade. Quite often, it is incidentally detected, when CT studies performed for clinical symptoms unrelated to the pancreas. Serous cystadenoma is a benign tumor, with no more than 10 cases of serous cystadenocarcinoma reported worldwide. Thus, in clinical practice there is no risk of malignant degeneration, which may direct clinical management of these tumors more toward follow-up.

The typical CT features of more common microcystic serous cystadenoma are multiple (usually more than six) small cysts that range from a few millimeters up to 2 cm in size, which tend to give the lesion an inhomogeneous, hypodense "pseudosolid" appearance at contrast-enhanced CT (SAHANI et al. 2005). Actually, there are no solid nodules in serous cystadenoma present, but the multitude of tiny septations and cyst walls may give

**Fig. 30.7a–c.** Serous cystadenoma. **a** Axial CT demonstrates a multicystic mass in the pancreatic head and neck, which (**b**) is better seen on the coronal MPR (*arrows*). **c** However, the internal structure of the lesion with multiple, small cysts is better appreciated on the axial T2-weighted MR image

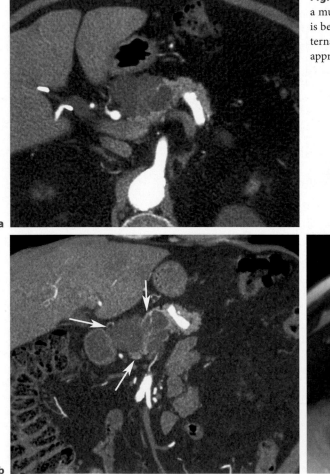

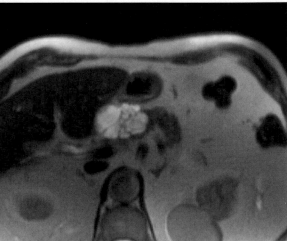

a pseudosolid appearance (Fig. 30.7). In case of equivocal CT, MRI will help to define the microcystic nature of the lesion (Fig. 30.7). In larger serous cystadenoma, central septations may have a sponge-like appearance with central, punctuate, or globular calcifications (MoRANA and GUARISE 2006). This helps to differentiate serous cystadenoma from ("macrocystic") mucinous cystadenoma with peripheral calcifications of cyst walls. The rare, oligocystic variant of serous cystadenoma presents with imaging features similar to mucinous cystadenoma, with a lobulated shape and several internal septations. In these cases, definitive diagnosis is usually based on EUS-guided aspiration biopsy or CT-guided core biopsy.

Further management of serous cystadenoma depends on tumor size. It has been shown that small tumors (up to 4 cm) tend to have a slow growth (mean growth rate: 0.12 cm per year), which renders follow-up reasonable (TSENG et al. 2005). However, for tumors larger than 4 cm in diameter, a mean growth rate of approximately 2 cm per year has been reported, which made some surgical groups recommend resection of this benign tumor, regardless of the presence or absence of symptoms.

## 30.4.2
## Mucinous Cystadenoma/Cystadenocarcinoma

Mucinous cystadenoma usually occur in women. In contrast to (the always benign) serous cystadenoma, mucinous tumors represent a histologic spectrum, ranging from adenoma, borderline tumor to non-invasive and invasive carcinoma. With advancing age, the histologic grade of the tumor tends to worsen. The CT appearance is always macrocystic (therefore the synonym

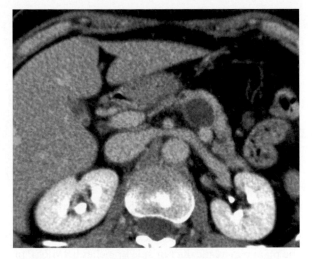

**Fig. 30.8.** Mucinous cystadenoma. The axial CT image shows a unilocular, thin-walled cyst. There was no history of pancreatitis in this patient, which renders diagnosis of a pseudocyst unlikely

*macrocystic cystadenoma*), either unilocular or multilocular. A unilocular cystic appearance is similar to a pseudocyst or the rare case of a simple cyst (Fig. 30.8). In the absence of imaging features typical for chronic pancreatitis, a history of pancreatitis is important to differentiate between pseudocyst and unilocular mucinous cystadenoma. Aspiration biopsy of the cyst definitely helps, because the cyst fluid in pseudocysts is rich in amylase, whereas mucinous cystadenoma aspirates will yield high tumor markers (carcinoembryonic antigen [CEA], cancer antigen [CA] 19-9, and CA 15-3). The tumor marker CEA in the cyst fluid is most specific for diagnosis of mucinous tumors (BRUGGE et al. 2004). The typical imaging features of mucinous cystadenoma are a multilocular, macrocystic appearance. Thick septa

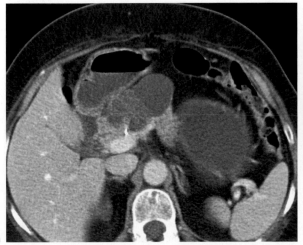

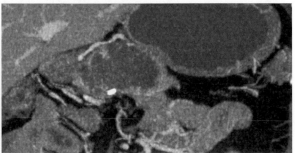

**Fig. 30.9a,b.** Mucinous cystadenoma recurrence. **a** The axial CT imaging shows a large cystic lesion, with one cyst exceeding 20 mm in diameter. There is a hyperdense clip present from previous surgery. **b** The coronal MIP image demonstrates the large cystic mass in the pancreatic head and body. Surgery confirmed recurrence of a benign mucinous cystadenoma

and solid papillary projections in the cyst wall or a partially solid appearance of the tumor are suggestive of malignant degeneration.

On CT, the typical features are a macrocystic appearance (>20-mm diameter of cysts) with thin septations (Fig. 30.9) (Schima et al. 2006). Cyst wall calcifications may be present (differential diagnosis: central, punctuate, or chunky calcifications in serous cystadenoma and parenchymal calcifications in chronic pancreatitis with pseudocyst). The septa may show a variable degree of enhancement. Septations are much better seen with T2-weighted MR imaging, but cyst wall calcifications will escape detection by MRI. Solid components display enhancement after iodine or gadolinium contrast agent. Demonstration of lack of communication with the main pancreatic duct or side branches by MRCP or ERCP helps to differentiate between mucinous cystadenoma/cystadenocarcinoma and intraductal papillary mucinous tumor (IPMT).

### 30.4.3
### Intraductal Papillary Mucinous Tumor

IPMT was first described in 1982 as a distinct entity. In the past few years, it has been described with increasing frequency, due to the revolution of thin-section MRI and, especially, MRCP. Another factor is the more widespread knowledge of this disease, which helps to avoid misclassifying IPMT as chronic pancreatitis. IPMT originates from the epithelium of the pancreatic main duct or branch ducts, growing carpet-like along the ductal system. Histologically, it represents a spectrum, ranging from benign dysplasia over borderline lesions to infiltrative carcinomas. Therefore, differentiating the benign IPMT from advanced malignant cases is important for deciding on the treatment plan. Small, benign IPMT can be followed-up, whereas borderline to invasive malignant lesions have to be treated with partial or total pancreatectomy. IPMT leads to mucin filling and duct dilatation (of the main duct or branch ducts). Subsequently, duct obstruction may clinically manifest as pancreatitis.

According of the type of duct involvement, IPMT are classified into three subtypes: (1) main-duct type with diffuse or segmental dilatation of the main pancreatic duct greater than 3 mm; (2) branch-duct type with unilocular or multilocular lesions, with a grape-like appearance; and (3) combined-type, in which both the main pancreatic duct and branch ducts are involved (Fig. 30.10) (Procacci et al. 1999; Taouli et al. 2000). Main-duct and combined types are at higher risk of malignant transformation. On CT, the most specific signs predictive for malignancy are main pancreatic duct dilatation greater than 10 mm, diffuse or multifocal involvement (Fig. 30.10), and calcified intraluminal content (Fukukura et al. 2000; Taouli et al. 2000). The presence of a bulging papilla (due to mucinous filling of the main duct) and solid, contrast-enhanced papillary proliferations in the duct are other signs suggestive of malignant groves (Fukukura et al. 2000; Procacci et al. 1999, 2001). Branch-duct-type IPMT is most often located in the uncinate process of the pancreas. The value of MDCT with 3D reconstructions lies in the vi-

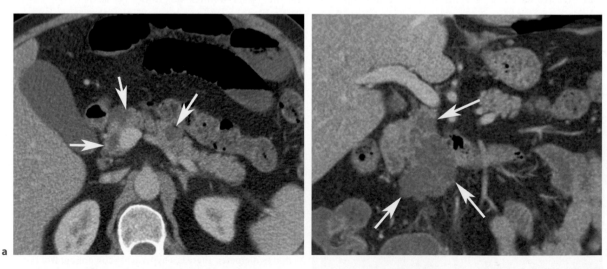

a                                                                      b

**Fig. 30.10a,b.** IPMT of the combined type. **a** Axial CT demonstrates multifocal enlargement of the main pancreatic duct (*arrows*). **b** The coronal MPR also demonstrates grape-like cystic lesion in the uncinate process, typical for an IPMT growing in the branch ducts and the main pancreatic duct. During surgery, an IPMT of borderline histology was resected

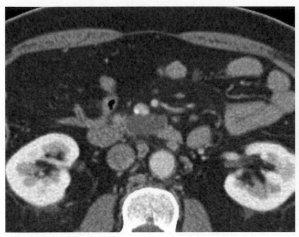 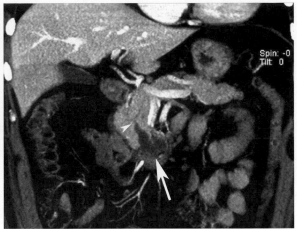

a | b

**Fig. 30.11a,b.** IPMT of the branch duct type. **a** The axial CT image shows a small cystic lesion in the uncinate process, which cannot be characterized further. **b** The coronal volume-rendered image demonstrates the communication of the cystic lesion (*arrow*) with the pancreatic duct system (*arrowhead*), indicative of an IPMT

sualization of the communication between the cystic lesion and the pancreatic ductal system (Fig. 30.11) (Sahani et al. 2006a).

There is international consensus (Tanaka et al. 2006) that an IPMT of the main-duct type or the combined type should be treated surgically, if possible. Likewise, large and symptomatic branch-duct-type IPMT should be resected. The low risk of malignancy in small (<30 mm); asymptomatic branch-duct type IPMT and their low tendency to grow warrant follow-up with cross-sectional imaging (Irie et al. 2004; Tanaka et al. 2006).

As mentioned, the most important differential diagnosis of a main-duct-type IPMT is chronic pancreatitis. The typical CT features indicative of IPMT are the bulging papilla, diffuse pancreatic duct dilatation without stricture, no circumscribed pancreatic duct stones, and solid contrast-enhanced nodules. Pancreatic gland atrophy may be present in IPMT and chronic pancreatitis as well, but pancreatic parenchyma classifications are almost always absent in IPMT.

### 30.4.4
### How Good is CT in Characterizing Cystic Lesions? How Aggressive Should Treatment Be in Small Cystic Lesions (≤3 cm)?

The increasing use of cross-sectional imaging of the abdomen has resulted in an increasing number of patients, who are labeled with the diagnosis of a cystic lesion of the pancreas. In contradiction to a widespread belief, the majority of these lesions are cystic neoplasms and not pseudocysts (Fernandez-del Castillo et al. 2003). Contrast-enhanced MDCT has a high accuracy, similar to that seen with MRI. The most significant limitation is that even small, morphologically benign appearing cysts maybe malignant (Visser et al. 2007). In the large study of Sahani et al. (2006b) on 86 cystic lesions 3 cm or smaller in diameter, the positive predictive value of unilocular cysts for prediction of benignity was 97%, which allows recommending follow-up in these lesions (Fig. 30.11). The presence of cyst septations was associated with borderline histology or in situ malignancy in 20%. In these patients, EUS-guided aspiration biopsy will decide on further treatment. In patients equivocal CT, MRI with MRCP will help to define the cystic nature of the lesion.

### 30.5
### Neuroendocrine Tumors

Neuroendocrine tumors (NET) of the pancreas are quite rare, accounting for not more than 1–5% of all pancreatic tumors (Noone et al. 2005). They arise from the endocrine pancreas. Frequently they have been referred to as "islet cell tumors," although this is a misnomer. Recently they were classified according the WHO proposal, which includes histopathologic and functional parameters (Rha et al. 2007). This new classification comprises a spectrum of well-differentiated endocrine tumors (with benign or uncertain biological behavior),

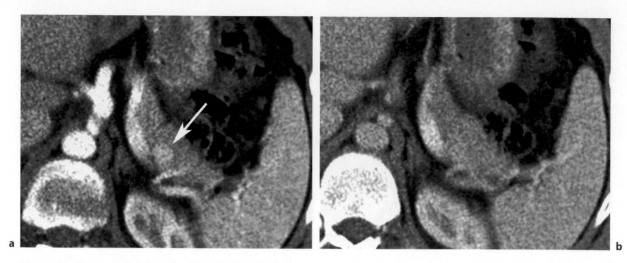

**Fig. 30.12a,b.** Insulinoma: superior visualization at arterial-phase CT. **a** Arterial-phase MDCT shows a small, typically hyperenhancing nodule in the pancreatic tail (*arrow*), which (**b**) is not seen in the venous-phase CT

which are functioning (i.e., hormone producing) or nonfunctioning, well-differentiated endocrine carcinoma with low malignancy potential and poorly differentiated endocrine carcinoma with a poor prognosis. This new classification of endocrine tumors may not be familiar to radiologists. Radiologically, one may be confronted with NET of the pancreas in two different scenarios: first, in patients, who present clinically with the diagnosis of a hormone-producing tumor (e.g., insulinoma, gastrinoma, VIPoma, somatostatinoma, glucagonoma, etc.). In these patients, the diagnosis is biochemically confirmed and the task of radiology is to localize the tumor. Second, patients with nonfunctioning (i.e., nonhormone hypersecreting) tumors may present clinically due to signs of local tumor spread such as jaundice. In these patients, cross-sectional imaging should suggest an alternative diagnosis to adenocarcinoma because of the different imaging features. CT and MRI (and EUS) should help to stage the tumor regarding local spread and the presence of metastases.

Multiphase contrast-enhanced CT for NET of the pancreas should always include an arterial-phase scan, because NET tends to be hypervascular, unless it is very large and partially necrotic.

The most common functioning NET is insulinoma, which tend to be equally distributed between the head, body, and tail. They are benign in 90% of cases and difficult to find because of their small size (approximately 90% are <2 cm in diameter) and often seen only in the arterial phase scan. With multiphase helical CT, 83% of insulinomas can be detected in retrospect (FIDLER et al. 2003). In the study of GOUYA et al. (2003), dual-

phase two-detector-row CT revealed 94% of insulinomas, comparable to the diagnostic value of EUS. Not surprisingly, the combined protocol of CT and EUS was most effective and showed all tumors (100%). The CT features insulinoma are a hyperenhancing nodule (Fig. 30.12). The value of MDCT with 3D reconstructions lies not only in the detection of insulinomas, but also in the surgical planning. Superficially located insulinomas distant to the main pancreatic duct may undergo enucleation, whereas tumors located deep in the parenchyma have to be resected together with a part of the gland (Fig. 30.13).

Gastrinomas are the second most common functioning NET. They are small, tend to be multiple, and are malignant in up to 60%. Ninety percent of gastrinomas are located in the "gastrinoma triangle" including the descending duodenum and the pancreatic head to the neck and the junction between the cystic and the common hepatic duct. In the older literature, CT detection rates were low, but now, state-of-the-art MDCT protocol will identify many gastrinomas, including small duodenal tumors (RAPPEPORT et al. 2006).

Glucagonoma, VIPoma, somatostatinoma, and nonfunctioning NET are almost always malignant. They present as large masses with moderate to strong enhancement (Fig. 30.14). The internal structure will be inhomogeneous with necrosis and cystic degeneration (RHA et al. 2007). Local tumor spread will lead to clinical symptoms, although pancreatic duct obstruction is rare (in comparison to adenocarcinoma). In well-differentiated endocrine carcinoma, metastases to the

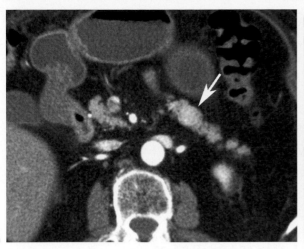

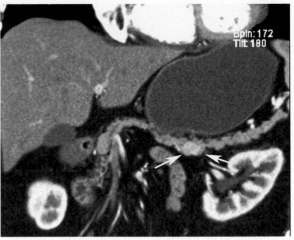

a

b

**Fig. 30.13a,b.** Insulinoma: importance of 3D-reconstructions for surgical planning. **a** Axial-contrast enhanced in CT in the arterial phase demonstrates small, hyperenhancing nodules in the pancreatic body, suggestive of insulinoma in a patient suf-fering from hypoglycemic attacks. **b** For surgical planning, the CPR along the pancreas is helpful: it demonstrates a superficial location of the insulinoma, which could be treated with enucle-ation instead of pancreatic tail resection

lymph nodes or liver are present in 70–80%. Metastatic spread to the liver with multiple tiny nodules may escape detection with CT. In these cases, MRI with liver-specific contrast agents is superior to CT for tumor staging. In general, contrast-enhanced MDCT and MRI are complementary methods in patients with suspected NET of the pancreas for reliable tumor localization and staging, which will obviate the need for intraoperative ultrasound.

## 30.6
## Pancreatic Metastases

The most common primary malignancies to seed metastases to pancreas are renal cell cancer, malignant melanoma, lung cancer, and breast cancer. Least commonly, adenoma carcinomas from other areas in the gastrointestinal tract will spread to the pancreas. Although once being thought of as a rare occurrence, pancreatic metas-

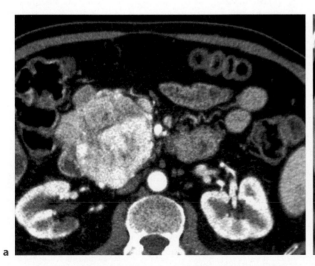

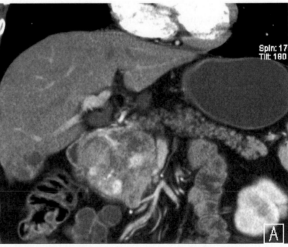

a

b

**Fig. 30.14a,b.** Malignant neuroendocrine tumor. **a** The axial CT image shows a large, inhomogeneous, partially hyper-vas-cular tumor in the pancreatic head. **b** The coronal MPR shows the tumor and the lack of pancreatic duct obstruction and sub-stantial pancreatic atrophy. There is a liver metastasis in the right lobe present. In adenocarcinoma, duct obstruction with gland atrophy of the body and tail would be expected

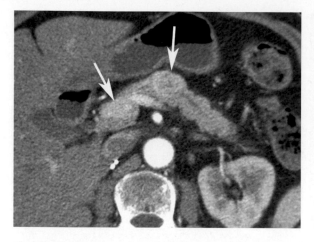

**Fig. 30.15.** Metastases from RCC. Axial contrast-enhanced CT typically shows more than one hyper-vascular tumor in the pancreas (*arrows*). CT features are similar to NET. Note that the right kidney has been resected

tases are not that rare in autopsy series. Recently, with the evolution of thin-section contrast-enhanced CT and MRI imaging, metastases in the pancreatic gland are found with increasing incidence (MERKLE et al. 1998; NG et al. 1999).

Differentiation between primary adenocarcinoma of the pancreas and metastases to the pancreas is important because of the different therapeutic strategies. For pancreatic metastases, systemic chemotherapy is sought. In rare cases, metastatic spread to the pancreas may be the first (and only) sign of systemic disease, and aggressive surgical therapy will result in prolonged survival (STANKARD and KARL et al. 1992) Pancreatic involvement may manifest as either a single pancreatic mass, multiple nodules, or diffuse swelling. The CT appearance of pancreatic metastases depends on the primary malignancy. Renal cell carcinoma (RCC) metastases enhance most conspicuously during early-phase scans with minimal tumor–pancreas contrast on delayed-phase scans. Metastases to the pancreas tend to be multiple (Fig. 30.15). Delineation of a hypervascular RCC metastasis to the pancreas in the arterial phase is often quite transient, similar to the contrast enhancement characteristics seen in insulinoma. According to our experience application of a high amount of contrast material (2 ml per kilogram body weight) with a flow rate of at least 4–5 ml s$^{-1}$ is crucial for the delineation of these masses.

As a stated previously, a variety of different tumors may metastasize to the pancreas. Melanoma metastases may show contrast enhancement similar to that seen in RCC, whereas lung and GI cancer tend to seed hypovascular, low-density metastases, similar to primary pancreatic adenocarcinoma.

## References

Alexakis N, Halloran C, Raraty M, Ghaneh P, Sutton R, Neoptolemos JP (2004) Current standards of surgery for pancreatic cancer. Br J Surg 91:1410–1427

Bluemke DA, Cameron JL, Hruban RH et al. (1995) Potentially resectable pancreatic adenocarcinoma: spiral CT assessment with surgical and pathologic correlation. Radiology 197:381–385

Boland GW, O'Malley ME, Saez M, Fernandez-del Castillo C, Warshaw AL, Mueller PR (1999) Pancreatic-phase versus portal vein-phase helical CT of the pancreas: optimal temporal window for evaluation of pancreatic adenocarcinoma. AJR Am J Roentgenol 172:605–608

Bronstein YL, Loyer EM, Kaur H et al. (2004) Detection of small pancreatic tumors with multiphasic helical CT. AJR Am J Roentgenol 182:619–623

Brugge WR, Lewandrowski KB, Lee-Lewandrowski E et al. (2004) Diagnosis of pancreatic cystic neoplasms: a report of the cooperative study group. Gastroenterology 126:1330–1336

DeWitt J, Deveraux B, Chriswell M et al. (2004) Comparison of endoscopic ultrasonography and multidetector computed tomography for detecting and staging pancreatic cancer. Ann Intern Med 141:753–763

Fernandez-del Castillo C, Targarona J, Thayer SP, Rattner DW, Brugge WR, Warshaw AL (2003) Incidental pancreatic cysts: clinicopathologic characteristics and comparison with symptomatic patients. Arch Surg 138:427–423; discussion, 433–424

Fidler JL, Fletcher JG, Reading CC et al. (2003) Preoperative detection of pancreatic insulinomas on multiphasic helical CT. AJR Am J Roentgenol 181:775–780

Fletcher JG, Wiersma MJ, Farrell MA et al. (2003) Pancreatic malignancy: value of arterial, pancreatic, and hepatic phase imaging with multi-detector row CT. Radiology 229:81–90

Freeny PC (2005) CT diagnosis and staging of pancreatic carcinoma. Eur Radiol 15(Suppl.):D96–D99

Fukukura Y, Fujiyoshi F, Sasaki M, Inoue H, Yonezawa S, Nakajo M (2000) Intraductal papillary mucinous tumors of the pancreas: thin-section helical CT findings. AJR Am J Roentgenol 174:441–447

Fukushima H, Itoh S, Takada A et al. (2006) Diagnostic value of curved multiplanar reformatted images in multislice CT for the detection of resectable pancreatic ductal adenocarcinoma. Eur Radiol 16:1709–1718

Goshima S, Kanematsu M, Kondo H et al. (2006) Pancreas: optimal scan delay for contrast-enhanced multi-detector row CT. Radiology 241:167–174

Gouya H, Vignaux O, Augui J et al. (2003) CT, endoscopic sonography, and a combined protocol for preoperative evaluation of pancreatic insulinomas. AJR Am J Roentgenol 181:987–992

Graf O, Boland GW, Warshaw AL, Fernandez-del Castillo C, Hahn PF, Mueller PR (1997) Arterial versus portal venous helical CT for revealing pancreatic adenocarcinoma: conspicuity of tumor and critical vascular anatomy. AJR Am J Roentgenol 169:119–123

Grenacher L, Klauss M, Dukic L et al. (2004) Hochauflösende Bildgebung beim Pankreaskarzinom: prospektiver Vergleich von MRT und 4-Zeilen-Spiral-CT. Fortschr Rontgenstr 176:1624–1633 (in German)

Hough TJ, Raptopoulos V, Siewert B, Matthews JB (1999) Teardrop superior mesenteric vein: CT sign for unresectable carcinoma of the pancreas. AJR Am J Roentgenol 173:1509–1512

Ichikawa T, Haradome H, Hachiya J et al. (1997) Pancreatic ductal adenocarcinoma: preoperative assessment with helical CT versus dynamic MR imaging. Radiology 202:655–662

Irie H, Honda H, Kaneko K, Kuroiwa T, Yoshimitsu K, Masuda K (1997) Comparison of helical CT and MR imaging in detecting and staging small pancreatic adenocarcinoma. Abdom Imaging 22:429–433

Irie H, Yoshimitsu K, Aibe H et al. (2004) Natural history of pancreatic intraductal papillary mucinous tumor of branch duct type: follow-up study by magnetic resonance cholangiopancreatography. J Comput Assist Tomogr 28:117–122

Klapman JB, Chang KJ, Lee JG, Nguyen P (2005) Negative predictive value of endoscopic ultrasound in a large series of patients with a clinical suspicion of pancreatic cancer. Am J Gastroenterol 100:2658–2661

Legmann P, Vignaux O, Dousset B et al. (1998) Pancreatic tumors: comparison of dual-phase helical CT and endoscopic sonography. AJR Am J Roentgenol 170:1315–1322

Lowenfels AB, Maisonneuve PM, Cavallini G et al. (1993) Pancreatitis and the risk of pancreatic cancer. New Engl J Med 328:1435–1437

Lowenfels AB, Maisonneuve P, DiMagno EP et al. (1997) Hereditary pancreatitis and the risk of pancreatic cancer. International Hereditary Pancreatitis Study Group. J Natl Cancer Inst 89:442–446

Lu DSK, Vedantham S, Krasny RM, Kadell B, Berger WL, Reber HA (1996) Two-phase helical CT for pancreatic tumors: pancreatic versus hepatic phase enhancement of tumor, pancreas, and vascular structures. Radiology 199:697–701

Lu DSK, Reber HA, Krasny RM, Kadell BM, Sayre J (1997) Local staging of pancreatic cancer: criteria for unresectability of major vessels as revealed by pancreatic-phase thin section helical CT. AJR Am J Roentgenol 168:1439–1443

McNulty NJ, Francis IR, Platt JF, Cohan RH, Korobkin M, Gebramaniam A (2001) Multi-detector row helical CT of the pancreas: effect of contrast-enhanced multiphasic imaging on enhancement of the pancreas, peripancreatic vasculature, and pancreatic adenocarcinoma. Radiology 220:97–102

Merkle EM, Boaz T, Kolokythas O, Haaga JR, Lewin JS, Brambs H-J (1998) Metastases to the pancreas. Br J Radiol 71:1208–1214

Morana G, Guarise A (2006) Cystic tumors of the pancreas. Cancer Imaging 6:60–71

Nakayama Y, Yamashita Y, Kadota M et al. (2001) Vascular encasement by pancreatic cancer: correlation of CT findings with surgical and pathologic results. J Comput Assist Tomogr 25:337–342

Ng CS, Loyer EM, Iyer RB, David CL, DuBrow RA, Charnsangavej C (1999) Metastases to the pancreas from renal cell carcinoma: findings on three-phase contrast-enhanced helical CT. AJR Am J Roentgenol 172:1555–1559

Noone TC, Hosey J, Firat Z, Semelka RC (2005) Imaging and localization of islet-cell tumours of the pancreas on CT and MRI. Best Pract Res Clin Endocrinol Metab 19:195–211

Procacci C, Megibow AJ, Carbognin G et al. (1999) Intraductal papillary mucinous tumor of the pancreas: a pictorial essay. Radiographics 19:1447–1463

Procacci C, Carbognin G, Biasiutti C, Guarise A, Ghirardi C, Schenal G (2001) Intraductal papillary mucinous tumors of the pancreas: spectrum of CT and MR findings with pathologic correlation. Eur Radiol 11:1939–1951

Prokesch R, Chow LC, Beaulieu CF, Bammer R, Jeffrey RB (2002) Isoattenuating pancreatic carcinoma at multi-detector row CT: secondary signs. Radiology 224:764–768

Prokesch RW, Chow LC, Beaulieu CF et al. (2002) Local staging of pancreatic carcinoma with multi-detector row CT: use of curved planar reformations-initial experience. Radiology 225:759–765

Rappeport ED, Hansen CP, Kjaer A, Knigge U (2006) Multidetector computed tomography and neuroendocrine pancreaticoduodenal tumors. Acta Radiol 47:248–256

Rha SE, Jung SE, Lee KL, Ku YM, Byun JY, Lee JM (2007) CT and MR imaging findings of endocrine tumor according to WHO classification. Eur J Radiol 62:371–377

Richter GM, Wunsch C, Schneider B et al. (1998) Hydro-CT in der Detektion und im Staging des Pankreaskarzinoms. Radiologe 38:279–286 (in German)

Sahani DV, Kadavigere R, Saokar A, Fernandez-del Castillo C, Brugge WR, Hahn PF (2005) Cystic pancreatic lesions: a simple imaging-based classification system for guiding management. Radiographics 25:1471–1484

Sahani DV, Kadavigere R, Blake M, Fernandez-Del Castillo C, Lauwers GY, Hahn PF (2006a) Intraductal papillary mucinous neoplasm of pancreas: multi-detector row CT with 2D curved reformations-correlation with MRCP. Radiology 238:560–569

Sahani DV, Saokar A, Hahn PF, Brugge WR, Fernandez-del Castillo C (2006b) Pancreatic cysts 3 cm or smaller: how aggressive should treatment be? Radiology 238:912–919

Schima W, Ba-Ssalamah A, Kolblinger C, Kulinna-Cosentini C, Puespoek A, Gotzinger P (2007) Pancreatic adenocarcinoma. Eur Radiol 17:638–649

Schima W, Függer R, Schober E et al. (2002) Diagnosis and staging of pancreatic cancer: comparison of mangafodipir-enhanced MRI and contrast-enhanced helical hydro-CT. AJR Am J Roentgenol 179:717–724

Schima W, Ba-Ssalamah A, Plank C et al. (2006) [Pancreas. Part II: tumors.]. Radiologe 46:421–437

Schueller G, Schima W, Schueller-Weidekamm C et al. (2006) Multidetector CT of pancreas: effects of contrast material flow rate and individualized scan delay on enhancement of pancreas and tumor contrast. Radiology 241:441–448

Stankard CE, Karl RC (1992) The treatment of isolated pancreatic metastases from renal cell carcinoma: a surgical review. Am J Gastroenterol 87:1658–1660

Tanaka M, Chari S, Adsay V et al. (2006) International consensus guidelines for management of intraductal papillary mucinous neoplasms and mucinous cystic neoplasms of the pancreas. Pancreatology 6:17–32

Taouli B, Vilgrain V, Vullierme M-P et al. (2000) Intraductal papillary tumors of the pancreas: helical CT with histopathologic correlation. Radiology 217:757–764

Trede M, Schwall G, Saeger H-D (1990) Survival after pancreatoduodenectomy. 118 consecutive resections without an operative mortality. Ann Surg 211:447–458

Tseng JF, Warshaw AL, Sahani DV, Lauwers GY, Rattner DW, Fernandez-del Castillo C (2005) Serous cystadenoma of the pancreas: tumor growth rates and recommendations for treatment. Ann Surg 242:413–419

Tublin ME, Tessler FN, Cheng SL, Peters TL, McGovern PC (1999) Effect of injection rate of contrast medium on pancreatic and hepatic helical CT. Radiology 210:97–101

Vargas R, Nino-Murcia M, Trueblood W, Jeffrey RBJ (2004) MDCT in pancreatic adenocarcinoma: prediction of vascular invasion and resectability using a multiphasic technique with curved planar reformations. AJR Am J Roentgenol 182:419–245

Visser BC, Yeh BM, Qayyum A, Way LW, McCulloch CE, Coakley FV (2007) Characterization of cystic pancreatic masses: relative accuracy of CT and MRI. AJR Am J Roentgenol 189:648–656

Warshaw AL, Fernandez-del Castillo C (1992) Pancreatic carcinoma. N Engl J Med 326:455–465

Yamada Y, Mori H, Kiyosue H, Matsumoto S, Hori Y, Maeda T (2000) CT assessment of the inferior peripancreatic veins: clinical significance. AJR Am J Roentgenol 174:677–684

Yanaga Y, Awai K, Nakayama Y et al. (2007) Pancreas: patient body weight tailored contrast material injection protocol versus fixed dose protocol at dynamic CT. Radiology 245:475–482

# Imaging of Colorectal Tumors with Multidetector Row CT

Andrea Laghi, Franco Iafrate and Cesare Hassan

A. Laghi MD
Department of Radiological Sciences, "Sapienza"-University of
Rome, Polo Pontino, I.C.O.T. Hospital, via Franco Fagiana 34,
04100 Latina, Italy

F. Iafrate MD
Department of Radiological Sciences, "Sapienza"-University of
Rome, Polo Pontino, I.C.O.T. Hospital, via Franco Fagiana 34,
04100 Latina, Italy

C. Hassan MD
Gastroenterology and Digestive Endoscopy Unit, "Nuovo
Regina Margherita" Hospital, via Emilio Morosini 30, 00153
Rome, Italy

## ABSTRACT

MDCT has a leading role in the diagnostic process of colorectal cancer (CRC), including early diagnosis (i.e., screening), staging, follow-up, and assessment of therapy response. Imaging protocols need to be tailored according to clinical requirements. Thus, CT colonography (CTC) is necessary for early diagnosis of CRC and polyps. Technical protocol needs preliminary bowel cleansing and air distension, although new developments include prepless approaches, without the use of laxative agents, and $CO_2$ automatic insufflation. Low-dose scanning protocols are routinely implemented for screening subjects, and image-reviewing software now offers new visualization tools that help decrease perceptual errors. CTC has a definite role in screening, being one of the official screening options suggested by major international societies. Contrast-enhanced MDCT, performed according to standard scanning protocols, is still the imaging modality of choice for staging and follow-up of CRC, although there is an emerging role of the hybrid PET–CT scanner, particularly in the follow-up. In addition, new information may arise from new PET–CT colonography examinations, whose role is still to be defined. Finally, in the assessment of therapy response, CT perfusion is required. CT perfusion offers functional information (blood flow, blood volume, mean transit time, and permeability surface), which correlate with tumor neoangiogenesis. Very preliminary results of few clinical studies using perfusion CT before and after radiochemotherapy treatment show a potential important clinical application in rectal cancer management. Monitoring the response to therapy may lead clinicians to customize treatment to the response of the individual patient, and reliable prediction of the response may improve patient selection and avoid nonproductive, costly treatments.

## Introduction

Colorectal cancer (CRC) is the second or third leading cause of cancer deaths across the develop world. CRC has been the most common form of cancer diagnosed in Europe since 2000, with an estimated 280,000 new cases per year (BOYLE and FERLAY 2005). Of these, 123,000 cases were diagnosed in men, while 135,000 were in women. The trend in CRC incidence from 1970 projected to 2006 showed a steady increase in all European countries, mainly because of an increase of the older population (SCHEIDEN et al. 2005; MALILA and HAKULINEN 2003). Such data are substantially different from what has been reported in the United States in the past decades. Indeed, the US long-term CRC incidence rate decreased by 1.8% per year through the period 1985–1995, thereafter stabilizing up to 2000 (RIES et al. 2000; WEIR et al. 2003). CRC death rates in the United States have been similarly declining from 1980 to 2000, with a 5-year survival rate around 60% (SANT et al. 2003). Nevertheless, CRC still ranks as the third cause of death in both men and women in the United States, ranking second in the whole of North America.

Besides population aging, incidence of CRC seems to be strictly related to several dietary and lifestyle factors of Western societies. Physical inactivity, excess body weight, a high-fat diet, high alcohol consumption, and smoking early in life have been shown to be consistent risk factors for CRC development in large epidemiological surveys.

Genetic susceptibility is of prime importance in colorectal carcinogenesis. Most of the population (75%) is at the same risk of developing CRC (i.e., average risk). However, people who have one first-degree relative with either a colorectal or an adenomatous polyp have approximately a twofold increased risk of colorectal cancer, and the risk begins approximately 10 years sooner (MITCHELL et al. 2005). A much higher lifetime risk of developing CRC–up to 90–100%–occurs in families affected by heritable colorectal cancer syndromes, such as hereditary nonpolyposis colorectal cancer (HNPCC) and familial adenomatous polyposis (FAP). Although rare, such syndromes account for 8% of the total CRC burden (BURT 1996; LYNCH and DE LA CHAPELLE 2003).

CT, since the very early era, has been extensively used in the evaluation of patients affected by CRC, primarily in staging and follow-up (BALTHAZAR et al. 1988; FREENY et al. 1986). However, it was with the advent of multislice technology that the role of CT has observed a great expansion, due to the development of novel techniques, such as CT colonography (CTC) (VINING and GELFAND 1994; TAYLOR et al. 2007) and CT perfusion (SAHANI et al. 2005). CTC has become in few years the second-best imaging modality among the colonic tests (PICKHARDT 2003) whereas CT perfusion, still under research investigation, is becoming an attractive method to monitor the response to therapy of rectal cancer. Thus, nowadays, diagnostic imaging and MDCT play a major role in CRC evaluation, covering the entire spectrum of the disease, from early diagnosis (i.e., screening) and diagnosis to staging, follow-up, and assessment of the response to therapy of rectal cancer.

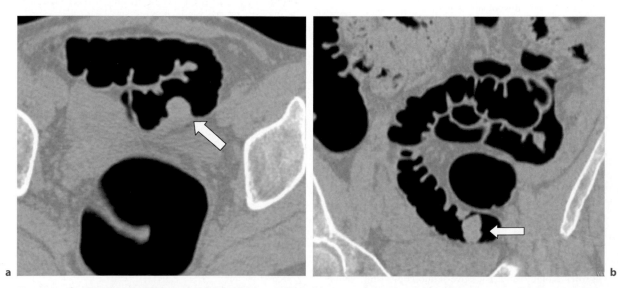

**Fig. 31.1a–f.** CTC showing pedunculated adenomatous polypoid lesion. **a, b** Axial and coronal multiplanar CT reformatted image obtain on supine position, showing a polypoid lesion (*arrow*) of the sigmoid. **c-d** *see next page*

## 31.2
## Technique

CT technique for a colon study should be tailored according to clinical indication. If MDCT is performed for staging of a known CRC and for follow-up, then a contrast-enhanced study of the abdomen and pelvis should be performed; no specific colon preparation is required, and the examination can be considered as a routine abdominal study. On the other hand, if a diagnosis of either a CRC or a precursor (adenomatous polyp) (Fig. 31.1) is concerned, then CTC is the exami-

nation of choice; it requires a meticulous preparation and a specific technical protocol. Finally, in the assessment of the response to therapy in the case of a rectal cancer, a different technical approach is needed, i.e., CT perfusion.

### 31.2.1
### MDCT of the Abdomen and Pelvis

The colon is usually examined as part of an upper and lower abdominal examination. Scan coverage should include the region from the diaphragm to the ischial tu-

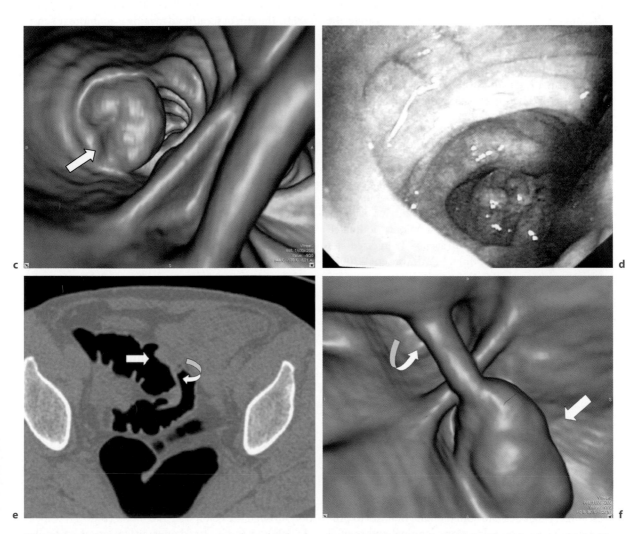

**Fig. 31.1a–f.** (*continued*) CTC showing pedunculated adenomatous polypoid lesion. **c,d** Three-dimensional threshold-rendered endoluminal CT colonograph and corresponding conventional endoscopic image showing the precise correlation between radiological and endoscopical aspect of the lesion

(*arrow*). **e** Axial prone image shows the lesion (*arrow*) is highly mobile, and suggests the presence of a stalk (*curved arrow*). **f** Prone endoluminal CT colonograph image, clearly shows the lesion (*arrow*) and its long pedicle (*curved arrow*)

berosities. When abdominal CT is performed to image the colon, colonic opacification might be considered, using oral administration of either a positive (iodinated or barium-based agents) or a neutral (hyperosmolar watery solutions or low-density barium agents) contrast medium the night before or at least 3 to 4 h before the study, to ensure that adequate contrast material reaches the colon (Doyle et al. 1993). In patients in whom limited rectosigmoid disease is suspected, the contrast material (positive, neutral, or also air in this case) can be gently administered via the rectum in order to facilitate evaluation of the bowel wall. A topogram can then be obtained to confirm filling of the entire colon before CT is performed. Another possible option is the administration of a water enema through the rectum (hydrocolon). It has been demonstrated to be effective in staging CRC improving the ability of CT to demonstrate the depth of tumor invasion of the colonic wall as well as the extension into the pericolonic fat (Gazelle et al. 1995; Hundt et al. 1999).

An optimal study of the abdomen and pelvis can be obtained with MDCT, 16 slices and over. A standard protocol should include a collimation no thicker than 3 mm, with overlapped image reconstruction in order to improve the quality of multiplanar reformations. Intravenous contrast administration should be performed in order to enable both colon and liver evaluation. For this reason, 2 ml per kilogram body weight (with an upper limit of 150 ml for patients weighing more than 75 kg) of nonionic iodinated contrast material should be intravenously injected at a flow rate of no less than 3 ml s$^{-1}$ (Yanaga et al. 2007). Image acquisition during the portal venous phase (65 to 70 s after the start of the injection) is optimal for liver imaging. Image analysis is usually performed on dedicated workstations on which different algorithms for 3D reconstructions are available, including MPR, MIP, and volume rendering.

## 31.2.2
## CT Colonography

CTC, also known as virtual colonoscopy, is an imaging modality, proposed by Vining and Gelfand in 1994 for the evaluation of the colonic mucosa in which thin-section spiral CT provides high-resolution 2D axial images, and CT data sets are edited offline in order to produce multiplanar reconstructions (coronal and sagittal images) as well as 3D endoscopic-like views. Workflow of CTC includes four different steps: (1) bowel cleansing, (2) patient preparation to scanning, (3) data acquisition, and (4) image analysis.

### 31.2.2.1
### Bowel Cleansing

Bowel cleansing is critical. To obtain optimal image quality, the patient's bowel should be free of stool or fluid residues, which might mimic an endoluminal mass lesion or alternatively may mask the presence of either a polyp or a colonic carcinoma. Different laxative regimens are used, with the final goal of minimizing the amount of fluid residues: this is the reason why the use of sodium phosphate or magnesium citrate is preferred over polyethylene glycol (Macari et al. 2001). Conventional bowel preparations can be used in conjunction with fecal/fluid tagging, i.e., the oral administration of a positive contrast agent, either barium or iodine, able to mark the colonic residues (Pickhardt and Choi 2003). The aim of fecal/fluid tagging is to improve sensitivity for lesions completely submerged by fluids on both prone and supine scans as well specificity, especially for small polyps, which can be easily misdiagnosed as tiny fecal residues.

Since bowel preparation is recognized as the most uncomfortable step in the workflow of a conventional colonoscopy as well as for CTC (Gluecker et al. 2003), in order to improve patient compliance, new reduced bowel preparation, or laxative-free study protocols, are under evaluation. Because of the presence of fecal/fluid residues, not completely removed by the absence of complete laxation, fecal tagging is mandatory. In terms of examination accuracy, several experiences have shown results similar to protocols including full bowel preparation (Iannaccone et al. 2004; McFarland and Zalis et al. 2004; Lefere et al. 2005; Dachman et al. 2007; Johnson et al. 2007).

### 31.2.2.2
### Patient Preparation for Scanning

Patient preparation for scanning consists of air insufflation, administration of an antiperistaltic drug, and intravenous injection of iodinated contrast medium, if required. Air insufflation is a critical step since collapsed bowel is another frequent cause of missed lesions at CTC. $CO_2$ represents a possible alternative to room air insufflation, due to the fact that $CO_2$ diminishes discomfort after the procedure, owing to quick resorption through the colon wall and blood (Bretthauer et al. 2002); in some cases better distension of particular segments (i.e., sigmoid and descending colon) has also been demonstrated (Burling et al. 2006).

The use of a spasmolytic agent (hyoscine butylbromide, Buscopan®, or glucagon) may provide better distension, especially in the sigmoid colon in the case of diverticular disease (TAYLOR 2003).

The use of intravenous injection of iodinated contrast medium is reserved to cases where evaluation of the extracolonic findings is needed (i.e., staging of CRC; patients under surveillance program), and it is performed with the acquisition of a contrast-enhanced supine scan during the portal venous phase (LAGHI et al. 2003).

### 31.2.2.3
### Data Acquisition

Data acquisition protocols are in continuous evolution, paralleling the progress of CT scanners. An important point, however, is that CTC can be performed on any MDCT scanner (four-slice or more) with excellent results; this is extremely important in the perspective of a widespread diffusion of the technique outside of referral or academic centers (HASSAN et al. 2008).

Acquisition protocols are now standardized, following the guidelines of the European Society of Gastrointestinal and Abdominal Radiology (ESGAR) CTC Working Group (TAYLOR et al. 2007). Effective slice width should be less than 3 mm, reaching 1 mm on 16 MDCT and over.

Another important issue is the containment of dose exposure, especially in the examinations performed for screening. In these cases, lowering the mA is the option of choice. For supine and prone nonintravenous-contrast-enhanced acquisition, a tube current of 100 mA or less and 50 mA or less, respectively, should be used. For contrast-enhanced scans, a tube current of 50 mA or less (non-contrast-enhanced prone acquisition) and 100–200 mA (contrast-enhanced supine acquisition) is optimal. Exact currents will be dependent on available CT technology (TAYLOR et al. 2007; LUZ 2007). Further improvements are represented by the support of automatic tube current modulation device, able to reduce the dose exposure of around 30–35% (GRASER et al. 2006).

### 31.2.2.4
### Image Analysis

Image analysis, obtained on dedicated offline workstations, is performed with either primary 2D or primary 3D approach. New visualization software is also available (i.e., "virtual dissection" and "unfolded cube" methods), which might improve reader confidence and speedup the reading process (JOHNSON 2006).

Software for automatic polyp detection (computed-assisted diagnosis [CAD]) is already available in the market. It offers the possibility to reduce interobserver variability as well perception errors, especially in inexpert readers (HALLIGAN 2006). The ideal paradigm of CAD integration into the workflow is still under discussion, with CAD as second reader as the most common approach (PETRICK 2008). However, more studies are needed to address this issue.

### 31.2.3
### CT Perfusion

CT perfusion is a noninvasive tool providing functional information on neoplastic tissue: in other words, it is a measurement of tumor neovascularity (neoangiogenesis) (GOH 2007). CT perfusion was first proposed in 1979, but technical limitations, such as poor temporal resolution, have limited the development (MILES and GRIFFITHS 2003). It is with the advent of MDCT, and in particular 64-slice scanners, that a radical change occurred, not only in temporal resolution (available already with MDCT scanners of previous generation), but especially in volume coverage.

CT perfusion consists of a cine-mode acquisition technique performed during dynamic intravenous injection of iodinated contrast medium (MILES 2003; SAHANI 2005). Volume coverage is essential in order to include the largest part of the tumor (or hopefully the entire lesion) within the acquired volume. For this reason, a great benefit derives from the use of 64-MDCT with 40-mm longitudinal coverage. Recently, the development of new devices has widened the volume covered by the scanner (up to 160 mm) by allowing a synchronized movement of the table during the data acquisition.

Nonionic iodinated contrast medium injection is performed at high flow rate (4 ml s$^{-1}$ or greater) with the start of the acquisition few seconds after the injection in order to have a full non-contrast-enhanced dataset.

Acquired data are postprocessed using dedicated software implemented on offline workstations. Perfusion analysis, now, can be performed using software based on deconvolution or compartmental model of analysis (SAHANI 2005). CT perfusion provides functional information about tumor neovascularity, represented by blood volume (milliliter per 100 g wet tissue), blood flow (milliliter per 100 g wet tissue per minute), mean transit time (seconds), and permeability surface area (milliliter per 100 g wet tissue per minute), that can be displayed as chromatic maps (Fig. 31.2).

Unfortunately, it seems that generalizability of the results is not possible, since tumor vascularity measurements obtained using different software based on different algorithms are not directly interchangeable (GOH

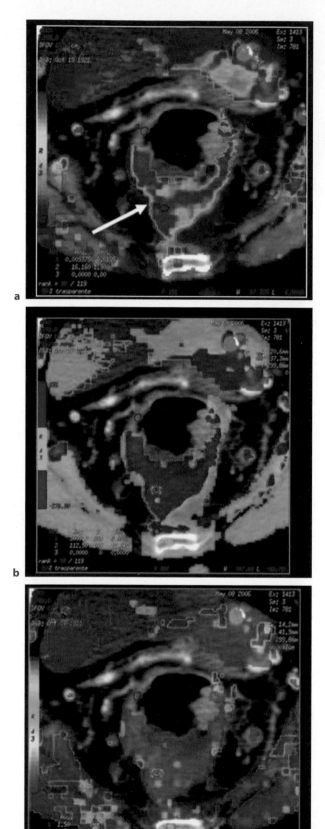

a

b

c

2007). This is a main problem if it is likely that functional imaging will be used to assess tumor response to treatment. In fact, cross-study comparisons will be very difficult and interpretation of data will be problematic as well.

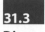
## 31.3
## Diagnosis

### 31.3.1
### Diagnosis of CRC

The diagnosis of CRC, in a symptomatic patient with typical symptoms, is usually performed with colonoscopy and biopsy. The use of a noninvasive imaging modality when the likelihood of disease is very high is useless and not cost-effective, since in most of the cases an invasive examination should be subsequently performed.

Sensitivity of colonoscopy for colon cancer either vegetating or stenosing is approximately 100%. However, up to 10% of colonoscopic examinations are technically difficult even for experienced colonoscopists (MARSHALL and BARTHEL 1993; ANDERSON et al. 1992). In addition to poor bowel preparation, an experienced colonoscopist may be unable to complete the colonoscopy and intubate the cecal pole for a variety of reasons (redundant colon; colonic spasm; severe diverticular disease; obstructing masses or strictures; and angulation or fixation of colonic loops, most commonly due to previous pelvic surgery). The reported rates of incomplete colonoscopy from various US and European series over the past 15 years range from 4 to 25% (ANDERSON et al. 1992; WINAWER et al. 1997; DAFNIS et al. 2000).

In the case of incomplete colonoscopy, CTC is the best imaging modality to evaluate the proximal colon, as indicated also by the statement of the American Gastroenterological Association on CTC (AGA CLINICAL PRACTICE and ECONOMICS COMMITTEE

◄ **Fig. 31.2a–c.** MDCT perfusion of rectal adenocarcinoma. Axial MDCT perfusion is a noninvasive tool, providing functional information about tumor neovascularity, represented by blood volume (milliliter per 100 g wet tissue) (**a**), blood flow (milliliter per 100 g wet tissue per minute) (**b**), mean transit time (seconds), and permeability surface area (milliliter per 100 g wet tissue per minute) (**c**), that can be displayed as chromatic maps

2006) (Fig. 31.3). It has been extensively demonstrated (JOHNSON et al. 2004; ROSMAN and KORSTEN 2007) that CTC is able to assess the entire colonic lumen before the obstruction in virtually all the cases, with accuracy in the detection of synchronous lesions, which is significantly higher than double-contrast barium enema (DCBE). DCBE suffers from different limitations: difficult opacification of proximal colon in the case of a highly stenosing lesion; lower sensitivity for polyps, even clinically significant (>10 mm) (JOHNSON et al. 2004); and poor patient compliance. Furthermore, CTC offers a simultaneous complete staging (local and distant) of the neoplastic lesion, if a contrast-enhanced examination is performed (Fig. 31.4).

## 31.3.2
## Early Diagnosis/Screening of CRC

Secondary prevention of CRC is based on two major considerations:

1. Early diagnosis of CRC is associated with a much better survival when compared with detection in an advanced stage. In fact, even after the introduction of effective chemotherapeutic agents for CRC treatment, the 5-year survival difference between early and late stages is still striking, falling from 96% for stage I to only 5% for stage IV (WONG et al. 2008).

2. Removal of premalignant lesions reduces the incidence of CRC and, therefore, its related mortality. In fact, according to the adenoma–carcinoma se-

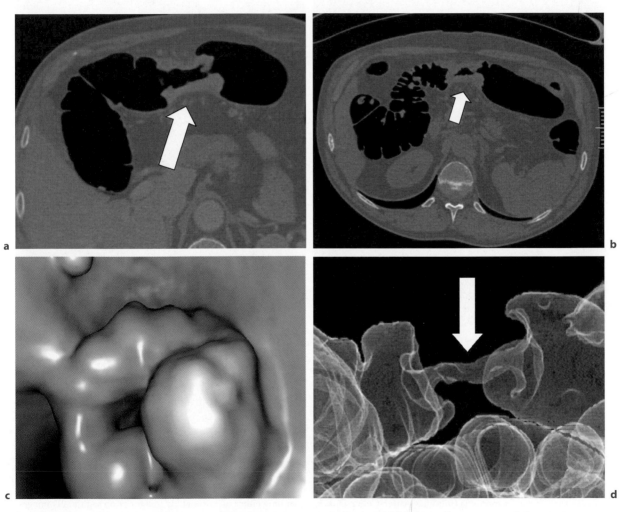

a    b    c    d

**Fig. 31.3a–d.** CTC showing circumferential adenocarcinoma of transverse colon. Stage B carcinoma (modified Astler-Coller-Dukes classification). **a,b** Axial 2D images obtained on supine and prone position showing a circumferential mass (*arrow*) of the transverse colon. **c,d** Intraluminal 3D image and volume-rendered image show only a small residual lumen (*arrow*).

Note the typical "apple-core" appearance of the carcinoma on the volume-rendered image. Because annular masses may be indistinguishable from incompletely distended segments of the colon on 3D images, correlation with the axial 2D images is often required for differentiation

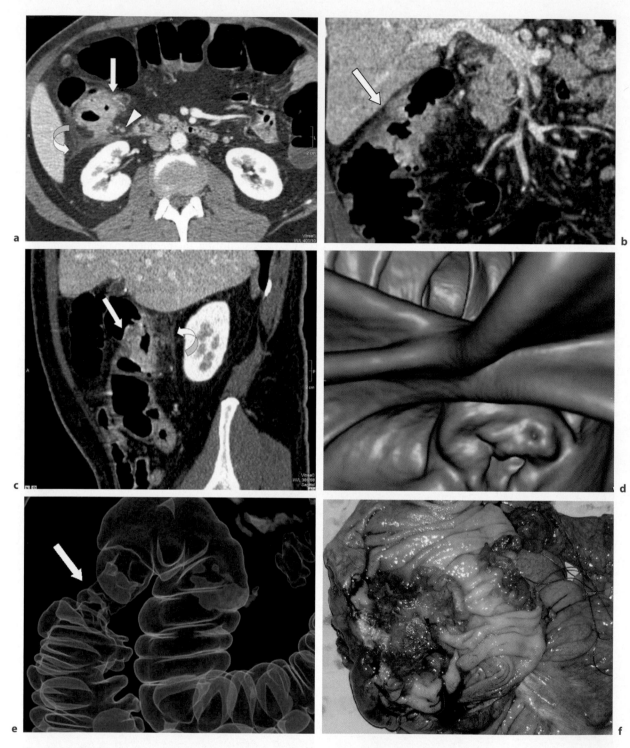

**Fig. 31.4a–f** CTC showing stenosing adenocarcinoma of hepatic flexure. Stage C carcinoma (modified Astler-Coller-Dukes classification). **a** Axial 2D image shows a huge mass (*arrow*) of hepatic flexure with evident involvement of pericolic fat tissue as well as anterior layer of renal fascia that is thickened (*arrowhead*). Pericolic enlarged lymph node (*curved arrow*), negative at histopathological examination is present within locoregional fat tissue. **b, c** The lesion (*arrow*) is well evaluable for surgical planning either on coronal 2D images or on sagittal 2D images, where thickening of anterior layer of renal fascia (*curved arrow*) is evident. Intraluminal 3D (**d**) and volume-rendered images (**e**) better depict the relationship between the lesion (*arrow*) and the hepatic flexure. **f** Surgical specimen obtained after right hemicolectomy

quence, most cases of CRC develop from benign adenomatous polyps. This concept is strongly supported by morphologic data, molecular biology, animal studies, and epidemiologic evidence (WINAWER 1997). Importantly, various clinical observations have clearly demonstrated that the removal of adenomatous polyps by endoscopic polypectomy is associated with a substantial reduction of incidence and mortality from CRC. However, no more than 1% of colonic adenomas will go on to become CRC (WINAWER et al. 1993). Thus, the concept of "advanced adenoma" has been developed, which is de-

fined as an adenomatous polyp measuring 10 mm or greater or one containing villous or dysplastic components at histologic examination (WINAWER and ZAUBER 2002) Certain polyps are recognized as being at a much higher risk than the others. In particular, those with high-grade dysplasia, diameter >1 cm, or villous component >25% are considered the main target of endoscopic screening (Fig. 31.5).

The evidence that CRC mortality was significantly reduced by fecal occult blood test in large randomized clinical trials (MANDEL 1993; HARDCASTLE 1996;

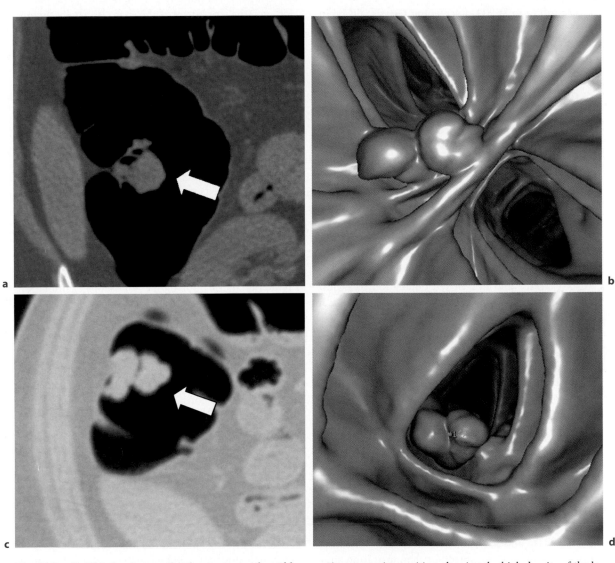

**Fig. 31.5a–d** CTC showing sessile adenomatous polypoid lesion of hepatic flexure. **a** Axial 2D image obtained on prone position showing a 1.5-cm sessile, polypoid lesion of hepatic flexure. **b** Corresponding 3D image shows endoscopical appearance of the lesion. **c** Axial 2D image obtained after turning patient on supine position, showing the high density of the lesion and how the lesion does not move, confirming diagnosis of solid lesion. **d** Corresponding 3D endoluminal image on supine position

KRONBORG 1996) and from flexible sigmoidoscopy in a well-designed case-control study (NEWCOMBE 1992) has led the most important scientific commissions - such as the US Preventive Services Task Force - to give, in the mid-1990s, a grade "A" recommendation that all men and women over 50 years should be screened for CRC (LIEBERMAN 1998). Moreover, cost-effective analyses have shown that CRC prevention compares favorably with other screening strategies such as breast and cervical cancers. More controversial is the debate over which screening technique to use, especially between stool-based tests and endoscopic or radiological procedures.

According to WHO, a screening test should be inexpensive, rapid, simple, and safe, requiring further evaluation in those with a positive test. No such test is available for CRC today, but CTC may fulfill the present requirements.

Three different large meta-analyses (HALLIGAN et al. 2005; MULHALL et al. 2005; ROSMAN and KORSTEN 2007) offer a good perspective of the performance of CTC, showing excellent sensitivity for colorectal cancer (over 95%) and clinically significant polyps (>10 mm: over 85%) and making this technique as the second best imaging test for the detection of colorectal lesions. Two recent large, multicenter trials have also tested the performance of CTC in comparison with conventional colonoscopy in respectively asymptomatic subjects at average risk, i.e., a typical screening population (the American College of Radiology Imaging Network [ACRIN] trials) and in a mixed population of asymptomatic subjects at higher-than-average risk and in patients referred for a positive fecal-occult blood test (FOBT) (Italian Multicentre Polyp Accuracy CTC [IMPACT] trial, an Italian multicenter study with collaboration of a single Belgian centre). Both the studies reported (data not yet published) per-patient sensitivity of 90% for polyps >10 mm and 78–84% for polyps larger than 6 mm; per-patient specificity was extremely high as well, over 85% independently of lesion size. In a preliminary screening project performed at the University of Wisconsin, Madison (KIM et al. 2007), after 2 years of recruitment over 3,000 subjects underwent CTC and over 3,000 conventional colonoscopies. Although no randomization between the two groups had been performed, the detection rate for advanced adenomas was 3.2% for CTC and 3.4% for conventional colonoscopy (not statistically significant), thus demonstrating similar results. However, no complications occurred in CTC group as opposed to seven perforations in colonoscopy examinations.

Compared with colonoscopy, CTC is definitely a safer test. Combining the results of different surveys,

perforation rate associated with CTC ranges between 0.03 and 0.009% (BURLING et al. 2006; PICKHARDT 2006; SOSNA et al. 2006), whereas it is around 0.1–0.2% for colonoscopy (GATTO et al. 2003). CTC complications were due to technical factors, such as the use of rigid catheter for bowel distension (now replaced by thin rubber devices), manual distension with air (now minimized by the use of an electronic pump delivering $CO_2$ and able to control pressure and volume), and inexpert personnel.

Patient compliance is still under debate, since colonoscopy is performed in most of the cases under sedation, without any pain suffered by the patient. However, the worst part of the exam is usually the preliminary bowel cleansing (GLUECKER et al. 2003). The advantage of CTC is the use of gentler preparation (now available) or unprepped examination (still under investigation). Furthermore, the pain related to colon distension by air may be minimized by the use of $CO_2$ delivered by an electronic pump with pressure and volume control. The use of $CO_2$ is also associated with a faster resorption, making the patient more comfortable immediately after the examination (BURLING et al. 2006).

Finally, before proposing a test for screening, cost-effectiveness needs to be demonstrated. Recent analysis on theoretical models concluded that CTC is the CRC screening strategy associated with the best cost-effectiveness ratio and the safest modality (HEITMAN et al. 2005; VIJAN et al. 2007). It has been calculated a decrease in the incidence of CRC of around 36.5%, with a reduction in the number of colonoscopy examinations of 76%, compared with a strategy using colonoscopy as a primary screening method; and with the further advantage of a significant decrease in colonoscopy-related complications (PICKHARDT et al. 2007).

Compared with other screening methods, CTC has the further advantage of the assessment of extracolonic organs. It may be considered a benefit in particular for the detection of unsuspected abdominal aortic aneurysm, which makes the method even more cost-effective than without the detection of extracolonic findings (HASSAN et al. 2008).

The main potential drawback of CTC is the exposure to ionizing radiations. However, this is not a major issue, since low-dose protocols are now routinely implemented, delivering a radiation dose of 4 to 6 mSv, which is twice the normal annual radiation exposure (2.6 mSv per year) (BRENNER and GEORGSSON 2005). It must be considered that CTC, in the case of a normal screening examination, has to be repeated every 5 to 7 years, and that airline personnel are annually exposed to around 4.0 mSv, without any recognized cancer-related problem (BALLARD et al. 2002).

## Staging

### 31.4.1
### Colon Cancer

Staging of CRC is essential, since survival rates depend on the stage of the disease (ACUNAS et al. 1990; KERNER et al. 1993; THOENI 1997). This information can then be used to deliver stage-specific treatment, with treatment more aggressive or palliation depending on the likely outcome of the treatments balanced against the morbidity of intensive therapy. The surgeon patholo-gist, and radiologist have complementary roles in the complete staging of those patients affected by colorectal carcinoma. The timing and nature of radiological input is variable and in part dependent on the mode of presentation.

CT has undeniable role in the staging of CRC determining if there is direct invasion of adjacent organs, enlargement of local nodes, or evidence of distant metastases. (Fig. 31.6) The accuracy of CT in the preoperative staging of colon cancer ranged from 48 to 77% (FREENY et al. 1986; BALTHAZAR et al. 1988), but this accuracy has largely increased with the use of MDCT and MDCT colonography. Recent studies reported accuracy from 83 to 94% for identifying tumor wall invasion and 80% for identifying regional lymph node involvement, using a combination of transverse and multiplanar reformatted images (FILIPPONE et al. 2004; KANAMOTO et al. 2007).

A routine use of CT in the preoperative management of CRC has been advocated (BARTON et al. 2002), showing that CT provides information for treatment planning in 37% of the cases (extended resections, blood units, consultations with other surgeons, intraoperative liver sonography), and it may alter the treatment in 19% of cases.

The major limitation of CT staging, even with MDCT, is the relatively inaccuracy in detecting metastatic lymph nodes. For this reason, preliminary studies have investigated the potential role of PET or PET–CT in staging of CRC. Unfortunately, only few studies are available, most of them with intrinsic bias in the comparison among different staging methods. However, no major differences in N staging were detected (ABDEL-NABI et al. 1998; MUKAI et al. 2000; KANTOROVA et al. 2003), although PET–CT was definitely better than was PET alone (SHIN et al. 2007). In a recent comparison between PET and MDCT (FURUKAWA et al. 2006), no statistically significant differences were observed between the two examinations, with PET modifying the

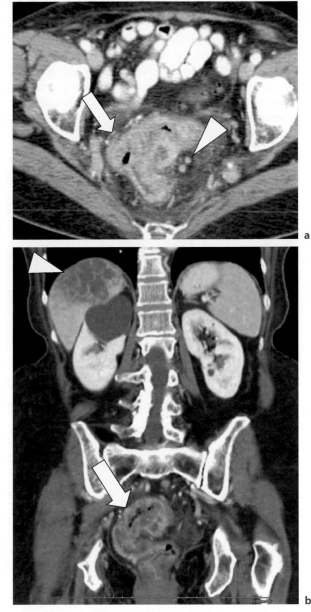

**Fig. 31.6a,b.** MDCT of sigmoid adenocarcinoma with distant metastases. **a** Axial 2D image obtained after intravenous administration of iodinated contrast showing a huge neoplastic mass (*arrow*) at rectosigmoid junction, involving pericolic fat tissue. Several enlarged lymph nodes (*arrowhead*) are present within mesorectum. **b** Coronal reformatted 2D image showing the craniocaudal extension of the neoplastic mass (*arrow*) as well as metastatic involvement of liver (*arrowhead*)

treatment in only 2% of the cases. On the other hand, in a study comparing PET–CT colonography and MDCT in TNM staging, a difference in favor of PET–CTC was demonstrated in 22% of the cases, all of them concerning distant metastases (M parameter), since no difference in N staging were demonstrated for a threshold for lymph node of 7 mm (VEIT-HAIBACH et al. 2006).

Thus, nowadays, the role of PET, or better PET–CT, in staging CRC should be recommended only in high-risk patients with increased tumor markers and no evidence of disease with other imaging modalities, in order to alter the treatment.

## 31.4.2
## Rectal Cancer

Staging of rectal cancer is relatively different from colon cancer. In fact, total mesorectal excision, with resection of the tumor together with surrounding mesorectal fat, is nowadays the surgically accepted treatment of choice for rectal cancer, as it is associated with a recurrence

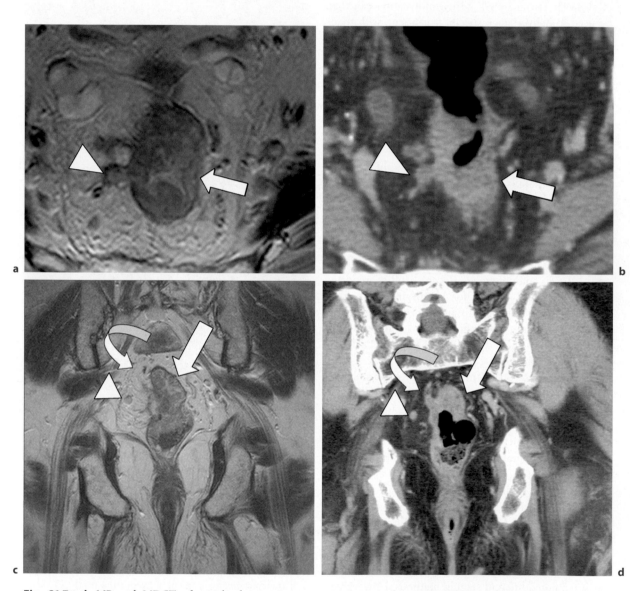

**Fig. 31.7a–d.** MR and MDCT of rectal adenocarcinoma. **a** Axial T2-weighted. Turbo spinecho (TSE) MR image showing rectal adenocarcinoma (*arrow*) with infiltration of the mesorectum (*arrowhead*) **b** Axial MDCT of same patient showing how in medium and high rectal cancer the high contrast between soft tissue density cancer and low-density mesorectal fat tissue allows good identification of the infiltration of the me-

sorectum, similar to MR. **c,d** Coronal T2-weighted TSE image and coronal reformatted MDCT image showing longitudinal extension of rectal adenocarcinoma (*arrow*) as well as enlarged lymph node (*arrowhead*) within the mesorectum, and relationship between tumor and mesorectal fascia (*curved arrow*)

rate of less than 10% without radiotherapy (MacFar- lane 1993; Peeters et al. 2007). In addition, this ther- apeutic approach demands accurate preoperative tumor staging, in particular the evaluation of spreading into mesorectal fat and of mesorectal fascia and the infiltra- tion of the sphincters. In fact, invasion of the mesorec- tal fascia will lead to pre- or postoperative radiotherapy in order to reduce the rate of recurrent lesions, whereas the invasion of the anal sphincter will change the surgi- cal intervention from anterior resection to abdomen– peritoneal amputation (Frileux et al. 2007).

The role of MDCT in rectal cancer staging is limited to some specific cases. In fact, in the case of superficial tumors (T1/T2), when the evaluation of different wall layers is mandatory, EUS is considered as the most accurate imaging modality, with an accuracy ranging between 64 and 94% (Holdsworth et al. 1988; Hulsmans et al. 1994). But for deeper tumors and for the evaluation of the involvement of mesorectal fat and fascia, MR imaging using a phased-array coil, or with a combination of phased-array and endorectal coil (Tatli 2006), is the examination of choice (Beets- Tan 2001; Iafrate 2006). Even better results are now obtained using 3-T MRI (Winter et al. 2007). However, characterization of nodal involvement is still disappointing, although MR has the potential benefit deriving from new lymph node–specific contrast agents, based on iron-oxide contrast material (Bellin et al. 1998, 2000).

MDCT with isotropic voxel and multiplanar refor- mations offers excellent views of the tumors in different planes providing an accurate overall staging, ranging between 71 and 93% (Matsuoka et al. 2003; Kulinna et al. 2004). The high contrast between soft tissue den- sity cancer and low-density mesorectal fat tissue allows good identification of the infiltration of the mesorec- tum, similar to MR, but only in the case of tumors of medium or high rectum where mesorectal fat is well represented (Fig. 31.7). For tumors of the low rectum, there is not enough intrinsic contrast to differentiate cancer from normal structure of anal canal. And this is confirmed by recent studies comparing 3-T MRI and MDCT, in which superiority of MRI in local staging is definitely demonstrated (Kim 2007).

## 31.5
## Follow-Up

The real issue of surveillance is the ability to identify as- ymptomatic recurrences after "curative" surgery, so that further treatment can be started and survival rate im-

proved. Unfortunately, despite the progress in surgical technique, recurrence of the disease occurs in more than a third of the cases (Sagar and Pemberton, 1996) and in around 80% of the cases, it is diagnosed within the first 2 years from surgery (Adloff et al. 1985). It may appear as local recurrence, hepatic disease, or extrahe- patic disease (mostly lymph nodes, but also lung, bones, etc., depending on the location of primary tumor). Fur- thermore, individuals with previous CRC cancer are at higher risk for metachronous tumors or adenomatous polyps (Neugut et al. 1996).

Thus, the strategy of the follow-up needs to cover different anatomical districts. The mainstay of most follow-up regimens is the serial measurement of CEA. Approximately 80% of patients have an elevated CEA at the time of the diagnosis, which usually returns to normal value after surgical resection. Failure to return to normal or a rising CEA suggests recurrent disease (Benson et al. 2000; Kievit 2002). Together with CEA, endoscopy and imaging represent the other two available techniques for the surveillance. Colonoscopy is the imaging modality of choice for the detection of metachronous tumors as well as adenomatous polyps (Rex et al. 2006), but it fails in the identification of ex- traluminal recurrence, very common at the level of the anastomosis.

CT, and in particular MDCT, still represents the first-line imaging modality in the follow-up for the iden- tification of hepatic and extrahepatic disease (Desch et al. 2005). Sensitivity for the detection of colorectal liver metastases larger than 1 cm in diameter reaches 94% (Scott et al. 2001), although performance drops off for lesions smaller than 1 cm. And in a recent comparison among PET–CT, contrast-enhanced MDCT, and SPIO- enhanced MRI, MDCT resulted as the method with the highest sensitivity for the detection of liver metastases, independently of lesion size (larger or smaller than 10 mm) (Rappeport et al. 2007).

However, an emerging role of PET and PET–CT has been demonstrated thanks to the promising results of several studies, showing high sensitivity (over 90%) and good specificity (in the range of 75–85%) in the follow- up of CRC (Huebner et al. 2000). Cost-effectiveness of a strategy combining PET and CT was found to be posi- tive for managing patients with elevated carcinoembry- onic antigen levels who were candidates for hepatic re- section (Park et al. 2001).

Thus, in those cases with raised tumor markers (i.e., CEA) and negative CT examination, or when a recur- rence is clinically highly suspicious and all the other examinations are inconclusive, PET–CT should be con- sidered the examination of choice (Manning et al. 2005).

In the rectum, the main clinical problem is the differential diagnosis between local recurrence and post-surgical fibrosis. Unfortunately, morphologic criteria are not sufficient to perform an accurate differential diagnosis, and even the advocated use of different signal intensity on MR imaging between recurrent tumor and fibrosis is reliable only several months after the therapy. This is another area where PET–CT may provide additional information although definite data are not yet available (SCHAEFER and LANGER 2007).

## 31.6
## Assessment of Therapy Response

Assessment of therapy response is an important, although difficult, target of diagnostic imaging. It is referred, in particular, to the evaluation of the response of rectal cancer after preoperative radiochemotherapy. Such therapy is useful for decreasing the tumor stage, to facilitate curative resection, and to decrease the rate of recurrence (PAHLMAN and GLIMELIUS 1995; SAHANI et al. 2005). However, now, there are no reliable methods to monitor the therapy, since all the available techniques (EUS, MRI and PET, or PET–CT) suffer from the same limitations: over-staging due to fibrotic reaction and inflammation of perirectal fat tissue due to the radiation therapy, and under-staging due to residual microscopic cancer foci beneath the normal rectal wall. Results from the literature are quite disappointing: EUS has an accuracy ranging between 44 and 72%, MRI between 47 and 54%, and PET or PET–CT between 56 and 80% (VANAGUNAS et al. 2004; ROMAGNUOLO et al. 2008; CHEN et al. 2005; KUO et al. 2005; HOFFMANN et al. 2002).

Furthermore, there are no methods able to offer prognostic information that predict which tumors will respond to chemo- and radiation therapy and those that will not. It would be very important in therapy planning to know a priori which patients may have a benefit from the treatment, since a different strategy might be used without wasting precious time.

A novel technique is now available, CT perfusion (see Sect. 31.2.3), which offers a measure of tumor neoangiogenesis. It provides functional information represented by blood volume, blood flow, mean transit time, and permeability surface area (Fig. 31.8). In tumors, compared with normal tissue, blood volume, blood flow, and permeability surface area are usually increased, whereas mean transit time (representing an indirect measure of arteriovenous shunts) is reduced because of the higher number of shunts compared with normal tissue (Fig. 31.9) (SAHANI et al. 2005).

Only few clinical studies using perfusion CT before and after radiochemotherapy treatment are avail-

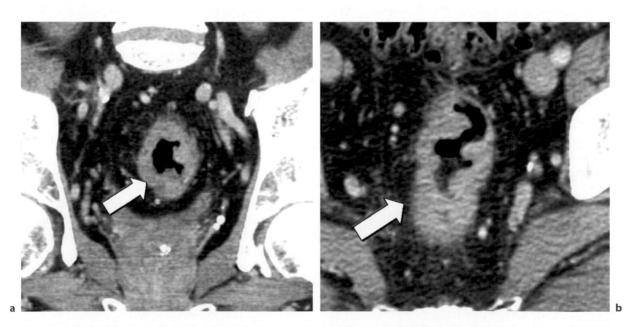

a b

**Fig. 31.8a–l.** MDCT of rectal adenocarcinoma before and after neoadjuvant chemoradiotherapy. **a,b** Axial and coronal MDCT of stenosing rectal cancer (*arrow*) before neoadjuvant chemo-radiotherapy. **c–l** *see next page*

able, but all of them are showing a potential important clinical application in rectal cancer management. Monitoring the response to therapy may lead clinicians to customize treatment to the response of the individual patient, and reliable prediction of the response may improve patient selection and avoid nonproductive, costly treatments (BELLOMI et al. 2007).

## 31.7
## Conclusion

In conclusion, MDCT still represents the imaging modality of choice in the evaluation of CRC, having a well-established role in staging and follow-up, an emerging

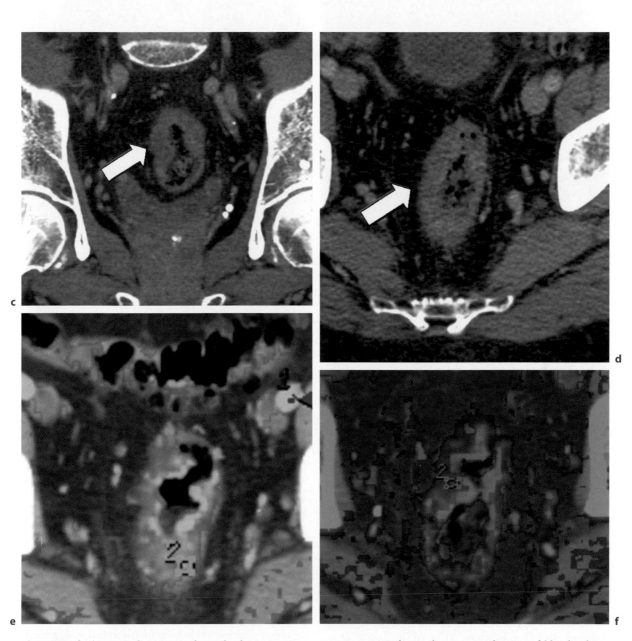

**Fig. 31.8a–l.** (*continued*) MDCT of rectal adenocarcinoma before and after neoadjuvant chemoradiotherapy **c,d** Axial and coronal MDCT of same lesion (*arrow*) obtained some months later after neoadjuvant chemoradiotherapy, showing only a mild volume reduction of the lesion. MDCT perfusion is a noninvasive tool, providing functional information about tumor neovascularity, showing a reduction of blood volume (milliliter per 100 g wet tissue), which is 9.4 ml/100 g before radiotherapy (**e**) and 7 ml/100 g after radiotherapy (**f**), Blood flow (milliliter per 100 g wet tissue per minute) is reduced from 28.5 (**g**) to 15.3 ml/100 g (**h**). **i–l** *see next page*

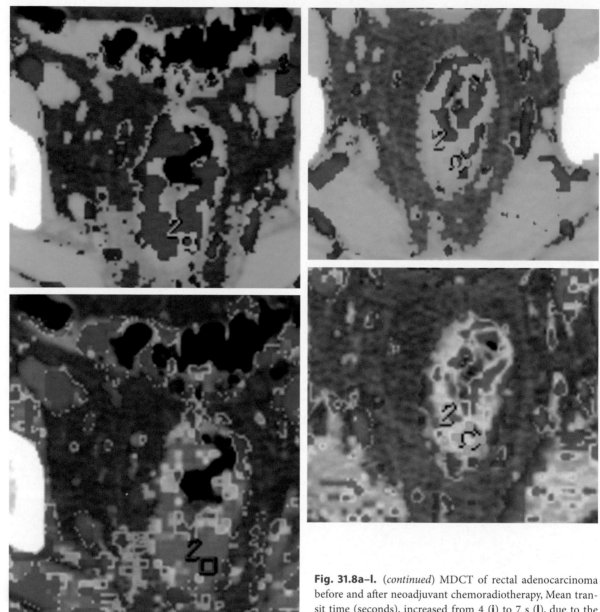

**Fig. 31.8a–l.** (*continued*) MDCT of rectal adenocarcinoma before and after neoadjuvant chemoradiotherapy, Mean transit time (seconds), increased from 4 (**i**) to 7 s (**l**), due to the presence of arteriovenous shunts

role in diagnosis and screening, and a future interesting role in the assessment of the response to therapy. To take advantages of the enormous potentials of the technology, imaging protocol should be tailored to the different clinical indications. Thus, in the case of staging and follow-up, a routine contrast-enhanced MDCT study is sufficient, whereas in the case of diagnosis and screening, CTC protocols are mandatory, and CT perfusion is the way to address the issues regarding the assessment of the response to therapy.

## References

Abdel-Nabi H, Doerr RJ, Lamonica DM et al. (1998) Staging of primary colorectal carcinomas with fluorine-18 fluorodeoxyglucose whole-body PET: correlation with histopathologic and CT findings. Radiology 206:755–760

Acunas B, Rozanes I, Acunas G et al. (1990) Preoperative CT staging of colon carcinoma (excluding the recto-sigmoid region). Eur J Radiol 11:150–153

Adloff M, Arnaud JP, Schloegel M et al. (1985) Factors influencing local recurrence after abdominoperitoneal resection for cancer of the rectum. Dis Colon Rectum 28:413–415

AGA Clinical Practice and Economics Committee (2006) Position of the American Gastroenterological Association (AGA) Institute on computed tomographic colonography. Gastroenterology 131:1627–1628

Anderson ML, Heigh RI, McCoy GA et al. (1992) Accuracy of assessment of the extent of examination by experienced colonoscopists. Gastrointest Endosc 38:560–563

Ballard TJ, Lagorio S, De Santis M (2002) A retrospective cohort mortality study of Italian commercial airline cockpit crew and cabin attendants, 1965–96. Int J Occup Environ Health 8:87–96

Balthazar EJ, Megibow AJ, Hulnick D et al. (1988) Carcinoma of the colon: detection and preoperative staging by CT. AJR Am J Roentgenol 150:301–306

Barton JB, Langdale LA, Cummins JS et al. (2002) The utility of routine preoperative computed tomography scanning in the management of veterans with colon cancer. Am J Surg 183:499–503

Beets-Tan RG, Beets GL, Vliegen RF et al. (2001) Accuracy of magnetic resonance imaging in prediction of tumour-free resection margin in rectal cancer surgery. Lancet 357:497–504

Bellin MF, Roy C, Kinkel K et al. (1998) Lymph node metastases: safety and effectiveness of MR imaging with ultrasmall superparamagnetic iron oxide particles—initial clinical experience. Radiology 207:799–808

Bellin MF, Beigelman C, Precetti-Morel S. (2000) Iron oxide-enhanced MR lymphography: initial experience. Eur J Radiol 34:257–264

Bellomi M, Petralia G, Sonzogni A, Zampino MG, Rocca A (2007) CT perfusion for the monitoring of neoadjuvant chemotherapy and radiation therapy in rectal carcinoma: initial experience. Radiology 244:486–93

Benson AB III, Choti MA, Cohen AM et al. (2000) National Comprehensive Cancer Network. NCCN Practice Guidelines for Colorectal Cancer. Oncology (Williston Park) 14:203–212

Boyle P, Ferlay J (2005) Cancer incidence and mortality in Europe, 2004. Ann Oncol 16:481–488

Brenner DJ, Georgsson MA (2005) Mass screening with CT colonography: should the radiation exposure be of concern? Gastroenterology 129:328–337

Bretthauer M, Thiis-Evensen E, Huppertz-Hauss G et al. (2002) NORCCAP (Norwegian colorectal cancer prevention): a randomised trial to assess the safety and efficacy of carbon dioxide versus air insufflation in colonoscopy. Gut 50:604–607

Burling D, Halligan S, Slater A, Noakes MJ, Taylor SA (2006) Potentially serious adverse events at CT colonography in symptomatic patients: national survey of the United Kingdom. Radiology 239:464–471

Burling D, Taylor SA, Halligan S et al. (2006) Automated colonic insufflation for multi-detector row CT colonography: distension and patient experience in comparison to manual carbon dioxide insufflation AJR Am J Roentgenol 186:96–103

Burt RW (1996) Familial risk and colorectal cancer. Gastroenterol Clin N Am 25:793–803

Chen CC, Lee RC, Lin JK, Wang LW, Yang SH (2005) How accurate is magnetic resonance imaging in restaging rectal cancer in patients receiving preoperative combined chemoradiotherapy? Dis Colon Rectum 48:722–728

Dachman AH, Dawson DO, Lefere P et al. (2007) Comparison of routine and unprepped CT colonography augmented by low fiber diet and stool tagging: a pilot study. Abdom Imaging 32:96–104

Dafnis G, Blomqvist P, Pahlman L et al. (2000) The introduction and development of colonoscopy within a defined population in Sweden. Scand J Gastroenterol 35:765–771

Desch CE, Benson AB III, Somerfield MR et al. (2005) American Society of Clinical Oncology. Colorectal cancer surveillance: 2005 update of an American Society of Clinical Oncology practice guideline. J Clin Oncol 23:8512–8519

Doyle GJ, O'Donnell SC, McDonald JR et al. (1993) Evaluation of "Gastromiro" for bowel opacification during computed tomography: comparison with diatrizoate and barium sulphate. Br J Radiol 66:681–684

Filippone A, Ambrosini R, Fuschi M et al. (2004) Preoperative T and N staging of colorectal cancer: accuracy of contrast enhanced multi-detector row CT colonography—initial experience. Radiology 231:83–90

Freeny PC, Marks WM, Ryan JA et al. (1986) Colorectal carcinoma evaluation with CT: preoperative staging and detection of postoperative recurrence. Radiology 158:347–353

Frileux P, Burdy G, Aegerter P et al. (2007) Surgical treatment of rectal cancer: results of a strategy for selective preoperative radiotherapy. Gastroenterol Clin Biol 31:934–940

Furukawa H, Ikuma H, Seki A et al. (2006) Positron emission tomography scanning is not superior to whole body multidetector helical computed tomography in the preoperative staging of colorectal cancer. Gut 55:1007–1011

Gatto NM, Frucht H, Sundarajan V et al. (2003) Risk of perforation after colonoscopy and sigmoidoscopy: a population-based study. J Natl Cancer Inst 95:230–236

Gazelle GS, Gaa J, Saini S et al. (1995) Staging of colon carcinoma using water enema CT. J Comput Assist Tomogr 19:87–91

Gluecker TM, Johnson CD, Harmsen WS et al. (2003) Colorectal cancer screening with CT colonography, colonoscopy, and double-contrast barium enema examination: prospective assessment of patient perceptions and preferences. Radiology 227:378–384

Goh V, Halligan S, Bartram CI (2007) Quantitative tumor perfusion assessment with multidetector CT: are measurements from two commercial software packages interchangeable? Radiology 242:777–782

Goh V, Padhani AR, Rasheed S (2007) Functional imaging of colorectal cancer angiogenesis. Lancet Oncol 8:245–255

Graser A, Wintersperger BJ, Suess C, Reiser MF, Becker CR (2006) Dose reduction and image quality in MDCT colonography using tube current modulation. Am J Roentgenol 187:695–701

Halligan S, Altman DG, Taylor SA et al. (2005) CT colonography in the detection of colorectal polyps and cancer: systematic review, meta-analysis, and proposed minimum data set for study level reporting. Radiology 237:893–904

Halligan S, Altman DG, Mallett S et al. (2006) Computed tomographic colonography: assessment of radiologist performance with and without computer-aided detection. Gastroenterology 131:1690–1699

Hardcastle JD, Chamberlain JO, Robinson MH et al. (1996) Randomised controlled trial of faecal-occult-blood screening for colorectal cancer. Lancet 348:1472–1477

Hassan C, Laghi A, Pickhardt PJ et al. (2008) Projected impact of colorectal cancer screening with computerized tomographic colonography on current radiological capacity in Europe. Aliment Pharmacol Ther 27:366–374

Hassan C, Pickhardt PJ, Laghi A et al. (2008) CT colonography to screen for colorectal cancer, extracolonic cancer, and aortic aneurysm: model simulation with cost-effectiveness analysis. Arch Intern Med 168:696–705

Heitman SJ, Manns BJ, Hilsden RJ et al. (2005) Cost-effectiveness of computerized tomographic colonography versus colonoscopy for colorectal cancer screening. CMAJ 173:877–881

Hoffmann KT, Rau B, Wust P, et al. (2002) Restaging of locally advanced carcinoma of the rectum with MR imaging after preoperative radio-chemotherapy plus regional hyperthermia. Strahlenther Onkol 178:386–92

Holdsworth PJ, Johnston D, Chalmers AG et al. (1988) Endoluminal ultrasound and computed tomography in the staging of rectal cancer. Br J Surg 75:1019–1022

Huebner RH, Park KC, Shepherd JE et al. (2000) A meta-analysis of the literature for whole-body FDG PET detection of recurrent colorectal cancer. J Nucl Med 41:1177–1189

Hulsmans FJ, Tio TL, Fockens P et al. (1994) Assessment of tumor infiltration depth in rectal cancer with transrectal sonography: caution is necessary. Radiology 190:715–720

Hundt W, Braunschweig R, Reiser M (1999) Evaluation of spiral CT in staging of colon and rectum carcinoma. Eur Radiol 9:78–84

Iafrate F, Laghi A, Paolantonio P et al. (2006) Preoperative staging of rectal cancer with MR imaging: correlation with surgical and histopathologic findings radiographics. 26:701–714

Iannaccone R, Laghi A, Catalano C et al. (2004) Computed tomographic colonography without cathartic preparation for the detection of colorectal polyps. Gastroenterology 127:1300–1311

Johnson CD, MacCarty RL, Welch TJ et al. (2004) Comparison of the relative sensitivity of CT colonography and double-contrast barium enema for screen detection of colorectal polyps. Clin Gastroenterol Hepatol 2:314–21

Johnson KT, Johnson CD, Fletcher JG, MacCarty RL, Summers RL (2006) CT colonography using 360-degree virtual dissection: a feasibility study. AJR Am J Roentgenol 186:90–95

Johnson KT, Carston MJ, Wentz RJ, Manduca A, Anderson SM, Johnson CD (2007) Development of a cathartic-free colorectal cancer screening test using virtual colonoscopy: a feasibility study. Am J Roentgenol 188:29–36

Kanamoto T, Matsuki M, Okuda J et al. (2007) Preoperative evaluation of local invasion and metastatic lymph nodes of colorectal cancer and mesenteric vascular variations using multidetector-row computed tomography before laparoscopic surgery. J Comput Assist Tomogr 31:831–839

Kantorova I, Lipska L, Belohlavek O et al. (2003) Routine $^{18}$F-FDG PET preoperative staging of colorectal cancer: comparison with conventional staging and its impact on treatment decision making. J Nucl Med 44:1784–1788

Kerner BA, Oliver GC, Eisenstat TE et al. (1993) Is preoperative computerized tomography useful in assessing patients with colorectal carcinoma? Dis Colon Rectum 36:1050–1053

Kievit J (2002) Follow-up of patients with colorectal cancer: numbers needed to test and treat. Eur J Cancer 8:986–999

Kim CK, Kim SH, Choi D et al. (2007) Comparison between 3-T magnetic resonance imaging and multi-detector row computed tomography for the preoperative evaluation of rectal cancer. J Comput Assist Tomogr 31:853–859

Kim DH, Pickhardt PJ, Taylor AJ et al. (2007) CT colonography versus colonoscopy for the detection of advanced neoplasia. N Engl J Med 357:1403–1412

Kronborg O, Fenger C, Olsen J, Jorgensen OD, Sondergaard O (1996) Randomised study of screening for colorectal cancer with faecal-occult-blood test. Lancet 348:1467–1471

Kulinna C, Eibel R, Matzek W et al. (2004) Staging of rectal cancer: diagnostic potential of multiplanar reconstructions with MDCT. Am J Roentgenol 183:421–427

Kuo LJ, Chern MC, Tsou MH, et al. (2005) Interpretation of magnetic resonance imaging for locally advanced rectal carcinoma after preoperative chemoradiation therapy. Dis Colon Rectum 48:23–28

Laghi A, Iannaccone R, Bria E et al. (2003) Contrast-enhanced computed tomographic colonography in the follow-up of colorectal cancer patients: a feasibility study. Eur Radiol 13:883–889

Lefere P, Gryspeerdt S, Marrannes J, Baekelandt M, Van Holsbeeck B (2005) CT colonography after fecal tagging with a reduced cathartic cleansing and a reduced volume of barium. Am J Roentgenol 184:1836–1842

Lieberman D (1998) How to screen for colon cancer. Annu Rev Med 49:163–72

Luz O, Buchgeister M, Klabunde M, Trabold T, Kopp AF, Claussen CD, Heuschmid M (2007) Evaluation of dose exposure in 64-slice CT colonography. Eur Radiology 17:2616–2621

Lynch HT, de la Chapelle A (2003) Hereditary colorectal cancer. N Engl J Med 348:919–932

Macari M, Lavelle M, Pedrosa I et al. (2001) Effect of different bowel preparations on residual fluid at CT colonography. Radiology 218:274–277

MacFarland EG, Zalis ME (2004) CT colonography: progress toward colorectal evaluation without catharsis. Gastroenterology 127:1623–1626

MacFarlane JK, Ryall RD, Heald RJ (1993) Mesorectal excision for rectal cancer. Lancet 341:457–460

Malila N, Hakulinen T (2003) Epidemiological trends of colorectal cancer in the Nordic countries. Scand J Surg 92:5–9

Mandel JS, Bond JH, Church TR et al. (1993) Reducing mortality from colorectal cancer by screening for fecal occult blood. Minnesota Colon Cancer Control Study. N Engl J Med 328:1365–1371

Manning K, Tepfer B, Goldklang G et al. (2007) Clinical practice guidelines for the utilization of positron emission tomography/computed tomography imaging in selected oncologic applications: suggestions from a provider group. Mol Imaging Biol 9:324–332

Marshall JB, Barthel JS (1993) The frequency of total colonoscopy and terminal ileal intubation in the 1990s. Gastrointest Endosc 39:518–520

Matsuoka H, Nakamura A, Masaki T et al. (2003) A prospective comparison between multidetector-row computed tomography and magnetic resonance imaging in the preoperative evaluation of rectal carcinoma. Am J Surg 185:556–559

Miles KA (2003) Perfusion CT for the assessment of tumour vascularity: which protocol? Br J Radiol 76:S36–S42

Miles KA, Griffiths MR (2003) Perfusion CT: a worthwhile enhancement? Br J Radiol 76:220–231

Mitchell RJ, Campbell H, Farrington SM et al. (2005) Prevalence of family history of colorectal cancer in the general population. Br J Surg 92:1161–1164

Mukai M, Sadahiro S, Yasuda S et al. (2000) Preoperative evaluation by whole-body $^{18}$F-fluorodeoxyglucose positron emission tomography in patients with primary colorectal cancer. Oncol Rep 7:85–87

Mulhall BP, Veerappan GR, Jackson JL (2005) Meta-analysis: computed tomographic colonography. Ann Intern Med 142:635–650

Neugut AI, Lautenback E, Abi-Rached B et al. (1996) Incidence of adenomas after curative resection for colorectal cancer. Am J Gastroenterol 91:2096–2098

Newcomb PA, Norfleet RG, Storer BE, Surawicz T, Marcus PM (1992) Screening sigmoidoscopy and colorectal cancer mortality. J Natl Cancer Inst 84:1572–1575

Pahlman L, Glimelius B (1995) The value of adjuvant radio(chemo)therapy for rectal cancer. Eur J Cancer 31:1347–1350

Park KC, Schwimmer J, Shepherd JE et al. (2001) Decision analysis for the cost-effective management of recurrent colorectal cancer. Ann Surg 233:310–319

Peeters KC, Marijnen CA, Nagtegaal ID et al. (2007) The TME trial after a median follow-up of 6 years: increased local control but no survival benefit in irradiated patients with resectable rectal carcinoma. Ann Surg 246:693–701

Petrick N, Haider M, Summers RM et al. (2008) CT colonography with computer-aided detection as a second reader: observer performance study. Radiology 246:148–156

Pickhardt PJ (2006) Incidence of colonic perforation at CT colonography: review of existing data and implications for screening of asymptomatic adults. Radiology 239:313–316

Pickhardt PJ, Choi JH (2003) Electronic cleansing and stool tagging in CT colonography: advantages and pitfalls with primary three-dimensional evaluation. Am J Roentgenol 181:799–805

Pickhardt PJ, Choi JR, Hwang I et al. (2003) Computed tomographic virtual colonoscopy to screen for colorectal neoplasia in asymptomatic adults. N Engl J Med 349:2191–2200

Pickhardt PJ, Hassan C, Laghi A et al. (2007) Cost-effectiveness of colorectal cancer screening with computed tomography colonography: the impact of not reporting diminutive lesions. Cancer 109:2213–2221

Rappeport ED, Loft A, Berthelsen AK et al. (2007) Contrast-enhanced FDG-PET/CT vs. SPIO-enhanced MRI vs. FDG-PET vs. CT in patients with liver metastases from colorectal cancer: a prospective study with intraoperative confirmation. Acta Radiol 48:369–378

Rex DK, Kahi CJ, Levin B et al. (2006) Guidelines for colonoscopy surveillance after cancer resection: a consensus update by the American Cancer Society and US Multi-Society Task Force on colorectal cancer. CA Cancer J Clin 56:160–167

Ries LA, Wingo PA, Miller DS et al. (2000) The annual report to the nation on the status of cancer, 1973–1997, with a special section on colorectal cancer. Cancer 88:2398–424

Romagnuolo J, Enns R, Ponich T et al. (2008) Canadian credentialing guidelines for colonoscopy. Can J Gastroenterol 22:17–22

Rosman AS, Korsten MA (2007) Meta-analysis comparing CT colonography, air contrast barium enema, and colonoscopy. Am J Med 120:203–210

Sagar PM, Pemberton JH (1996) Surgical management of locally recurrent rectal cancer. Br J Surg 83:293–304

Sahani DV, Kalva SP, Hamberg LM et al. (2005) Assessing tumor perfusion and treatment response in rectal cancer with multisection CT: initial observations. Radiology 234:785–792

Sant M, Aareleid T, Berrino F, Bielska Lasota M, Carli PM, Faivre J, Grosclaude P et al. (2003) EUROCARE-3-survival of cancer patients diagnosed 1990–94—results and commentary. Ann Oncol 14:v61–v118

Schaefer O, Langer M (2007) Detection of recurrent rectal cancer with CT, MRI and PET/CT. Eur Radiol 17:2044–2054

Scheiden R, Pescatore P, Wagener Y et al. (2005) Colon cancer in Luxembourg: a national population-based data report, 1988–1998. BMC Cancer 5:52

Scott DJ, Guthrie JA, Arnold P et al. (2001) Dual phase helical CT versus portal venous phase CT for the detection of colorectal liver metastases: correlation with intraoperative sonography, surgical and pathological findings 56:235–242

Shin SS, Jeong YY, Min JJ et al. (2007) Preoperative staging of colorectal cancer: CT vs. integrated FDG PET/CT. Abdom Imaging 33:270–277

Sosna J, Blachar A, Amitai M et al. (2006) Colonic perforation at CT colonography: assessment of risk in a multicenter large cohort. Radiology 239:457–463

Tatli S, Mortele KJ, Breen EL et al. (2006) Local staging of rectal cancer using combined pelvic phased-array and endorectal coil MRI. J Magn Reson Imaging 23:534–540

Taylor S, Laghi A, Lefere P, Halligan S, Stoker J (2007) European society of gastrointestinal and abdominal radiology (ESGAR): Consensus statement on CT colonography. Eur Radiol 17:575–579

Taylor SA, Halligan S, Goh V et al. (2003) Optimizing colonic distention for multi-detector row CT colonography: effect of hyoscine butylbromide and rectal balloon catheter. Radiology 229:99–108

Thoeni RF (1997) Colorectal cancer: radiologic staging. Radiol Clin North Am 35:457–485

Vanagunas A, Lin DE, Stryker SJ. (2004) Accuracy of endoscopic ultrasound for restaging rectal cancer following neoadjuvant chemoradiation therapy. Am J Gastroenterol 99:109–112

Veit-Haibach P, Kuehle CA, Beyer T et al. (2006) Diagnostic accuracy of colorectal cancer staging with whole-body PET/CT colonography. JAMA 296:2590–2600

Vijan S, Hwang I, Inadomi J et al. (2007) The cost-effectiveness of CT colonography in screening for colorectal neoplasia. Am J Gastroenterol 102:380–390

Vining DJ, Gelfand DW (1994) Non-invasive colonoscopy using helical CT scanning. 3D reconstruction and virtual reality. Syllabus of the 23rd Annual Meeting Society of gastrointestinal Radiologists, Maui, Hawaii, 13–18 February 1994

Weir HK, Thun MJ, Hankey BF et al. (2003) Annual report to the nation on the status of cancer, 1975–2000, featuring the uses of surveillance data for cancer prevention and control. J Natl Cancer Inst 95:1276–1299

Winawer SJ, Zauber AG (2002) The advanced adenoma as the primary target of screening. Gastrointest Endosc Clin N Am 12:1–9

Winawer SJ, Zauber AG, May Nah Ho et al. (1993) Prevention of colorectal cancer by colonoscopic polypectomy. N Engl J Med 329:1977–1981

Winawer SJ, Fletcher RH, Miller L et al. (1997) Colorectal cancer screening: clinical guidelines and rationale. Gastroenterology 112:594–642

Winter L, Bruhn H, Langrehr J et al. (2007) Magnetic resonance imaging in suspected rectal cancer: determining tumor localization, stage, and sphincter-saving resectability at 3-Tesla-sustained high resolution. Acta Radiol 48:379–387

Wong SK, Jalaludin BB, Morgan MJ et al. (2008) Tumor pathology and long-term survival in emergency colorectal cancer. Dis Colon Rectum 51:223–230

Yanaga Y, Awai K, Nakayama Y et al. (2007) Pancreas: patient body weight tailored contrast material injection protocol versus fixed dose protocol at dynamic CT. Radiology 245:475–482

# Urogenital Tumors

Peter Hallscheidt

## CONTENTS

## ABSTRACT

With the advances in CT, temporal and spatial resolution constantly improves. With the introduction of MDCT scanners, imaging of the whole body in an early arterial phase with a reconstructed slice thickness of 1 mm and less became technically feasible. 3D reconstructions allow an artifact-free multiplanar reconstruction of these high-resolution CT datasets. With the development of new MRI technologies like parallel imaging, higher field strength, and the use of designated coils, image quality is improving. In the wide field of urogenital tumors, the different imaging modalities offer different advantages and are limited in some indications. Additionally, the traditional use of established imaging modalities and traditional staging methods like excretory urography (EU) and digital rectal examination limit the use of modern cross-sectional imaging with its excellent staging results. The improvements of imaging quality for urogenital tumors will influence the pre- and postoperative workup of patients. In some tumor entities, the results are discussed controversial in the literature, so further studies have to compare modern with traditional diagnostic methods.

P. Hallscheidt, MD
Department of Diagnostic Radiology, Heidelberg University,
INF 110, 69120 Heidelberg, Germany

### 32.1

## Transitional Cell Carcinoma
## of the Urinary Bladder and the Ureter

### 32.1.1
### Pathogenesis and Incidence

Transitional cell carcinoma (TCC) of the upper and lower urinary tract usually occurs in the sixth and seventh decades.

Risk factors are male gender, smoking, coffee drinking, anatomic abnormalities like obstructions or horseshoe kidney, and exposition to chemical carcinogens like aniline, aromatic amine, and benzidine, as the metabolites of these substances are excreted into the urinary tract.

Patients with a high consumption of analgesics like phenacetin have an elevated risk of developing TCC. Human papilloma virus as well as Balkan endemic nephropathy have also been suggested risk factors for TCC. In up to 5% of the cases, the patients present with bilateral TCC. Up to 13% of patients with TCC develop metastases in the upper urinary tract.

Transitional cancer is usually located in the urinary bladder and is diagnosed by means of cystoscopy. Up to 20% of urothelial carcinomas develop in the upper urinary tract, with 25% of these tumors being located in the upper tract of the ureter. The vast majority of the upper-tract TCC are superficial tumors and of low stage. Only about 15% of the upper-tract carcinomas are infiltrating tumors. The patients usually present with hematuria, and in a third of the patients, flank pain and acute renal colic is present.

Metastases are typically located in the liver, bone, and the lungs.

### 32.1.2
### Imaging TCC

A patient with hematuria requires complete diagnostic workup of the kidney and the complete urinary tract to exclude calculi. The guidelines of the American Urological Association (AUA) suggest cytological analysis, analysis of the urine and cystoscopy as well as excretory urography (GROSSFELD et al. 2001).

In cases with positive findings in the urine, cytology, such as selective lavage or brush biopsies, have to be performed.

Retrograde pyelography (RP), EU, and ultrasonography as well as computed tomographic urography (CTU) are the available diagnostic modalities.

MRI with its capability of gadolinium-enhanced 3D MR angiography and urography is increasingly used for delineation of TCC.

MR techniques like MR angiography and urography have an improved spatial and temporal resolution and are therefore increasingly used for the workup of the urinary tract and the kidneys.

CTU has a higher detection rate for ureter calculi and renal parenchyma masses (ALBANI et al. 2007) compared to EU. Even for the lower urinary tract, CTU has similar detection rates as cystoscopy (PARK et al. 2007).

As lesions in the parenchyma can cause hematuria, EU cannot exclude a tumor in the renal parenchyma; so additional imaging studies like contrast-enhanced CT or MRI have to be performed (GRAY et al. 2002).

### 32.1.2.1
### EU

EU is the most frequent used modality to exclude TCC. EU is a noninvasive method to workup the anatomy and pathology of the upper and in some cases, of the lower urinary tract. TCC can be diagnosed as a filling defect in the contrast-enhanced collecting system. A filling defect within a dilated calyx may cause an amputation of the calyx. A tumor in the ureter is usually diagnosed as a single or multiple ureter-filling defect(s), sometimes with an obstruction and dilatation of the renal pelvis. In these cases, the obstruction in the ureter can cause reduced excretion rates, with no or low contrast medium concentration in the ureter, causing difficulties in delineating the tumor. The same limitation is given in patients with nonfunctioning kidneys. In these cases, CTU clearly shows its superiority to diagnose the tumor.

### 32.1.2.2
### RP

RP is usually performed during cystoscopy in patients with hematuria. It is an invasive method and considered the gold standard for detection of TCC, as an additional cytological test can be performed. RP is also limited in cases in which an obstruction is present, as distal to this obstruction, no evaluation of the urothelium is possible. However, RP as well as EU cannot demonstrate the extension of the tumor into the surrounding tissue, and therefore staging of TCC is impossible.

### 32.1.2.3
### MRI

MRI still is not routinely used for detection and staging TCC. Although the improvements in imaging quality and the development of fast sequences MR imaging, CT still is the gold standard in cases with TCC. With multiplanar imaging, MRI in the coronal plane images the kidney, the ureter, and the bladder in thin slices. However, in MRI, TCC has almost isointense signal in T1- and T2-weighed images. In contrast-enhanced scans, TCC shows low enhancement of the tumor. In the excretory phase, a T1-weighted MR urography can be performed. A dynamic acquisition at different time intervals allows detecting tumors even in an obstructed ureter, in which the excretion is delayed. 3D reconstructions help to detect tumors of the urinary tract.

But as the spatial resolution is poor compared to modern multislice CT scanner, TCC of the upper and lower tract are still difficult to detect.

### 32.1.2.4
### MDCT

MDCT is a well-established method to delineate and stage TCC. With the introduction of multislice CT scanners, single-breath coverage with thin-slice reconstruction of the whole urinary tract is possible (Figs. 32.1, 32.2). The detection rate for upper and lower urinary tract tumors is comparable to RP and cystoscopy, with sensitivity for the upper urinary tract of up to 92%, and similar sensitivity for the lower tract (PARK et al. 2007; Fig. 32.3). With a better detection rate and the multifocal nature of TCC, CTU replaces EU for detection of TCC (ALBANI et al. 2007). In this study, the usefulness of CT for evaluation of patients with hematuria was evaluated.

The sensitivity in finding the origin of the hematuria was 94.1%, compared with 50% by EU. The hematuria was caused by calculi, renal pelvic masses, bladder masses, prostate masses, or inflammatory disorders. In

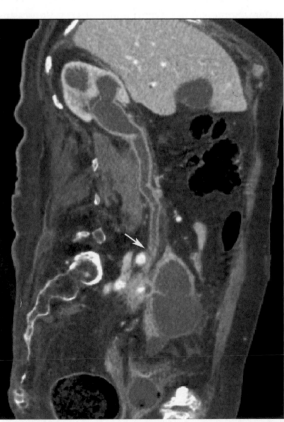

**Fig. 32.1.** Sagittal reconstructed CT data set with a tumor of the right ureter (*arrow*), causing obstruction of the right pelvis and the proximal right ureter. CT with its high spatial resolution enables the detection of the tumor

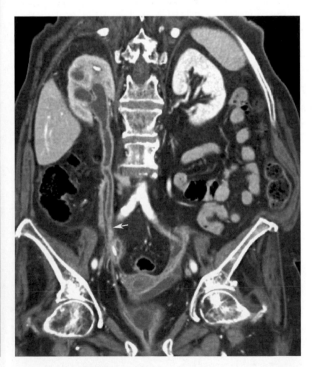

**Fig. 32.2.** Coronal reconstruction with delineation of the complete ureter with a slightly dilatation and an additional stone in the distal ureter

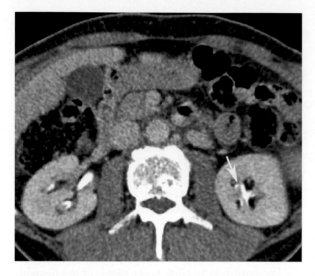

**Fig. 32.3.** Filling defect in the upper pole of the left kidney in the nephrographic phase. Histopathology showed tubulointerstitial injury of the left kidney in the upper pole calyx

a study by PARK et al. (2007), the accuracy to determine bladder lesions in patients with hematuria of CTU compared to cystoscopy was evaluated (Fig. 32.4a,b). One hundred eighteen patients underwent cystoscopy and CTU. The sensitivity and specificity for detection of bladder lesions was 89–92% and 88–97% in a per-lesion analysis. However, CTU has its limitation in detecting small bladder lesion with a diameter of less than 10 mm, with a sensitivity of 80–83% for these lesions.

Additionally CTU for evaluation of the urinary bladder is better tolerated in a higher percentage and gives additional information about the surrounding structures and the extension of the tumor, as well as the status of the lymph nodes and the distant metastases. Another advantage of CTU is that the complete urinary tract can be evaluated in order to exclude tumors of the upper tract with one CTU (Fig. 32.5).

CTU usually will be performed in three phases. A nonenhanced scan will be done from the upper pole of the kidneys to the symphysis to exclude calculi. An enhanced scan in the corticomedullary phase (usually with a delay of about 30 s) allows detecting renal parenchyma lesions and gives information about the intra- and extrarenal vascular situation. The third phase is performed in the nephrographic phase, with a delay of more than 200 s. In this phase, the urothelium can be evaluated. Moreover, tumors of the urinary bladder can be detected in this phase. The axial images can be postprocessed with volume rendering and thick- and thin-slap reconstructions, allowing demonstrating the extension of a lesion and multifocal tumors (Figs. 32.1, 32.2). In contrast to EU, CT is not dependent on contrast medium in the ureter or bladder, as the enhancement of the tumor allows its detection.

TCC is diagnosed as a filling defect in the excretory system. Some studies even published very impressing staging results for TCC (FRITZ et al. 2006). Usually TCC demonstrates delayed enhancement compared to the renal parenchyma. In some cases, because of its early enhancement, the TCC shows a similar enhancement as RCC, making the differential diagnosis difficult.

The CT not only allows detecting the TCC, but also allows staging the tumor, as the lymph nodes, the bones, and the other organs are scanned and can be evaluated for staging.

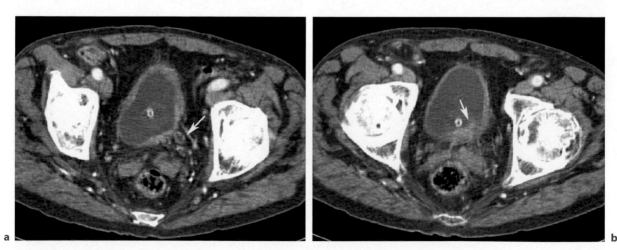

**Fig. 32.4.** **a** Dilated left ureter (*arrow*) and a slight thickening of the wall of the bladder. **b** Carcinoma of the urinary bladder with infiltration of the left ostium (*arrow*) and consecutive dilatation of the left ureter (**a**)

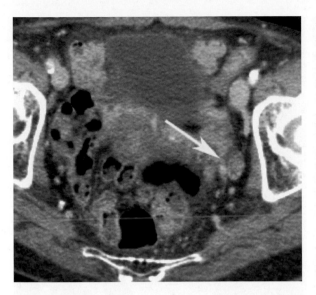

**Fig. 32.5** TCC in the distal left ureter (*arrow*) with dilatation of the left ureter

## 32.2
## Renal Cell Carcinoma

### 32.2.1
### Pathogenesis and Incidence

RCC is the third most common genitourinary tumor and accounts for 3% of all malignancies in adults. The tumor usually is detected in older patients. Some known risk factors for renal cell carcinoma are von Hippel-Lindau disease and smoking. With the increased use of ultrasound, MRI and CT, the detection rate of carcinomas in an asymptomatic state is increasing. These incidentally detected tumors usually have smaller size, lower tumor stage, and better survival rates of the patients.

### 32.2.2
### Imaging RCC

### 32.2.2.1
### MRI

MRI allows data acquisition with a very good soft tissue contrast and multiplanar image acquisition, especially in patients with extensive tumor with invasion of the inferior vena cava. MRI determines cranial extension of the thrombus much more effectively than does single-slice CT. Before the introduction of MDCT scanners, MRI used to be the image modality of choice for

delineation of tumor thrombus (KALLMAN et al. 1992). MDCT scanners are able to generate multiplanar reconstructions with a high resolution, with similar staging results for MDCT and MRI for staging RCC with extension of the thrombus into the inferior vena cava (HALLSCHEIDT et al. 2004, 2005). MRI allows, in contrast to CT, detection of the pseudocapsule of the tumor in patients with small RCC. For nephron-sparing surgery, the infiltration into the perinephric fat has to be excluded, and the presence of a pseudocapsule enables the possibilities to perform nephron-sparing surgery in these small tumors (PRETORIUS et al. 1999). MR imaging showed results more superior than CT in detecting cystic RCC, as the better soft tissue contrast detects enhancement even in thin cystic septa or walls (ISREAL and BOSNIAK 2004).

In differential diagnosis of solid renal lesions, MRI and MDCT have similar advantages. The diagnosis of an angiomyolipoma can be made with MDCT and MRI, whereas both modalities have limitations in oncocytomas.

### 32.2.2.2
### MDCT

MDCT allows similar staging results as MRI, especially in extensive tumors (Fig. 32.6). In earlier studies, single-slice CT and MRI have similar staging capabilities for limited RCC. The introduction of MDCT allowed improving the staging accuracy of extensive tumors with tumor–thrombus of the inferior vena cava (Fig. 32.7a,b). Although MDCT provides images with a high spatial

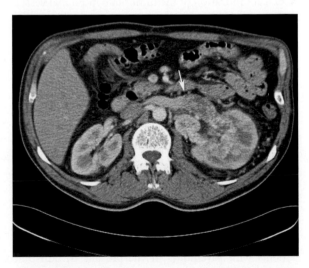

**Fig. 32.6.** Extensive RCC with tumor thrombus in the left distended renal vein (*arrow*). The extension of the tumor is difficult to define

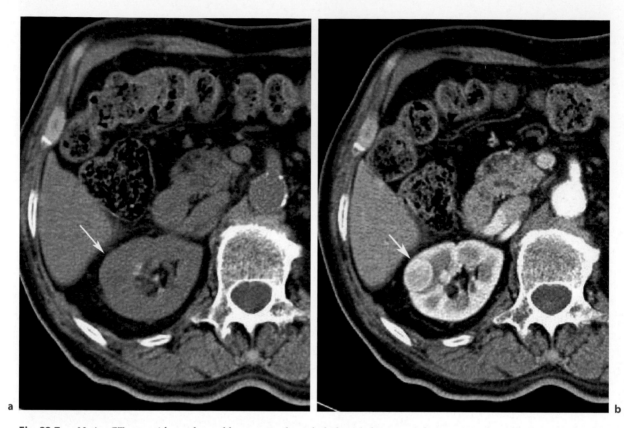

**Fig. 32.7. a** Native CT scan with not detectable tumor in the right kidney (*white arrow*). **b** Contrast enhanced CT scan in an early arterial phase with a small RCC in the upper pole of the right kidney (*white arrow*)

resolution and MPR, its role in planning nephron-sparing surgery is, like in MRI, still limited. Despite the high spatial resolution, it remains an unsolved problem to detect infiltration of the tumor into intrarenal vessels and the renal pelvis (HALLSCHEIDT et al. 2006).

## 32.3
## Carcinoma of the Prostate

### 32.3.1
### Pathogenesis and Incidence

Despite improvements in screening and therapy of prostate cancer, it still is the most common malignancy in men. The use of prostate-specific antigen (PSA) has led to an early detection of the carcinomas, with a lower tumor stage and a better survival. Today, only 5% of the patients with carcinoma of the prostate demonstrate with distant metastases and only 2% with lymph nodes metastases at initial diagnosis (SOH et al. 1997). De-

pending on the tumor stage and the grade of the tumor, a wide variety of treatment possibilities are available ranging from watchful wait to radical surgery or focal ablative therapies like cryoablation, radiofrequency ablation, or focused ultrasound.

### 32.3.2
### Imaging Carcinoma of the Prostate

#### 32.3.2.1
#### Transrectal Ultrasound

Transrectal ultrasound is the imaging modality most widely used and is used as biopsy guidance in patients with suspected prostate cancer. Usually prostate cancer presents as a hypoechogenic area and additionally to systematic sampling of the prostate, further core biopsies can be performed in these suspected hypoechogenic areas. The number of the routinely obtained cores is growing from 6 to 10 or 12, or even 24, with a higher detection rate (TAKENAKA et al. 2006). For staging, transrectal ultrasound is generally considered insufficient. Although the extracapsular extension or the infiltration into the seminal vesicles can be predicted in up to 80% (SCARDINO et al. 1989), in lower tumor stages transrectal ultrasound is less useful.

### 32.3.2.2
### MRI

MRI currently is used for local cancer detection in cases with elevated PSA levels and negative core biopsies. The use of an endorectal coil improves the spatial resolution (Fig. 32.8a). 3-T scanners have improved signal-to-noise ratio, offering similar staging results without endorectal coil. Additional techniques like spectroscopic imaging and dynamic contrast enhanced imaging of the prostate help to detect carcinomas in the transitional zone (ZAKIAN et al. 2003). As MRI has the ability to detect extracapsular extension and seminal vesicles (SALA et al. 2006) and staging accuracies of up to 93%, MR imaging of the prostate is increasingly used for preoperative workup in patients with cancer of the prostate.

### 32.3.2.3
### MDCT

MDCT plays a role in staging in patients with newly diagnosed prostate cancer, but for the local tumor staging of the prostate or detection of the tumor, CT has limited value due to its reduced soft tissue contrasts (Fig. 32.8b). CT of the abdomen and pelvis is recommended for patients with a PSA levels greater than 20 ng ml$^{-1}$ or a Gleason score greater than 7, or a local tumor stage of a least T3. Sensitivity for staging lymph nodes in prostate cancer varies between 25 and 78% and has a specificity 67 and 97% (WOLF et al. 1995), depending on the used diameter of the suspected lymph nodes. CT also is used to detect and follow-up bone metastases and to estimate the stability of lytic and blastic bone lesions.

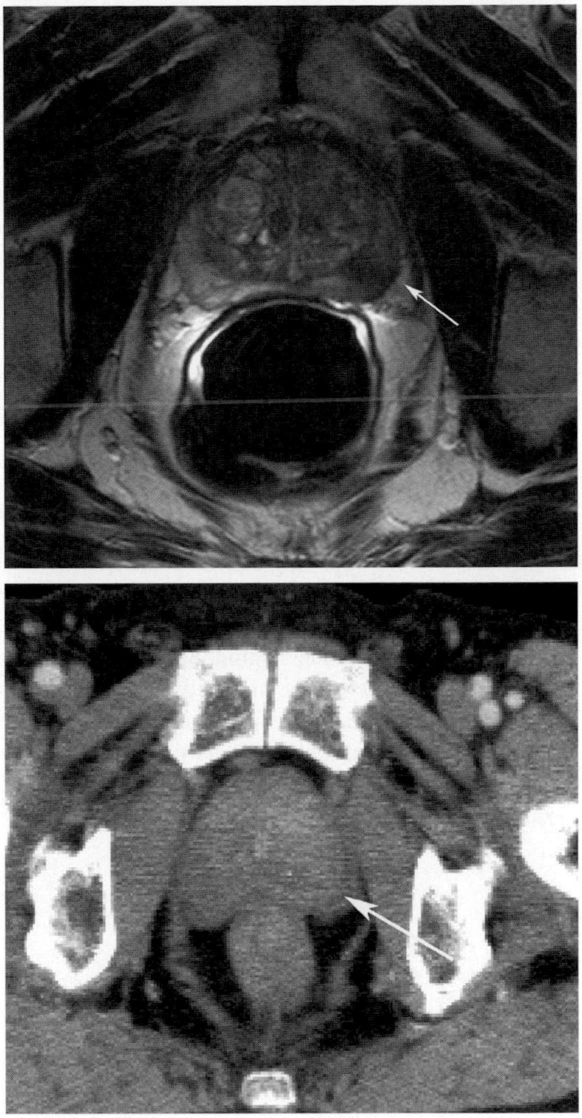

**Fig. 32.8. a** T2 weighted MR scan with a hypodense area in the peripheral zone of the prostate (T2a) (courtesy of Dr. Zechmann, German Cancer Research Center, Heidelberg, Germany). **b** CT scan of the patient (**a**) with a reduced soft tissue contrast. The tumor cannot be detected in this contrast enhanced CT scan (*arrow*)

## 32.4
## Seminomas and Non-Seminomatous Tumors

### 32.4.1
### Pathogenesis and Incidence

Patients with seminomas are usually aged between 20 and 50, accounting for 40% of testicular neoplasm.

Non-seminomatous tumors contain teratocarcinomas, embryonal cell tumors, teratomas, and choriocarcinomas. Peak incidence is in the ages of 20 to 30.

CT is routinely used for staging of the chest, the abdomen, and the pelvis in patients with seminomas and non-seminomatous germ cell tumor.

MRI is used for local tumor detection, with usually an isointense signal on T1-weighted images and a hypointense signal on T2-weighted images. Local tumor staging is done histopathologically.

## 32.4.2
## Imaging Seminomas and Non-Seminomatous Tumors

MRI and CT are used for staging regional and retroperitoneal lymph nodes.

Accuracy for preoperative staging of retroperitoneal lymph nodes with incremental CT in ranged from 67 to 81% in earlier studies. Especially in stage 1 patients with non-seminomatous germ cell tumor, a high rate of false-negative CT findings have been reported up to 44%. With the introduction of MDCT, the motion misregistration has been reduced, and a better intravenous contrast has been achieved reducing the rate of false-negative lymph node staging. Still, CT and MRI have difficulties to detect the histopathological positive lymph node, causing false-positive findings.

In the follow-up of these younger patients, the MRI with a lack of radiation should be used to exclude retroperitoneal and iliac lymph nodes.

## 32.5
## Endometrial Cancer

### 32.5.1
### Pathogenesis and Incidence

Endometrial cancer is the fourth most common cancer. In Western industrial nations, it is the most common gynecologic malignancy. Ninety-five percent of cases occur in women older than 40 years. As the risk factor the estrogen stimulation without progesterone is know. Endometrial cancer usually is staged surgically by the International Federation of Gynecology and Obstetrics (FIGO) staging system. In limited preoperative FIGO staging by conventional procedures, the extension of the tumor is underestimated in 23% of the cases (HRICAK et al. 1991). The FIGO system has better results for early stages, but it has inaccuracies in advanced stages and does not address nodal involvement. The percentage of invasion of the myometrium is essential for the tumor staging and prognosis. Other risk factors are the histological subtype and grade and nodal involvement. Infiltration of more than 50% of the thickness of the myometrium (IC) has a significantly higher percentage

of lymph node metastasis than infiltration of less than 50%.

Preoperative workup of these tumors allows predicting, whether a lymph node dissection is necessary or not.

### 32.5.2
### Imaging Endometrial Cancer

#### 32.5.2.1
#### Transvaginal Ultrasound

Transvaginal ultrasound (TVUS) is a widely accepted method to evaluate patients with abnormal genital bleeding. The diagnosis of an endometrial cancer is made by hysteroscopy-guided biopsy. The surgical procedures included hysterectomy in early stages with or without pelvic lymphadenectomy and radiochemotherapy in extensive tumors.

#### 32.5.2.2
#### MRI

MRI has very good staging results and is currently the staging method of choice (KINKEL et al. 1999; HRICAK et al. 1991). Sensitivity and specificity for staging the myometrial extension of the tumor are in a recently published meta-analysis 92 and 90%, respectively, for MRI. In particular, the sagittal MR images allow an evaluation of the tumor. MRI not only allows an evaluation of the myometrial invasion, but also cervical infiltration and nodal metastases. MRI is a one-stop shop examination allows a high overall staging accuracy of 80–90% (KINKEL et al. 1999).

#### 32.5.2.3
#### CT

Despite the improvements of CT technology, staging capabilities for endometrial carcinoma are limited. In a study published by HARDESTY et al. (2001), sensitivity and specificity for evaluation of the depth of myometrial invasion was 83 and 42%, respectively. The ability of helical CT to evaluate the presence of cervical invasion is also limited with a sensitivity of 25% and a specificity of 70%.

Even with the use of helical CT, it is a less sensitive and less specific modality compared with MRI.

## 32.6
# Cervical Cancer

### 32.6.1
### Pathogenesis and Incidence

Cervical carcinoma is the third most common gynecological tumor, accounting for 2% of female cancers. The presence of a high-risk papilloma virus infection seems to be mandatory for development of a carcinoma.

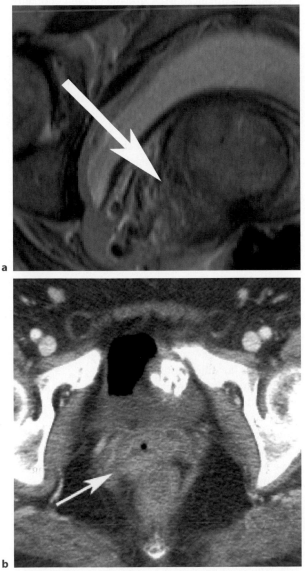

**Fig. 32.9. a** T2-weighted MR scan showing cervical cancer with infiltration into the right parametric space (arrow). **b** Same patient in a contrast-enhanced CT scan. Due to the reduced soft tissue contrast, the infiltration of the parametric space (**a**) cannot be clearly delineated

For staging of cervical carcinomas, infiltration of the rectum and the urinary bladder, as well as the infiltration of the pelvic floor and the sidewalls of the pelvis has to be excluded. Resection of the tumor is planned in patients with a tumor limited to the cervix without infiltration of the parametrium.

Recurrent tumors after surgery are seen as a soft tissue mass in the region of the vaginal vault, usually with involvement of the adjacent parametrium. After radiotherapy, the tumor is seen as a mass within the cervix. The involvement of the pelvic floor or the sidewalls is essential for planning resection of primary and recurrent tumors.

### 32.6.2
### Imaging Cervical Cancer

In a multicenter study (ACRIN 6651/GOG 183), MR imaging allowed very good tumor delineation of the cervical carcinoma even in early stages. Tumor visualization was significantly more superior with MR than in CT, with a mean AUC of 0.77 for MRI and 0.58 for CT. Detection of parametrial infiltration also was significantly better in MRI than in CT, with a mean AUC of 0.62 for CT and 0.68 for MRI.

For staging advanced cancers (stage IIB or higher), CT had a sensitivity of 0.28 and a specificity of 0.9, whereas MRI had a sensitivity of 0.47 and a specificity of 0.79. The positives predictive values were low for both modalities, with an average of 0.55 for CT and 0.36 for MRI (HRICAK et al. 2007). CT and MRI had a high negative predictive value stage IIb cervical cancer.

The staging results for both modalities were quite low. These results suggest that CT and MRI are imperfect for the evaluation of the cervical cancer, and further technical improvements have to be made.

## 32.7
# Ovarian Cancer

### 32.7.1
### Pathogenesis and Incidence

Despite the efforts in screening and advances in imaging, today 70% of all ovarian carcinomas are diagnosed in an advanced tumor stage, causing a high mortality. Recently, imaging has become an integral part of initial patient management with a more individualized patient care. About 1.5% of women develop ovarian cancer. Ovarian cancer is the fifth most frequent female cancer. Among the gynecological cancers, it has the highest morbidity and mortality. Sixty percent of all cancers are found in women older than 65 years. Prognostic factors are the initial tumor stage, high age, and large tumor volumes. A direct correlation between tumor stage and 5-year survival rate has been documented (HOLSCHEIDER and BEREK 2000).

The staging of ovarian cancer is defined by the extent of the tumor and the location of the disease diagnosed during an initial staging laparotomy. Still today, FIGO as well as TNM staging are based upon the intraoperative findings.

CT and MRI have widely gained acceptance for preoperative tumor staging. Cross-sectional imaging modalities have replaced conventional imaging studies like barium enema and EU.

## 32.7.2
## Imaging Ovarian Cancer

### 32.7.2.1
### MRI

MRI staging accuracies range between 78 and 88% (WOODWARD et al. 2002). The role of MRI in staging ovarian cancer has several limitations. Longer examination times, higher costs, and lower spatial resolution and problems to cover the complete abdomen have made MRI an alternative imaging modality in patients with contraindications for CT or unclear findings in CT.

### 32.7.2.2
### CT

CT currently has a staging accuracy of 53–92% (Yoshida). It is the staging modality of choice. The high resolution of MDCT scanners gives information about the size of the tumor, its extension, localization of peritoneal implants, and lymph node enlargement.

*Local tumor extension.* Invasion of the pelvic sidewalls, direct invasion into the muscular pelvic sidewalls, or the invasion of the sidewall vessels has to be excluded. Infiltration of the rectosigmoid and the urinary bladder should be excluded.

*Peritoneal spread.* Peritoneal seeding is caused by distribution of tumor cells into the normal peritoneal fluid. Peritoneal metastases are usually nodular soft tissue lesions or plaque-like thickening of the parietal or visceral peritoneum. They usually show moderate enhancement. Diagnosing small peritoneal implants can be difficult, with very low detection rates for CT (COAK-

LEY et al. 2002). The presence of ascites gives a hint for peritoneal spread. Still, CT and MRI have limitations in detecting small-size peritoneal metastasis.

*Lymphatic tumor spread.* The main location of tumor spread in ovarian cancer is the ovarian vessels, the common iliac vessels, and the para-aortic lymph nodes. The threshold for diagnosing a metastatic lymph node is about 1 cm, with a sensitivity of about 40% and a specificity of about 90% (TEMPANY et al. 2000).

*Hematogenous dissemination.* Metastases are found in the bones, the lung, and the kidneys. However, liver metastases are only found in about 1% of the patients.

Contrast-enhanced MDCT is the imaging modality of choice for staging ovarian cancer. It provides essential information for surgery planning and allows patient-specific management.

In cases of typical findings of ovarian cancer, the tumor extent is crucial for treatment and surgery planning. Imaging is not competitive to surgical staging but provides complementary information for planning surgery and helps to prevent under-staging. Even in patients undergoing neo-adjuvant chemotherapy, imaging can help to predict the resectability of the residual tumor (QAYYUM et al. 2005).

## 32.8
## Conclusion

The kidneys, ureter, urinary bladder, as well as the female and male reproductive organs together form the urogenital system. The different parts of this system contribute many different carcinomas. For these entities different diagnostic modalities have be established to diagnose the different tumors.

Hematuria is the initial symptom for TCC located in the kidneys, the ureter, and the urinary bladder. A source of hematuria is located in 40% in the excretory urography and in over 90% in computerized tomographic urography (ALBANI et al. 2007). Cystoscopy and CTU show similar detection rates for urinary bladder cancer.

MRI shows very good results in staging prostate cancer, with correct staging results in up to 90%. Additional techniques like spectroscopy and perfusion allow improving the specificity. Sonography is the diagnostic modality of choice in case of testicular cancer; CT or MRI is performed to rule out retroperitoneal lymph nodes.

MRI could improve staging in preoperative workup of endometrium and cervical cancer. Especially in cervical cancer, MRI showed superior staging results compared to the FIGO staging system (HRICAK et al. 2007).

In cases of ovarian tumors, MRI allows a better differentiation of benign and malign tumors. Additional information about the extension of the tumor and the T stadium is given in one MRI.

# References

Akin O, Sala E, Moskowitz CS, Kuroiwa K, Ishill NM, Pucar D, Scardino PT, Hricak H (2006) Transition zone prostate cancers: features, detection, localization, and staging at endorectal MR imaging. Radiology 239:784–792

Albani JM, Ciaschini MW, Streem SB, Herts BR, Angermeier KW (2007) The role of computerized tomographic urography in the initial evaluation of hematuria. J Urol 177:644–648

Coakley FV, Choi PH, Gougoutas CA, Pothuri B, Venkatraman E, Chi D, Bergman A, Hricak H (2002) Peritoneal metastases: detection with spiral CT in patients with ovarian cancer. Radiology 223:495–499

Forstner R, Hricak H, Powell CB, Azizi L, Frankel SB, Stern JL (1995) Ovarian cancer recurrence: value of MR imaging. Radiology 196:715–720

Fritz GA, Schoellnast H, Deutschmann HA, Quehenberger F, Tillich M (2006) Multiphasic multidetector-row CT (MDCT) in detection and staging of transitional cell carcinomas of the upper urinary tract. Eur Radiol 16:1244–1252

Gray Sears CL, Ward JF, Sears ST, Puckett MF, Kane CJ, Amling CL (2002) Prospective comparison of computerized tomography and excretory urography in the initial evaluation of asymptomatic microhematuria. J Urol 168:2457–2460

Grossfeld GD, Wolf JS, Litwin MS et al. (2001) Evaluation of asymptomatic microscopic hematuria in adults: the American Urologic Association vest practice policy recommendations. Part II: patient evaluation, cytology, voided markers, imaging, cystoscopy, nephrology evaluation, and follow-up. Urology 57:604–610

Hallscheidt PJ, Bock M, Riedasch G, Zuna I, Schoenberg SO, Autschbach F, Soder M, Noeldge G (2004) Diagnostic accuracy of staging renal cell carcinomas using multidetector-row CT and MRI: a prospective study with histopathological correlation. JCAT 2004 28:333–338

Hallscheidt PJ, Fink C, Soder M, Pomer S, Zuna I, Noeldge G, Kauffmann G (2005) Preoperative staging of renal cell carcinoma with inferior vena cava thrombus using multislice CT and MRI: prospective study with histopathological correlation: JCAT 29:64–68

Hallscheidt P, Wagener N, Gholipour F, Aghabozorgi N, Dreyhaupt J, Hohenfellner M, Haferkamp A, Pfitzenmeier J (2006) Multislice CT in planning nephron-sparing surgery in a prospective study with 76 patients: comparison of radiological and histopathological findings in the infiltration of renal structures. JCAT 30:869–874

Hardesty LA, Sumkin JH, Hakim C, Johns C, Nath M (2001) The ability of helical CT to preoperatively stage endometrial carcinoma. AJR Am J Roentgenol 3:603–606

Holschneider CH, Berek JS (2000) Ovarian cancer: epidemiology, biology, and prognostic factors. Semin Surg Oncol 19:3–10

Hricak H, Rubinstein LV, Gherman GM, Karstaedt N (1991) MR imaging evaluation of endometrial carcinoma: results of an NCI cooperative study. Radiology 179:829–832

Hricak H, Gatsonis C, Coakley FV, Snyder B, Reinhold C, Schwartz LH, Woodward PJ, Pannu HK, Amendola M, Mitchell DG (2007) Early invasive cervical cancer: CT and MR imaging in preoperative evaluation—ACRIN/GOG comparative study of diagnostic performance and interobserver variability. Radiology 245:491–498

Israel GM, Bosniak MA (2004) MR imaging of cystic renal masses. Magn Reson Imaging Clin N Am 3:403–412

Kallman DA, King BF, Hattery RR, Charboneau JW, Ehman RL, Guthman DA, Blute ML (1992) Renal vein and inferior vena cava tumor thrombus in renal cell carcinoma: CT, US, MRI and vena cavography. J Comput Assist Tomogr 16:240–247

Kinkel K, Kaji Y, Yu KK, Segal MR, Lu Y, Powell CB, Hricak H (1999) Radiologic staging in patients with endometrial cancer: a meta-analysis. Radiology 212:711–718

Oyen RH, Van Poppel HP, Ameye FE, Van de Voorde WA, Baert AL, Baert LV (1994) Lymph node staging of localized prostatic carcinoma with CT and CT-guided fine-needle aspiration biopsy: prospective study of 285 patients. Radiology 190:315–322

Park SB, Kim JK, Lee HJ, Choi HJ, Cho KS (2007) Hematuria: portal venous phase multi detector row CT of the bladder—a prospective study. Radiology 245:798–805

Pretorius ES, Siegelman ES, Parvati Ramchandani, Cangiano T, Banner MP (1999) Renal neoplasms amenable to partial nephrectomy. MR Imaging Radiol 212:28–34

Qayyum A, Coakley FV, Westphalen AC, Hricak H, Okuno WT, Powell B (2005) Role of CT and MR imaging in predicting optimal cytoreduction of newly diagnosed primary epithelial ovarian cancer. Gynecol Oncol 96:301–306

Sala E, Eberhardt SC, Akin O, Moskowitz CS, Onyebuchi CN, Kuroiwa K, Ishill N, Zelefsky MJ, Eastham JA, Hricak H (2006) Endorectal MR imaging before salvage prostatectomy: tumor localization and staging. Radiology 238:176–183

Scardino PT, Shinohara K, Wheeler TM, Carter SS (1989) Staging of prostate cancer. Value of ultrasonography. Urol Clin N Am 16:713–734

Soh S, Kattan MW, Berkman S, Wheeler TM, Scardino PT (1997) Has there been a recent shift in the pathological features and prognosis of patients treated with radical prostatectomy? J Urol 157:2223–2224

Takenaka A, Hara R, Hyodo Y, Ishimura T, Sakai Y, Fujioka H, Fujii T, Jo Y, Fujisawa M (2006) Transperineal extended biopsy improves the clinically significant prostate cancer detection rate: a comparative study of 6 and 12 biopsy cores. Int J Urol 13:10–14

Tempany CM, Zou KH, Silverman SG, Brown DL, Kurtz AB, McNeil BJ (2000) Staging of advanced ovarian cancer: comparison of imaging modalities—report from the Radiological Diagnostic Oncology Group. Radiology 215:761–767

Wolf JS Jr, Cher M, Dall'era M, Presti JC Jr, Hricak H, Carroll PR (1995) The use and accuracy of cross-sectional imaging and fine needle aspiration cytology for detection of pelvic lymph node metastases before radical prostatectomy. J Urol 153:993–999

Woodward PJ, Hosseinzadeh K, Saenger JS (2004) From the archives of the AFIP: radiologic staging of ovarian carcinoma with pathologic correlation. Radiographics 24:225–246

Yoshida Y, Kurokawa T, Kawahara K, Tsuchida T, Okazawa H, Fujibayashi Y, Yonekura Y, Kotsuji F (2004) Incremental benefits of FDG positron emission tomography over CT alone for the preoperative staging of ovarian cancer. AJR Am J Roentgenol 182:227–233

Zakian KL, Eberhardt S, Hricak H, Shukla-Dave A, Kleinman S, Muruganandham M, Sircar K, Kattan MW, Reuter VE, Scardino PT, Koutcher JA (2003) Transition zone prostate cancer: metabolic characteristics at 1H MR spectroscopic imaging—initial results. Radiology 229:241–247

# PET–CT in Oncology

Gerald Antoch

CONTENTS

**ABSTRACT**

Hardware-based image fusion with an integrated PET–CT scanner overcomes typical limitations of morphology and function alone. PET–CT using $^{18}$F-2-Fluoro-2-deoxy-D-glucose (FDG) as a radionuclide has been found of benefit over both imaging procedures acquired separately when it comes to tumor staging of different malignant diseases. However, there are also limitations of the combined imaging approach. Inflammation or tissue regeneration may be difficult to differentiate from malignancy, based on an increase in FDG-uptake. Furthermore, FDG-PET–negative tumors may be missed if the CT is not acquired in a diagnostic manner. Apart from focusing on state-of-the-art CT as part of the PET–CT scan, alternative radionuclides will improve tumor detection even in typically FDG-PET–negative lesions. This chapter covers the technical basics of PET–CT and addresses its value and limitations in clinical oncology.

## 33.1
## Introduction

For assessment of patients with malignant diseases, morphological and functional imaging procedures have been available. While CT provides mainly morphological data on a tumor in question, PET can assess functional aspects of a lesion. However, both imaging modalities have their limitations if they are acquired separately; morphology alone has been found inferior to functional imaging when assessing lymph nodes for metastatic spread (HABERKORN and SCHOENBERG 2001; TOLOZA et al. 2003). Furthermore, characterization of parenchyma lesions may be difficult if based on morphological data alone. Functional imaging with

G. ANTOCH, MD
Department of Diagnostic and Interventional Radiology and Neuroradiology, University Hospital Essen, Hufelandstrasse 55, 45127 Essen, Germany

PET can provide these functional data that are lacking in CT. However, in PET alone there is only limited anatomical information available. Accurate localization of a lesion within a certain organ, or even within a segment of an organ, can be extremely difficult on PET alone. This is the case when $^{18}$F-2-fluoro-2-deoxy-D-glucose (FDG) is administered as a radioactive tracer, but even more if imaging is performed with a highly specific radionuclide (Fig. 33.1) (WEBER et al. 1999; DIEDERICHS et al. 2000). Thus, correlation of PET with CT must be considered mandatory. Retrospective image fusion of CT and PET data sets has been performed to overcome these limitations of morphology and function. Retrospective software-based image fusion works nicely in static organs, such as the head and skull. However, thoracic and abdominal image fusion has been hampered by organ shift due to differences in patient positioning and breathing-associated misalignment (TOWNSEND 2001). In addition, retrospective image fusion can be time-consuming, making it impractical in daily clinical routine if performed on a regular basis.

Hardware-based image fusion with an integrated PET–CT scanner overcomes these limitations. Accurately fused morphological and functional data sets are available immediately after the examination, without the need to manually fuse the images. FDG-PET–CT has been found of benefit over both imaging procedures acquired separately when it comes to tumor staging of different malignant diseases (BAR-SHALOM et al. 2003; LARDINOIS et al. 2003; ANTOCH et al. 2004). However, there are also limitations of the combined imaging approach. This chapter covers the technical basics of PET–CT and addresses its value and limitations in clinical oncology.

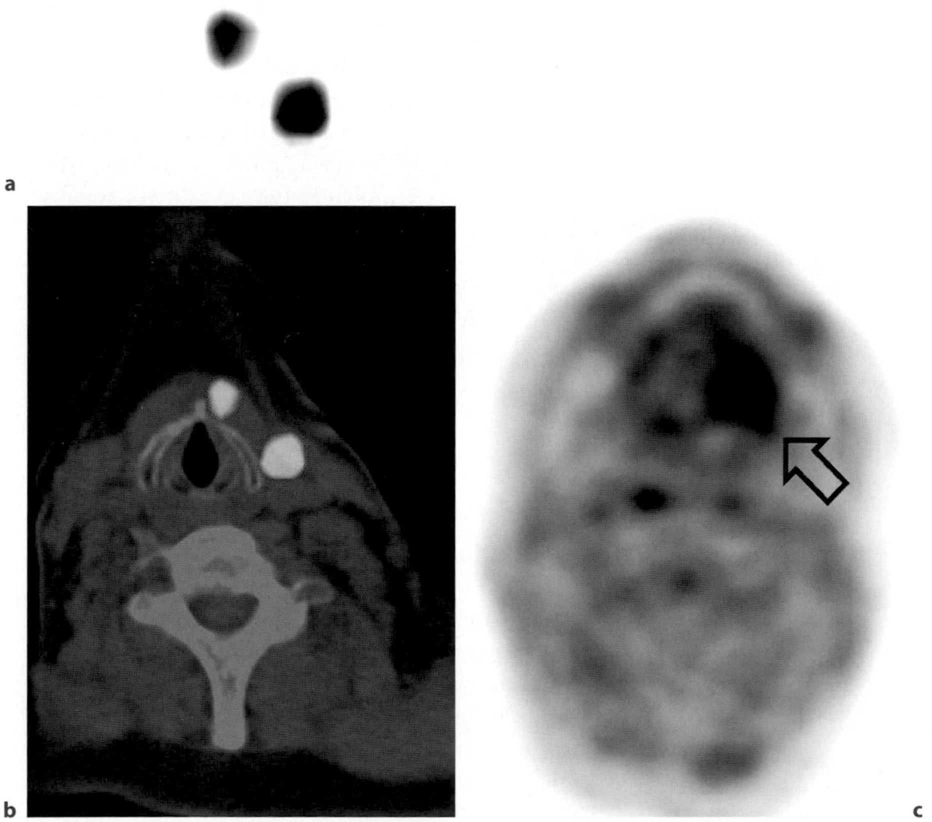

**Fig. 33.1a-c.** $^{124}$I–PET in a patient with differentiated thyroid cancer following thyroidectomy (**a**). There is no anatomical background, as $^{124}$I is highly specific for thyroid tissue. Fusion with anatomical data is mandatory for correct localization of $^{124}$iodine uptake (**b**). FDG as a nonspecific radionuclide provides some limited anatomical data, which allows localization of the area of increased tracer uptake (*arrow*) within the left base of the tongue (**c**).

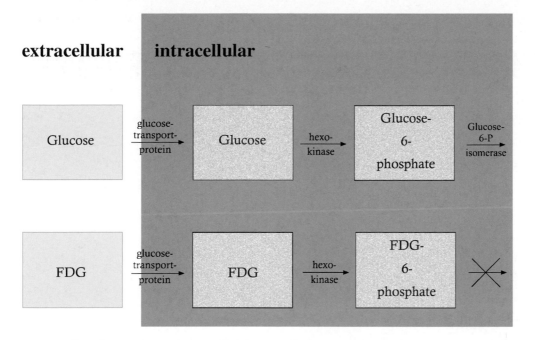

**Fig. 33.2.** $^{18}$F-2-fluoro-2-deoxy-D-glucose (*FDG*) is actively taken up by glucose transport proteins into the cell. Within the cell, FDG is metabolized to FDG-6-phosphate, which is metabolically trapped

## Technical Basics of PET–CT

### 33.2.1
### Radionuclides

A radioactively labeled tracer is administered to the patient for PET scanning. Most PET and PET–CT studies in oncology are performed with FDG, which is injected intravenously 60–90 min before the examination. FDG is a glucose analog, which is taken up by cells through glucose-transport proteins. Once taken up into the cell, FDG is metabolized to FDG-6-phosphate. FDG-6-phosphate, however, is not a substrate of hexokinase and is trapped within the cell (Fig. 33.2). Radioactive decay of $^{18}$F, a positron emitter with a half-life of 109 min, leads to release of two 511-keV gamma rays, which travel in opposite directions (Fig. 33.3). These gamma rays are detected by photoluminescent PET crystals.

Depending on their glucose metabolism, different organs are represented by different FDG uptake. The brain, the heart, and the liver have physiologically very high glucose metabolism. Many tumors are characterized by an increase in glucose metabolism. These tumors can be detected as "hot spots" on an FDG-PET–CT. Inflammatory processes and tissue regeneration after an operation or an interventional procedure may cause interpretative problems. Both, inflammation and tissue regeneration are characterized by increased glucose metabolism, leading to increased FDG uptake.

However, not all tumors are characterized by an increase in glucose metabolism. Table 33.1 provides an overview of tumors that are frequently FDG-PET positive, and others that may not be. In FDG-PET–neg-

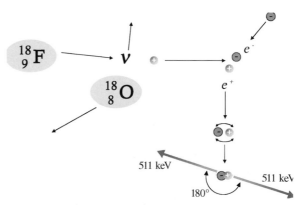

**Fig. 33.3.** Imaging principle of FDG-PET: $^{18}$F decays to $^{18}$O by emission of a positron (e$^+$) and a neutrino (ν). The positron annihilates with an electron (e$^-$), releasing two 511-keV gamma rays, which travel in opposite directions. These gamma rays are detected by two photoluminescent PET crystals and are followed by computer-based calculation of the point of origin

**Table 33.1** Tumors frequently FDG-PET positive (*left column*) and tumors in which FDG-PET may only be of limited value (*right column*)

| Tumors frequently FDG-PET positive | Tumors often FDG-PET negative |
| --- | --- |
| Head and neck | Neuroendocrine tumors |
| Differentiated thyroid cancer | Hepatocellular carcinoma |
| NSCLC | RCC |
| CRC | Prostate cancer |
| Stomach/GIST | |
| Malignant melanoma | |
| Breast cancer | |
| CUP | |
| Lymphoma | |

NSCLC non-small-cell lung cancer,

RCC renal cell cancer,

GIST gastrointestinal stromal tumours,

CUP cancer of unknown primary

ative tumors, alternative tracers may be an option. Many radionuclides have been developed and implemented in clinical routine. Some examples are [11]C-choline for prostate cancer (FARSAD et al. 2005), [68]Ga-DOTA-D-Phe1-Tyr3-octreotide (DOTATOC) for neuroendocrine tumors (HOFMANN et al. 2001), or [124]I for differentiated thyroid cancer (FREUDENBERG et al. 2004a). None of these new and often-specific tracers can, however, currently replace FDG as the workhorse in functional oncological imaging. However, further development and implementation of new PET tracers in clinical routine will increase the number of PET–CT indications.

## 32.2.2
## PET–CT

Commercially available PET–CT scanners are based on the imaging principle described by BEYER et al. (2000). Two separate scanners, a CT and a PET, are installed in series. A single examination table serves both imaging components of the PET–CT (Fig. 33.4). The patient is positioned on the examination table; this is followed by acquisition of the CT, and then by acquisition of the PET. In between the two scans, the patient remains in the same position on the examination table. This assures that morphological and functional data sets can be accurately fused after image acquisition. Patient motion in between the two scans or motion of internal organs may result in different positions of an organ or a lesion

during CT and PET. This event may result in inaccurate co-registration of CT and PET. In the event of image misregistration, software-based manual adjustment may be performed.

Apart from organ movement and patient motion, inaccuracies in image co-registration may result from differences in image acquisition with CT and PET. CT data are acquired with continuous table movement over a very short period, typically allowing coverage of a

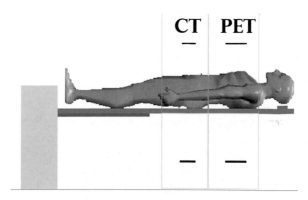

**Fig. 33.4** Principle of PET–CT imaging: CT and PET are installed in series. A single examination table serves both the CT and the PET. After positioning the patient on the examination table, CT data are acquired first followed by acquisition of the PET. Since the patient is in the same position on the examination table during CT and PET, both data sets can be accurately fused following the examination

large axial scan range in a single breath-hold. However, PET is performed discontinuously over several bed positions, each with an axial field of view of approximately 15 cm. Per bed position, the examination time may range from 1 to 5 min, depending on the amount of tracer applied and depending on the image quality desired. To cover a field-of-view from head to the upper thighs, examination times range between 10 and 30 min. Thus, PET imaging is performed with shallow breathing. These differences in breathing while acquiring the CT data and the PET data may cause inaccuracies in image fusion. Both data sets can be fused most accurately, if the CT is acquired in expiration breath-hold (GOERRES et al. 2002; BEYER et al. 2003).

Differences between PET–CT systems apply to the number of detector rows with which the CT component is equipped. Currently, up to 64 detector rows have been integrated in PET–CT. For the PET component, different detector materials have been available. The three most common detector materials are bismuth germanate (BGO), lutetium oxyorthosilicate (LSO), and gadolinium oxyorthosilicate (GSO). All available PET–CT systems are equipped with a full-ring PET detector (360° coverage). The size of each detector crystal defines the spatial resolution of the tomograph, which may range from 2 to 5 mm.

Image evaluation of PET is performed both qualitatively and quantitatively. The reader assesses the PET data for regions of focally increased tracer uptake (qualitative image analysis). A region of interest is drawn around a hot spot on PET, offering quantitative analysis of the tracer activity in that area. Quantitative PET data are typically reported as standardized uptake values (SUV):

$$SUV = \frac{\text{activity concentration of lesion (MBq ln}^{-1})}{\text{injected activity (MBq)/patient weight (g)}}$$

The SUV may be normalized for patient weight (as shown above) or patient body surface area. However, a potential benefit of the SUV as compared with qualitative image analysis alone has been discussed controversially. The SUV may be used to differentiate benign from malignant lesions (KANG et al. 2004; RASMUSSEN et al. 2004), but the overlap of SUV values between these two entities often generates false diagnoses (KEYES 1995). Therefore, in most institutions, the SUV is currently used as an add-on to qualitative image analysis, while qualitative image analysis represents the backbone for the correct diagnosis. The SUV does, however, provide an invaluable tool in patients undergoing PET imaging for follow-up of tumor therapy. With the pretherapeutic

SUV as a basis, a decrease in the SUV can indicate tumor response to a certain therapy.

PET annihilation quanta are attenuated by body tissue when travelling from the point of origin to the PET detectors. The extent of attenuation may be influenced by many factors, such as potential obesity of the patient. To account for the attenuation of the PET quanta, PET data sets need to be attenuation corrected. In PET–CT scanning, the CT data can be used for attenuation correction of the PET quanta. CT represents transmission images (as opposed to the PET emission images) that are attenuated when passing through the patient. This information on CT attenuation can be used for attenuation correction of the PET data. However, based on their energy of 70–140 keV, the CT X-rays are attenuated stronger by structures of high density (e.g., contrast agents or metal implants) than are the PET annihilation quanta at 511 keV. This stronger attenuation of CT as compared with PET may cause inaccuracies in the calculation of the attenuation coefficients for PET, leading to artifacts and inaccuracies in PET tracer quantification. While artifacts may be clinically relevant if they are mistaken for true tracer uptake, inaccuracies in tracer quantification have been found of no clinical relevance (DIZENDORF et al. 2003; NAKAMOTO et al. 2003). An artifact typically appears as a region of apparently increased tracer uptake in co-registration with an area of high attenuation on CT (ANTOCH et al. 2002, 2004; GOERRES et al. 2002; HALPERN et al. 2004). Potential artifacts only appear very infrequently, if the CT protocol is optimized for PET–CT. Adapting the CT protocol to the needs of PET requires using as little positive contrast agents as possible. As described above, these positive contrast agents increase the risk of PET artifacts caused through high CT attenuation. While there are no alternatives to positive intravenous contrast agents, water-equivalent oral contrast agents should be administered for intestinal distension rather than barium or iodine. These water-equivalent agents do not increase attenuation on CT, thus avoiding PET artifacts (ANTOCH et al. 2004). Sometimes, however, it may be difficult to differentiate an artifact from an area of true tracer uptake in PET. In these cases, non-attenuation-corrected PET images should be assessed in addition to the attenuation-corrected data sets (Fig. 33.5).

In PET–CT, both PET and CT add to the radiation exposure of the patient. For PET, the radiation exposure depends on the radionuclide applied. A PET examination with FDG typically results in a radiation exposure of approximately 7 mSv for 350 MBq of FDG injected. In addition, there is radiation exposure from the CT component. The dose from CT strongly depends on the CT protocol. If CT is performed mainly for anatomical

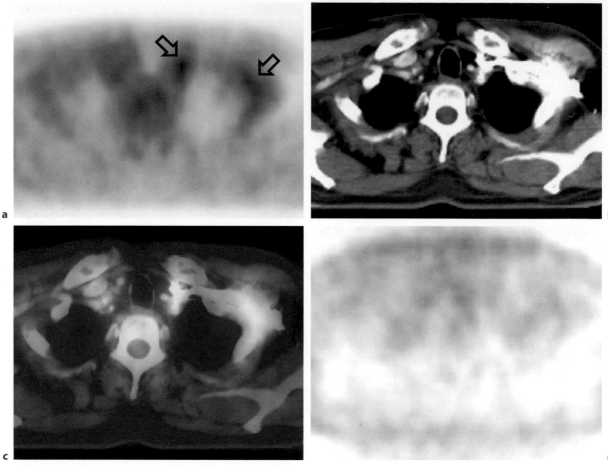

**Fig. 33.5a–d.** Contrast-associated PET artifact: apparent focal tracer uptake in the left axilla on PET (*arrow* in **a**). The corresponding CT demonstrates high-attenuation contrast material in the left axillary vein (**b**). Apparent focal tracer uptake can be identified as an artifact when fusing CT with PET (**c**). On non-attenuation corrected images, the artifact is not detected (**d**)

correlation rather than additional diagnostic information, then low-dose CT from head to the upper thighs will add approximately 3–5 mSv to the exposure from PET. However, if the CT is performed in a diagnostic manner, then full-dose CT acquisition results in an additional radiation exposure of approximately 15 mSv (Brix et al. 2005). Thus, in the setting of diagnostic CT imaging, a whole-body (head to upper thighs) PET–CT examination results in a radiation exposure of more than 20 mSv. Therefore, the indication for diagnostic CT as part of the PET–CT has to be made cautiously (Table 33.2).

**Table 33.2** PET–CT indications in which a contrast-enhanced CT component may be of benefit (*left column*) and in which diagnostic contrast-enhanced CT may not be required as part of the PET–CT (*right column*)

| Intravenous contrast | No intravenous contrast |
| --- | --- |
| Tumor staging | Contrast-enhanced CT available |
| Follow-up | Therapy response assessment |
| Radiation therapy planning | |

## 33.3
# Accuracy of PET–CT in Oncology

While PET imaging has been available since the 1980s, PET–CT was first introduced into clinical routine in 2001. Thus, there are many data on PET available from the literature, while data on PET–CT are still scarce for some tumor entities. Depending on the indication and the radionuclide, data on PET imaging may also apply to PET–CT.

### 33.3.1
# Indications in Oncology

### 33.3.1.1
# PET–CT for Tumor Staging

For tumor staging, accurate localization of a lesion must be considered of utmost importance. Several studies have been published on the accuracy of FDG-PET–CT for tumor staging of different tumors. The first two larger series (Bar-Shalom et al. 2003; Antoch et al. 2004) included a variety of different tumor entities. In their series of 204 patients, Bar-Shalom et al. reported additional findings with FDG-PET–CT as compared with separate image evaluation of FDG-PET and CT in 49% of patients. These additional findings led to a change in patient management in 14% of patients compared with CT and PET assessed side by side. Our own data on 260 patients with different oncological diseases (Antoch et al. 2004) found an accuracy of 84% for assessment of the TNM stage with FDG-PET–CT. As compared with

CT alone, patient management was altered in 15% of cases, compared with FDG-PET alone in 17% of cases, and compared with FDG-PET and CT read side by side in 6% of cases. Initiation of a stage-adapted therapy is known to improve patient survival for a variety of malignant tumors (Smythe 2001; Cerny and Giaccone 2002; Forastiere et al. 2001). Thus, FDG-PET–CT may affect the patient's prognosis by altering patient management.

There are numerous studies available from the literature that cover the accuracy of FDG-PET for staging of *lymphoma*. Sensitivities for detection of viable disease range between 80 and 90%, with specificities of 69–99% (Bohuslavizki et al. 2000; Brucerius et al. 2006). The tumor stage was altered at initial staging in 36% of patients compared with a conventional imaging algorithm including CT imaging (Brucerius et al. 2006). Raanani et al. (2006) compared FDG-PET–CT with CT alone for staging of Hodgkin's disease (HD) and non-Hodgkin's lymphoma (NHL). The authors report upstaging of patients with HD in 32% and in those with NHL in 31% of cases compared with CT. The patients were down-staged in 15% and 1% for HD and NHL, respectively. Patient management was altered by FDG-PET–CT in 45% of patients in this study. Considering the fact that treatment of lymphoma and the patients' prognoses strongly depend on the tumor stage, this higher accuracy for lymphoma staging must be considered clinically relevant. Currently there is only one study comparing FDG-PET–CT with separately acquired CT and FDG-PET in the setting of primary lymphoma patients (Hernandez-Maraver et al. 2006). The authors report an increase in the tumor stage in 11 of 47 patients with FDG-PET–CT as compared with

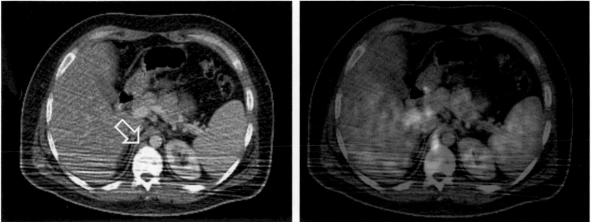

a                                                                                                                b

**Fig. 33.6a,b.** Male patient with abdominal NHL. Small retrocrural lymph node not suspected to be malignant based on its small size on CT (**a**). FDG-PET–CT demonstrates focal FDG uptake within this lymph node, upstaging the patient from stage II to stage III

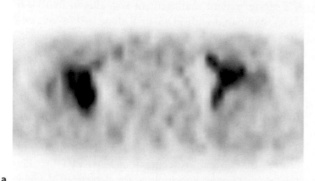

a

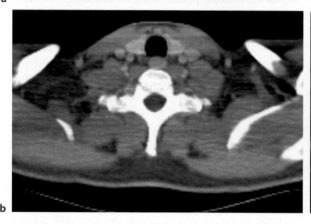

b

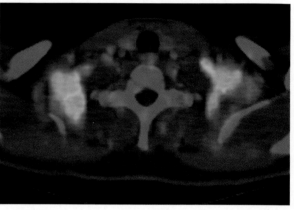

c

**Fig. 33.7a–c.** Extensive FDG uptake in the supraclavicular region on FDG-PET (**a**). The corresponding CT does not show any pathology (**b**). When fusing PET with CT, FDG uptake in supraclavicular brown fat becomes obvious (**c**).

both imaging procedures assessed side by side (Fig. 33.6). Based on these staging results, a change in patient management occurred in 15% of patients in this study.

Therefore, PET and PET–CT have a substantial impact on diagnostic accuracy and patient management (TATSUMI et al. 2005; HUTCHINGS et al. 2006; RAANANI et al. 2006).

FDG-PET has been found of higher accuracy than CT when staging *head and neck tumors*, with sensitivities of up to 90% for detection of lymph node metastases (KUTLER et al. 2006). There are, however, some limitations to PET in the head and neck region. Physiologically increased tracer uptake in salivary glands or in muscles of the head and neck may be difficult to interpret without anatomical correlation. In addition, activation of brown fat may be challenging (Fig. 33.7). Thus, correlation with anatomy as provided by PET–CT will be helpful. VEIT-HAIBACH et al. (2007) detected a significant improvement when assessing the TNM stage of head and neck tumors with FDG-PET–CT as compared with CT alone and CT viewed side by side with PET. This difference was based mainly on more accurate assessment of the T stage and the N stage, rather than the M stage.

Detection of the primary tumor in CUP has been an important indication of FDG-PET. The median survival for patients with CUP may increase from 12 to 23 months if the primary tumor is detected and treated specifically (RABER et al. 1991). Detection rates between 24% and 53% have been reported for FDG-PET (RESKE and KOTZERKE 2001). These substantial differences in the detection rates result mainly from differences in the definition of the term CUP. If defined correctly, a CUP is diagnosed if no tumor can be detected with morphological cross-sectional imaging and blind nasopharyngeal biopsies have been negative. In this setting, detection rates are low, even with FDG-PET and FDG-PET–CT (Fig. 33.8). GUTZEIT et al. (2005) retrospectively evaluated with FDG-PET–CT 45 patients with cervical CUP. In 15 patients (33%), the primary tumor could be detected with FDG-PET–CT, and in 30 patients (67%), no primary tumor site was found. In this study, CT alone found the primary tumor in 8 patients (18%), PET alone in 11 patients (24%), and CT read side by side with PET in 13 patients (29%). While PET–CT was able to outperform the other imaging modalities in this study, these differences did not prove to be of statistical significance.

*Non-small cell lung cancer* (NSCLC) has been one of the most important indications for FDG-PET imaging. Tumor staging in NSCLC patients strongly benefits from anatomical correlation of the PET data with CT. Several studies have demonstrated improved TNM-staging of NSCLC patients with FDG-PET–CT (AN-

TOCH et al. 2003; LARDINOIS et al. 2003; HALPERN et al. 2005; SHIM et al. 2005). This advantage relates to more accurate T staging with improved differentiation of the tumor from an adjacent atelectasis, and, even more important, more accurate N staging as compared with CT alone. SHIM et al. (2005) report correct staging of the

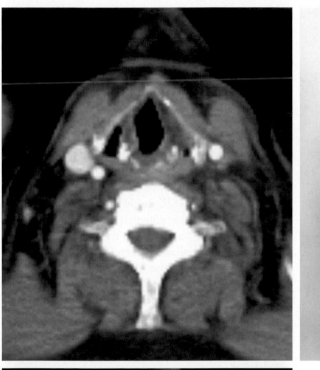

a

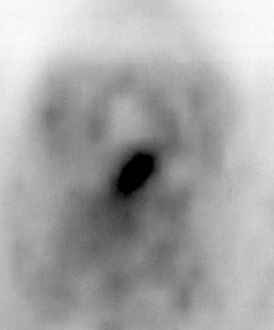

b

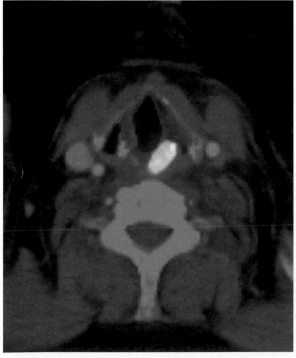

c

**Fig. 33.8a–c.** Male patient with cervical lymph node metastases (not shown) of unknown primary. Unremarkable CT without tumor detection (**a**). Focal FDG uptake on PET indicating malignant disease (**b**). By fusion of PET with CT, the primary tumor can be localized in the left dorsal larynx (**c**).

primary tumor in 86% of patients with FDG-PET–CT as compared with only 79% of patients with CT alone. The sensitivities, specificities, and accuracies for detection of nodal disease were 85, 84, and 84% with PET–CT, and 70, 69, and 69% with CT, respectively.

The *solitary pulmonary nodule* is another major indication for FDG-PET imaging. In this setting, FDG-PET is used to differentiate between a benign and a malignant lesion. In a solitary pulmonary nodule, potential FDG uptake supports the diagnosis of a malignant lesion, whereas an FDG-PET–negative lesion may be followed-up (REINHARDT et al. 2006). However, even in the case of FDG negativity, close imaging follow-up remains necessary, as there are FDG-PET–negative tumors. Lesion size is an important factor when it comes to using FDG-PET and PET–CT for assessment of pulmonary lesions. Small pulmonary lesions (<1 cm) may appear PET-negative even though they take up FDG. This is caused by breathing-induced "smearing" of FDG-uptake.

*Breast cancer* patients may be staged with FDG-PET–CT. The primary focus of the examination will be the N stage and the M stage rather than local tumor assessment. Though specific FDG-PET protocols and PET–CT protocols have been developed to evaluate the primary breast tumor (KUEHL et al. 2007), the high sensitivity of mammography and MR mammography coupled with the high soft tissue contrast of MR obviate the need to locally assess a breast lesion with PET–CT. CRIPPA et al. (1998) reported an overall sensitivity, specify, and accuracy for detection of lymph node metastases and distant metastases of 85, 91, and 89%, respectively, when assessing breast cancer patients with FDG-PET. Literature on primary staging of breast cancer with FDG-PET–CT is scarce. Theoretically, more accurate lesion localization with PET–CT should increase the staging accuracy compared with FDG-PET. TATSUMI et al. (2006) reported on a more accurate staging accuracy of FDG-PET–CT as compared with CT alone. Compared with PET, more lesions could be definitely defined as malignant or benign with PET–CT. Compared with PET alone, PET–CT may reduce the number of false-positive findings by identifying areas of mild FDG uptake in brown fat as benign (ROUSSEAU et al. 2006).

Staging of *CRC* can be performed with FDG-PET–CT. So far, FDG-PET and FDG-PET–CT have mainly been used for M staging of patients with colorectal tumors. FDG-PET has been found of higher diagnostic accuracy than CT imaging when assessing the M stage of patients with CRC. However, there are limitations of FDG-PET and FDG-PET–CT when it comes to detection of distant metastases. As described above,

small pulmonary lesions may appear FDG-PET negative due to smearing of FDG uptake. The same applies to small liver lesions. Since PET data are acquired during shallow breathing, small lesions may appear FDG-PET negative, even though they take up the radioactive tracer. In fact, MRI has been found of higher diagnostic accuracy than FDG-PET–CT for liver metastases (ANTOCH et al. 2003). By optimizing the CT component of the PET–CT, small liver lesions may be detected on CT that are negative on PET. These lesions should be followed-up to exclude distant metastases. The value of FDG-PET in assessment of locoregional lymphatic spread has been discusses controversially. While some authors report an only limited value of FDG-PET and PET–CT in the setting of N staging (SUN et al. 2008), others report the opposite (GEARHART et al. 2006). The sensitivity does, however, not seem to be high enough to obviate the need for surgical lymph node resection in FDG-PET–negative nodes after primary tumor resection. Implementation of a tumor-specific PET–CT protocol including whole-body PET–CT and PET–CT colonography has the potential to improve both, assessment of the N stage and the T stage, offering an all-in-one imaging approach (VEIT-HAIBACH et al. 2006; VEIT et al. 2006). However, there are only limited data available on this new imaging concept, and further studies are necessary to define the actual accuracy of PET–CT-colonography.

### 33.3.1.2
### PET–CT for Therapy Assessment

Assessment of tumor therapy has been challenging with morphological imaging procedures alone. Traditional morphological response criteria, such as the Response Criteria in Solid Tumors (RECIST) or criteria published by WHO rely on a reduction in tumor size as the sign for therapy response. However, tumor size reduction often requires time to develop. Functional imaging modalities have been found of benefit over morphology alone when it comes to early therapy assessment. A decrease in FDG uptake on PET typically precedes the decrease in tumor size, thus offering early characterization of a patient in responder versus nonresponder (Fig. 33.9). Many studies have been published demonstrating a benefit of FDG-PET over CT or other morphological imaging procedures when it comes to therapy assessment. The question arises whether PET–CT may be able to outperform PET alone in the setting of therapy response evaluation. When characterizing a tumor as "responding" or "nonresponding" one has to acknowledge that all lesions have already been accurately localized on

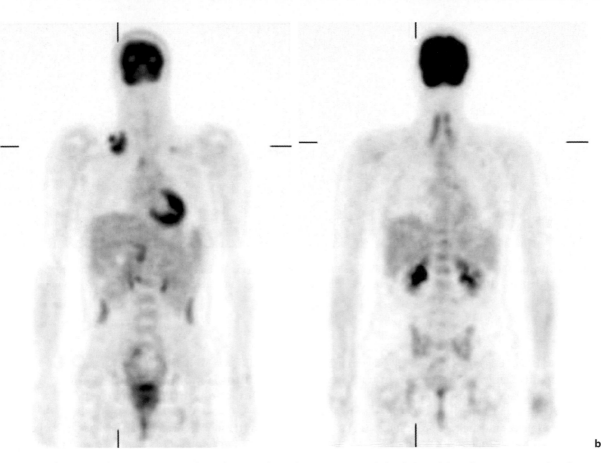

a

b

**Fig. 33.9a,b.** Manifestation of NHL in the right supraclavicular region start of the therapy (**a**). Follow-up image after three cycles of chemotherapy demonstrates complete metabolic response (**b**)

a staging examination performed before the start of the therapy. This obviates the need for just another anatomical localization in the setting of therapy assessment. The question to be answered seems rather, "Does PET-tracer uptake decrease as a sign of tumor response, or does it not?" This question can be perfectly answered with PET alone. Therefore, no advantage of PET–CT over PET alone can be expected when comparing the two imaging procedures for therapy assessment. As expected, nearly all studies on PET–CT in the setting of therapy response either found no difference between FDG-PET–CT and FDG-PET or did not even compare the two (Veit 2006; Cerfolio, et al. 2005; Pottgen et al. 2006). There is only one study that was able to document an advantage of the additional anatomical information as compared with FDG-PET alone: Sironi et al. (2004) report an advantage of FDG-PET–CT over PET alone in the setting of ovarian cancer after therapy. In this series, the advantage of the additional anatomical data results from the clinical setting. Therapy assessment was coupled with the question for potential tumor resection. If the tumor

residual was resectable, then PET–CT was able to accurately localize the tumor residual and, therefore, guide the surgeon to the tumor.

When discussing radiation therapy, fusion of anatomical data with function may improve the definition of the radiation target volume (Ciernik et al. 2003; van Baardwijk et al. 2006). Both an increase and a decrease in the target volume have been described with FDG-PET and FDG-PET–CT as compared with CT alone. Differentiation of viable tumor from adjacent atelectasis is a major reason for a decrease in the target volume based on FDG-PET and PET–CT (Ciernik et al. 2003). More accurate assessment of locoregional lymph nodes with functional data has an effect on the target volume, either increasing or decreasing it (Ashamalla et al. 2005). In the case of radiotherapy with a curative intent, the dose to nontumor tissue has been the dose-limiting factor. In patients with NSCLC, the use of FDG-PET–CT can effectively reduce the radiation exposure of nontumor tissue, allowing a radiation dose escalation (De Ruysscher et al. 2005; van der

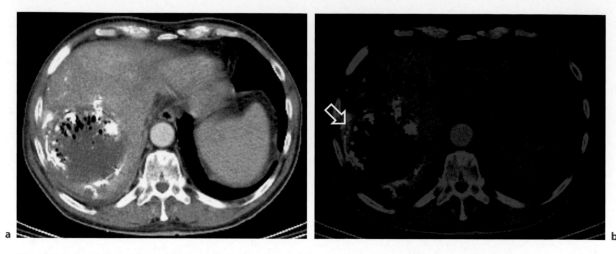

**Fig. 33.10a,b.** Male patient with hepatocellular carcinoma following chemo-embolization. CT (**a**) did not detect any residual disease. FDG-PET–CT (**b**) revealed a small area of residual tumor (*arrow*) in the lateral aspect of the embolized tumor

WEL et al. 2005). Further studies will have to assess if more accurate target volume definition translates into improved patient prognosis.

FDG-PET and FDG-PET–CT can be of benefit in interventional radiological procedures (Fig. 33.10). Compared with CT alone, PET and PET–CT have been found of higher accuracy when assessing the liver for residual disease after radiofrequency ablation (RFA) of liver metastases (BARKER et al. 2005). However, a substantial number of false-negative cases caused by very small tumor residuals must be kept in mind. These small tumor residuals, not visible on CT or PET, lead to early tumor recurrence and require a close follow-up of patients (VEIT et al. 2006). Other authors report promising results when following-up patients with liver metastases undergoing therapy with application of $^{90}$Y microspheres (LEWANDOWSKI et al. 2005).

If FDG-PET and FDG-PET–CT are used for therapy assessment, then false-positive findings due to therapy-induced tissue regeneration and inflammatory reaction may occur. Regenerating tissue and inflammatory changes go along with an increase in glucose metabolism, and this increased FDG uptake may be difficult to differentiate from viable tumor. This problem applies specifically to radiation therapy and interventional radiological procedures. The right time to perform FDG-PET after tumor therapy has been discussed controversially. While early PET–CT after interventional radiological procedures (day 1 after the intervention) seems to be of benefit (VOGT et al. 2007), a 4- to 8-week interval is currently recommended between the end of radiation therapy and the PET–CT scan.

### 33.3.1.3
### PET–CT for Tumor Follow-Up and Detection of Tumor Recurrence

In many tumors, recurrence can be detected earlier with functional imaging data as compared with morphology. In addition, differentiation of residual and/or recurrent disease from nonviable tissue after therapy may be more easily accomplished with PET imaging. PET–CT offers the advantage of accurate anatomical localization of a recurrent tumor site, which aids therapy planning if surgery, interventional therapy, or radiation therapy is an option. STRUNK et al. (2005) report a higher accuracy of fused FDG-PET–CT in the setting of following-up CRC as compared with PET alone and CT viewed side by side with PET. COHADE et al. (2003) report an increase in the accuracy of staging/restaging from 78% for FDG-PET alone to 89% for FDG-PET–CT. This increase in accuracy results from more accurate lesion localization and from better differentiation of a lesion from the urinary bladder. HAUG et al. (2007) report a significant improvement of the number of detected breast cancer metastases in patients with rising tumor markers, if assessed with FDG-PET–CT as compared with CT alone and to PET alone. Anatomical correlation of focal tracer uptake improves differentiation of a hot spot into malignant or benign: while focally increased tracer uptake within a lymph node or the bone suggests metastatic disease, tracer uptake in the esophagus may be caused by therapy-induced esophagitis.

However, in tumors that are treated with further systemic therapy rather than surgery, interventional procedures, or radiation therapy accurate characterization of the site of a lesion may not be of clinical relevance. FREUDENBERG et al. (2004). In their study on lymphoma report a patient-based sensitivity of 78% for CT alone, 86% for FDG-PET alone, 93% for CT and FDG-PET read side by side, and 93% for combined FDG-PET–CT. FDG-PET–CT imaging was found to be superior to CT alone, with additional benefit over FDG-PET only in patients planned for local tumor therapy.

# References

Antoch G, Freudenberg, LS et al. (2002) Focal tracer uptake: a potential artifact in contrast-enhanced dual-modality PET–CT scans. J Nucl Med 43:1339–1342

Antoch G, Stattaus J et al. (2003) Non-small cell lung cancer: dual-modality PET–CT in preoperative staging. Radiology 229:526–533

Antoch G, Vogt FM et al. (2003) Whole-body dual-modality PET–CT and whole-body MRI for tumor staging in oncology. JAMA 290:3199–3206

Antoch G, Freudenberg, LS et al. (2004) To enhance or not to enhance? $^{18}$F-FDG and CT contrast agents in dual-modality $^{18}$F-FDG PET–CT. J Nucl Med 45(Suppl):56S–65S

Antoch G, Kuehl H et al. (2004) Dual-modality PET–CT scanning with negative oral contrast agent to avoid artifacts: introduction and evaluation. Radiology 230:879–885

Antoch G, Saoudi N et al. (2004) Accuracy of whole-body dual-modality fluorine-18-2-fluoro-2-deoxy-D-glucose positron emission tomography and computed tomography (FDG-PET-CT) for tumor staging in solid tumors: comparison with CT and PET. J Clin Oncol 22:4357–4368

Ashamalla H, Rafla S et al. (2005) The contribution of integrated PET–CT to the evolving definition of treatment volumes in radiation treatment planning in lung cancer. Int J Radiat Oncol Biol Phys 63:1016–1023

Baardwijk, A. van, B. G. Baumert et al. (2006) The current status of FDG-PET in tumour volume definition in radiotherapy treatment planning. Cancer Treat Rev 32:245–260

Bar-Shalom R, Yefremov N et al. (2003) Clinical performance of PET–CT in evaluation of cancer: additional value for diagnostic imaging and patient management. J Nucl Med 44:1200–1209

Barker DW, Zagoria RJ et al. (2005) Evaluation of liver metastases after radiofrequency ablation: utility of $^{18}$F-FDG PET and PET–CT. AJR Am J Roentgenol 184:1096–1102

Beyer T, Antoch G et al. (2003) Dual-modality PET–CT imaging: the effect of respiratory motion on combined image quality in clinical oncology. Eur J Nucl Med Mol Imaging 30:588–596

Beyer T, Townsend DW et al. (2000) A combined PET–CT scanner for clinical oncology. J Nucl Med 41:1369–1379

Bohuslavizki KH, Klutmann S et al. (2000) Correlation of $^{18}$F FDG-PET and histological findings in patients with malignant melanoma. J Nucl Med 41:302P

Brix G, Lechel U et al. (2005) Radiation exposure of patients undergoing whole-body dual-modality $^{18}$F-FDG PET–CT examinations. J Nucl Med 46:608–613

Brucerius J, Herkel C et al. (2006) $^{18}$F-FDG PET and conventional imaging for assessment of Hodgkin's disease and non-Hodgkin's lymphoma. An analysis of 193 patient studies. Nuklearmedizin 45:105–110

Cerfolio RS, Bryant AS et al. (2005) The accuracy of endoscopic ultrasonography with fine-needle aspiration, integrated positron emission tomography with computed tomography, and computed tomography in restaging patients with esophageal cancer after neoadjuvant chemoradiotherapy. J Thorac Cardiovasc Surg 129:1232–1241

Cerny T, Gillessen S (2002) Advances in the treatment of non-Hodgkin's lymphoma. Ann Oncol 13:211–216

Ciernik IF, Dizendorf E et al. (2003) Radiation treatment planning with an integrated positron emission and computer tomography (PET–CT): a feasibility study. Int J Radiat Oncol Biol Phys 57:853–863

Cohade C, Osman M et al. (2003) Direct comparison of F-FDG PET and PET–CT in patients with colorectal carcinoma. J Nucl Med 44:1797–1803

Crippa F, Agresti R et al. (1998) Prospective evaluation of fluorine-18-FDG PET in presurgical staging of the axilla in breast cancer. J Nucl Med 39:4–8

De Ruysscher D, Wanders S et al. (2005) Effects of radiotherapy planning with a dedicated combined PET-CT-simulator of patients with non-small cell lung cancer on dose limiting normal tissues and radiation dose-escalation: a planning study. Radiother Oncol 77:5–10

Diederichs CG, Staib L et al. (2000) Values and limitations of $^{18}$F-fluorodeoxyglucose-positron-emission tomography with preoperative evaluation of patients with pancreatic masses. Pancreas 20:109–116

Dizendorf E, Hany TF et al. (2003) Cause and magnitude of the error induced by oral CT contrast agent in CT-based attenuation correction of PET emission studies. J Nucl Med 44:732–738

Farsad M, Schiavina R et al. (2005) Detection and localization of prostate cancer: correlation of C-choline PET–CT with histopathologic step-section analysis. J Nucl Med 46:1642–1649

Forastiere A, Koch W et al. (2001) Head and neck cancer. N Engl J Med 345:1890–1900

Freudenberg LS, Antoch G et al. (2004a) Value of $^{124}$I-PET–CT in staging of patients with differentiated thyroid cancer. Eur Radiol 14:2092–2098

Freundenberg LS, Antoch G et al. (2004b) FDG-PET–CT in restaging of patients with lymphoma. Eur J Nucl Med Mol Imaging 31:325–329

Gearhart SL, Frassica D et al. (2006) Improved staging with pretreatment positron emission tomography/computed tomography in low rectal cancer. Ann Surg Oncol 13:397–404

Goerres GW, Hany TF et al. (2002) Head and neck imaging with PET and PET–CT: artefacts from dental metallic implants. Eur J Nucl Med Mol Imaging 29:367–370

Goerres GW, Kamel E et al. (2002) Accuracy of image coregistration of pulmonary lesions in patients with non-small cell lung cancer using an integrated PET–CT system. J Nucl Med 43:1469–1475

Gutzeit A, Antoch G et al. (2005) Unknown primary tumors: detection with dual-modality PET–CT—initial experience. Radiology 234:227–234

Haberkorn U, Schoenberg SO (2001) Imaging of lung cancer with CT, MRT and PET. Lung Cancer 34(Suppl):S13–S23

Halpern BS, Dahlbom M et al. (2004) Cardiac pacemakers and central venous lines can induce focal artifacts on CT-corrected PET images. J Nucl Med 45:290–293

Halpern BS, Schiepers C et al. (2005) Presurgical staging of non-small cell lung cancer: positron emission tomography, integrated positron emission tomography/CT, and software image fusion. Chest 128:2289–2297

Haug AR, Schmidt GP et al. (2007) F-18-fluoro-2-deoxyglucose positron emission tomography/computed tomography in the follow-up of breast cancer with elevated levels of tumor markers. J Comput Assist Tomogr 31:629–634

Hernandez-Maraver D, Hernandez-Navarro F et al. (2006) Positron emission tomography/computed tomography: diagnostic accuracy in lymphoma. Br J Haematol 135:293–302

Hofmann M, Maecke H et al. (2001) Biokinetics and imaging with the somatostatin receptor PET radioligand Ga-DOTA-TOC: preliminary data. Eur J Nucl Med 28:1751–1757

Hutchings M, Loft A et al. (2006) Position emission tomography with or without computed tomography in the primary staging of Hodgkin's lymphoma. Haematologica 91:482–489

Kang W, Chung J et al. (2004) Differentiation of mediastinal FDG uptake observed in patients with non-thoracic tumours. Eur J Nucl Med Mol Imaging 31:202–207

Keyes J (1995) SUV: standard uptake of silly useless value? J Nucl Med 36:1836–1839

Kuehl H, Veit P et al. (2007) Can PET–CT replace separate diagnostic CT for cancer imaging? Optimizing CT protocols for imaging cancers of the chest and abdomen. J Nucl Med 48(Suppl):45S–57S

Kutler DI, Wong RJ et al. (2006) The current status of positron-emission tomography scanning in the evaluation and follow-up of patients with head and neck cancer. Curr Opin Otolaryngol Head Neck Surg 14:73–81

Lardinois D, Weder W et al. (2003) Staging of non-small-cell lung cancer with integrated positron-emission tomography and computed tomography. N Engl J Med 348:2500–2507

Lewandowski RJ, Thurston KG et al. (2005) $^{90}$Y microsphere (TheraSphere) treatment for unresectable colorectal cancer metastases of the liver: response to treatment at targeted doses of 135–150 Gy as measured by $^{18}$F-fluorodeoxyglucose positron emission tomography and computed tomographic imaging. J Vasc Interv Radiol 16:1641–1651

Nakamoto Y, Chin BB et al. (2003) Effects of nonionic intravenous contrast agents at PET–CT imaging: phantom and canine studies. Radiology 227:817–824

Pottgen C, Levegrun S et al. (2006) Value of 18F-fluoro-2-deoxy-D-glucose-positron emission tomography/computed tomography in non-small-cell lung cancer for prediction of pathologic response and times to relapse after neoadjuvant chemoradiotherapy. Clin Cancer Res 12:97–106

Raanani P, Shasha Y et al. (2006) Is CT scan still necessary for staging in Hodgkin and non-Hodgkin lymphoma patients in the PET–CT era? Ann Oncol 17:117–122

Raber MN, Faintuch J et al. (1991) Continuous infusion 5-fluorouracil, etoposide and cis-diamminedichloroplatinum in patients with metastatic carcinoma of unknown primary origin. Ann Oncol 2:519–520

Rasmussen I, Sorensen J et al. (2004) Is positron emission tomography using $^{18}$F-fluorodeoxyglucose and $^{11}$C-acetate valuable in diagnosing indeterminate pancreatic masses? Scand J Surg 93:191–197

Reinhardt MJ, Wiethoelter N et al. (2006) PET recognition of pulmonary metastases on PET–CT imaging: impact of attenuation-corrected and non-attenuation-corrected PET images. Eur J Nucl Med Mol Imaging 33:134–139

Reske SN, Kotzerke J (2001) FDG PET for clinical use: results of the 3rd German Interdisciplinary Consensus Conference, Onko-PET III. Eur J Nucl Med. 28:1707–1723

Rousseau C, Bourbouloux E et al. (2006) Brown fat in breast cancer patients: analysis of serial F-FDG PET/CT scans. Eur J Nucl Med Mol Imaging 33:785–791

Shim SS, Lee KS et al. (2005) Non-small cell lung cancer: prospective comparison of integrated FDG PET–CT and CT alone for preoperative staging. Radiology 236:1011–1019

Sironi S, Messa C et al. (2004) Integrated FDG PET–CT in patients with persistent ovarian cancer: correlation with histologic findings. Radiology 233:433–440

Smythe WR (2001) Treatment of stage I and II non-small-cell lung cancer. Cancer Control 8:318–325

Strunk H, Bucerius J et al. (2005) Combined FDG PET–CT imaging for restaging of colorectal cancer patients: impact of image fusion on staging accuracy. Rofo 177:1235–1241

Sun L, Wu N et al. (2008) Colonography by CT, MRI and PET–CT combined with conventional colonoscopy in colorectal cancer screening and staging. World J Gastroenterol. 14:853–863

Tatsumi M, Cohade C et al. (2005) Direct comparison of FDG PET and CT findings in patients with lymphoma: initial experience. Radiology 237:1038–1045

Tatsumi M, Cohade C et al. (2006) Initial experience with FDG-PET–CT in the evaluation of breast cancer. Eur J Nucl Med Mol Imaging 33:254–262

Toloza EM, Harpole L et al. (2003) Noninvasive staging of non-small cell lung cancer: a review of the current evidence. Chest 123(Suppl): 137S–146S

Townsend DW (2001) A combined PET–CT scanner: the choices. J Nucl Med 42:533–534

Veit P, Antoch G et al. (2006) Detection of residual tumor after radiofrequency ablation of liver metastasis with dual-modality PET–CT: initial results. Eur Radiol 16:80–87

Veit P, Kuhle C et al. (2006) Whole body positron emission tomography/computed tomography (PET–CT) tumour staging with integrated PET–CT colonography: technical feasibility and first experiences in patients with colorectal cancer. Gut 55:68–73

Veit-Haibach P, Kuehle CAet al. (2006) Diagnostic accuracy of colorectal cancer staging with whole-body PET–CT colonography. JAMA 296:2590–2600

Veit-Haibach P, Luzcak C et al. (2007) TNM staging with FDG-PET–CT in patients with primary head and neck cancer. Eur J Nucl Med Mol Imaging 34:1953–1962

Vogt FM, Antoch G et al. (2007) Morphologic and functional changes in nontumorous liver tissue after radiofrequency ablation in an in vivo model: comparison of $^{18}$F-FDG PET–CT, MRI, ultrasound, and CT. J Nucl Med 48:1836–1844

Weber WA, Avril N et al. (1999) Relevance of positron emission tomography (PET) in oncology. Strahlenther Onkol 175:356–373

Wel van der A, Nijsten S et al. (2005) Increased therapeutic ratio by $^{18}$FDG-PET CT planning in patients with clinical CT stage N2-N3M0 non-small-cell lung cancer: a modeling study. Int J Radiat Oncol Biol Phys 61:649–655

# PET and PET–CT in Neuroendocrine Tumors

**34**

Gabriele Pöpperl

**ABSTRACT**

Several molecular features of neuroendocrine tumors (NET), like their ability to metabolize glucose ($^{18}$F-FDG), to express somatostatin receptors ($^{68}$Ga-labeled somatostatin analogs) or to decarboxylate amine precursors ($^{18}$F-DOPA or $^{11}$C-HTP) can be addressed by specific PET probes. The lack of anatomic information when using such highly specific PET tracers requires exact morphologic correlation, which now is offered by hybrid PET–CT scanners. The broad histopathologic variety of NET demands an individual diagnostic workup tailored to the patient's pathology. While $^{18}$F-FDG should be preserved for less differentiated tumors, amine precursors and somatostatin analogs will be implemented in the diagnostic process of well-differentiated NET, with the latter being extremely useful to select patients for peptide-receptor radionuclide therapy. This chapter offers a comprehensive overview on literature data for PET imaging of NET, using these different radiopharmaceuticals.

G. Pöpperl MD, PD
Department of Nuclear Medicine, Ludwig-Maximilians-University of Munich, Munich University Hospitals, Marchioninistrasse 15, 81377 Munich, Germany

## 34.1
## Introduction

NET constitute a heterogeneous group of neoplasms originating from tissues derived from the embryonic neural crest, neuroectoderm, and endoderm. In consequence, they may occur at various organ sites. Preferred locations, however, are the pancreas and gastrointestinal tract, followed by the lungs. Other locations like the skin, adrenal glands, thyroid, or urogenital tract are rare (Jensen 2000). The incidence of NET is generally considered low; however, since many of them do not cause any symptoms, it might be expected that some of the patients are not diagnosed during their lifetimes, and that the true incidence of NET may be somewhat higher. Traditionally, NET have been divided according to their location into foregut, midgut, and hindgut tumors. The most recent WHO guidelines now classify NET into well-differentiated neuroendocrine tumors, well-differentiated neuroendocrine carcinomas, and poorly differentiated neuroendocrine carcinomas, regardless of their origin (KLOPPEL et al. 2004). The distinction between these three groups relies on clinical and pathological data such as biological behavior, presence of metastases, presence of hormonal symptoms, histological differentiation, proliferation index (Ki-67 index), tumor size, and invasion of the muscularis propria or adjacent organs. The clinical behavior of NET varies widely, ranging from benign and low-grade, to high-grade malignancy and can be partly predicted on the basis of clinicopathological criteria. The majority of the NET have low growth rates, with survival times longer than other gastrointestinal malignancies; some NET, however, are highly aggressive and very malignant. Tumor growth in patients even with metastasized NET, also is not uniform; they can exhibit long periods of spontaneous tumor standstill or reveal exploding growth. The overall 5-year-survival rate for NET is about 67%. NET may be also classified according to the presence or absence of clinical symptoms. The most common symptoms of functional active tumors are diarrhea, flushing, abdominal pain, or hormone-specific symptoms which, in general, lead to an earlier diagnosis compared with nonfunctioning tumors, which are most often detected not until a late-metastasized stage of disease because of the mass effect of the tumor.

Besides clinical features and biochemical tumor markers such as chromogranin A, neuron-specific enolase, serotonin, or other specific tumor markers like, e.g., gastrin, diagnosis of NET is based on imaging modalities. CT is the most widely used imaging tool for localization and staging of NET. MDCT has markedly improved image quality by providing rapid scan times (reducing movement artifacts), accurate contrast medium bolus tracking (ensuring optimal timing of biphasic scans), and the ability to reformat the images in thin slices (multiple anatomical planes). MRI is useful especially in cervical manifestations, intracranial or spinal lesions, liver metastases and for the detection of bone marrow involvement. However, based on morphological methods alone, diagnosis and staging of NET and their metastases may be difficult, since the lesions frequently are small and located at variable anatomical locations. Therefore, functional imaging modalities

that provide the possibility of whole-body scans in a single study have great impact on patient management by optimizing the staging of the disease, visualization of small occult tumors, and evaluation of eligibility for somatostatin analog treatment.

NET cells are characterized by their ability to take up and concentrate amine precursors such as dihydroxy-phenylalanine (DOPA) and hydroxytryptophane (HTP) and to produce amines and peptides, for which reason they were also classified as amine precursor uptake and decarboxylation (APUD) cells. They may also express different peptide hormone receptors (like somatostatin receptors) or transporters at their cell membrane. These uptake mechanisms and the presence of peptide receptors and transporters constitute the basis for the use of specific radiolabeled ligands for imaging of neuroendocrine tumors.

Radionuclide imaging based on planar scintigraphy and single-photon emission tomography (SPECT) has been widely used for the diagnosis of NET. However, during the last years, PET using $^{18}$F-FDG has evolved as powerful method in oncology. The recent introduction of hybrid systems, providing a PET and CT scanner in the same device, and the development of more specific radiopharmaceuticals like radiolabeled amine precursors or somatostatin analogs, led to several advantages in the diagnosis of NET.

This chapter provides an overview on the different radiopharmaceuticals that are used for PET and imaging of NET.

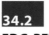

## 34.2
## FDG-PET

FDG is the most commonly used radiopharmaceutical for PET imaging. It is taken up via a glucose transporter, phosphorylated, and trapped in the cell according to its metabolic rate. Many malignant tumors show increased FDG uptake compared with normal tissue. Therefore, FDG-PET is used for the differentiation of malignant from benign lesions, for the detection of unknown primaries in case of unclear metastases, for tumor staging and restaging, for diagnosis of tumor recurrence, and for monitoring treatment response. Many studies in different tumor types have been performed, presenting with high overall sensitivities and specificities, resulting in a modification of therapeutic management based on PET results in about one third of patients.

The diagnostic value of FDG-PET for imaging NET, however, is limited and depends on the grade of differentiation, proliferation activity, and aggressiveness of the tumors (ADAMS et al. 1998b). Well-differentiated and slow-growing tumors, which compose the majority of NET, show no or only minor FDG uptake. Positive FDG uptake of gastroenteropancreatic tumors correlated with the proliferation index (Ki-67) and was seen only in less well-differentiated tumors with high proliferative activity (ADAMS 1998a; BELHOCINE et al. 2002) and also in metastasizing medullary thyroid cancer (MTC) associated with rapidly increasing CEA levels (ADAMS 1998a). For MTC patients with postoperatively elevated tumor marker levels, FDG-PET was more sensitive and superior in localizing lymph node involvement than were the other imaging modalities (CT, MRI, and metaiodobenzylguanidine [MIBG] scintigraphy), especially in the cervical, supraclavicular, and mediastinal lymphatic regions (SZAKALL, JR., et al. 2002). In a multicenter retrospective study including a relatively large number of 85 MTC patients comparing FDG-PET to conventional radiological methods

(CT, MRI) and nuclear medicine modalities, FDG-PET also showed the highest lesion detection probability for MTC tissue, with a sensitivity of 78% and specificity of 79% (DIEHL et al. 2001). In other studies, a heterogeneity of tracer uptake in various lesions of NET with multiple tumor sites was described (PASQUALI 1998) as was the so-called "flip-flop phenomenon" showing high FDG uptake in somatostatin receptor negative parts of the tumor and vice versa, suggesting that FDG and somatostatin analogs show different degrees of differentiation in the heterogeneous NET. Figure 34.1a shows a representative example of a patient with less well-differentiated liver metastases of a neuroendocrine carcinoma of the pancreas (primary resected) and Fig. 34.1b of a patient with a well-differentiated metastasized NET, showing positive uptake of metastases with the specific tracers but no positive FDG uptake.

A study on FDG-PET in the subgroup of pheochromocytomas showed that many pheochromocytomas

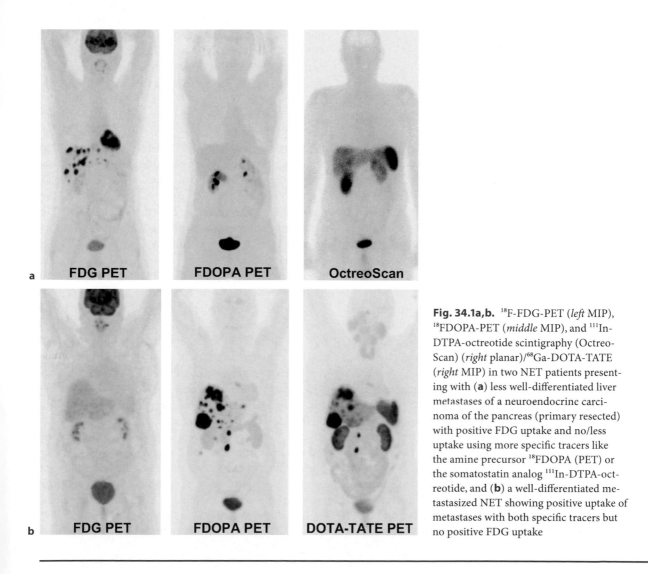

a    **FDG PET**    **FDOPA PET**    **OctreoScan**

b    **FDG PET**    **FDOPA PET**    **DOTA-TATE PET**

**Fig. 34.1a,b.** [18]F-FDG-PET (*left* MIP), [18]FDOPA-PET (*middle* MIP), and [111]In-DTPA-octreotide scintigraphy (Octreo-Scan) (*right* planar)/[68]Ga-DOTA-TATE (*right* MIP) in two NET patients presenting with (**a**) less well-differentiated liver metastases of a neuroendocrine carcinoma of the pancreas (primary resected) with positive FDG uptake and no/less uptake using more specific tracers like the amine precursor [18]FDOPA (PET) or the somatostatin analog [111]In-DTPA-octreotide, and (**b**) a well-differentiated metastasized NET showing positive uptake of metastases with both specific tracers but no positive FDG uptake

accumulate FDG. Uptake, however, was also found in a greater percentage in malignant than in benign pheochromocytomas, and FDG-PET seemed to be especially useful in detecting those pheochromocytomas that fail to concentrate radioiodinated MIBG. The latter is a norepinephrine analog that is highly sensitive for catecholamine-secreting tumors (SHULKIN et al. 1999) and that can be used for gamma camera imaging (planar scintigraphy and SPECT, labeled with iodine-123) as well as for radionuclide therapy (labeled with iodine-131).

In general, therefore, it is suggested to use FDG-PET only in patients with fast-growing NET and (if applicable) high proliferation rate, who show negative findings in more specific investigations such as somatostatin-receptor scintigraphy (SRS) or MIBG scintigraphy. Furthermore, it seems to be useful in staging and follow-up of MCT patients and in malignant pheochromocytomas.

## 34.3
## PET Using Amine Precursors

Based on the concept of APUD, the $^{11}$C- and $^{18}$F-labeled amine precursors L-DOPA and 5-HTP have been utilized for imaging of NET.

One of the first studies was performed in 1993, using 5-HTP in seven patients with histopathologically verified neuroendocrine tumors and liver metastases, indicating that 5-HTP can be used to visualize serotonin-producing neuroendocrine tumors, and that it seems to be of value to monitor the effects of treatment, possibly also as an early predictive test of the outcome of treatment (ERIKSSON et al. 1993). These findings were confirmed in a larger group of patients presenting with high 5-HTP uptake in neuroendocrine gastrointestinal tumors, allowing improved visualization compared with CT. Furthermore, linear regression analyses showed a clear correlation ($r = 0.907$) between changes in urinary 5-hydroxyindole acetic acid and changes in the transport rate constant for 5-HTP during medical treatment (ORLEFORS et al. 1998). Another study from the same group evaluating $^{11}$C-labeled L-DOPA and 5-HTP in the diagnosis of pancreatic endocrine tumors somewhat restricted the indication for these tracers, since they showed that these techniques can be a valuable complement to CT in demonstration of functional pancreatic endocrine tumors, in particular, glucagonomas, but are less useful in detection of nonfunctional tumors (AHLSTROM et al. 1995). Results of L-DOPA and 5-HTP correlated well, even though 5-HTP showed

a somewhat-higher uptake in some patients. In a study more recent, 5-HTP-PET was performed in a serious of 42 NET patients, showing that PET is sensitive, especially in imaging small lesions, such as primary tumors, and in the majority of patients was able to detect more tumor lesions compared with conventional SRS and CT (ORLEFORS et al. 2005). The same group examined the effect of pretreatment with carbidopa, a peripheral inhibitor of aromatic amino acid decarboxylase (AADC), which converts 5-HTP to serotonin (5-hydroxytryptamine [5-HT]), and showed that premedication significantly improves 5-HTP-PET image quality by decreasing the renal excretion and increasing the tumor uptake and, therefore, facilitates detection of NET lesions (ORLEFORS et al. 2006).

Even more data are available on the amine precursor L-DOPA. Both, $^{11}$C-labeled and $^{18}$F-labeled L-DOPA have been used in a number of studies imaging NET. As already mentioned, $^{11}$C-L-DOPA allowed visualization of 50% of tumors in the first clinical study, but failed to detect nonfunctioning tumors or very small insulinomas. HOEGERLE et al. (2001) compared $^{18}$F-L-DOPA with FDG-PET, conventional SRS, and morphological methods in 17 patients with gastrointestinal carcinoid tumors. Overall sensitivities were 65% for FDOPA-PET, only 29% for FDG-PET, 57% for conventional SRS, and 73% for the morphologic imaging modalities. Although the morphologic procedures were most sensitive for organ metastases, FDOPA-PET enabled best localization of primary tumors and lymph node staging. In another study in 23 patients with advanced NET, FDOPA-PET was also superior to SRS and even performed better than did CT in bone lesions (BECHERER et al. 2004). In a more recent prospective study, FDOPA-PET with carbidopa pretreatment was compared with SRS, CT, and combined SRS and CT in 53 patients with a metastatic carcinoid tumor. In this study, FDOPA-PET detected more lesions, regions more positive, and more lesions per region than combined SRS and CT. In region-based analysis, sensitivity of FDOPA-PET was 95% versus 66% for SRS, 57% for CT, and 79% for combined SRS and CT. The authors state that, if these results will be confirmed by other studies, FDOPA-PET could replace SRS (KOOPMANS et al. 2006). However, all these studies compare FDOPA-PET with conventional SRS, not with PET using $^{68}$Ga-labeled somatostatin analogs. Comparative PET studies using amine precursors in comparison to somatostatin analogs have to be awaited. Further, MONTRAVERS et al. (2006) point out the importance of precise histological characterization of NET to optimize imaging strategy. In a sample of 30 patients, they demonstrated that sensitivity and accuracy of FDOPA-PET was only high in well-differentiated carcinoid tumors

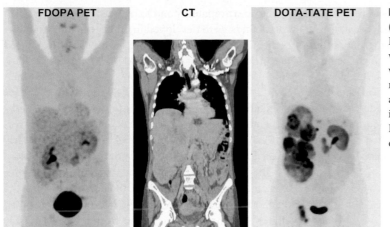

**Fig. 34.2.** [18]FDOPA-PET (*left* MIP), CT (*middle* selected coronal slice), and [68]Ga-DOTA-TATE PET (*right* MIP) of a patient with liver and lymph node metastases of a well-differentiated NET with negative immunohistochemical detection of serotonin and normal serum serotonin levels, showing no increased uptake of metastases on FDOPA-PET but highly increased uptake on DOTA-TATE-PET

with positive immunohistochemical detection of serotonin, while FDOPA-PET showed a very low sensitivity of only 25% in noncarcinoid tumors without immunohistochemical detection of serotonin. Interestingly, sensitivity of conventional SRS did not differ between both groups. FDOPA-PET, therefore, was proposed to be useful only in secretory carcinoid tumors. A representative example is shown in Fig. 34.2.

Furthermore, FDOPA-PET seems to have a promising role in patients with gastroenteropancreatic NET, with negative or inconclusive findings at conventional morphological or conventional SRS (AMBROSINI et al. 2007), where it could help to detect the primary tumor or other unsuspected lesions in the majority of patients.

In addition, various subentities of NET were investigated separately using FDOPA. FDOPA-PET, for example showed 100% sensitivity and specificity for detection of pheochromocytomas in a small group of 14 patients (HOEGERLE et al. 2002) and seemed to be also highly sensitive for the detection of glomus tumors (HOEGERLE et al. 2003). Therefore, this method was

supposed to have potential as a screening method for glomus tumors in patients with proven mutations of the succinate dehydrogenase subunit D gene, causing predisposition of the development of glomus tumors and other paragangliomas. Carbidopa pretreatment was shown to enhance the sensitivity for adrenal pheochromocytomas and extra-adrenal abdominal paragangliomas by increasing the tumor-to-background ratio of tracer uptake (TIMMERS et al. 2007). The sensitivity of FDOPA-PET for metastases of paraganglioma, however, appeared to be limited (TIMMERS et al. 2007). In medullary thyroid carcinoma, FDOPA-PET was also reported to be a useful supplement to morphological diagnostic imaging, which showed the highest overall sensitivity. PET, however, improved lymph node staging and enabled a more specific diagnosis of primary tumor and local recurrence (HOEGERLE et al. 2001). A representative result for the improved diagnosis of recurrence in a patient following thyroidectomy for MTC and presenting with elevated calcitonin levels is shown in Fig. 34.3.

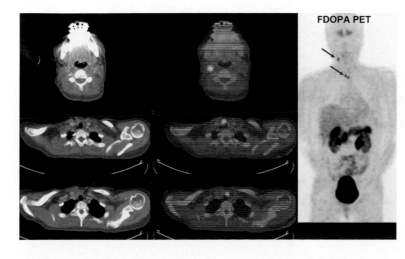

**Fig. 34.3.** [18]FDOPA images (CT on the *left*, fused images in the *middle*, and whole-body PET [MIP] on the *right*) of a patient after thyroidectomy for medullary thyroid carcinoma (6 years ago), actually presenting with elevated calcitonin levels. PET shows pathologically increased uptake in a normal sized cervical lymph node (*upper row*) and in two lesions within the thyroid bed. Surgery confirmed local recurrence of MTC and lymph node metastasis in this patient. Calcitonin levels normalized following surgery

Promising results for FDOPA-PET were also obtained in patients with insulinoma and negative CT, MRI, and ultrasound results. For this subgroup, somatostatin receptor imaging is less useful, since insulinomas express the latter only in about 50%. Preoperative FDOPA imaging seemed to be a method of choice for the detection of beta-cell hyperplasia in adults and was recommended for the detection of insulinoma or beta-cell hyperplasia in patients with confirmed hyperinsulinemic hypoglycemias when other diagnostic workup is negative (KAUHANEN et al. 2007).

## 34.4
### PET Using Somatostatin Analogs

For about the last 15 years SRS has been a well-established technique for functional imaging of NET. To date, five human somatostatin receptor subtypes (hsst1–hsst5) are known, showing differences in their expression on NET and their affinity for somatostatin analogs. Most of NET express hsst2, which is mainly addressed by the diagnostically used somatostatin analogs so far.

The first and most common used somatostatin analog for functional imaging using planar gamma camera scintigraphy and SPECT was [111]In-DTPA-octreotide, which is commercially available (OctreoScan®). Results have shown high sensitivities and specificities for the detection of primary and metastasizing NET (KWEKKEBOOM and KRENNING 2002). In a recent study in 63 patients with histological diagnosis of NET, SRS accuracy was 95% for well-differentiated neuroendocrine tumors, 86% for well-differentiated neuroendocrine carcinomas, and 60% for poorly differentiated neuroendocrine carcinomas (CIMITAN et al. 2003). To enhance image quality and availability and to reduce costs, [99mTc]-labeled compounds were developed in 2000, which have shown higher image quality compared with the [111]In-labeled ones (DECRISTOFORO et al. 2000, GABRIEL et al. 2003, 2005). However, the spatial resolution of SRS, even when SPECT is performed, is comparably low (1.5–2 cm for [111]In and 1–1.5 cm for [99mTc]), and quantification is difficult and not routinely performed. The better spatial resolution (about 0.5 cm) and ease of quantification clearly favors PET compared with conventional scintigraphy.

The possibility to label somatostatin analogs with [68]Ga, therefore, revolutionized the role of PET in the diagnostic workup of NET. [68]Ga is a metallic positron emitter, which can be produced from a [68]Ge/[68]Ga generator and may become easily available in the nuclear medicine department independent of an onsite cyclotron. [68]Ga has a physical half-life of 68 min, which is compatible with the pharmacokinetics of most radiopharmaceuticals of low molecular weight such as antibody fragments, peptides, aptamers, or oligonucleotides. Another step forward was the development of somatostatin analogs with higher affinities to the hsst2 or with improved affinity also for the other hsst subtypes, especially hsst 3 and 5. Table 34.1 summarizes the affinity profiles ($IC_{50}$) of the three most commonly used [68]Ga-labeled DOTA-octapeptides for hsst 1–5. Furthermore, attempts have been made, to use [18]F for labeling of somatostatin analogs (MEISETSCHLÄGER et al. 2006).

First clinical results using [68]Ga-DOTA-TOC-PET in eight patients with histologically confirmed carcinoid tumors PET resulted in high tumor-to-nontumor contrast and identified 100% of 40 lesions predefined by CT and/or MRI and detected >30% additional lesions, whereas conventional [111]In-octreotide planar and SPECT imaging identified only 85% (HOFMANN et al.

**Table 34.1** Affinity profiles of the most frequently used DOTA-octapeptides for PET imaging given for the human somatostatin receptor subtypes hsst 1–5

| Peptide | hsst subtype | | | | |
|---|---|---|---|---|---|
| | hsst1[a] | hsst2[a] | hsst3[a] | hsst4[a] | hsst5[a] |
| [68]Ga-DOTA-TOC | >10,000 | 2.5 ± 0.5 | 613 ± 140 | > 1,000 | 7321 |
| [68]Ga-DOTA-NOC | >10,000 | 1.9 ± 0.4 | 40.0 ± 5.8 | 260 ± 74 | 7.2 ± 1.6 |
| [68]Ga-DOTA-TATE | >10,000 | 0.20 ± 0.04 | > 1,000 | 300 ± 140 | 377 ± 18 |

Adapted from ANTUNES et al. 2007

[a]$IC_{50}$ values given in nmol l$^{-1}$ (mean±SEM)

2001). In another small patient group, PET seemed to be superior, especially in detecting small tumors or tumors bearing only a low density of somatostatin receptors (KOWALSKI et al. 2003). In a very recent prospective study by Gabriel et al. [68]Ga-DOTA-TOC-PET was compared with conventional scintigraphy and dedicated MDCT in 84 patients (GABRIEL et al. 2007). PET (true positive [TP] in 69 patients, true negative [TN] in 12 patients, false positive [FP] in 1 patient, and false negative [FN] in 2 patients) resulted in a sensitivity of 97%, a specificity of 92%, and an accuracy of 96%. PET showed higher diagnostic efficacy compared with SPECT (TP in 37 patients, TN in 12 patients, FP in 1 patient, and FN in 34 patients) and diagnostic CT (TP in 41 patients, TN in 12 patients, FP in 5 patients, and FN in 26 patients). This difference was statistically significant ($P < 0.001$). However, the combined use of PET and CT showed the highest overall accuracy. Most clinical applications have used DOTA-TOC so far. Comparative data on [68]Ga-DOTA-TATE-PET, which shows a higher affinity to hsst2 (ANTUNES et al. 2007) and, therefore, would expect to show a higher uptake in hsst2-positive NET compared with [68]Ga-DOTA-TOC, are still lacking. Clinical data are very limited and only available for a very small sample size of neuroectodermal tumors like paraganglioma or pheochromocytoma (WIN et al. 2007), showing a positive uptake in four of five tumors. A representative example of a [68]Ga-DOTA-TATE examination in a patient with a small well-differentiated NET of the pancreas is given in Fig. 34.4.

Another somatostatin analog, DOTA-NOC, with higher affinity to the receptor subtypes 3 and 5 was recently presented (WILD et al. 2005). An intra-individual comparison of [68]Ga-DOTA-NOC and [68]Ga-DOTA-TATE in a patient with metastases of a neuroendocrine pancreatic carcinoma demonstrated that the broader somatostatin receptor subtype profile of DOTA-NOC may be of clinical relevance as a significantly higher uptake of this radiopeptide was found, compared with the high-affinity but hsst2-selective radiopeptide DOTA-TATE. In addition, very small lesions were detected when using DOTA-NOC as compared with DOTA-TATE (ANTUNES et al. 2007).

In a recent study of MEISETSCHLÄGER et al. (2006), one of the first [18]F-labeled PET tracers Gluc-Lys([18]F-FP)-TOCA for somatostatin receptor imaging was evaluated in patients with hsst-positive tumors and compared with the conventional SRS using [111]In-DTPA-octreotide. The biokinetics and diagnostic performance of the new tracer were superior to [111]In-DTPA-octreotide and—as far as can be derived from the literature—seemed to be comparable with [68]Ga-DOTA-TOC. In a recent prospective study, Gluc-Lys([18]F-FP)-TOCA, CT and the image fusion of PET and CT (PET–CT) were assessed in the detection of metastases from gastrointestinal neuroendocrine tumors. In 31 patients PET, venous-dominant (VD) contrast-enhanced CT, and PET-CT showed a lesion-by-lesion–based overall detection rate for liver metastases ($n = 858$) of 90.8% ($P < 0.001$), 73.9% ($P < 0.001$), and 100%. PET, VD CT, and PET-CT showed an overall detection rate for lymph node metastases ($n = 193$) of 93.8% ($P < 0.001$), 64.8% ($P < 0.001$), and 100%, and for osseous metastases ($n = 567$) of 98.6% ($P < 0.005$), 40.7% ($P < 0.001$), and 100%. PET as single modality revealed most liver, lymph node, and osseous metastases. The combination of molecular/

**DOTA-TATE PET**

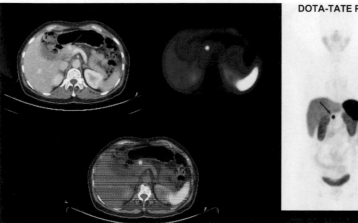
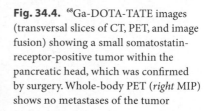

**Fig. 34.4.** [68]Ga-DOTA-TATE images (transversal slices of CT, PET, and image fusion) showing a small somatostatin-receptor-positive tumor within the pancreatic head, which was confirmed by surgery. Whole-body PET (*right* MIP) shows no metastases of the tumor

metabolic with anatomical/morphological information improves the diagnostic accuracy for the detection of metastases in comparison to any single imaging modality (SEEMANN 2007).

Beside the diagnostic impact of in vivo somatostatin-receptor imaging for tumor localization and staging of disease, PET-CT imaging using these recently introduced $^{68}$Ga- or $^{18}$F-labeled compounds may be especially valuable for selecting patients for radiopeptide therapy (RPT). The latter approach is based on the administration of the same peptides, however, labeled with therapeutic nuclides such as yttrium-90 or lutetium-177 (FORRER et al. 2007) for treatment of inoperable metastasized NET. Another very interesting aspect will be to monitor this type of treatment with regard to response rates. One example for treatment monitoring

with using $^{68}$Ga-labeled somatostatin analogs is shown in Fig. 34.5.

## Conclusion

With the introduction of hybrid scanners, this combined morphological and functional imaging approach has been one of the fastest-growing techniques. The lack of anatomic information, especially when highly specific PET tracers as in NET are used, requires exact anatomic correlation, which now is offered by hybrid scanners. Although data on imaging of NET using the above-mentioned radiopharmaceuticals are still sparse,

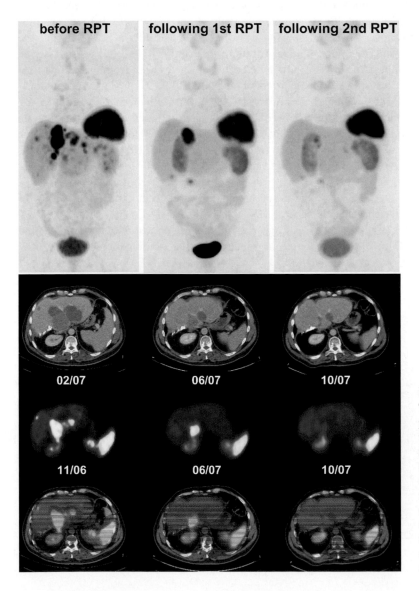

**Fig. 34.5.** Follow-up $^{68}$Ga-DOTA-TATE-PET, CT, and fused images of a patient with metastasized carcinoid of the rectum (primary resected). Baseline investigations (PET and CT done separately with an interval of 4 months) show extensive liver metastases. Follow-up investigations (performed in parallel on a hybrid scanner) after the first and second cycle of radiopeptide therapy using $^{90}$Y-DOTA-TATE show a marked decrease of uptake in PET as well as a shrinkage of metastases on CT

the preliminary data are very promising and fully justify further investigations in this field. The better spatial resolution of PET clearly argues for a replacement of planar scintigraphy and SPECT.

Concerning the various tracers, the broad variety of NET demands for a diagnostic workup which is tailored to the specific patient's pathology. FDG-PET, in general, should only be applied to patients with poorly differentiated, highly proliferative NET associated with rapidly increasing tumor markers. Promising data exist especially for NET with high Ki-67 expression, for metastasized medullary thyroid carcinomas and malignant pheochromocytomas.

For all other indications in NET, [68]Ga or [18]F-labeled somatostatin analogs will mainly enhance diagnostic workup and will probably become the tracers of first choice in this tumor entity. The development of somatostatin analogs with broader range of receptor affinity will potentially further improve this approach. Furthermore, this method and the ease of quantification will contribute to a more precise evaluation of patients eligible for specific therapy like biotherapy with somatostatin analogs or peptide receptor radionuclide therapy.

The field of application for amine precursors such as [18]F- and [11]C-labeled L-DOPA or 5-HTP has to be further investigated. These tracers could potentially be applied as first-line molecular imaging probes in pheochromocytomas/paragangliomas and also in medullary thyroid carcinomas. Furthermore, these tracers may play a promising role in somatostatin receptor negative tumors with positive immunohistochemical detection of serotonin as well as in insulinomas.

# References

Adams S, Baum RP, Hertel A et al. (1998a) Metabolic (PET) and receptor (SPECT) imaging of well- and less well-differentiated tumours: comparison with the expression of the Ki-67 antigen. Nucl Med Commun 19:641–647

Adams S, Baum R, Rink T et al. (1998b) Limited value of fluorine-18 fluorodeoxyglucose positron emission tomography for the imaging of neuroendocrine tumours. Eur J Nucl Med 25:79–83

Ahlstrom H, Eriksson B, Bergstrom M et al. (1995) Pancreatic neuroendocrine tumors: diagnosis with PET. Radiology 195:333–337

Ambrosini V, Tomassetti P, Rubello D et al. (2007) Role of [18]F-dopa imaging in the management of patients with [111]In-pentetreotide negative GEP tumours. Nucl Med Commun 28:473–477

Antunes P, Ginj M, Zhang H et al. (2007) Are radiogallium-labeled DOTA-conjugated somatostatin analogs superior to those labeled with other radiometals? Eur J Nucl Med Mol Imaging 34:982–993

Becherer A, Szabo M, Karanikas G et al. (2004) Imaging of advanced neuroendocrine tumors with [18]F-FDOPA-PET. J Nucl Med 45:1161–1167

Belhocine T, Foidart J, Rigo P et al. (2002) Fluorodeoxyglucose positron emission tomography and somatostatin receptor scintigraphy for diagnosing and staging carcinoid tumours: correlations with the pathological indexes p53 and Ki-67. Nucl Med Commun 23:727–734

Cimitan M, Buonadonna A, Cannizzaro R et al. (2003) Somatostatin receptor scintigraphy versus chromogranin A assay in the management of patients with neuroendocrine tumors of different types: clinical role. Ann Oncol 14:1135–1141

Decristoforo C, Mather SJ, Cholewinski W et al. (2000) 99mTc-EDDA/HYNIC-TOC: a new [99m]Tc-labeled radiopharmaceutical for imaging somatostatin receptor-positive tumours; first clinical results and intra-patient comparison with [111]In-labeled octreotide derivatives. Eur J Nucl Med 27:1318–1325

Diehl M, Risse JH, Brandt-Mainz K et al. (2001) Fluorine-18 fluorodeoxyglucose positron emission tomography in medullary thyroid cancer: results of a multicentre study. Eur J Nucl Med 28:1671–1676

Eriksson B, Bergstrom M, Lilja A et al. (1993) Positron emission tomography (PET) in neuroendocrine gastrointestinal tumors. Acta Oncol 32:189–196

Forrer F, Valkema R, Kwekkeboom DJ et al. (2007) Neuroendocrine tumors. Peptide receptor radionuclide therapy. Best Pract Res Clin Endocrinol Metab 21:111–129

Gabriel M, Decristoforo C, Donnemiller E et al. (2003) An intrapatient comparison of [99m]Tc-EDDA/HYNIC-TOC with [111]In-DTPA-octreotide for diagnosis of somatostatin receptor-expressing tumors. J Nucl Med 44:708–716

Gabriel M, Decristoforo C, Kendler D et al. (2007) [68]Ga-DOTA-Tyr3-octreotide PET in neuroendocrine tumors: comparison with somatostatin receptor scintigraphy and CT. J Nucl Med 48:508–518

Gabriel M, Muehllechner P, Decristoforo C et al. (2005) [99m]Tc-EDDA/HYNIC-Tyr(3)-octreotide for staging and follow-up of patients with neuroendocrine gastro-entero-pancreatic tumors. Q J Nucl Med Mol Imaging 49:237–244

Hoegerle S, Altehoefer C, Ghanem N et al. (2001) [18]F-DOPA positron emission tomography for tumour detection in patients with medullary thyroid carcinoma and elevated calcitonin levels. Eur J Nucl Med 28:64–71

Hoegerle S, Altehoefer C, Ghanem N et al. (2001) Whole-body [18]F dopa PET for detection of gastrointestinal carcinoid tumors. Radiology 220:373–380

Hoegerle S, Ghanem N, Altehoefer C et al. (2003) [18]F-DOPA positron emission tomography for the detection of glomus tumours. Eur J Nucl Med Mol Imaging 30:689–694

Hoegerle S, Nitzsche E, Altehoefer C et al. (2002) Pheochromocytomas: detection with [18]F DOPA whole body PET—initial results. Radiology 222:507–512

Hofmann M, Maecke H, Borner R et al. (2001) Biokinetics and imaging with the somatostatin receptor PET radioligand [68]Ga-DOTATOC: preliminary data. Eur J Nucl Med 28:1751–7

Jensen RT (2000) Carcinoid and pancreatic endocrine tumors: recent advances in molecular pathogenesis, localization, and treatment. Curr Opin Oncol 12:368–77

Kauhanen S, Seppanen M, Minn H et al. (2007) Fluorine-18-L-dihydroxyphenylalanine ([18]F-DOPA) positron emission tomography as a tool to localize an insulinoma or beta-cell hyperplasia in adult patients. J Clin Endocrinol Metab 92:1237–1244

Kloppel G, Perren A, Heitz PU (2004) The gastroenteropancreatic neuroendocrine cell system and its tumors: the WHO classification. Ann N Y Acad Sci 1014:13–27

Koopmans KP, de Vries EG, Kema IP et al. (2006) Staging of carcinoid tumours with [18]F-DOPA PET: a prospective, diagnostic accuracy study. Lancet Oncol 7:728–734

Kowalski J, Henze M, Schuhmacher J et al. (2003) Evaluation of positron emission tomography imaging using [[68]Ga]-DOTA-D Phe(1)-Tyr(3)-Octreotide in comparison to [[111]In]-DTPAOC SPECT. First results in patients with neuroendocrine tumors. Mol Imaging Biol 5:42–48

Kwekkeboom DJ, Krenning EP (2002) Somatostatin receptor imaging. Semin Nucl Med 32:84–91

Meisetschläger G, Poethko T, Stahl A et al. (2006) Gluc-Lys([[18]F]FP)-TOCA PET in patients with SSTR-positive tumors: biodistribution and diagnostic evaluation compared with [[111]In]DTPA-octreotide. J Nucl Med 47:566–573

Montravers F, Grahek D, Kerrou K et al. (2006) Can fluorodihydroxyphenylalanine PET replace somatostatin receptor scintigraphy in patients with digestive endocrine tumors? J Nucl Med 47:1455–1462

Orlefors H, Sundin A, Ahlstrom H et al. (1998) Positron emission tomography with 5-hydroxytryprophan in neuroendocrine tumors. J Clin Oncol 16:2534–2541

Orlefors H, Sundin A, Garske U et al. (2005) Whole-body [11]C-5-hydroxytryptophan positron emission tomography as a universal imaging technique for neuroendocrine tumors: comparison with somatostatin receptor scintigraphy and computed tomography. J Clin Endocrinol Metab 90:3392–3400

Orlefors H, Sundin A, Lu L et al. (2006) Carbidopa pretreatment improves image interpretation and visualisation of carcinoid tumours with [11]C-5-hydroxytryptophan positron emission tomography. Eur J Nucl Med Mol Imaging 33:60–65

Pasquali C, Rubello D, Sperti C et al. (1998) Neuroendocrine tumor imaging: can [18]F-fluorodeoxyglucose positron emission tomography detect tumors with poor prognosis and aggressive behavior? World J Surg 22:588–592

Seemann MD (2007) Detection of metastases from gastrointestinal neuroendocrine tumors: prospective comparison of [18]F-TOCA PET, triple-phase CT, and PET–CT. Technol Cancer Res Treat 6:213–220

Shulkin BL, Thompson NW, Shapiro B et al. (1999) Pheochromocytomas: imaging with 2-[fluorine-18]fluoro-2-deoxy-D-glucose PET. Radiology 212:35–41

Szakall S Jr, Esik O, Bajzik G et al. (2002) [18]F-FDG-PET detection of lymph node metastases in medullary thyroid carcinoma. J Nucl Med 43:66–71

Timmers HJ, Hadi M, Carrasquillo JA et al. (2007) The effects of carbidopa on uptake of [6-18]F-fluoro-L-DOPA in PET of pheochromocytoma and extraadrenal abdominal paraganglioma. J Nucl Med 48:1599–1606

Wild D, Macke HR, Waser B et al. (2005) 68Ga-DOTANOC: a first compound for PET imaging with high affinity for somatostatin receptor subtypes 2 and 5. Eur J Nucl Med Mol Imaging 32:724

Win Z, Al-Nahhas A, Towey D et al. (2007) 68Ga-DOTATATE PET in neuroectodermal tumours: first experience. Nucl Med Commun 28:359–363

## 35

# Role of MDCT in Bone Tumors, Metastases, and Myeloma

Andrea Baur-Melnyk and Maximilian F. Reiser

## CONTENTS

### ABSTRACT

Bone marrow malignancies are primarily subject for MR diagnostics, since MRI can directly display the bone marrow components. The role for MDCT is on the one hand to show the matrix of a bone tumor and on the other hand to evaluate the extension of osseous destructions and to assess the fracture risk. More and more whole-body exams are performed in patients with multifocal metastases or multiple myeloma.

### 35.1

## MDCT in Primary Bone Tumors and Metastases

Plain radiography remains the first imaging technique for evaluation of skeletal tumors. In most cases, radiographs provide features resulting in the most probable histopathologic prediction. On the other hand, x-rays might be false negative in osteolyses (Edelstyn et al. 1967). Edelstyn et al. showed in experimental studies of the spine that in cancellous bone 50–75% of the bony thickness in the beam axis of the vertebral body must be destroyed until it can be seen on lateral radiographs. The detection rate was even less accurate on anterior–posterior radiographs. A small break in the cortex was apparent much earlier, especially when it is tangential to the x-ray beam.

MDCT is an important modality for the diagnosis and for preoperative planning of bone tumors. With the introduction of MDCT, especially 16-row (or more) scanners a very thin collimation of ~0.7 mm became possible. Therefore, small details and especially the tra-

A. Baur-Melnyk MD, PD
Ass. Prof. of Radiology, Department of Clinical Radiology, Munich University Hospitals, Ludwig-Maximilians-University, Marchioninistrasse 15, 81377 Munich, Germany

M. F. Reiser MD
Director, Institute of Clinical Radiology, Munich University Hospitals, Ludwig-Maximilians-University, Marchioninistrasse 15, 81377 Munich, Germany

becular network can be visualized. Images can be reconstructed in the orthogonal planes as well as oblique and curved planes, so that MDCT can now be viewed at as a real multiplanar modality. The exact location and extent of osseous destructions can be determined, which is important for the assessment of the fracture risk and for planning of surgery (Fig. 35.1). MRI is superior in precisely visualizing the extent of tumor infiltration and tumor margins within the marrow cavity and within the soft tissues (ZIMMER et al. 1985). The relationship to neural and vascular structures as well as to articular surfaces is of utmost importance for the determination of the resectability of a tumor and eligibility for limb salvage surgery, respectively.

MDCT may also be of value in the differentiation of benign and malignant bone tumors by showing the matrix of a lesion, without superimposition of adjacent structures. The measurement of Hounsfield units permits differentiation of solid (30–100 HU) and cystic lesions (HU ~0–10), as well as intratumoral bleeding (HU ~50–70) and calcifications (HU ~250–1,000). The particular site of the tumor as displayed by CT in combination with clinical data and the age of the patient is sometimes characteristic for a certain entity. CT readily demonstrates the zone of transition, which is usually narrow in benign and broad in aggressive lesions. Moreover, cortical and periosteal reactions are depicted without superimpositions (Figs. 35.2, 35.3).

Sometimes nontumoral lesions like stress fractures may mimic a bone tumor, especially in MRI, where strong bone marrow edema and contrast enhancement may be misleading (WOERTLER 2003; GOULD et al. 2007; Fig. 35.4). In those cases, CT may demonstrate subtle cortical fracture lines, which allows exclusion of

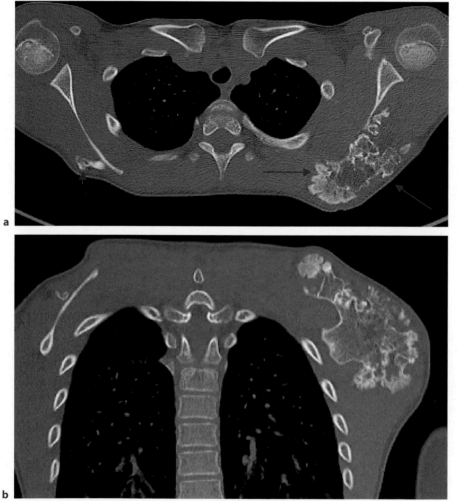

**Fig. 35.1. a** Axial CT image and **b** coronal reconstruction of an 11-year-old boy with Ollier's disease and multiple osteochondromas of the skeleton. A large osteochondroma is located at the left scapula (*arrows*). Note also a small osteochondroma the right scapula (*small arrow*). Due to the thin slices and the possibility of multiplanar reconstructions, the exact location can be determined for planning of surgery

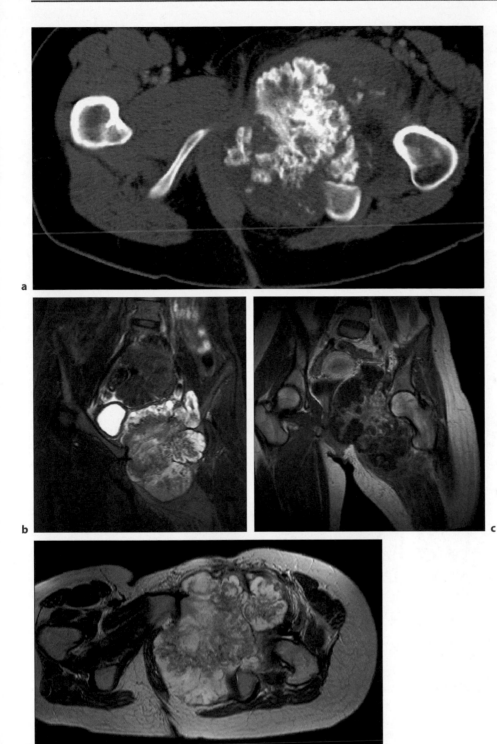

**Fig. 35.2. a** Axial CT images of a 22-year-old female with a large tumor originating from the left pubic bone. Typical cauliflower like calcifications within the para-osseal soft tissue tumor. Dedifferentiated osteochondroma (chondrosarcoma grade II) of the pubic bone. **b** Coronal STIR, **c** coronal T1-weighted SE post-gadolinium. **d** Axial T2-weighted TSE, same patient. The STIR image (**b**) and the axial T2-weighted TSE image allow delineation the soft tissue tumor components from the surrounding normal tissue. Postcontrast (**c**) an inhomogeneous enhancement of the tumor is found

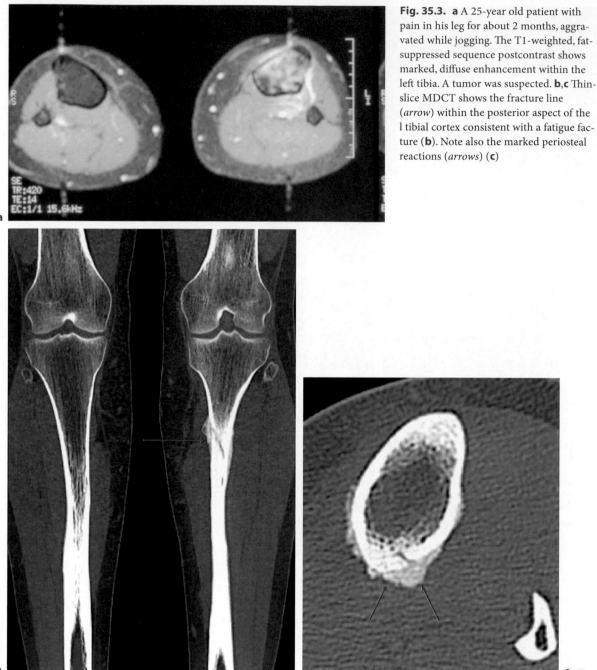

malignant bone tumor. Stress fractures may be due to insufficiency fractures (abnormal bone, normal load) or as fatigue fractures (normal bone, abnormal load). The detailed history of the patient (e.g., sports, jogging) may contribute important clues for the diagnosis.

With MDCT, even subtle intratumoral calcifications are displayed with high sensitivity, which remain unde-

tected in MRI (Fig. 35.5). The morphology and the location of calcifications may offer important diagnostic information for the differential diagnosis (Figs. 35.6, 35.7). Chondromatous tumors typically contain calcifications (Littrell et al. 2004). In enchondromas, central, popcorn-like calcifications are detected in many cases, whereas bone marrow infarcts show a serpiginous pe-

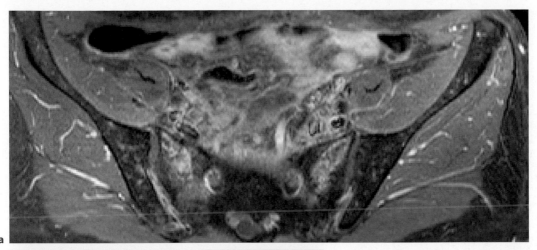

a

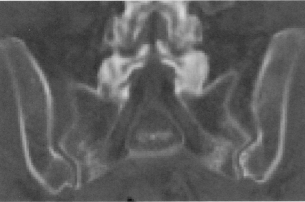

b

**Fig. 35.4. a** T1-weighted image postcontrast with fat saturation shows bilateral diffuse enhancement within the sacral wings. Since the patient preciously had a carcinoma of the uterus and because of increased uptake in the bone scan, bony metastases were suspected. **b** CT shows serpiginous sclerosis within the sacrum parallel to the sacroiliac joint typical for sacral insufficiency fractures. The patient had previously received radiation therapy of the pelvis, which is known to result in local osteoporosis with weakening of the bone. The patient was followed-up, and bisphosphonates were administered

a,b                                                                                                                                c

**Fig. 35.5. a** A 52-year-old male with increasing swelling and pain of his left ankle. Osteosarcoma with aggressive growth and extensive intraosseous and paraosseous bone formation. **b,c** In MRI, a large tumor arising from the distal tibia with an extensive soft tissue component is depicted. The central hypointensity is due to massive calcification. Radiography and CT are highly indicative for the diagnosis of an osteosarcoma, while MRI enables precise assessment of soft tissue and bone marrow extension in (**b**) coronal T1-weighted SE and (**c**) coronal STIR sequences

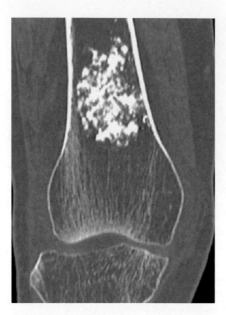

**Fig. 35.6.** Coronal reconstruction of a MDCT dataset in an 81-year-old female with a large enchondroma of the femur. Typical popcorn-like calcifications within the marrow cavity, no osseous destructions or periosteal reactions indicative of malignancy are visualized. The diagnosis of a benign enchondroma was proven by biopsy

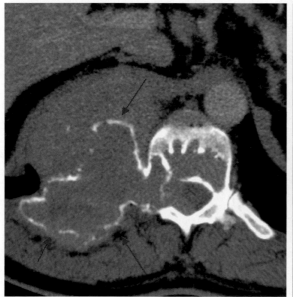

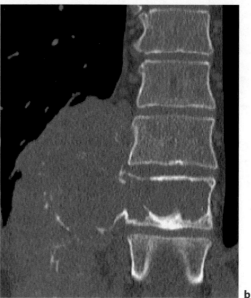

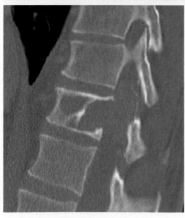

**Fig. 35.7.** **a** Axial CT, **b** coronal reconstruction, and **c** sagittal reconstruction of the spine of a 43-year-old male with pain in the thoracic spine. A large expansile bone tumor is present at the right side of T12. The tumor affects the right pedicle, the costotransversal joint, the vertebral body, and the posterior portion of the 12th rib. Note also the large soft tissue mass, which shows a sort of neocorticalis (*arrows*): A giant cell tumor

ripheral rim of calcification (FLEMMING and MURPHEY 2000). Aneurysmal bone cysts commonly exhibit a layering with sedimented blood in a mixed cystic and solid tumor surrounded by a small rim of sclerosis (PARMAN and MURPHEY 2000; KEENAN and BUI-MANSFIELD 2006). Some tumors, such as osteosarcomas may have a bone-forming matrix (Fig. 35.5). Skeletal metastases of various primary tumors, such as prostate and breast cancer may also be osteoblastic (RESNICK 2002).

A sclerotic border of a bony lesion is more obvious with MDCT than with radiograms. The presence or absence of such a sclerotic border may allow narrowing the differential diagnosis. Chondroblastomas, nonossifying fibromas, and fibrous dysplasia typically are surrounded by a sclerotic rim, while eosinophilic granulomas and osteolytic metastases are not (Fig. 35.8; GOULD et al. 2007).

MDCT is the most accurate imaging method for the diagnosis of osteoidosteoma (KRANSDORF 1991). Using reconstruction of thin slices the nidus of osteoid osteome (usually <1 cm) is readily detected as a round circumscribed lytic lesion. It is usually located in the

bony cortex, with extensive surrounding sclerosis and/or periosteal bone formation. The nidus may be calcified in about 50% of cases, noncalcified in about a third of the patients, and sometimes it can be completely calcified. In x-rays, the surrounding sclerosis may often mask the nidus, which is pathognomonic for osteoidosteoma (Fig. 35.9). With MRI, a marked reactive edema may also mask the nidus. In postoperative imaging, CT is the method of choice in assessing either complete removal or recurrence, respectively.

## 35.2
## Whole-Body MDCT in Multiple Myeloma

Primarily myeloma infiltrates the bone marrow. Complex biochemical mechanisms and the secretion of osteoclast-activating factors lead to bony destructions. MDCT is the method of choice in the depiction of bony destruction. Whole-body MDCT replaces the radiographic skeletal survey (Fig. 35.10; BAUR-MELNYK et al. 2005). As compared with radiographic examinations, MDCT has a significantly higher sensitivity in the detection of bony destruction, both of cortical and cancellous bone, and can be performed within a shorter examination time (1–2 min). Scanners with 16 and more detector rows are suitable for this kind of whole-body MDCT. Due to the high contrast of bone to soft tissue, a low-dose protocol can be used (~100 mA, 120 kV) so that radiation dose can be limited (~4 mSv). Raw data sets should be reconstructed in 3- to 4-mm axial slices, sagittal slices of the spine, and coronal slices for the

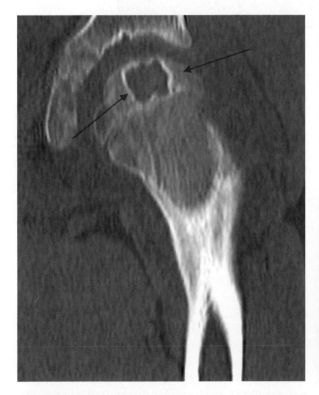

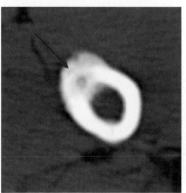

**Fig. 35.8.** An 11-year-old female with hip pain. With MDCT, a circumscribed osteolysis with surrounding sclerosis in the left epiphysis of the femur is detected. In combination with the age of the patient, this is a typical finding of a chondroblastoma (biopsy proven)

**Fig. 35.9.** A 19-year-old male with an osteoidosteoma in the left femur. The nidus (*arrow*) is located in the anteromedial aspect of the cortex. It is osteolytic with subtle central calcification. Note the marked surrounding reactive sclerosis. It was successfully treated with CT-guided radiofrequency ablation

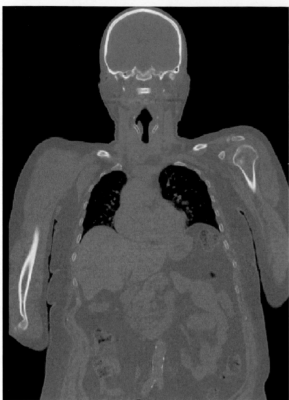

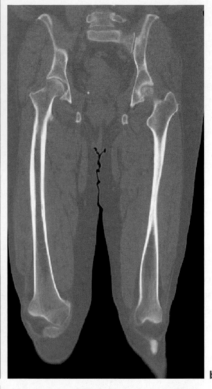

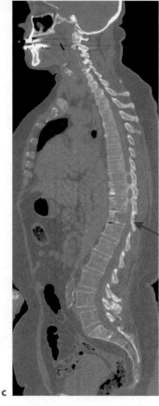

**Fig. 35.10.** **a** Coronal upper parts, **b** coronal lower parts, and **c** sagittal spine images of whole-body MDCT of a patient with multiple myeloma. A 64-detector-row CT, low-dose protocol with 120 kV, 100 mA, and anatomic tube current modulation. Large destruction of T11 body is evident (*arrow*)

whole body, and separately for the upper (skull/thorax/arms) and the lower parts (pelvis, legs).

Bony destructions in multiple myeloma are usually well circumscribed and have a narrow zone of transition. They usually have Hounsfield units of soft tissue density (~40–80 HU). The bony destructions in multiple myeloma involve predominantly the trabecular bone. When these tumor foci grow, the cortical bone is also affected, with cortical destructions and eventually soft tissue expansion (Fig. 35.11). In the skull, the osteolyses manifest as punched-out lesions, which are situated within the tabula externa and interna. Differential diagnosis includes choroid plexus enlargement. However, those show up with contiguity to the subarachnoid space. In the diaphyses of the long tubular bones, where only sparse trabecular bone is present, early osteolyses may be missed when only looking at the bone window. Circumscribed areas with soft tissue density (>30–40 HU) within the normal fatty marrow (negative HU values) are highly suspicious for myeloma manifestations. Comparison with the contralateral side may be helpful in evaluating marrow involvement. Cortical scalloping in the long bones may be visible on axial or reformatted coronal or sagittal images. Rib lesions are often overlooked since the ribs are small structures and signs of

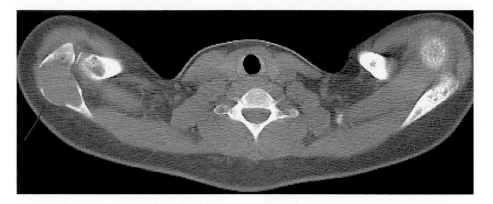

**Fig. 35.11** A 36-year old female patient with multiple myeloma, with involvement of the right acromion. The tumor results in an expansion and destruction of the cortex (*arrow*)

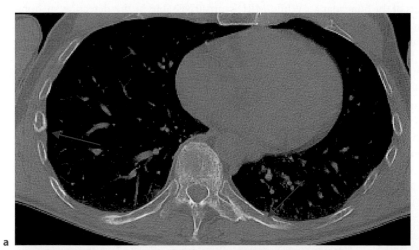

**Fig. 35.12a,b** Bone and soft-tissue windows of a patient with multiple myeloma (*arrows*). In the bone window, endosteal scalloping, focal enlargement, and a cortical fracture as signs of myeloma infiltration in two ribs are found (**a**). In the soft tissue window (with enlarged image), the higher density of the tumor is visible (**b**)

a

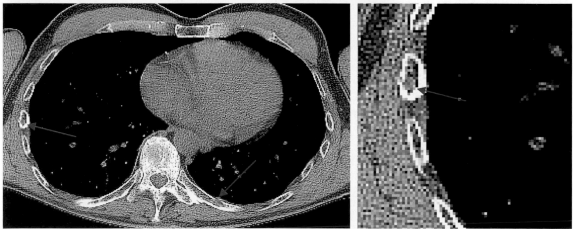

b

involvement may be subtle. Focal enlargement of a particular rib with soft tissue density within the lesion is indicative of myeloma involvement. The cortex may be normal or thinned (Fig. 35.12). If the tumor continues to grow, then a pathological fracture may result. Careful examination of every rib is necessary in order not

to overlook a rib lesion. The shoulder girdle with its complex structures (acromion, coracoid process, etc.) is another predilection site.

In cases with diffuse bone marrow infiltration, inhomogeneous osteoporosis can be detected with MDCT. However, as in X-ray diagnostics, this is often hard to distinguish from senile or perimenopausal osteoporosis. In those cases, MRI should be performed, which can demonstrate neoplastic bone marrow infiltration in the absence of bony destruction (BAUR et al. 2004).

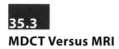

## MDCT Versus MRI

MDCT is more sensitive than radiography is in the diagnosis of skeletal metastases and myeloma manifestations (MAHNKEN et al. 2002; SCHREIMAN et al. 1985). However, MDCT is less sensitive than MRI. Unlike MDCT, MRI allows to visualize tumor infiltration, which results in replacement of normal components of the bone marrow, such as fat and hematopoietic cells. Metastases, primary bone tumors, as well as bone marrow malignancies usually originate from the bone marrow, and during the course of their natural history, progress by involving the spongy and eventually the cortical bone. This takes some time, and a certain amount of bone has to be destructed before it becomes visible in CT imaging. In the current literature, only few studies exist that

directly compare MDCT and MRI. In our own study, comparing metastases to the spine with both methods, MRI was significantly more sensitive than 16-detector-row CT was (Fig. 35.13; BUHMANN-KIRCHHOFF et al. 2008). We also found whole-body MRI more sensitive than whole-body MDCT in patients with multiple myeloma, and this superior sensitivity resulted in 27% of the patients in the assignment to a different stage of disease (BAUR-MELNYK et al. 2008).

## MDCT for Fracture Risk Assessment

While MRI is unsurpassable in the detection of bone marrow infiltration, it does not allow for precise assessment of bone destruction, which is predictive for the risk of fracture. In order to prevent for potentially catastrophic pathologic fracture, it is most important to assess the fracture risk and initiate prophylactic stabilization, if required. MDCT is most useful in the precise assessment of the extent of bony destructions and thereby in the prediction of fracture risk.

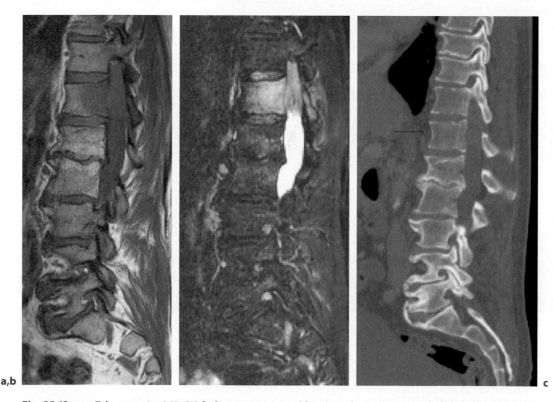

**Fig. 35.13a–c.** False-negative MDCT finding in a 64-year-old male with metastases to the T12 body. With MRI, a large metastasis, hypointense on T1-weighted SE images (**a**) and hyperintense on STIR images (**b**) was detected. With MDCT, no osseous destructions were found (*arrows*) (**c**)

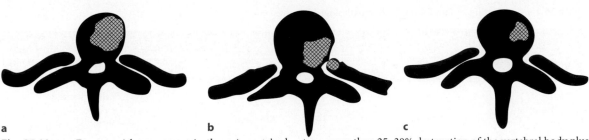

| a | b | c |

**Fig. 35.14a–c.** Fracture risk assessment in thoracic vertebral bodies (T1–10). Examples: **a** Impending fracture: more than 50–60% destruction of the vertebral body, **b** impending fracture: more than 25–30% destruction of the vertebral body plus destruction of the costovertebral joint, **c** no impending fracture. Osteolyses in the vertebral body of 20% is noted

There exist major differences between the thoracic (T1–10) and thoracolumbar vertebral bodies (T11–L5), since the rib cage serves as a stabilizer of the thoracic vertebral column. Four factors have to be determined: (1) percentage of osteolyses in the vertebral body, (2) presence of involvement of the pedicles, (3) posterior elements, and (4) costovertebral joint involvement at the thoracic spine (TANEICHI et al. 1997).

Fracture risk assessment in vertebral bodies:

- >50% Destruction of thoracic (T1–10) vertebral bodies
- >25% Destruction of thoracic vertebral bodies plus costovertebral destruction
- >35% Destruction of thoracolumbar (T11–L5) vertebral bodies
- >20% Destruction of thoracolumbar (T11–L5) plus pedicle/posterior elements

A vertebral body is at risk of fracture in the thoracic spine if more than 50% of the vertebral body is missing or if more than 25% of osseous destruction of the vertebral body is combined with a destruction of the costovertebral joint (see above; Fig 35.14). In the lumbar spine, a vertebral body is at risk of fracture if more than 35% of the body is destroyed or if a more than 20% de-

struction of the body is combined with involvement of the posterior elements/pedicles (see above; Fig 35.15).

Numerous studies have been undertaken to identify metastatic lesions in tubular bones, which are at risk of fracture. However, most of these studies lack a well-performed statistical basis. One of the most reliable risk analyses for fractures of the tubular bones was performed by Mirels, who proposed a classification system (MIRELS 2003; DAMRON et al. 2003). It includes four risk factors: (1) location, (2) lesion type, (3) pain, and (4) lesion size. To every risk factor, 1–3 points are allotted. Scores range from 4 to 12 points. The fracture risk increases exponentially when a sum score more than 8 points is obtained (Table 35.1). A score of 8 is suggestive of an impending fracture (probability of a fracture 15%), while a score of 9 is found to be diagnostic for a fracture (probability of a fracture 33%; no false positives in this group). When a score of 7 or less is obtained, the probability of a fracture is low (5%). Such a lesion can be treated conservatively. In patients with a score of at least 9, prophylactic surgery is recommended. If the sum is 8, then an individual decisions should be made.

VAN DER LINDEN et al. (2004) emphasized the importance of cortical involvement in femoral metastases. This is best done using MDCT. In a multivariate analy-

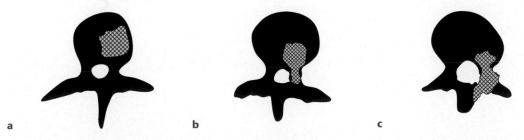

| a | b | c |

**Fig. 35.15a–c.** Fracture risk assessment in lumbar vertebral bodies (T11–L5). **a** Impending fracture: more than 35–40% destruction of the vertebral body, **b** impending fracture: more than 20–25% destruction of the vertebral body plus pedicle destruction, **c** no impending fracture: 10% destruction of the vertebral body plus pedicle and posterior elements destruction

**Table 35.1** Mirels' rating system for impending pathologic fractures

| Criteria | Score | | |
|---|---|---|---|
| | 1 | 2 | 3 |
| Site | Upper limb | Lower limb | Peritrochanteric |
| Pain | Mild | Moderate | Funtional[a] |
| Lesion | Sclerotic | Mixed | Lytic |
| Diameter | <⅓ | ⅓–⅔ | >⅔ |

With a score of more than 9, an impending fracture can be assumed

[a] Pain aggravated by limb function

sis of reported risk factors in the literature, two factors were significant in predicting fractures. First, "axial cortical involvement," which represents the length of cortical involvement in head-to-feet direction. Axial cortical involvement of >3 cm was predictive of fracture. Second, "circumferential cortical involvement" (on axial slices) >50% was predictive of fracture. Similar findings have been reported by FIDLER et al. (1981) in a study on metastases of long bones evaluated by radiography. Pathological fractures were unlikely (2.3% fractures) when less than 50% of the cortex were destroyed, likely (60% fractures) when more than 50% were destroyed,

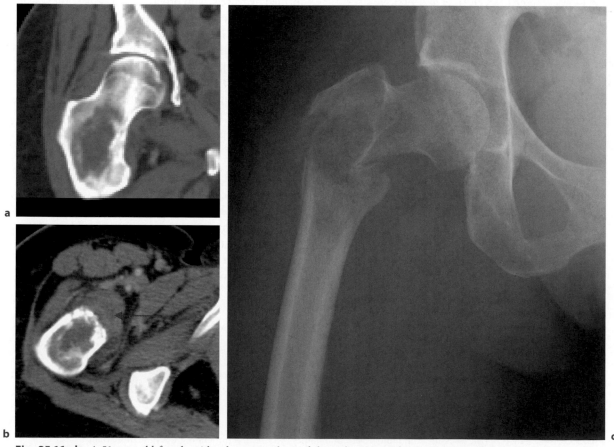

**Fig. 35.16a,b.** A 51-year-old female with a large osteolysis of the right intertrochanteric region. The cortex is destructed on the medial side (*arrow*). (High risk for fracture!) **c** 1 week after the first examination, the femur fractured while the patient was hospitalized

and most likely (80% fractures) when more than 75% were destroyed (Fig. 35.16).

It has to be mentioned that in all cases, individual circumstances have to be considered before prophylactic surgery is performed in order not to over-treat patients with only limited life-expectancy. Radiological parameters can hereby support therapeutic decisions.

# References

Baur A, Bartl R, Pellengahr C, Baltin V, Reiser MF (2004) Neovascularization of bone marrow in patients with diffuse multiple myeloma: a correlative study of MR-imaging and histopathologic findings. Cancer 101:2599–2604

Baur-Melnyk A, Buhmann S, Dürr HR, Reiser M (2005) Role of MRI for the diagnosis and prognosis of multiple myeloma. Eur J Radiol 55:56–64

Baur-Melnyk A, Buhmann S, Becker C, Schoenberg SO, Lang N, Bartl R, Reiser MF (2008) Whole-body-MRI versus whole-body MDCT for the staging of patients with multiple myeloma. AJR Am J Roentgenol 190:1097–1104

Buhmann-Kirchhoff S, Becker C, Duerr HR, Reiser M, Baur-Melnyk A (2008) Detection of osseous metastases of the spine: Comparison of high resolution multi-detector CT with MRI. Eur Radiol (in press) doi: http://dx.doi.org/10.1016/j.ejrad.2007.11.039

Damron TA, Morgan H, Prakash D, Grant W, Aronowitz J, Heiner J (2003) Critical evaluation of Mirels' rating system for impending pathologic fractures. Clin Orthop Relat Res 415(Suppl):S201–S207

Edelstyn GA, Gillespie PJ, Grebbell FS (1067) The radiological demonstration of osseous metastases: experimental observations. Clin Radiol 18:158–162

Fidler M (1981) incidence of fracture through metastases in long bones. Acta Orthop Scand 52:623

Flemming DJ, Murphey MD (2000) Enchondroma and chondrosarcoma. Semin Musculoskelet Radiol 4:59–71

Gould CF, Ly JO, Lattin GE, Beall DP, Sutcliff JB (2007) Bone tumor mimics: avoiding misdiagnosis. Curr Probl Diagn Radiol 36:124–141

Keenan S, Bui-Mansfield LT (2006) Musculoskeletal lesions with fluid-fluid level: a pictorial essay. J Comput Assist Tomogr 30:517–524

Kransdorf MJ, Stull MA, Gilkey FW, Moser RP Jr (1991) Osteoid osteoma. Radiographics 11:671–679

Linden YM van der, Dijkstra PDS, Kroon HM, Lok JJ, Noordijk EM, Leer JWH, Marijnen CA (2004) Comparative analysis of risk factors for pathological fracture with femoral metastases. J Bone Surg Br 86:566–573

Littrell LA, Wenger DE, Wold LE, Bertoni F, Unni KK, White LM, Kandel R, Sundaram M (2004) Radiographic, CT and MR imaging features of dedifferentiated chondrosarcomas: a retrospective review of 174 de novo cases. Radiographics 24:1397–1409

Mahnken AH, Wildberger JE, Gehbauer G et al. (2002) Multidetector CT of the spine in multiple myeloma: comparison with MR imaging and radiography. Am J Roentgenol 178:1429–1436

Mirels H (2003) Metastatic disease in long bones: a proposed scoring system for diagnosing impending pathologic fractures. 1989. Clin Orthop Relat Res 415(Suppl):S4–S13

Parman LM, Murphey MD (2000) Alphabet soup: cystic lesions of bone. Semin Musculoskelet Radiol 4:89–101

Resnick D (2002) Diagnosis of bone and joint disorders. Tumors and tumor like lesions, 4th edn. Saunders, Philadelphia, pp 3743–4352

Schreiman JS, McLeod RA, Kyle RA, Beabout JW (1985) Multiple myeloma: evaluation by CT. Radiology 154:483–486

Taneichi H, Kaneda K, Takeda N, Abumi K, Satoh S (1997) Risk factors and probability of vertebral body collapse in metastases of the spine. Spine 22:239–245

Woertler K (2003) Benign bone tumors and tumor-like lesions: value of cross-sectional imaging. Eur Radiol 13:1820–1835

Zimmer WD, Berquist TH, McLeod RA et al. (1985) Bone tumors: magnetic resonance imaging versus computed tomography. Radiology 155:709–718

ANNO GRASER and MICHAEL MACARI

## CONTENTS

A. GRASER, MD
Department of Clinical Radiology, Ludwig-Maximilians-University of Munich, University of Munich Hospitals, Marchioninistrasse 15, 81377 Munich, Germany

M. MACARI, MD
Department of Radiology, New York University Medical Center, 560 1st Avenue, New York, NY 10016, USA

## ABSTRACT

Since the introduction of a dual source CT scanner, several dual energy applications operating the two tubes of the scanner at different potentials have been described. The simultaneous acquisition of images at 80 and 140 kVp allows for material differentiation and subtraction of iodine from the dataset. Clinical use of this technique enhances diagnostic capabilities of abdominal MDCT.

## 36.1
## Introduction

Technological advances including helical and multidetector row acquisition as well as dose modulation continuously increase the clinical applications and diagnostic value of CT (HOUNSFIELD 1995; JOHNSON et al. 2007; GENANT and BOYD 1997; GOLDBERG et al. 1982). A recent technological advance in CT has been the introduction of a dual-source CT scanner. On this scanner, two X-ray tubes can be operated at different tube potentials, making dual energy (DE) scanning possible. DE scanning implies simultaneously acquiring data sets at two different photon spectra in a single CT acquisition (CANN et al. 1982; CHIRO et al. 1979).

The first available system is the Siemens Somatom Definition (Siemens Medical Systems, Forchheim, Germany, Fig. 36.1; FLOHR et al. 2006). There are three main advantages of this system when compared with a single-source CT scanner. First, the tubes can be used in unison at equal tube potentials, permitting increased photon flux in larger patients. Second, since an image can be acquired using 90° of gantry rotation rather than 180°, temporal resolution can be increased by a factor of 2 when using the two tubes at identical kVp levels.

Using this technique, a temporal resolution of 83 ms is possible. Third, and most important for abdominal applications, the system can be used such that the tubes operate at different tube potentials. For all applications described in this chapter, tube currents used were 80 and 140 kVp, as these lead to maximum density differences between different materials and therefore allow for optimum material differentiation.

By scanning at different photon energies, differences in material composition can be detected, based on differences in photon absorption. This technique exploits attenuation differences of materials with large atomic numbers like iodine. For example, the attenuation of iodine will be much greater at 80 than at 140 kVp. Importantly, based on the reconstruction of complete 80 and 140 kVp image data sets from the raw data, virtual noncontrast (VNC) data sets and virtual angiographic data sets can be generated utilizing various DE postprocessing algorithms based on three-material decomposition principles. In the abdomen, the three materials usually analyzed are soft tissue, fat, and iodine (JOHNSON et al. 2007).

The potential applications of dual energy CT (DECT) when evaluating the abdomen are numerous. Generation of VNC images may obviate the routine need for noncontrast acquisitions. That is, a single contrast-enhanced acquisition can yield both contrast-enhanced and noncontrast CT data. This is of importance when evaluating the liver, adrenal glands, and kidneys and may be utilized to decrease radiation exposure to patients. Furthermore, differences in attenuation of data acquired at 80 and 140 kVp may be beneficial in the diagnosis of inflammatory and ischemic bowel disease or poorly vascularized tumors such as pancreatic cancer. Finally, the attenuation of vessels is substantially greater when acquired at 80 as opposed to 140 kVp. This may improve vessel detection and evaluation at CT angiography and at the same time, allow a smaller amount of iodinated contrast material to be administered. The purpose of this chapter is to review our initial experience with the technical aspects, potential clinical applications, as well as current limitations of DECT scanning when evaluating the abdomen and pelvis.

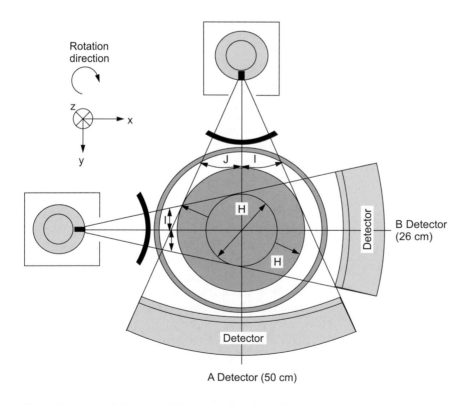

**Fig. 36.1.** Technical drawing of the dual source dual detector CT system. Detector "*A*" with standard 50 cm FOV and detector "*B*" with reduced 26 cm FOV are mounted in the gantry at a 90° angle

## Technical Considerations

The first report on DECT scanning was in 1977 (GENANT and BOYD 1977). Initial investigations of DE were in bone mineral analysis, quantification of hepatic iron and calcium in pulmonary nodules, and for the differentiation of various tissues (GENANT and BOYD 1977; GOLDBERG et al. 1982; CANN et al. 1982; CHIRO et al. 1979). Despite initial promising results, clinical utilization of DE scanning was abandoned. At that time, two separate consecutive CT scans needed to be acquired. Neither helical nor MDCT were available, and thus long acquisition times were required leading to motion misregistration, high image noise due to scattered radiation at low kVp settings, and excessive radiation exposure.

The development of a dual-tube, dual-detector CT system (Somatom Definition) in 2006 has led to increased investigation and now utilization of DE scanning. This system consists of two X-ray tubes mounted in one gantry at a 90° angle from each other (FLOHR et al. 2006). For each tube, a 64-element detector is present: the "A" detector, which is equal in size to a standard detector (50 cm) used in a single-source 64-slice system, and the "B" detector, which also has a 64-slice design, but with a reduced FOV of 26 cm (see Fig. 36.1) (FLOHR et al. 2006). This detector array provides high spatial resolution of isotropic 0.38 mm edge-length voxels and allows a rapid acquisition of a large $z$-axis volume.

The two X-ray tubes of the scanner can be operated at identical tube potentials to provide an increase in temporal resolution for cardiac examinations (JOHNSON et al. 2006) or photon flux in obese patients (JOHNSON et al. 2007). Alternatively they can be operated at two different tube energies potentially allowing differentiation various tissues based on different photon absorption rates at high and low kVp settings (JOHNSON et al. 2007).

A limitation of DECT in the abdomen and pelvis is that the smaller size of the B detector (26 cm) will prevent imaging of the entire FOV in larger patients. Therefore, patients may have to be positioned off center if the location of pathology is known and it is in the periphery of the FOV (see Sect. 35.5.1). It is important to center the scanner table with the patient in the center of the FOV in the $x$- (right/left) as well as in the $y$- (anterior/posterior) axes. Therefore, it is mandatory to acquire both anterior/posterior and lateral topograms to make sure that the scanner table is not positioned too high or too low in the gantry ($y$-axis of the patient). Moreover, objects at the outer periphery of the B detector may be unable to undergo optimal postprocessing due to the technical specifications of the postprocessing algorithm. In detail, adjacent volume elements (voxels) have to be used for calculation of the DE properties of any voxel within the FOV. Therefore, the reconstructed DE FOV will be about 5 mm smaller than the actual B detector FOV. In the periphery of the FOV, no color-coded images or VNC images are available.

## CT Dose and Image Noise

Since the 80 kVp X-ray photons have a lower energy than a standard acquisition at 120 kVp, image noise will substantially increase in large patients. In order to minimize image noise, the mA needs to be increased. To minimize patient exposure to ionizing radiation, abdominal DECT protocols operate using an online dose modulation system (CareDOSE 4D, Siemens Medical Solutions, Forchheim, Germany) that adapts the tube current to the patients anatomy (GRASER et al. 2006). The image quality reference mA values are set to 400 mA on the B tube and 96 mA on the A tube, thereby splitting the energy between the two tubes. These settings take into account that higher mA values on the A tube would lead to increased image noise on the B detector due to scatter radiation. On the B tube, technical limitations prevent mA values over 600 mA. The calculated effective patient doses for abdominal scans will range from 4.5 to 12.5 mSv, which is similar to the effective dose of a standard abdominal CT acquisition using 120 kVp with 250 mA (GRASER et al. 2008).

For abdominal imaging, DECT acquisitions should employ a collimation of 14 × 1.2 mm rather than 64 × 0.6 mm, as the latter configuration will cause very high image noise on the B detector images. Since a reconstructed slice thickness below 1.2 mm is usually not required for most applications in the abdomen, this typically does not represent a significant limitation in terms of spatial resolution. However, the data acquired are not isotropic in the $x$, $y$, and $z$ dimensions.

DECT is not recommended for patients whose body mass index is >30. In morbidly obese patients, the two tubes could both be operated at 120 kVp, which will help to decrease image noise in these very large patients. The system can be used to scan patients with a body weight of up to 500 lbs (220 kg). In this instance, the maximum mA value will be 750 on both tubes at 120 kVp.

36.4
## 36.4
### Image Generation and Postprocessing

Each DE acquisition can generate the following types of data: pure 80 kVp data, pure 140 kVp data, and a weighted average 120 kVp data set, which is a composition of 70% from the A (high kV) and 30% from the B (low kV) tube. Using a slider bar, this relation can be manually adjusted on a DE workstation, and we found that in larger patients image quality can be improved using a 50:50 ratio. In addition, using DE postprocessing software based on the DE index of materials in the scan range, VNC CT data, an iodine data set, and a color-coded data set that shows iodine distribution over the VNC CT data can be generated (Fig. 36.2).

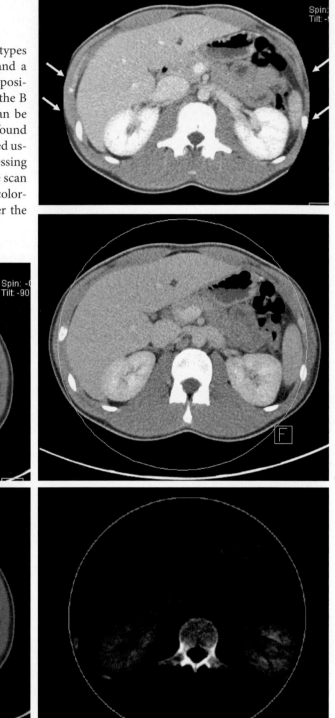

**Fig 36.2a–g.** Image data generated from a dual energy acquisition. **a** Axial CT image obtained at 80 kVp and 400 mA. In this slim patient, only the left lateral abdominal wall is not included in the 26 cm FOV (*arrows*). **b** Axial CT image obtained at 140 kVp and 96 mA. Note the entire abdomen is included in the standard 50-cm FOV. **c** Axial CT image obtained with weighted average of 80 and 140 kVp data sets. This image equals a 120-kV image from a standard CT scan. The *yellow line* represents the B detector FOV. **d** VNC image. Note the slightly increased image noise and FOV of the B detector (*yellow line*)

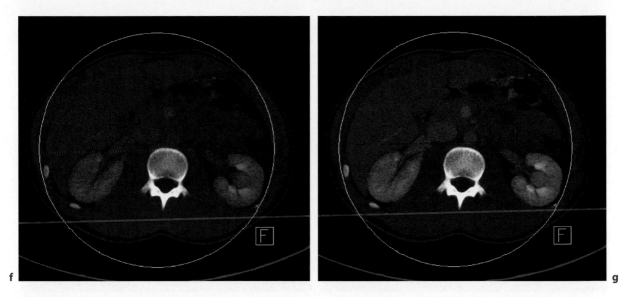

f                                                                                                          g

**Fig 36.2a–g.** (*continued*) **f,g** Image data generated from a dual energy acquisition

## 36.5
### Applications in the Abdomen

#### 36.5.1
#### DE Imaging of Renal Masses

Assessment of renal masses is based upon enhancement and requires an NCCT and contrast-enhanced acquisition to be performed (SZOLAR et al. 1997; BIRNBAUM et al. 1996). Currently, noncontrast (NC) CT images are acquired prior to the injection of iodinated contrast agent in order to allow for baseline density measurements of the renal mass and to evaluate for calcification and fat. The most important criterion for the differentiation of benign from malignant masses is the presence of enhancement in a lesion (ISRAEL and BOSNIAK 2005).

Utilizing DECT, a VNC CT image can be generated, and this data may be used for baseline density measurements, thereby making a true noncontrast scan unnecessary and saving radiation. This is especially useful in cases of incidentally detected renal lesions with high attenuation on a contrast-enhanced CT. The main differential diagnosis considered here is hyperdense cysts and renal mass. Preliminary data show that there is good correlation between VNC and true noncontrast CT Hounsfield units of the renal parenchyma (GRASER 2007). In a study conducted at our institutions, we found mean density values of 30.8±4.0 (true NC) and 31.6±7.1 (VNC) HU ($P = 0.26$). No statistical differences in density were also found in liver parenchyma and psoas muscle, underlining the stability of HU numbers measured on VNC images (GRASER 2007).

DE scanning can be used for the differentiation of high-density cysts from solid renal masses (Fig. 36.3). Using DE postprocessing software, the contrast agent can be digitally subtracted from the image. This can be done because the DE index of iodine is significantly different from the DE index of soft tissue and fat. The DE data can also be used to generate a color-coded image that shows the distribution of iodine within the scan field. This color-coded display is very sensitive to subtle enhancement and can aid in assessing enhancement. In our experiences, high-density renal cysts with a density greater than the renal parenchyma (e.g., 60 HU for a hemorrhagic cyst) will be reliably identified and characterized based on measured HU values, as those correlate well between NCCT and VNC datasets. This underlines the ability of the algorithm to deal with different high-density materials in the presence of iodine.

Off-center positioning of the patient may be beneficial for imaging the kidneys if the site of the lesion is known, for example, a lesion detected on ultrasound. As stated above, the smaller FOV of the B detector can be a limiting factor in abdominal imaging, depending on the body size of the patient. In patients with suspected or

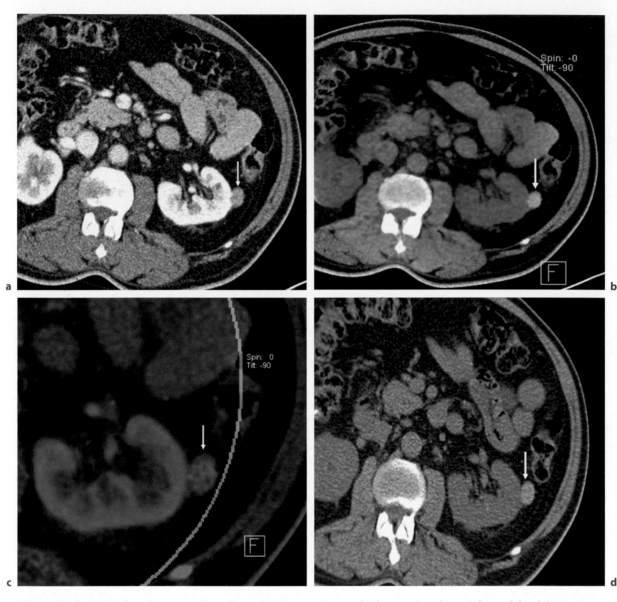

**Fig 36.3a–d.** DECT for characterization of renal masses. **a** Axial contrast-enhanced CT image of the upper abdomen in a 75-year-old male. Weighted average DECT image showing a hyperdense lesion in the left kidney (*arrow*) measuring 75 HU. **b** Virtual noncontrast image at the same slice position shows the lesion (*arrow*) has high density (70 HU). **c** Color-coded DECT image showing that the lesion (*arrow*) does not enhance. Note in this large patient the periphery of the abdomen is not included in the B detector FOV (*yellow circle*). **d** True NC image in same patient shows the lesion has high-density, measuring 72 HU. This case demonstrates how a virtual noncontrast image can be used if a true NCCT is unavailable

known renal masses, the patient can be shifted slightly to the contralateral side, thus ensuring that the entire kidney with the mass is included in the B detector FOV. Due to the nonisotropic data, we found that lesions smaller than 5 mm in size cannot be reliably characterized due to partial volume averaging effects and pseudoenhancement.

## 36.5.2
## DE Imaging of Urinary Calculi

When evaluating the patient with flank pain and suspected urinary stones, NC low-dose MDCT is the most accurate imaging technique (Boulay et al. 1999; Smith et al. 1995). It provides the exact location of calculi within the renal parenchyma, the ureter, and the urinary bladder and can aid treatment decisions based on the size and location of the stone (POLETTI et al. 2007; KLUNER et al. 2006). Metabolic evaluation of patients with chronic recurrent calculi is often performed in an attempt to identify an underlying metabolic abnormality (PARK 2007; MOE 2006). While MDCT can identify patients with urinary tract stones, it cannot reliably predict stone composition. The characterization of urinary stones can be important for treatment decisions. Stones consisting predominantly of uric acid can be treated with oral medication (alkalinization) rather than endoureteral extraction or extracorporeal shock-wave lithotripsy (ESWL).

Studies have demonstrated that the chemical composition of calculi can be partially determined by CT in vitro, but this differentiation is more complicated and less reliable in vivo (HILLMAND et al. 1984; MOSTAFAVI et al. 1998; NAKADA et al. 2000; ALKADHI et al. 2007). Using DECT, the chemical characterization of stones is possible based on their characteristic DE index. DE postprocessing software algorithms assume a mixture of water, calcium, and uric acid for every voxel and color codes voxels that show a DE behavior similar to calcium in blue and one that is similar to uric acid in red (Fig. 36.4). Voxels that show a linear density behavior at

both tube potentials remain grey. Using DECT differentiation of pure uric acid, mixed uric acid, and calcified stones is possible (GRASER ET AL. 2008). Furthermore, the differentiation of struvite and cystine is possible by adapting the slope of the three-material decomposition algorithm (GRASER ET AL. 2008).

In order to maintain a low radiation exposure, a standard NC low-dose MDCT scan of the entire abdomen and pelvis using a single-source technique (tube potential, 120 kV; collimation, 64 × 0.6 mm; reference mA, 40; dose modulation) can be utilized. Subsequently, a focal DE acquisition of the anatomical region containing the stone can be performed. Limiting the DE acquisition will substantially decrease radiation exposure. However, this approach requires the radiologist or trained technologist to evaluate the initial data set while the patient is still on the scanner in order to determine the presence and location of stones. Based on this assessment, a localized DE scan can be planned.

### 36.5.3
### DE Imaging of Hematuria

Another potential application for DECT is the evaluation of patients with hematuria. Hematuria may be

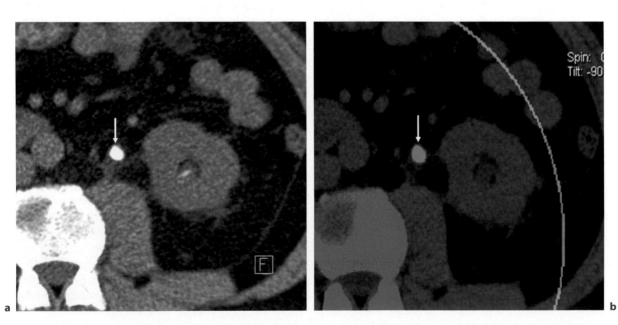

**Fig. 36.4a,b.** DECT to differentiate urinary renal stone composition. **a** Axial low-dose, single-energy NCCT image shows an 8-mm stone in the proximal ureter in a 45-year-old male with acute flank pain. **b** DECT in the same patient and same slice position. The color-coded display from the DE postprocessing workstation shows the composition of the stone (*arrow*). *Red* indicates that the calculus consists of uric acid

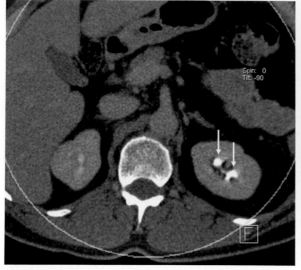
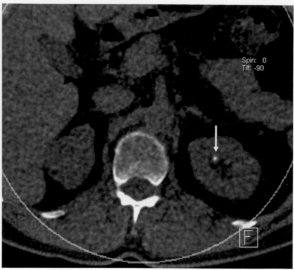

**Fig. 36.5a,b.** DECT for the evaluation of hematuria. **a** Axial weighted average DECT image in the urographic phase shows contrast agent in the left renal collecting system (*arrows*) in a 63-year-old male imaged for evaluation of hematuria. **b** In the same patient, VNC CT image at the same slice position identifies a 4-mm stone in the anterior left collecting system (*arrow*). The stone becomes visible only after subtraction of iodine from the image

caused by stone disease, renal or urothelial tumors, as well as a variety of other inflammatory conditions of the urinary tract. There is controversy on how to best image the patient with hematuria. While there is no radiation with MR, MR imaging has a major limitation in not being able to confidently depict stones. There are numerous CT protocols for evaluating hematuria, which usually include an NCCT, a nephrographic phase (100–120 s), and a urographic phase (5–7 min postinjection). While these three acquisitions are important when evaluating the patient with hematuria, the acquisition imparts a large radiation dose to the patient.

In order to minimize radiation exposure to the patient with hematuria, the number of acquisitions obtained after the administration of intravenous contrast can be reduced. As in CT of renal masses, DECT helps to reduce the number of acquisitions. If the DE acquisition is performed during the delayed urographic phase of enhancement, then excreted contrast agent can be electronically removed from the renal pelvis and ureters, thus allowing for evaluation of the presence of urinary stones that would otherwise be obscured by the dense contrast material (Fig. 36.5) (ALKADHI et al. 2007). Therefore an NCCT acquisition may be eliminated. Moreover, if a split-bolus technique is used, then a single contrast-enhanced acquisition yielding both nephrographic and urographic data (as well as virtual NCCT data) may be potentially all that is required to evaluate the patient with hematuria.

## 36.5.4
### DECT After Abdominal Aortic Aneurysm Repair

Traditionally, patients who undergo endovascular repair of abdominal aortic aneurysms (AAA) are evaluated using a multiphase CT protocol (MITA et al. 2000). NC, arterial-, and venous-phase acquisitions have been utilized for optimization of the detection of possible complications including endoleaks (ROZENBLIT et al. 2003). The possibility to eliminate the arterial phase without loss of diagnostic information with a dose saving of up to 36.5% of the total radiation has been shown feasible (MACARI et al. 2006). Using this protocol, an NCCT and acquisition are acquired. The NCCT typically cannot be omitted because it demonstrates calcifying thrombus in the lumen of the aneurysm. Without the NCCT data, differentiation of calcifying thrombus from an endoleak may be difficult or impossible. The typical appearance of an endoleak is a blush of contrast agent in the aneurysm sac. DECT can provide information about high-density material within the thrombosed lumen of the aneurysm by generating a virtual NCCT data set and can therefore potentially eliminate the standard NCCT acquisition. This can substantially reduce radiation exposure (Fig. 36.6). In addition, since the attenuation of iodine is greater at 80 than at 120/140 kVp, the possibility that small endoleaks will be easier seen at 80 kVp exists.

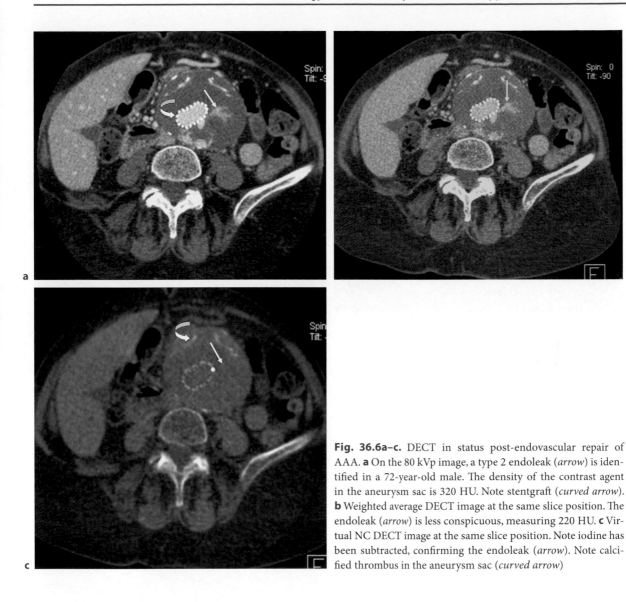

**Fig. 36.6a–c.** DECT in status post-endovascular repair of AAA. **a** On the 80 kVp image, a type 2 endoleak (*arrow*) is identified in a 72-year-old male. The density of the contrast agent in the aneurysm sac is 320 HU. Note stentgraft (*curved arrow*). **b** Weighted average DECT image at the same slice position. The endoleak (*arrow*) is less conspicuous, measuring 220 HU. **c** Virtual NC DECT image at the same slice position. Note iodine has been subtracted, confirming the endoleak (*arrow*). Note calcified thrombus in the aneurysm sac (*curved arrow*)

## 36.5.5
## DECT of Adrenal Adenomas

In up to 5% of patients undergoing contrast-enhanced abdominal CT, an incidental adrenal mass is discovered (KOROBKIN et al. 1996). In order to differentiate a lipid-rich adrenal adenomas from pheochromocytomas and other masses such as metastases, patients have to either undergo additional NCCT or chemical-shift MR imaging (ISRAEL et al. 2004). The diagnostic criterion at NCCT that is used to make the diagnosis of adrenal adenoma is low mean attenuation of the lesion <10–15 HU, which is caused by the presence of intracellular fat (ISRAEL et al. 2004). In cases with higher attenuation at NCCT, MRI utilizing opposed-phase imaging may be helpful in confirming the diagnosis of adenoma, since it appears to be somewhat more sensitive to the presence of intracytoplasmic fat (PROKESCH et al. 2002a). However, by acquiring abdominal CT with a DE acquisition, VNC CT data sets can be generated. If an adrenal mass is incidentally detected during contrast enhanced CT of the abdomen, then VNC data can be used to determine its density (Fig. 36.7). Currently, all patients who undergo adnominal CT on the DE scanner at our institution have routine virtual NCCT data sets sent to the PACS. This enables an assessment of both adrenal and renal masses incidentally discovered at CT.

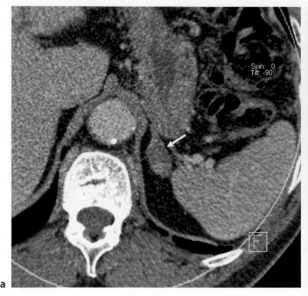

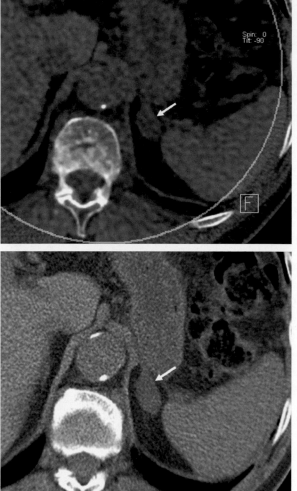

**Fig 36.7a–c.** DECT for adrenal mass characterization. **a** Axial weighted average DECT image in a 68-year-old male shows 2.1-cm solid mass (*arrow*) in left adrenal gland. The density of the mass is 45 HU. **b** Virtual noncontrast image at the same slice position shows the mass is hypoattenuating, measuring 5 HU (*arrow*). This is most consistent with an adrenal adenoma. **c** The true NC image at the same slice position confirms the low density of the mass (*arrow*), measuring 5 HU

## 36.5.6
## DECT of Pancreatic Tumors

Pancreatic adenocarcinoma typically appears as hypodense mass at CT. The low attenuation is primarily due to fibrosis and desmoplasia within the tumor. Dual-phase imaging of the pancreas performed during the pancreatic phase (approximately 40 s) and portovenous phases of enhancement at CT optimizes detection pancreatic neoplasms (PROKESCH et al. 2002a). The tumor usually appears more conspicuous during the pancreatic as opposed to the venous phase of enhancement because of the fibrosis and desmoplasia within the tumor.

In the setting of pancreatic adenocarcinoma, MDCT allows depiction of the tumor, visualization of the peripancreatic vessels, lymph nodes, and distant metastases, allowing for high accuracy in staging (PROKESCH et al. 2002b). However, occasionally it may be difficult to detect pancreatic adenocarcinoma even utilizing dual phase imaging. One study showed that in up to 11% of cases, pancreatic adenocarcinoma is isoattenuating to the surrounding parenchyma on both the pancreatic and the venous phases of the acquisition (PROKESCH et al. 2002a). Another study demonstrated that upon retrospective review, patients with proven pancreatic adenocarcinoma who had undergone prior CT had subtle findings at the initial CT that suggested the diagnosis

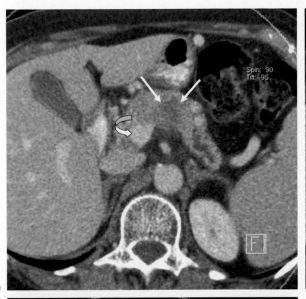

a

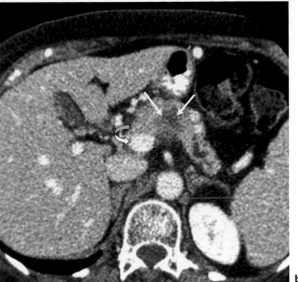

b

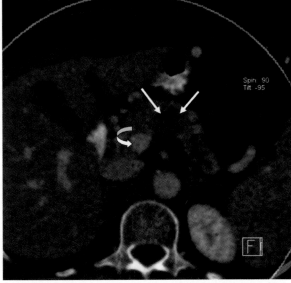

c

**Fig. 36.8a–c.** DECT in imaging of pancreatic masses. **a** Axial weighted average DECT image in a 72-year-old female patient shows marked dilatation of the pancreatic duct due to a 2.5 cm hypoattenuating mass (*arrow*). The mass measures 60 HU, the surrounding normal pancreatic parenchyma 89 HU. Note the superior mesenteric vein (SMV) (*curved arrow*). **b** An 80 kVp image from DECT scan at same slice position shows greater conspicuity of the mass (*arrows*) that measures 81 HU, while the density of the surrounding pancreas is 155 HU. Note increased density of SMV (*curved arrow*). **c** Color-coded DECT image at same slice position shows excellent delineation of the mass (*arrows*) and provides information on reduced iodine uptake. SMV (*curved arrow*)

(Gangi et al. 2004). In most cases the neoplasm was not seen, but a dilated pancreatic duct was present.

Since the normal pancreas enhances vividly during the pancreatic phase and contains much more iodine than a pancreatic adenocarcinoma, DE scanning may improve detection and allow a more accurate assessment of the size of the tumor compared with non-DE acquisitions. We have noted that pancreatic adenocarcinoma may be more conspicuous when viewed with low (80) kVp data sets than at 120 or 140 kVp (Fig. 36.8). This is related to the differences in the amount of iodine within these different tissues. These characteristics may prove to be helpful in the detection of tumors that show enhancement patterns similar to the normal paren-

chyma of the gland. The potential for dose reduction is also possible. Two separate acquisitions may no longer be needed if indeed tumor conspicuity is maintained during the portal venous phase of imaging when viewed at 80 kVp, thus potentially eliminating the need for the pancreatic phase of enhancement.

## 36.5.7
## DECT of the Small Bowel

CT enterography is performed with neutral oral contrast and a rapid bolus of intravenous contrast to facilitate imaging of the small bowel. It is utilized to visualize

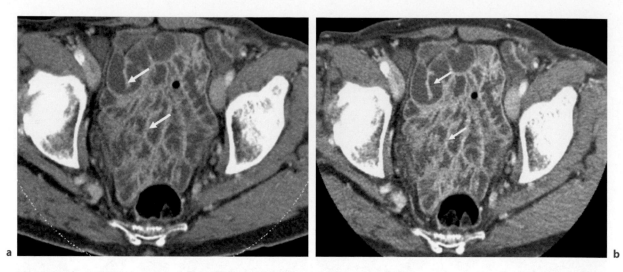

**Fig. 36.9a,b.** DECT in imaging of the small bowel. **a** Axial weighted average DECT image in 78-old-male shows normal small bowel mucosa (*arrows*) of the jejunum. **b** An 80-kV image at same slice position shows marked increase in attenuation of the mucosa (*arrows*) of the small bowel

various pathologic conditions affecting the small bowel including obscure gastrointestinal bleeding, Crohn's disease, and various inflammatory and ischemic conditions (Macari et al. 2007). Neutral oral contrast agents are used to distend the small bowel. After the administration of a rapid bolus of intravenous contrast the degree of enhancement and enhancement pattern is easily seen (Macari et al. 2007; Megibow et al. 2006). In the setting of Crohn's disease, increased enhancement of the bowel wall has been shown to correlate with the histologic degree of inflammation (Bodily et al. 2006). On standard CT images acquired at 120 kVp, it can be difficult to discriminate between physiological and abnormal enhancement of the small bowel wall. Since low-kVp images display greater density of contrast agent than do standard images, DECT might help to determine the presence of subtle inflammation when data are viewed at 80 kVp (Fig. 36.9). Similarly in patients with suspected small bowel ischemia, differences in enhancement between poorly perfused ischemic small bowel and adjacent normal segments may be accentuated.

## 36.6
## Limitations

Despite the numerous clinical opportunities that dual-source DECT allows, several important limitations exist. As previously stated, the B tube has a smaller FOV than does the standard FOV with the A tube. Moreover,

the very peripheral part of the FOV of the B tube cannot be utilized for DE postprocessing. Therefore, in large/wide patients, the periphery of the patient will not be included in the field. While this does not affect the overall image quality of the exam, it does affect the ability to exploit the benefits of DE in these regions.

This FOV limitation will not be a problem for the aorta, pancreas, adrenal glands, or small bowel. However, it may be problematic for some renal masses. As stated above, if a known renal mass is to be imaged, then the patient can be positioned eccentrically in the scanner to take advantage of the DE capabilities. In addition, the ability to tag fecal material with iodine and electronically remove it based on its iodine content by CT colonography will be of limited value in the ascending and descending colons since these segments are often out of the B detector FOV.

Eighty-peak-kilovoltage data sets inherently have more noise than images acquired at 120 or 140 kVp. As a result, DE acquisitions are ineffective in obese patients or patients with very large abdomens. Also related to the noise in the scan, data should not be acquired with the thinnest detector configuration. On the current scanner a detector configuration of 1.2 mm is used as opposed to 0.6 mm. For most abdominal applications, this is not a severe limitation, as data can be reconstructed at 1.2 mm thickness, allowing reasonable z-axis resolution for multiplanar reformatting and volume rendering. Finally, radiation dose to the patient theoretically can be increased using a DE acquisition. However, utilizing the protocol discussed earlier in this review a typical DECT scan of the abdomen results in an effective dose similar to a routine standard CT of the abdomen performed without a DE technique. Moreover, the potential to decrease the overall radiation exposure to patients by eliminating the routine acquisition of NCCT data is a major benefit of DECT.

## 36.7
## Conclusion

DECT has several potential applications in abdominal imaging. First, VNC CT data sets are useful in many ways. They can be use to assess for hepatic steatosis, determine baseline density measurements in renal and adrenal masses, and to differentiate calcium and iodine in patients status post AAA repair. Using DECT, the composition of various kidney stones is possible, thus aiding in treatment decisions. Low-kVp images from the B detector provide increased conspicuity of hypoattenuating masses in the pancreas, and color-coded images may aid in the detection of small tumors. Moreover, if tumor conspicuity is maintained during portovenous phase imaging, then the pancreatic phase may be eliminated thus reducing radiation exposure to patients. In addition, the low-80-kVp images may aid in visual assessment of small bowel enhancement and hence perfusion.

For all clinical applications, collimation should be 14 × 1.2 mm in order to avoid excess image noise. Careful patient positioning will greatly improve image quality and help to overcome technical limitations. Continued research with DECT will help to determine the optimal utilization and indications of this new technology.

## References

Alkadhi H et al. (2007) Dual-energy contrast-enhanced computed tomography for the detection of urinary stone disease. Invest Radiol 42:823–829

Birnbaum BA, Jacobs JE, Ramchandani P (1996) Multiphasic renal CT: comparison of renal mass enhancement during the corticomedullary and nephrographic phases. Radiology 200:753–758

Bodily KD, Fletcher JG, Solem CA et al. (2006) Crohn disease: mural attenuation and thickness at contrast-enhanced CT enterography—correlation with endoscopic and histologic findings of inflammation. Radiology 238:505–516

Boulay I, Holtz P, Foley WD, White B, Begun FP (1999) Ureteral calculi: diagnostic efficacy of helical CT and implications for treatment of patients. AJR Am J Roentgenol 172:1485–1490

Cann CE, Gamsu G, Birnberg FA, Webb WR (1982) Quantification of calcium in solitary pulmonary nodules using single- and DECT. Radiology 145:493–496

Chiro GD, Brooks RA, Kessler RM et al. (1979) Tissue signatures with dual-energy computed tomography. Radiology 131:521–523

Flohr TG, McCollough CH, Bruder H et al. (2006) First performance evaluation of a dual-source CT (DSCT) system. Eur Radiol 16:256–268

Gangi S, Fletcher JG, Nathan MA et al. (2004) Time interval between abnormalities seen on CT and the clinical diagnosis of pancreatic cancer: retrospective review of CT scans obtained before diagnosis. AJR Am J Roentgenol 182:897–903

Genant HK, Boyd D (1977) Quantitative bone mineral analysis using dual-energy computed tomography. Invest Radiol 12:545–551

Goldberg HI, Cann CE, Moss AA, Ohto M, Brito A, Federle M (1982) Noninvasive quantitation of liver iron in dogs with hemochromatosis using DECT scanning. Invest Radiol 17:375–380

Graser A (2008) DECT in the assessment of renal masses: can dual-energy virtually unenhanced images replace noncontrast scanning? Radiology (in press)

Graser A, Wintersperger BJ, Suess C, Reiser MF, Becker CR (2006) Dose reduction and image quality in MDCT colonography using tube current modulation. AJR Am J Roentgenol 187:695–701

Graser A, Johnson TR, Bader M et al. (2008) DECT characterization of urinary calculi: initial in vitro and clinical experience. Invest Radiol 43:112–119

Hillman BJ, Drach GW, Tracey P, Gaines JA (1984) Computed tomographic analysis of renal calculi. AJR Am J Roentgenol 142:549–552

Hounsfield GN (1995) Computerized transverse axial scanning (tomography): Part I. Description of system. Br J Radiol 68:H166–H172

Israel GM, Bosniak MA (2005) How I do it: evaluating renal masses. Radiology 236:441–450

Israel GM, Korobkin M, Wang C, Hecht EN, Krinsky GA (2004) Comparison of unenhanced CT and chemical shift MRI in evaluating lipid-rich adrenal adenomas. AJR Am J Roentgenol 183:215–219

Johnson TR, Nikolaou K, Wintersperger BJ et al. (2006) Dual-source CT cardiac imaging: initial experience. Eur Radiol 16:1409–1415

Johnson TR, Krauss B, Sedlmair M et al. (2007) Material differentiation by DECT: initial experience. Eur Radiol 17:1510–1517

Kluner C, Hein PA, Gralla O et al. (2006) Does ultra-low-dose CT with a radiation dose equivalent to that of KUB suffice to detect renal and ureteral calculi? J Comput Assist Tomogr 30:44–50

Korobkin M, Francis IR, Kloos RT, Dunnick NR (1996) The incidental adrenal mass. Radiol Clin North Am 34:1037–1054

Macari M, Chandarana H, Schmidt B, Lee J, Lamparello P, Babb J (2006) Abdominal aortic aneurysm: can the arterial phase at CT evaluation after endovascular repair be eliminated to reduce radiation dose? Radiology 241:908–914

Macari M, Megibow AJ, Balthazar EJ (2007) A pattern approach to the abnormal small bowel: observations at MDCT and CT enterography. AJR Am J Roentgenol 188:1344–1355

Megibow AJ, Babb JS, Hecht EM et al. (2006) Evaluation of bowel distention and bowel wall appearance by using neutral oral contrast agent for multidetector row CT. Radiology 238:87–95

Mita T, Arita T, Matsunaga N et al. (2000) Complications of endovascular repair for thoracic and abdominal aortic aneurysm: an imaging spectrum. Radiographics 20:1263–1278

Moe OW (2006) Kidney stones: pathophysiology and medical management. Lancet 367:333–344

Mostafavi MR, Ernst RD, Saltzman B (1998) Accurate determination of chemical composition of urinary calculi by spiral computerized tomography. J Urol 159:673–675

Nakada SY, Hoff DG, Attai S, Heisey D, Blankenbaker D, Pozniak M (2000) Determination of stone composition by noncontrast spiral computed tomography in the clinical setting. Urology 55:816–819

Park S (2007) Medical management of urinary stone disease. Expert Opin Pharmacother 8:1117–1125

Poletti PA, Platon A, Rutschmann OT, Schmidlin FR, Iselin CE, Becker CD (2007) Low-dose versus standard-dose CT protocol in patients with clinically suspected renal colic. AJR Am J Roentgenol 188:927–933

Prokesch RW, Chow LC, Beaulieu CF et al. (2002a) Local staging of pancreatic carcinoma with multidetector row CT: use of curved planar reformations initial experience. Radiology 225:759–765

Prokesch RW, Chow LC, Beaulieu CF, Bammer R, Jeffrey RB Jr (2002b) Isoattenuating pancreatic adenocarcinoma at multidetector row CT: secondary signs. Radiology 224:764–768

Rozenblit AM, Patlas M, Rosenbaum AT et al. (2003) Detection of endoleaks after endovascular repair of abdominal aortic aneurysm: value of unenhanced and delayed helical CT acquisitions. Radiology 227:426–433

Smith RC, Rosenfield AT, Choe KA et al. (1995) Acute flank pain: comparison of noncontrast-enhanced CT and intravenous urography. Radiology 194:789–794

Szolar DH, Kammerhuber F, Altziebler S et al. (1997) Multiphasic helical CT of the kidney: increased conspicuity for detection and characterization of small (< 3-cm) renal masses. Radiology 202:211–217

# Intervention

## 37

Christoph G. Trumm and Ralf-Thorsten Hoffmann

## CONTENTS

## ABSTRACT

CT-guided percutaneous biopsies are performed in patients with a known primary tumor, to rule out metastatic malignancy, to establish the final diagnosis, or to differentiate between tumor necrosis and potential vital tumor tissue in residual lesions after therapy. CT-guided aspiration, punch, and drill biopsy may be performed in essentially every organ system and location, and overall complication rates are low. Given an experienced operator, using repeated single-shot CT-fluoroscopic (CTF) acquisitions for needle positioning, in comparison to sequential CT guidance, CTF can markedly reduce both the in-room time and radiation dose for the patient. Improved availability and imaging quality of CT, modified techniques of percutaneous drainage, and more effective antibiotic regimens have made CT-guided drainage a common means for percutaneous therapy of abscesses and abnormal fluid collections, representing a dramatic improvement of patient care during the last 20 years. Primary and postoperative fluid collections in nearly every organ system and multiple locations can now be safely treated percutaneously. In a collective of severely ill patients, the instant postoperative detection and consecutive therapy of abscesses under CT guidance have resulted in reduced morbidity and mortality and have helped to reduce length of hospital stay and hospital costs.

C. G. Trumm, MD
Department of Clinical Radiology, Ludwig-Maximilians-University of Munich, University of Munich Hospitals, Marchioninistrasse 15, 81377 Munich, Germany

R.-T. Hoffmann
Department of Clinical Radiology, Ludwig-Maximilians-University of Munich, University of Munich Hospitals, Marchioninistrasse 15, 81377 Munich, Germany

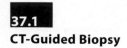

## CT-Guided Biopsy

### 37.1.1
### Introduction

Image-guided percutaneous biopsy using ultrasound (US) and CT is widely established as safe method for differentiation of benign and malignant masses while MR imaging was only introduced as guidance method in the mid-1990s. Most of the procedures are performed in patients with a known primary tumor, to rule out metastatic malignancy, to establish the final diagnosis, or to differentiate between tumor necrosis and potential vital tumor tissue in residual lesions after therapy. Success rates of an individual institution depend on the number of samples obtained, the size of the lesion, the organ in which the biopsy is performed, the experience of the local pathologist staff, the available imaging equipment and—first and foremost—the skills of the operator.

### 37.1.2
### Patient Preparation and Aftercare

Most image-guided biopsies can be performed on an outpatient basis. Informed patient consent including possible conscious sedation after detailed explanation of potential complications should be obtained at least 24 h before the intervention. A coagulation disorder should be ruled out by taking platelet levels (>50,000/mm³), partial thromboplastin time ([PTT] <50 s), prothrombin time ([PT] >50%) and international normalized ratio ([INR] ≤1.5) in all patients, especially if the lesion is located in the depth of the chest and abdomen. In case the patient has taken nonsteroidal anti-inflammatory drugs inhibiting platelet aggregation (e.g., acetylic salicylic acid), a core biopsy should be postponed by 7 days. In absence of any abnormalities regarding platelet levels, PTT, and PT, a fine-needle biopsy (≥20 G) may be performed because the risk of hemorrhage due to nonsteroidal anti-inflammatory drugs alone is low (Table 37.1) (CARDELLA et al. 2003).

The majority of CT-guided biopsies can be performed under local anesthesia. Children, incompliant adult patients, or biopsies of deep abdominal lesions (e.g., pancreatic masses) represent potential exceptions. In those selected cases, sufficient analgosedation can be reached by intravenous administration of benzodiazepines, e.g., midazolam (1 mg per dose; given in two to four doses) for anxiolysis and opioids, e.g., Fentanyl (0.02 mg per dose; given in one to five doses) for analgesia. If analgosedation is used, then the patient should be monitored during the whole procedure, using pulse oximetry. The nurse or radiology technician is responsible for keeping the patient compliant while the radiologist can concentrate on the procedure. Before the in-

**Table 37.1.** Contraindications for CT-guided biopsy

| Condition | Comment |
|---|---|
| Uncorrectable coagulation disorder | |
| Platelets are < 50,000/mm³ | Preprocedural platelet transfusion may be necessary |
| INR > 1.5 | Usually due to coumarins or liver disease; coumarin withdrawal takes a few days to reverse INR. INR can also be reversed by vitamin K or fresh frozen plasma |
| PT (quick) < 50% | |
| PTT > 50 s | Usually prolonged secondary to heparin or heparin-like drugs. These agents generally have short half lives and can be quickly reversed |
| Intake of platelet inhibitors < 24 h before the intervention | Clinical assessment should be made as to whether to proceed or reschedule the biopsy |
| Massive ascites | |
| Adiposity in combination with small cirrhotic liver (transjugular or surgical biopsy recommended) | |
| Incompliant patients | |
| Absence of a safe pathway from the skin to the target site | |

tervention, the patient should be placed in a stable and comfortable position. Depending on the lesion location supine, prone, or lateral decubitus position are most commonly used.

For correlation, pre-, peri-, and postinterventional CT or MR images should be obtained in the same position during the respiratory cycle, preferably during expiration. Preparation of the skin area overlying the entry point of the biopsy needle includes shaving (if necessary), sterile draping, and skin disinfection.

After CT-guided biopsy, patients are kept in the ward with vital signs observed every 15 min for 1 h. In high-risk patients, observation can be continued beyond this time, for example, with checking of vital signs every 30 min for 3 h. After lung biopsy, the patient should lie with the puncture site down for 2 h. The two pleural layers are compressed by the weight of the lung itself, and further air leakage through the pleural defect is minimized. Chest radiographs (posteroanterior) are obtained 2 and 4 h after the intervention, to rule out delayed pneumothorax. If the chest radiograph in erect position after 2 h shows a small pneumothorax, then a further chest X-ray should be obtained after 4 h. In cases of pneumothorax and patient symptoms, air aspiration or a chest tube should be inserted for treatment.

### 37.1.3
### Sequential and CTF Guidance

CT as guiding method is especially suitable for lesions located deep under the skin surface that are not or not easily depictable via US (e.g., deep retroperitoneal, pelvic, and thoracic lesions). With some exceptions, such as liver lesions isodense to normal parenchyma in the nonenhanced CT scan, CT usually provides excellent visualization of the target lesion for biopsy, and differentiation from adjacent organs. It is generally preferable not to schedule a biopsy procedure at the same time as the first diagnostic scan. If available, recent outside films not older than 2 weeks or a separate preceding diagnostic study should be used for selection of target lesions for biopsy and planning of the access pathway. Two different techniques of CT guidance can be utilized.

**Sequential CT guidance.** For planning of the access route, a CT scan of the region of interest is performed first. The preliminary scan can be performed without contrast, if a recent diagnostic study is available and the lesion is easily visible. In the chest, a nonenhanced CT scan ($\leq$3-mm slice thickness) is also sufficient for detection of intrapulmonary lesions suitable for aspira-

tion or punch biopsy. For suspect masses in the mediastinum and abdomen (intra- and retroperitoneal), a contrast-enhanced CT scan is necessary for clear differentiation of parenchymal organs, intestines, and blood vessels. Focal lesions within parenchymal organs are usually visualized during venous phase (scan delay: 50–70 s). An additional arterial phase (scan delay: ~30 s) scan should be obtained if arteries are present along the access path (e.g., parasternal access: internal mammary artery) and in hypervascularized lesions (e.g., hepatocellular carcinoma, metastases of renal cell carcinoma).

For defining the skin entry point of the biopsy needle, a radiopaque grid is placed on the skin of the patient. The patient is positioned in the prone, supine, or lateral decubitus position, depending on the shortest distance from the skin surface to the lesion. Then the CT scan is performed covering the region of interest. Grid systems are either commercially available or a homemade grid of several 4- to 5-French catheters that are cut into a length of 15–30 cm, and taped together at intervals of 1 cm, can be used. After the planning CT scan (with the grid system taped on the skin of the patient) has been performed, the slice position showing both the lesion and the potential in-plane access route, or the intended needle entry point only (double-oblique access), is chosen. The distance from the skin level of the needle entry point to the lesion is measured. The CT table is moved to the position of choice for biopsy, and the needle entry point can be marked with a felt pen, using the grid as well as the centering laser light beam.

After skin disinfection, local anesthesia using 10–20 ml of 1–2% lidocaine hydrochloride is applied in the subcutaneous fat and down to the capsule of parenchymal organs (e.g., the liver) or down to the periosteum of bones, using a 22-G needle that additionally marks the entry point and intended angle of the biopsy needle. After a small skin incision with a scalpel and CT rescanning with the local anesthesia needle in the skin entry point to confirm the correct position, the biopsy needle is inserted parallel to the local anesthesia needle. Thereafter repeated CT scans covering a short range above and below the needle entry point (e.g., 3–5 cm along the z-axis) are performed, and the angulation of the needle is adapted to interfering anatomical structures if necessary. The use of multislice spiral CT (MSCT) with its inherent ability to simultaneously acquire several sections is beneficial for this purpose, as it omits the need for multiple scans above and below the needle entry point. The direction of the needle in relation to the lesion can be easily detected using the streak artifact at the needle tip. Finally, the needle is inserted into the edge of the lesion for tissue sampling.

**CTF guidance.** Since the introduction of CTF with faster image reconstruction on MSCT scanners, real-time visualization nearly comparable to US is available. Cross-sectional CT images are reconstructed at reduced spatial resolution and updated continually at a rate of up to 10 frames per second by using a high-speed array processor (Carlson et al. 2001). In contrast to the grid-based technique using repeated nonenhanced CT scans covering the volume of interest, the needle is visualized on an in-room monitor. The operator can dynamically adjust the needle position under single-shot or continuous CTF until the lesion is reached. The main advantages are a substantial reduction of in-room time for both the patient and the operator, and real-time visualization of critical anatomical structures along the trajectory like vessels during needle insertion. This technique is particularly helpful in cases of incompliant patients who are unable to cooperate, e.g., to hold their breath, or in regions with persistent motion, as may be found close to the heart and diaphragm. In contrast to conventional CT guidance, the main disadvantage is a radiation exposure of the operator (Silverman et al. 1999). The use of a grab handle for holding the needle helps to avoid the direct exposure of the operator's hand to the radiation beam during CTF. As important advantages of this technique, patient absorbed radiation dose and in-room time can be significantly reduced by 94 and 32%, respectively (Carlson et al. 2001).

## 37.1.4
## CT-Guided Aspiration Biopsy

Percutaneous fine-needle aspiration biopsy (FNAB) is a well-established method to obtain an aspirate with a thin needle (≥20 G), which usually provides enough material to confirm or rule out malignancy by cytologic analysis. In most cases, a histological diagnosis is not possible due to an insufficient amount of material.

### 37.1.4.1
### Indications

FNAB is suitable for tissue sampling of pulmonary lesions as well as neck lesions (e.g., lymph nodes) and abdominal lesions, given a known primary tumor in combination with suspected metastases of the liver, lymph nodes, etc. In abdominal lesions, FNAB is preferable where a direct access is precluded by surrounding organs. It is generally considered insufficient if the primary tumor is unknown.

### 37.1.4.2
### Materials

FNABs are performed with 20- to 25-G needles (small gauge) including various commercially available needle types and needle tip designs. The needle tip is either sharp beveled (e.g., Chiba or spinal needle) or cutting (Turner needle: 45° bevel tip with cutting edge; Franseen needle: three-pronged needle tip; Westcott needle: slotted side opening proximal to the needle tip; E-Z-EM needle: trough cut in the needle tip) (Lee 2004; Fig. 37.1). Coaxial biopsy sets consist of an outer guide needle in combination with a smaller aspiration needle. Typical needle combinations for coaxial FNAB are 23/20- or 22/19-G sets (Table 37.2).

### 37.1.4.3
### Technique

#### 37.1.4.3.1
#### General Considerations

FNAB can be performed by solely using the fine needle, applying a coaxial approach, or using a tandem technique. The first technique is characterized by the straightforward puncture of the target lesion. This technique has some disadvantages including limited controllability. The coaxial technique is characterized by a combination of two needles. A thicker, shorter needle is inserted down to the anterior edge of the lesion. Then a thinner, longer needle is introduced through the first needle. Multiple samples can be taken using the thinner needle without several punctures. If necessary, the larger needle can be pulled back and its angle changed

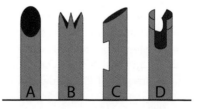

**Fig. 37.1.** The most common fine needle types: Turner (*A*), Franseen (*B*), Westcott (*C*), and E-Z-EM (*D*) needle. The Turner needle is characterized by a 45° bevel with a cutting edge. The Franseen needle has a three-pronged tip. The Westcott needle contains a side-cutting trough close to its tip. The E-Z-EM needle shows a trough cut within the needle tip (schematic according to Lee 2004)

**Table 37.2.** Commercially available needles for CT-guided aspiration biopsy (exemplary selection of different manufacturers and needles)

| Needle type (manufacturer) | Diameter (gauge) | Length (cm)[a] |
|---|---|---|
| Chiba (Boston Scientific, Natick, Mass., USA) | 22 | 6, 8 |
| Franseen (Boston Scientific) | 18, 20, 22 | 6, 8 |
| Coaxial lung biopsy set, Greene type (Boston Scientific) | 22 | 6 |
| Chiba (Cook Medical, Bloomington, Ind., USA) | 18–23, 25 | 5, 10, 15, 20 |
| Spinal needles (Cook Medical) | 18, 20, 22 | 10, 15 |
| CHIBA-NEEDLE-ULTRA (Somatex, Teltow, Germany) | 19.5, 22 | 9, 12, 15, 22, 28 |
| Chiba (E-Z-EM, Lake Success, N.Y., USA) | 18, 20, 22 | 10, 15, 20 |
| PercuCut cut-biopsy needle with keyhole cutting edge (E-Z-EM) | 18, 19.5, 21 | 5, 10, 15 |

[a]Not all diameter-length combinations may be available

in order to reach different areas of the lesion. With the tandem technique, first a single reference needle is introduced into the lesion. Then further needles are introduced in tandem, i.e., parallel to the first needle, without having to guide them separately.

After measuring the appropriate needle length in the planning scan, preparation of the chosen entry site, and local anesthesia, the fine needle is inserted to the lesion under image control, i.e., repeated nonenhanced short CT scans or CTF sequences triggered by the operator. As soon as the needle has been introduced into the lesion, the trocar is removed and a 10- or 20-ml Luer-Lok syringe is connected to the proximal end of the needle, and suction is applied. The aspirated volume ranges between 3 and 5 ml for most biopsies, and should be reduced (1–2 ml) in hypervascularized lesions in order to avoid aspiration of larger amounts of blood. During application of suction, the needle is moved back and forth within the lesion for 10–15 s, or until the hub of the syringe fills with blood. Before removing the needle from the lesion, the suction is stopped in order to avoid aspiration of further tissue, potentially confusing cytologic evaluation of the sample.

If a cytopathologist is in the room during the biopsy procedure, then he or she can give an initial statement if the tissue sample is sufficient for evaluation, or if further samples have to be taken. Otherwise, the aspirated material is spread on a glass slide and immediately fixated with alcohol. An additional blood clot should be ob-

tained and fixated in formalin, as this will significantly increase sensitivity for malignancy (WILDBERGER et al. 2003).

### 37.1.4.3.2
### Special Considerations

**Lung.** The advantages of CT-guided lung biopsy are that the lung parenchyma and not inflated areas at the puncture site are visualized, which can be used as access path to the lesion, substantially reducing the risk of pneumothorax. Local anesthesia is applied subcutaneously. Then a coaxial needle can be inserted through the parietal pleura under suspended respiration. The operator can adjust the needle direction by withdrawing the coaxial needle to the periphery of the lung (without removing the needle outside the pleura). If the coaxial technique is used, then the outer coaxial needle is inserted 2–3 mm into the edge of the lesion, providing stability during coaxial biopsies. Then the inner biopsy needle is introduced and at least two samples obtained (Fig. 37.2).

**Mediastinum.** Biopsies in the mediastinum have to be performed with special respect to vascular structures (Fig. 37.3). For planning of the biopsy procedure, a contrast-enhanced CT is performed in order to rule out vascular abnormalities like aneurysms, and to visualize

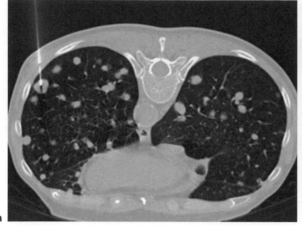

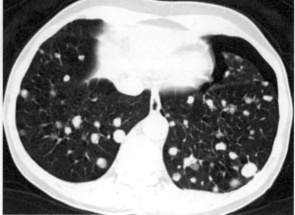

**Fig. 37.2a,b.** Patient (prone position) with multiple lung metastases. A subpleural nodule in the left lower lobe was chosen for aspiration biopsy under CT-fluoroscopic guidance with a 19-G (10 cm) needle (**a**). Postinterventional CT (supine position) showed a small pneumothorax that did not require therapy after further follow-up with X-ray (**b**). Cytology revealed pulmonary metastases of an adenocarcinoma (sigmoid colon)

the mediastinal vessels. For sampling lesions in the anterior mediastinum, an anterior parasternal approach is usually chosen. The internal mammary artery and vein that are located approximately 1 cm beside the sternum have to be avoided. Additionally, the access path through the mediastinal fat can be widened by injection of sterile saline through a 22-G needle. When the lesion is located in the posterior mediastinum, the paravertebral space can also be distended using sterile saline.

**Liver.** Depending on the experience of the operator and availability of an interventional CT unit, the majority of liver biopsies can also be performed under US guidance. If lesions in the dome of the liver cannot be visualized with US, then a CT/CTF-guided (double) oblique approach may be preferable (crossing the costophrenic sulcus should be avoided). Gantry angulation may help to access high liver lesions. Before introducing the bi-

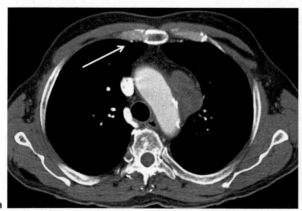

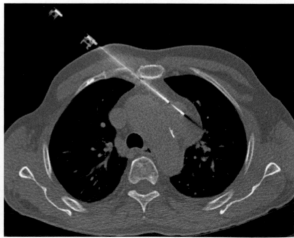

**Fig. 37.3a,b.** Patient (supine position) with a para-aortal mass in the upper mediastinum. The preinterventional CT (arterial phase) showed the right internal mammary artery and vein (*arrow*) next to the sternum (**a**). First sterile saline was injected with a 22-G needle for widening of the parasternal space. Then an 18-G (13 cm) Tru-Cut biopsy needle was introduced under CTF guidance. Note the typical black streak artifact along the needle pathway (**b**). Histopathology revealed a mesenchymal tumor

opsy needle into the liver parenchyma, the capsule has to be infiltrated with local anesthetic. During penetration of the liver capsule, the patient should be asked not to breathe. Passing normal liver tissue before entering the lesion reduces the risk of relevant subcapsular or intraparenchymal bleeding occurring after the puncture due to self-tamponade. The sample should normally be taken from the edge of the liver mass where the vital tumor tissue is located (Fig. 37.4).

**Pancreas.** Typically, the pancreas is surrounded by various organs like the stomach, liver, transverse colon, kidney, or major vessels. In particular, needle biopsy of small suspect masses in the pancreatic head is therefore usually regarded as technically sophisticated, and CT guidance preferred instead of ultrasound (Fig. 37.5). For differentiation of the tumor from surrounding normal parenchyma or inflammation, a contrast-enhanced CT scan obtained in an arterial phase should generally be performed prior to the intervention. The most common access route is from an anterior approach and often

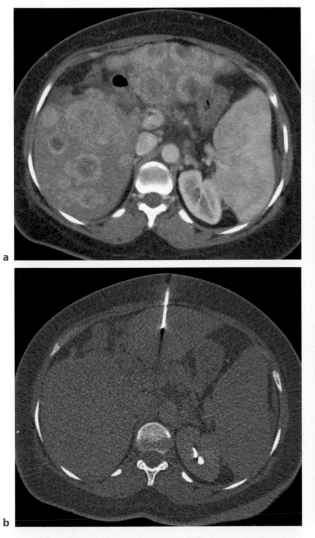

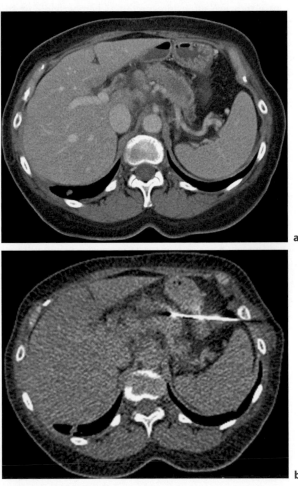

**Fig. 37.4a,b.** Patient (supine position) with multiple hepatic rim–enhancing lesions in both liver lobes (preinterventional CT, venous phase) (**a**). An easy-to-access lesion in segment 3 was chosen for Tru-Cut biopsy with a 16-G (10 cm) needle under CTF guidance (**b**). Histopathology revealed hepatic metastases of gall bladder carcinoma

**Fig. 37.5a,b.** Patient (supine position) with suspect pancreatic mass and pulmonary metastases. Preinterventional CT (venous phase) showed a hypodense area in the pancreatic body and tail (**a**). An intercostal left lateral access path between the spleen and the smaller gastric curvature was chosen for Tru-Cut biopsy with an 18-G (13 cm) needle under CTF guidance (**b**). Histopathology revealed a pancreatic adenocarcinoma

traverses gastrointestinal structures and the mesenteric vessels increasing the general risk of the procedure. In difficult-to-access lesions, the stomach or the small intestines may be punctured with a 20- to 22-G needle. Given an immunocompetent patient, FNAB traversing the GI tract or the liver has been shown to be technically acceptable in many studies (BRANDT et al. 1993; ELVIN et al. 1990; LÜNING et al. 1985; MUELLER 1993). The colon should generally not be penetrated, even with a small-gauge needle in order to avoid superinfection, especially if cystic pancreatic lesions containing fluid are sampled (MUELLER 1993). Transhepatic, transsplenic, and para-/transcaval approaches have also been described (BRANDT et al. 1993).

**Kidney.** Biopsies of the kidney are rarely performed because they are often interpreted as hemorrhagic or inconclusive, and most solid renal masses are surgically removed. Exceptional indications for biopsy are suggested lymphoma and metastasis to the kidney from another primary tumor, since these conditions are usually not treated surgically. The usual access route under CT guidance is posterior or lateral while the renal hilum should be avoided.

**Adrenal Glands.** Due to the anatomic localization in the upper retroperitoneum, the access path for biopsy is relatively sophisticated while several approaches are possible:

- The right lateral transhepatic approach (right adrenal gland: through right liver lobe, supine position)
- The left anterior transhepatic approach (left adrenal gland: through left liver lobe, supine position)
- The angled prone approach (both adrenals: subcostal approach in a 45° angle, prone position)
- The lateral decubitus approach (the patient side with the adrenal lesion is placed next to the table preventing full expansion of the ipsilateral pulmonary recesasus while the overlying lung is fully expanded).

**Retroperitoneum.** Biopsies of retroperitoneal lesions are usually performed under CT guidance. With the most common posterior approach, the needle passes through or parallel to the psoas muscle (Fig. 37.6). Small-gauge needles are only necessary using an anterior approach.

**Pelvic Lesions.** While transrectal and transvaginal biopsies are routinely guided using ultrasound, the access routes for CT-guided biopsy in the pelvis include:

- The transgluteal approach through the greater sciatic foramen

- The presacral approach through the gluteal cleft
- The anterior approach (Fig. 37.7).

For the transgluteal approach, the patient is placed in prone position. The needle is introduced from the buttock through the greater sciatic foramen into the deep pelvis as close to the coccygeal bone as possible in order to avoid puncture of the sciatic nerve.

### 37.1.4.4
### Results

#### 37.1.4.4.1
#### Lung

In pulmonary lesions, FNAB has been reported to have diagnostic accuracy and sensitivity rates of more than 93% (SWISCHUK et al. 1998) and 95% (KLEIN et al. 1996; LAURENT et al. 2000), respectively. While several authors reported accuracy rates of less than 75% for lesions 1 cm or smaller (LI et al. 1996; TSUKADA et al. 2000; vanSONNENBERG and CASOLA 1988), respiratory gating (TOMIYAMA et al. 2000) and CTF (IRIE et al. 2001) have contributed to improve success rates. The study of IRIE et al. (2001) showed a reduction of procedure time using CTF ($n$ = 79 biopsies with 29 lesions <1.5 cm), while accuracy was not improved for the subset of patients with lesions ≤1 cm.

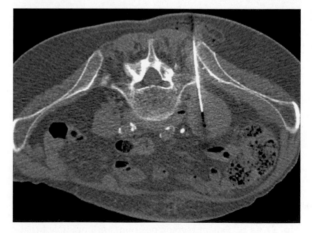

**Fig. 37.6.** Patient (prone position) with suspect mass of the right psoas muscle. A posterior paravertebral (5th lumbar vertebra) access was chosen for Tru-Cut biopsy with an 18-G (13 cm) needle under CTF guidance. Histopathology revealed metastasis of ovarian carcinoma

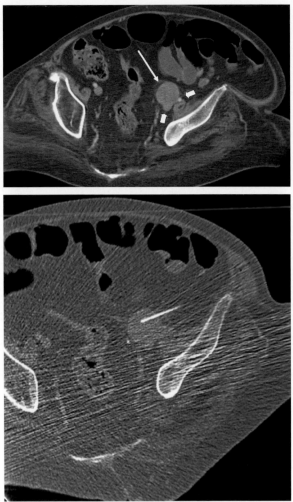

**Fig. 37.7a,b.** Patient (supine position) with a history of diffuse large B-cell lymphoma (DLCL). Preinterventional CT showed a moderately enhancing nodule (*large arrow*) next to the iliac vessels (*small arrows*) (**a**). The 18-G (13 cm) Tru-Cut biopsy needle was introduced under CTF guidance next to the left iliac crest through the peritoneal fat (**b**). Histopathology revealed recurrence of DLCL

### 37.1.4.4.2
### Mediastinum

In 89 patients undergoing CT-guided mediastinal FNAB for lung cancer staging (50, with 39 without core biopsy of lymph nodes >1.5-cm short-axis diameter) before mediastinoscopy, ZWISCHENBERGER et al. (2002) reported diagnostic success (cancer cell type, sarcoidosis, or caseating granulomas) in 78% of the cases, while only in 9 patients lymph nodes (paraesophageal, pulmonary ligament, parasternal, and para-aortic) could not be accessed.

### 37.1.4.4.3
### Liver

FNAB in the abdomen with both US and CT guidance has been described as safe and technically successful procedure by several authors (FERRUCCI et al. 1980; MEMEL et al. 1996; SMITH 1991; WELCH et al. 1989). CT-guided FNAB of liver lesions has been reported to have sensitivity rates of 92% and specificity rates of 96% (LÜNING et al. 1984).

### 37.1.4.4.4
### Kidney

Most renal masses can be characterized with high accuracy by noninvasive imaging alone, and a solid non-fat-containing or complex renal mass should be considered a renal cell carcinoma until proven otherwise. Metastases to the kidney are usually small and multifocal or perinephric. Lymphomatous involvement of the kidneys also usually occurs in the setting of disseminated disease and is characterized by typical CT patterns like multiple small masses, spread from retroperitoneal disease, diffuse infiltration, and perinephric encasement. In a study by LECHEVALLIER et al. (2000), CT-guided renal biopsy of 63 patients had an overall accuracy of 89%. Biopsy material was not sufficient for analysis in 15 patients (21%). Unsuccessful biopsy was related to lesion size: biopsy was unsuccessful in 11 of 30 tumors (37%) of 3 cm or less, versus 4 of 43 (9%) of tumors greater than 3 cm.

### 37.1.4.4.5
### Adrenal Glands

Incidentally discovered adrenal masses (incidentalomas) are relatively frequent. Adrenal incidentalomas exceeding 1 cm in size are found in 1–5% of the patients undergoing chest or abdominal CT for unrelated reasons. The risk of malignancy in patients with nonfunctioning adrenal masses is between 3.5 and 34% (LUMACHI et al. 2001). Since the development of dedicated MRI imaging techniques for differentiation of adrenal masses, adrenal biopsy is performed only in exceptional cases, and benign adrenocortical nodules are the most common lesion to be found with FNAB (>40%). LUMACHI et al. (2003) performed a study in order to compare the usefulness of FNAB cytology, CT, and MR imaging in patients with nonfunctioning adrenal masses. Including 34 patients with adrenal masses incidentally discovered in a CT scan, the authors found a sensitivity and specificity of 100% for the combination of both MR imaging and FNAB. The authors recommended performing image-guided FNAB in all patients with non-functioning adrenal masses of 2 cm or more in size.

#### 37.1.4.4.6
#### Retroperitoneum and Pelvis

Nahar Saikia et al. (2002) performed 242 aspiration biopsies of deep-seated thoracic, abdominal, and retroperitoneal lymph nodes under US (*n* = 216) and CT (*n* = 26) guidance, respectively. Diagnostic accuracy rate was 86%.

### 37.1.4.5
### Complications

In the lung, apart from pneumothorax (16–44.6%) and consecutive thoracostomy tube insertion, complication rates for image-guided FNAB are low (Laurent et al. 2000; Swischuk et al. 1998; vanSonnenberg et al. 1988). Factors increasing the risk of pneumothorax are a small lesion size (Cox et al. 1999; Fish et al. 1988; Kazerooni et al. 1996), an increasing depth of the lesion, several passes through the pleura, and an underlying pulmonary disease (Poe et al. 1984; Quon et al. 1988). Pulmonary hemorrhage and hemoptysis are observed in up to 1.4 and 1.7% of the procedures, respectively (Arslan et al. 2002). Air embolism is also a rare complication of thoracic FNAB, resulting from a direct communication between a pulmonary vein and atmospheric air. The patient should receive 100% oxygen and lie in the left lateral decubitus position with the head down in order to prevent cerebral embolism.

Complication rates of FNAB in the abdomen are very low. In the meta-analysis including literature data and results of questionnaires distributed in North American and European hospitals in the 1980s, Smith (1991) found mortality rates between 0.006% (63,108 biopsies) and 0.031% (16,381 biopsies) in the United States, and between 0.008 and 0.018% in European hospitals. Leading causes of death reported in Europe (*n* = 33) were hemorrhage after liver biopsy (17/21) and pancreatitis after pancreas biopsy (5/6). Frequency of needle tract seeding was in a range between 0.003 and 0.009% in the four questionnaires. In hepatocellular carcinoma, given a high positive predictive value of suspicious imaging findings alone (Torzilli et al. 1999), percutaneous biopsy has a limited role. Common

risks include intraperitoneal bleeding and needle-tract tumor implantation. As far as vascular structures are concerned, many studies have shown that the transgression of vessels, especially low-pressure veins, does not significantly elevate the complication rate (Ferrucci et al. 1980; Smith 1991; Welch et al. 1989).

### 37.1.4.6
### Key Points

- Histopathologic analysis is not possible.
- Suitable technique in patients with a known primary tumor.
- Needle diameter 20–25 G with standard needle lengths of 5–20 cm.
- Needle should be introduced in coaxial or tandem technique.
- Cytologic sample obtained through back-and-forth movement of needle within lesion under manual aspiration.
- Sampling of hypervascularized lesions without aspiration.
- Transgression of bowels possible if direct access to lesion is precluded.

### 37.1.5
### CT-Guided Punch Biopsy

In comparison to aspiration biopsy, the punch biopsy (synonymous with *core biopsy*) technique is performed either with spring-activated cutting needles (Tru-Cut) in combination with a biopsy gun or with manually activated cutting needles. This technique allows for obtaining cores of tissue with an intact histological structure that facilitates a precise histological diagnosis or immunohistochemical analysis.

### 37.1.5.1
### Indications

Large-gauge automated needle biopsies (14–19 G) are traditionally performed in patients without a known primary tumor, in cases of potential lymphoma, and after inconclusive FNAB. Due to the varying availability of a cytopathologist and results that are comparable to FNAB (or even better), in most radiological departments punch biopsy has meanwhile been established as the primary technique of choice.

### 37.1.5.2
### Materials

In comparison to the aspiration technique, core-biopsy needles are defined by diameters of 14–19 G (large gauge), and usually by the combination with a spring-activated Tru-Cut system. The Tru-Cut biopsy needle is characterized by a trough at the distal end. First, the biopsy gun fires the inner needle into the lesion, and a core of tissue falls into the trough. Then, the outer needle cuts the sample lying in the trough out of the surrounding tissue and captures the sample, which can be safely removed through the outer needle or with the whole system (Fig. 37.8). When an automated Tru-Cut system is used for biopsy, the localization of the needle tip next to the lesion should be documented before taking the sample. Usually at least two samples are taken for histological evaluation and instantly put into 10% formalin. Different manufacturers offer either disposable all-in-one systems, or the combination of disposable biopsy needles of various diameters and lengths (up to 30 cm) with a standard multi-use gun (Table 37.3). The main advantage is cost reduction. With respect to histopathological evaluation, the advantages of the core biopsy system are that the amount of obtained tissue is more or less constant while the sample keeps its histological structure. In contrast to manually handled large-gauge biopsy systems, the automated mechanism ensures a

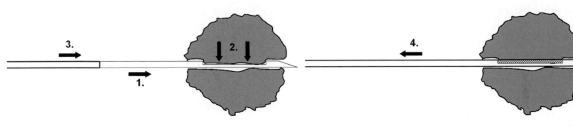

**Fig. 37.8.** Schematic fig. illustrating the automated Tru-Cut biopsy technique: The inner needle (characterized by a trough at its end) is fired into the target lesion by the biopsy gun (*1*). A core of tissue falls into the trough (*2*). The outer needle slides across the trough and thereby cuts out the specimen (*3*). Finally, the specimen can be safely removed with the inner needle or with the whole system (*4*)

**Table 37.3.** Commercially available needles for CT-guided punch biopsy (exemplary selection of different manufacturers and needles)

| Needle type (manufacturer) | Diameter (G) | Length (cm)[a] |
|---|---|---|
| Tru-Cut manual biopsy needle (Allegiance, McGaw Park, Ill., USA) | 14, 18 | 7, 11, 15 |
| Temno semiautomated biopsy system, adjustable cutting length (Allegiance)[b] | 14–22 | 6, 9, 11, 15, 20, 48 |
| PercuCut self-aspirating type cut needle (E-Z-EM) | 18, 19.5, 21 | 5, 10, 15 |
| Easy Core automated biopsy system (Boston Scientific) | 15, 18, 20 | 10, 15, 21, 25 |
| Magnum reusable core biopsy gun with disposable biopsy needles (Bard Biopsy, Tempe, Ariz., USA)[b] | 12–20 | 10, 13, 16, 20, 25, 30 |
| Max Core disposable automated biopsy needle (Bard Biopsy) | 14, 16, 18, 20 | 10, 16, 20, 25 |
| Monopty disposable core biopsy system (Bard Biopsy) | 12, 14, 16, 18, 20 | 10, 16, 20 |
| Quick Core automated biopsy needle with spring (Cook Medical)[b] | 14, 16, 18, 19, 20 | 6, 9, 15, 20 |
| Biopsy-Handy (Somatex)[b] | 14–20 | 10, 15, 20 |
| Semiautomated biopsy device SABD (Pflugbeil, Zorneding, Germany) | 14–21 | 11.5, 15, 20 |

[a]Not all diameter-length combinations may be available

[b]Coaxial needles available

quick procedure with the biopsy needle in the patient only for a short period.

### 37.1.5.3
### Technique

Before introduction of the biopsy needle, local anesthesia is applied with a 22-G needle. In children, the elderly, and anxious patients, intravenous anxiolysis and sedation may be used. During the intervention, cardiorespiratory monitoring is needed in case of conscious sedation. After local anesthesia, a small skin incision is made at the intended needle entry point. The rest of the puncture procedure is performed in an identical manner as described in Sect. 37.1.4.3.

### 37.1.5.4
### Results

#### 37.1.5.4.1
#### Lung

ANDERSON et al. (2003) performed a study to determine diagnostic accuracy comparing fine-needle aspiration with core biopsies of 195 pulmonary lesions in 182 patients, and found a significantly higher diagnostic yield of the core biopsy technique (93%) compared with FNAB (78%). The authors concluded that core biopsy should be the method of choice, especially if a dedicated cytopathologist is not available.

#### 37.1.5.4.2
#### Abdomen

In contrast to FNAB, histological classification of liver masses is only possible with larger core-biopsy systems in most cases, as true-positive findings increase from 84 to 98% (PAGANI 1983). Regarding the ability to differentiate samples obtained with either 14- or 18-G needles, no significant difference was found between both large-gauge needle types (HAAGE et al. 1999). Automated cutting needles have additionally contributed to increase the accuracy of the histological sample (HOPPER et al. 1993). In case of poor visualization of liver lesions in the nonenhanced CT scan, correlation between the liver lesion and anatomical landmarks can be used for verifying the correct position of the biopsy needle. In addition, interventional MR imaging has the potential to reveal lesions that are poorly visible in CT and US, providing results comparable to

CT guidance: 87–94% sensitivity, 90–100% specificity, and 85–93% accuracy (SALOMONOWITZ 2001; ZANGOS et al. 2003).

For CT-guided core biopsies conducted in intra-abdominal organs (liver, pancreas) the study by WUTKE et al. (2001) showed sensitivity, specificity, and accuracy values of 88.4, 100, and 90.4%, respectively.

#### 37.1.5.4.3
#### Retroperitoneum and Pelvis

In their analysis of 180 CT-guided coaxial core biopsies, WUTKE et al. (2001) reported markedly higher diagnostic utility rates for non-organ related retroperitoneal (88%) than liver and pancreatic lesions (66%). Overall sensitivity, specificity, and accuracy rates were 91.1, 100, and 93.3%, respectively (WUTKE et al. 2001).

### 37.1.5.5
### Complications

The study of ANDERSON et al. (2003) (see Sect. 37.1.5.4.) showed an initial pneumothorax rate after the biopsy of 30%, which was reduced to 18% after a 4-h follow-up. Only 2% of the patients developed clinical symptoms requiring further therapy with a chest tube. Separated pneumothorax rates according to the biopsy technique were 35% (FNAB) and 16% (core biopsy), respectively.

In a large retrospective multicenter study by PICCININO et al. (1986) including 68,276 liver biopsies with a Tru-Cut system, a complication rate of only 0.4% was found. Deaths after liver biopsy were rarely observed, usually due to hemoperitoneum in patients with malignant disease or cirrhosis. The rate of tumor cell seeding after percutaneous tumor puncture of hepatocellular carcinoma (HCC) has been reported to be in the range between 1% (LLOVET et al. 2001) and 5% (TAKAMORI et al. 2000). In biopsy of subcapsular lesions, the rate can even increase up to 12% (LLOVET et al. 2001).

### 37.1.5.6
### Key Points

- Needle diameter 12–19 G.
- Standard needle lengths 5–20 cm.
- Spring-activated Tru-Cut needle is common standard.
- Sample is usually sufficient for histopathological analysis.
- Needle must not transgress bowels.

## 37.1.6
## CT-Guided Drill Biopsy

During the past decades, surgical (open) biopsy of musculoskeletal tumors could be gradually replaced by image-guided (closed) biopsy techniques (BICKELS et al. 1999). Main advantages of image-guided percutaneous biopsy in the musculoskeletal system are reduced morbidity and costs. FNAB is often limited in bone tumors given an inadequate ability to sample the tissue matrix while core biopsy reaches accuracy rates of 68–100% (PRAMESH et al. 2001).

### 37.1.6.1
### Indications

Indications for image-guided percutaneous bone biopsy are bone metastases and primary bone tumors. The biopsy is performed to verify that a suspicious bone lesion is indeed a metastasis, or in order to detect the primary tumor. In patients with breast cancer, hormone sensitivity of a metastatic bone lesion can be important for adequate therapy. In suspected primary bone tumors, biopsy is only exceptionally performed for histological evaluation with respect to the intended therapy. Special attention should be given to potential tumor seeding, and the access path for biopsy carefully planned together with the surgeon responsible for resection (SCHWEITZER et al. 1996). Another indication for percutaneous bone biopsy is suspected osseous infection with microorganisms that have to be identified before antibiotic therapy. Common contraindications are an uncorrectable coagulopathy and potential soft tissue infection with the danger of superinfection of the bone.

### 37.1.6.2
### Materials

A variety of bone biopsy needles are available, ranging from sharp-threaded, drilling-type 17-G needles to large-bore 8-G needles (Table 37.4). For sclerotic or osteoplastic bone lesions of the spine, it is advantageous to collect as much material as possible, because these lesions are often difficult to adequately decalcify for diagnostic workup. Therefore, for sclerotic bone lesions, bone biopsy needles of 11 G or larger are usually best.

**Table 37.4.** Commercially available needles for CT-guided drill biopsy (exemplary selection of different manufacturers and needles)

| Needle type (manufacturer) | Diameter (G) | Length (cm)[a] |
|---|---|---|
| Ackermann biopsy needle set (Cook Medical) | 14<br>14 | 9.7, 11<br>17.2, 18.5 |
| Elson biopsy needle set (Cook Medical) | 14 (with 22-G introducer and 12-G coaxial needle) | 17.1, 18.3 |
| Geremia vertebral biopsy set (Cook Medical) | 16 (with 22-G introducer needle) | 15 |
| Myers biopsy needle set (Cook Medical) | 14 | 10 |
| Spi-Cut biopsy needle (Somatex)[b] | 12.5, 14 | 5, 10, 15, 20 |
| Ostycut Bone biopsy needle (Bard Biopsy)[b] | 14–17 | 5, 7.5, 10, 12.5, 15 |
| Bonopty coaxial biopsy system eccentric drill penetration set (Radi Medical Systems, Uppsala, Sweden) | 14 | |
| PercuCut bone biopsy needle (E-Z-EM) | 17 | 5, 7.5, 10, 12.5, 15 |
| PercuCut coaxial sheath cut-biopsy needle with keyhole cutting edge (E-Z-EM) | 19.5 | 15 |
| Laredo trephine needle | 8 | |

[a]Not all diameter-length combinations may be available

[b]Removal of sample under aspiration

### 37.1.6.3
### Technique

In comparison to MR imaging, CT is inexpensive and easily available in most institutions. Therefore, most bone biopsies are performed under CT guidance. First, a CT scan is performed in order to visualize the bone lesion, and the needle entry point and access path are chosen. In cases of superficial bone biopsies without potential interference with vascular and nerve structures along the access path, a nonenhanced CT scan is usually sufficient for planning of the access route. Vessels, nerves, visceral, and articular structures should be avoided. Depending on the localization of the bone lesion, different approaches are available:

- Vertebral body (Fig. 37.9): depending on the vertebral level, the access path is anterior (cervical spine), transpedicular or intercostovertebral (thoracic spine), and transpedicular or posterolateral (lumbar spine).
- Pelvis: an anterior, lateral, or posterior approaches (avoiding the femoral and sacral nerve plexus and the sacral canal) are used.
- Peripheral long tubular bones: an approach orthogonal to the cortical bone is used. This reduces the risk of the biopsy needle gliding off the cortex. The shortest possible access path should be chosen in order to avoid critical structures like vessels and nerves.

- Flat bones (ribs, sternum, scapula): an oblique approach angle of 30–60° is chosen, which provides more material for biopsy, and helps to protect the underlying structures behind the flat bone.

The whole procedure has to be carried out under strictly sterile conditions to avoid osseous infection with subsequent osteomyelitis. Percutaneous drill biopsy is usually performed under local anesthesia or analgosedation (in incompliant patients), whereas pediatric bone biopsy represents an exception requiring general anesthesia. Local anesthesia is applied from the skin level down to the periosteum of the intended entry point of the biopsy needle with a 22-G needle. Leaving the anesthetic needle in the skin by detaching the syringe from the needle with the needle along the intended trajectory course saves time in subsequent needle placements. The initial anesthetic needle serves as a relative directional marker on both the images and the skin, and longer needles can subsequently be placed with positional readjustments as necessary so that the final needle can be placed in tandem (or coaxial) fashion relative to the target zone. The biopsy needle is introduced through the cortical bone under intermittent CT/CTF control verifying the correct needle direction. The needle containing the sample is completely removed, and the sample fixed in 10% formalin. In cases of suspected infection, the specimen is not fixed but directly put into a sterile container for microbiological analysis. Osteolyses char-

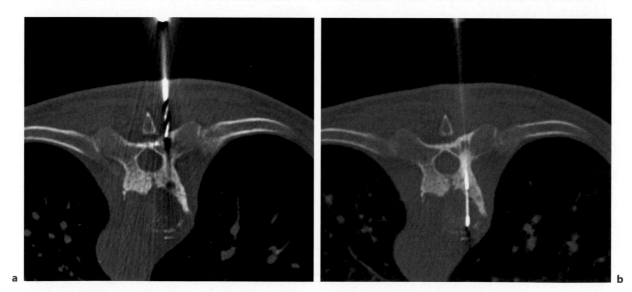

a                                                                    b

**Fig. 37.9a,b.** Patient (prone position) with major osteolysis (anterior two thirds) of lower thoracic vertebra showing osteosclerosis of the posterior third and both pedicles. First transpedicular access was obtained with a surgical manual drill (**a**).

Then the soft tissue sample was taken with an 18-G (13 cm) Tru-Cut biopsy needle under CTF guidance (**b**). Histopathology revealed a spinal metastasis of prostate carcinoma

acterized by a soft tissue core are directly sampled using a 16- or 18-G Tru-Cut biopsy needle. Depending on the thickness of the cortical bone and the degree of sclerosis surrounding the bone lesion, either a surgical hammer in combination with the bone biopsy needle (e.g., 14 G, Somatex Spi-Cut, Teltow, Germany), an 8-G trephine needle (e.g., Laredo type), a dedicated bone penetration set (e.g., Bonopty, Radi Medical Systems, Uppsala, Sweden), or a manual drill can be used in order to penetrate the cortex.

### 37.1.6.4
### Results

In comparison to conventional CT guidance, the advantage of CTF is the online visualization, the excellent resolution of bone, and the surrounding soft tissue and the possibility to target even small lesions (DALY and TEMPLETON 1999). The very good resolution of bone and soft tissue is furthermore able to reduce the amount of complications due to misplacement of the needle.

JELINEK et al. (2002) reported their results in 110 primary bone tumors that were sampled under CT and fluoroscopic guidance, respectively. Correct final diagnosis could be obtained by biopsy in 88% of the patients, while the only minor complication was a small hematoma (0.9% complication rate). The efficacy of CT-guided percutaneous biopsy in the management of spinal bone lesions has also been evaluated extensively (RENFREW et al. 1991).

### 37.1.6.5
### Complications

When biopsies are performed in thoracic lesions, the operator should always be cautious of a possible pneumothorax; at the end of the procedure, either a follow-up CT scan or an expiratory chest radiograph should be obtained to rule out a pneumothorax. A chest tube kit should be available before biopsy of the thoracic spine.

In bone lesions that are assumed to be extremely hypervascularized such as suspected metastases of renal cell carcinoma, a digital subtraction angiography may have to be obtained prior to biopsy. Transarterial embolization or direct puncture of the lesion with injection of absorbable gelatin sponge or polyvinyl alcohol particles helps to prevent serious hemorrhage when samples of the lesion are taken.

When pushing or drilling a needle through very dense bone, and when vital structures such as the aorta, the carotid artery, or the vertebral artery are located

just beyond the target zone along the trajectory path, the operator may want to use a détente technique, with one hand pushing the needle toward the target and the other hand grasping the needle shaft to provide a counteraction force in order to prevent piercing beyond the target area into vital structures if resistance to the needle should suddenly give way.

### 37.1.6.6
### Key Points

- Needle diameter 8–19 Gauge.
- Needle lengths 5–20 cm.
- Strictly sterile conditions mandatory during the whole biopsy procedure.
- Primary bone tumors: needle pathway should lie within the surgical resection area.
- Access angle should be chosen according to type of bone (tangential access in flat bones, orthogonal access in tubular bones).
- Access to the spine: anterior/anterolateral in the cervical, intercostovertebral/transpedicular in the thoracic, transpedicular/posterolateral in the lumbar spine.
- Needle insertion with a handgrip or a surgical hammer.
- Hand drill preferable for access to lesions with a sclerotic rim/thickened cortical bone.

## 37.2
## CT-Guided Drainage

### 37.2.1
### Introduction

Percutaneous drainage is defined as the placement of a catheter using imaging guidance to provide continuous drainage of a fluid collection. This includes localization of the collection, and placement and maintenance of the drainage catheter. This may be performed during a single session or as a staged procedure during multiple sessions.

### 37.2.2
### Indications

The indication for percutaneous drainage of (non)inflammatory fluid collections should always be discussed in a multidisciplinary team, i.e., between the radiologist and the referring physicians, surgeons, etc. Common indications are abscess and empyema, less common indications lymphocele, bilioma, urinoma, hematoma, necrosis, pseudocyst, and pleural effusion with clinical signs of superinfection or showing continuous enlargement. In comparison to surgical therapy, percutaneous drainage is less invasive and expensive, and can be performed without general anesthesia in most cases. In addition to the contraindications summarized in Sect. 37.1.2 for CT-guided biopsy (see Table 37.1), a specific contraindication for CT-guided percutaneous drainage is the absence of a circumscript fluid collection (e.g., peritonitis, phlegmonous inflammation).

### 37.2.3
### Patient Preparation and Aftercare

Informed patient consent including possible conscious sedation after detailed explanation of potential complications should be obtained at least 24 h before the intervention. As the decision for percutaneous drainage usually derives from a septic constellation of blood counts in combination with an abscess clinically suspected or proven by means of postoperative follow-up imaging, a 24 h interval cannot be guaranteed in many cases. The patient should undergo prophylactic intravenous antibiotic therapy according to prior blood culture results. In patients with negative blood culture tests, broad-spectrum antibiotics like vancomycin and metronidazole are appropriate. Preparation of the intended entry point of the drainage catheter includes sufficient sterile draping (especially to guarantee that the guide wire will remain sterile during the whole procedure if the Seldinger technique is used), skin disinfection, and local anesthesia with a 22-G needle using 10–20 ml of lidocaine. After successful placement of the drainage catheter in the interventional radiology unit, the patient is sent back to the ward where the catheter bag is left to drainage by gravity. The drainage should be irrigated several times per day with sterile saline by the nursing staff in order to avoid clogging.

### 37.2.4
### Materials

Preinterventional imaging should elucidate in which compartment the fluid collection is located (intra- vs. retroperitoneal, intraparenchymal vs. subcapsular, intramuscular, pleural vs. mediastinal vs. intrapulmonal, etc.), whether the fluid collection shows signs of potential infection (rim-enhancement, gas bubbles),

and which access path is suitable for safe percutaneous drainage.

For image guidance, US offers the advantages of missing radiation exposure, real-time visualization, cost-effectiveness, and availability even in small institutions. The operator should have a high level of experience in US-guided interventional procedures. Pleural effusion and empyema, as well as superficially located abdominal and circumscript intraparenchymal abscesses, can be drained under US guidance. As a major drawback, visualization of critical anatomical structures is not sufficient in patients with adiposity. In contrast, CT allows the detection, instant evaluation of a suitable access path, and placement of a drainage catheter at the time of the diagnostic CT scan. Typical indications for CT-guided percutaneous drainage are iliopsoas, retroperitoneal, deep abdominal, and pelvic abscesses. Sequential CT guidance or CT-fluoroscopy can be alternatively utilized for CT guidance of drainage procedures (see Sect. 37.1.3.).

A variety of different catheter models is commercially available. Most of them are characterized by a pigtail configuration and sump or non-sump designs, respectively. Sump catheters have a double lumen: the outer lumen prevents a blocking of the catheter side holes if they lie next to the abscess wall. Common diameters of drainage catheters suitable for intra-abdominal abscesses are 12–14 French. Larger catheters (≥16–28 French) are necessary only in exceptional cases like peripancreatic abscesses and hematomas where the fluid collection may be characterized by a higher viscosity. In the chest, large non-sump catheters are preferable in order to avoid kinking due to expiratory excursions. In loculated abscesses, e.g., pleural empyema or small presacral abscesses, smaller catheters (8–10 French) are used in order to safely place all side holes within the fluid collection. Locking pigtail catheters are commonly used in combination with a transrectal or transvaginal access in order to avoid dislodging of the catheter.

### 37.2.5
### Technique

The two common techniques for insertion of a drainage catheter are (Table 37.5):
1. The Seldinger technique
2. The Trocar technique

**Seldinger technique.** First, an 18-G long-dwell sheath is inserted into the fluid collection, followed by a 0.035/0.038-in. guide wire, which is consecutively coiled within the abscess cavity. Another possible combination is a 22-G needle and a 0.018-in.guide wire. The intended access path of the drainage catheter is additionally dilated with fascial dilators of an increasing diameter up to 2-French larger than the drainage catheter. Finally, the drainage catheter is introduced over the guide wire. It is important to ensure that all side holes of the drainage catheter lie within the fluid collection.

Trocar technique. First, a reference needle is inserted into the fluid collection. Then, a drainage catheter containing a sharp stylet is introduced parallel to the reference needle to the intended depth. Sufficient incision and dissection of the skin and the subcutaneous tissue with a scalpel or surgical forceps are crucial; otherwise, the drainage catheter may be stuck subcutaneously. When the tip of the drainage penetrates the abscess wall, the operator usually feels the initial resistance suddenly giving in. The central stylet is removed, and the drainage catheter aspirated in order to verify a correct position. If pus or fluid can be aspirated, then the operator disengages and stabilizes the trocar with one hand while pushing the catheter into the cavity with the other. Afterwards, the complete fluid is aspirated using a three-way stopcock and a drainage bag. In cases of highly viscous fluid, sterile saline can be injected until the aspirated fluid gets clear. Finally, the catheter is sutured to the skin, or fixed with a dedicated fixation device. A follow-up CT scan is performed immediately after drainage placement in order to ensure that no further abscess collections are present.

### 37.2.5.1
### Special Considerations

#### 37.2.5.1.1
#### *Abdominal Fluid Collections*

**Subdiaphragmatic Abscess.** Most subdiaphragmatic abscesses occur postoperatively after pancreatic, gastric, or biliary surgery. For a strictly extrapleural approach, a technically more sophisticated double-oblique access is often necessary, given the pleural attachments at the level of the 12th rib posteriorly, the 10th rib laterally, and the 8th rib anteriorly.

**Retroperitoneal Abscess.** Abscesses in the retroperitoneum occur in patients with spondylodiscitis (Fig. 37.10) or acute spinal osteomyelitis, with Crohn's disease, or via hematogenous spreading. CT-guided drainage is usually required due to the deep location. Given an involvement of both, the psoas and iliacus muscle, one drainage catheter placed in the iliacus muscle is sufficient if a communication between both compartments is present. Otherwise, a separate drainage catheter is introduced into the psoas abscess.

**Hepatic Abscess.** Nowadays, most hepatic abscesses are seen in patients after liver or biliary surgery. CT imaging may reveal a heterogeneous appearance with more solid and liquid areas or even septae (Fig. 37.11). With respect to the costophrenic sulcus, the approach is ante-

**Table 37.5.** Advantages and disadvantages of the Trocar and the Seldinger techniques

| Advantages of the Trocar technique | Disadvantages of the Trocar technique |
| --- | --- |
| • Stiffness of catheter-cannula-stylet combination allows better directional control of the drainage catheter when traversing large muscular structures<br>• No serial dilation is required<br>• Placement in one step is possible<br>• Faster placement of drainage catheter compared to Seldinger technique is possible | • In case of malposition, repositioning of the catheter is usually not possible. Reinsertion of the drainage is necessary |
| **Advantages of the Seldinger technique** | **Disadvantages of the Seldinger technique** |
| • In difficult-to-access and deep abdominal/pelvic fluid collections, the direction of the guiding needle can be exactly controlled with respect to adjacent neurovascular structures and bowels | • Time-consuming<br>• Guide-wire is sometimes not visualized entirely in the axial CT image. Guide-wire kinking can complicate insertion of the catheter–cannula combination |

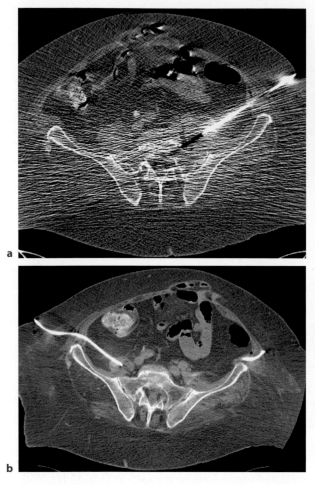

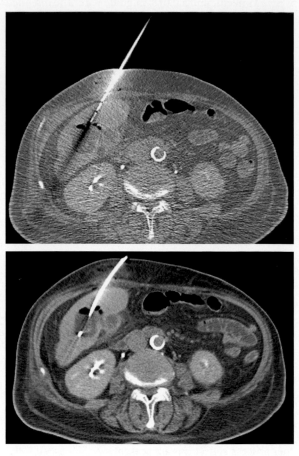

**Fig. 37.10a,b.** Patient with spondylodiscitis and bilateral psoas abscesses. With a lateral approach along the iliac crest (**a**), an 8-French drainage catheter was placed in both abscesses under CTF guidance using the Trocar technique (**b**)

**Fig. 37.11a,b.** Patient with chronic cholecystitis who developed a hepatic abscess adjacent to the gallbladder. An 8-French drainage catheter was directly inserted from an anterior approach under CT fluoroscopy (**a, b**). Elective surgery of the abscess after repeated drainage procedures revealed a perforated gallbladder maintaining the inflammatory process

rior or lateral, and intercostal or subcostal. Abscesses in the dome of the liver are accessed with a double oblique approach. In superficial intraparenchymal abscesses, a small bridge of normal liver tissue provides additional stabilization of the drainage catheter.

**Renal Abscess.** Indications for percutaneous drainage of renal fluid collections are perinephric and large intrarenal abscesses, as well as small intrarenal abscesses not responding to antibiotic therapy. Another indication are infected urinomas, which are treated by a single percutaneous drainage, or in combination with additional nephrostomy when a communication between the urinoma and the urinary collecting system persists.

**Splenic Abscess.** Because the spleen is a highly vascularized organ, splenic abscess drainage is not (or only exceptionally) performed in most institutions. The drainage catheter (maximum diameter of 8–10 French) should pass as little normal splenic parenchyma as possible.

### 37.2.5.1.2
### Pancreatic Fluid Collections

Pancreatic abscesses are often multilocular while the abscess content is highly viscous, requiring large drainages (≥20–30 French). For safe placement of those large drainages, the Seldinger technique should be used (Fig. 37.12).

Pancreatic necrosis occurs in patients with severe acute pancreatitis detected through perfusion defects in the contrast-enhanced CT. Therapeutic method of choice is surgical necrosectomy; percutaneous drainage is not suitable. On the other hand, the differentiation of sterile from infected pancreatic necrosis is done by percutaneous sampling of the necrotic pancreatic parenchyma with a small-gauge needle (20 G).

Indications for drainage of pancreatic pseudocysts are a diameter of more than 5 cm or an ongoing enlargement, pain, suspected infection, and obstruction of the GI or biliary tract. Preinterventional contrast-enhanced CT performed in an arterial and venous phase enables the operator to differentiate clearly surrounding organs and vessels. A transgastric approach may be chosen for placement, which can be later used for transgastric stent placement (internal drainage) between the pseudocyst and the stomach. In case the pseudocyst communicates with the pancreatic duct, duration of percutaneous drainage may take up to 8–12 weeks.

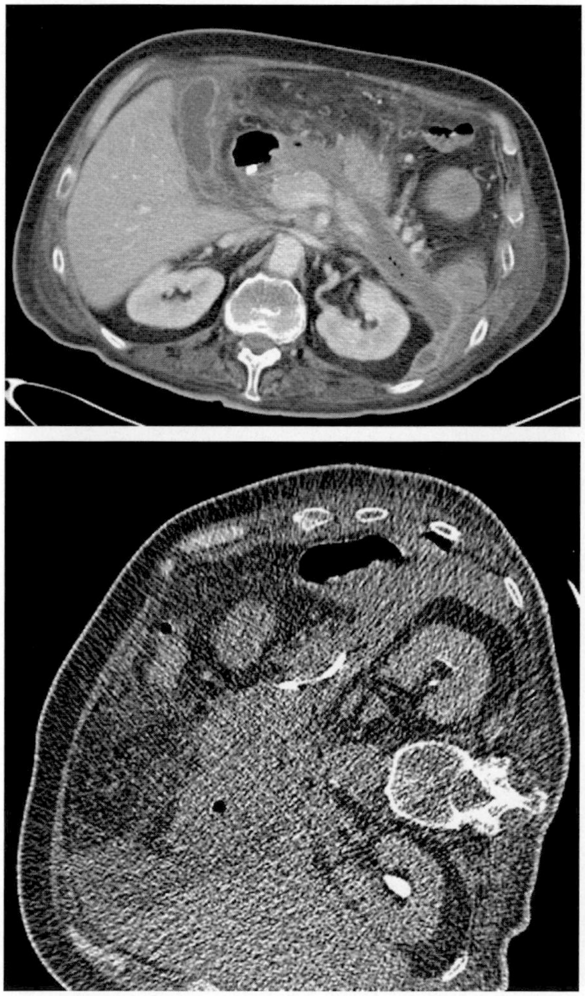

### 37.2.5.1.3
### Pelvic Abscesses

Depending on the location of a pelvic fluid collection, different access paths determined by the surrounding pelvic ring are suitable: the presacral approach (patient in prone position) is especially useful in patients who develop a presacral abscess after an abdominoperineal resection (Fig. 37.13). Using a slight (double) angula-

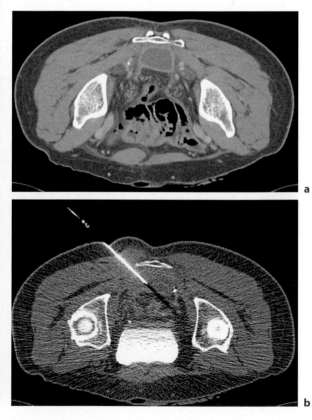

**Fig. 37.12a,b.** Patient who had undergone resection of the pancreatic tail and developed an abscess in the resection area postoperatively (**a**). The Seldinger technique was used for placement of an 8-French drainage catheter within the fluid collection (**b**)

**Fig. 37.13a,b.** Patient (prone position) with a fever showing a presacral fluid collection 10 days after abdominoperineal rectum resection (**a**). An 8-French drainage catheter was inserted using the Seldinger technique. **b** Guide wire being introduced through an 18-G sheath under CT fluoroscopy

tion, the needle is inserted through the gluteal cleft below the coccygeal bone. For deep pelvic abscesses, a transgluteal access through the greater sciatic foramen (patient in prone position) in combination with the Seldinger technique is preferable. The operator has to pay special attention to the sciatic nerve, which is located close to the ischial tuberosity. The trajectory of the small 20-G needle has to stay close to the sacrum. Afterwards, a large drainage catheter can be inserted without affection of the sciatic nerve. Abscesses in the rectouterine or rectovesical pouch may be treated from a transvaginal and transrectal approach under endocavitary US guidance only.

### 37.2.5.1.4
### Thoracic Fluid Collections

The majority of pleural fluid collections are drained under US guidance (therapeutic thoracocentesis,) while CT is required for safe access to lung and mediastinal

abscesses. Therapeutic thoracocentesis can be combined with diagnostic thoracocentesis in patients with suspected infection or malignancy within the pleural space.

**Pleural Effusion.** The basic indication for drainage of pleural fluid collections is dyspnea in patients with malignant pleural effusions, while benign parapneumonic effusions are drained only exceptionally. Thoracocentesis can be performed with a small intravenous cannula as a temporary solution, or a small drainage catheter (8 French) using either the Seldinger or Trocar technique. The drainage catheter is connected to a three-way-stopcock and a sterile evacuated bottle that drains the effusion continuously.

**Empyema.** While blind surgical drainage may often result in a placement of the chest tube within the pleural space outside a pleural empyema, CT guidance is especially preferable for drainage of loculated empyemas (Fig. 37.14). For optimal access, the patient is placed in

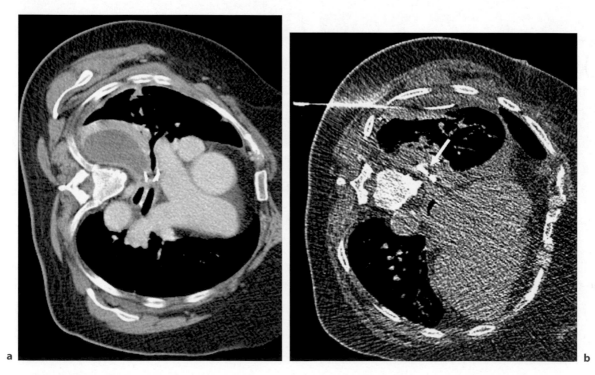

**Fig. 37.14a,b.** Patient (left lateral decubitus position) with a fever who had undergone resection of several mediastinal lymph nodes, and showed two loculated pleural fluid collections of the right lung postoperatively (**a**). An 8-French drainage catheter was inserted into both fluid collections (Seldinger technique). **b** The first drainage already within paramediastinal fluid collection (*arrow* empyema), and the guide wire inserted through an 18 Gauge sheath into the lateral fluid collection (sterile pleural effusion)

a right or left lateral decubitus, supine, or prone position. In order to prevent clogging of the catheter due to the high viscosity of the pus, and to avoid catheter kinking caused by the respiratory excursions, some authors recommend large drainage catheters ($\geq$20 French). On the other hand, the complete coiling of a pigtail drainage and placement of all side holes within a small loculated empyema requires smaller drainage diameters of 8–12 French. With the combination of the Seldinger technique and CT guidance, even small paramediastinal empyemas lying in the depth of the thorax are accessible. After successful catheter placement, the drainage is sutured to the skin and connected to an underwaterseal pleural drainage bottle. Several separate catheter insertions may be necessary to drain multiple loculated empyemas.

**Mediastinal Abscess.** Mediastinal abscesses are most often seen after cardiac surgery. Especially if a parasternal access is necessary, the preinterventional planning CT is performed in an arterial and a venous phase in order to visualize the internal mammary artery and vein. To avoid a pneumothorax, drainage placement has to be conducted after dissection of the parasternal soft tissue, using sterile saline. With respect to the large mediastinal vessels, CT guidance and the Seldinger technique are preferred for safe catheter placement.

## 37.2.6
## Results

### 37.2.6.1
### Abdomen

HASHIMOTO et al. (1995) reported 56 cases of pyogenic liver abscesses: 39 and 10 patients underwent CT-guided drainage or simple aspiration without drainage, respectively. Six patients were treated with open operative drainage, while one patient with advanced cancer only received antibiotics. Five of 39 patients had to undergo operation after primary percutaneous drainage (87% success rate). Overall mortality rate was 12.5% (7/56).

Due to autopsy results, the incidence of splenic abscesses is estimated to be between 0.2 and 0.7% (PARIS 1994). Underlying disorders are infection, emboli, trauma, recent surgery, malignant hematologic conditions, and immunosuppression. In the past, antibiotic therapy and splenectomy were the only available treatments. While mortality rates of surgical drainage range between 13 and 28% (LUCEY et al. 2002), several authors

underlined the technical feasibility and safety of CT-guided drainage of splenic abscesses (KANG et al. 2007; LUCEY et al. 2002; THANOS et al. 2002). Success rates of percutaneous splenic drainage reported in the literature are between 60 and 77% (QUINN 1986; LERNER 1984; GASPARINI 1994).

According to LEE (2004), success rates of pancreatic abscess drainage range between 32% (infected necrosis) and 90% (pancreatic abscess). For complete drainage, often large and multiple catheters are required.

Indications for percutaneous drainage of necrotizing pancreatitis are stabilization of critically ill patients prior to surgical debridement, a treatment with a primary curative intention, and a postoperative treatment of pseudocysts when surgical therapy alone has not, or only partially, been successful (SEGAL et al. 2007). Typical locations are the lesser sac, the anterior pararenal space, or other parts of the retroperitoneum. Due to the high viscosity of the fluid collections resulting from pancreatic necrosis, minimum diameter of drainages necessary is 12–14 French. In patients with sterile pancreatic necrosis, CT scans of the abdomen are repeated every 7–10 days to look for complications. When aspirating these sterile fluid collections, traversing of the small and large bowels must be avoided in order to prevent superinfection. GOUZI et al. (1999) published a 15% mortality and 70% success rate of percutaneous drainage (average three 24-French double-lumen drainage catheters per patient) in 32 patients with severe acute necrotizing pancreatitis.

In a large retrospective analysis, SPIVAK et al. (1998) found that surgical therapy of pancreatic pseudocysts had been superior to percutaneous drainage: a third of their 77 patients undergoing percutaneous drainage finally required major salvage procedures like pancreatic debridement, cystogastrostomy, cystojejunostomy, cystectomy, or external drainage. Percutaneous drainage of superinfected pseudocysts can at least postpone surgical therapy significantly. Catheters between 8 and 12 French are usually sufficient for drainage. Pseudocysts with communication to the pancreatic duct may take several weeks to months for complete drainage.

### 37.2.6.2
### Retroperitoneum and Pelvis

CANTASDEMIR et al. (2003) reported their experience with CT-guided percutaneous drainage in 21 patients with iliopsoas abscesses, which were technically successful in 21/22 cases. Nineteen and three procedures were performed with the Trocar and Seldinger techniques, respectively. Three cases of recurrence could successfully be managed with antibiotic therapy or needle aspiration alone. The study by HARISINGHANI et al. (2003) including 154 deep pelvic abscesses in 140 patients showed complete resolution in 96% of the cases (134/140), without necessary subsequent surgery. Origins of the abscesses were predominantly postoperative fluid collections, followed by diverticulitis, Crohn's disease, perforating appendicitis, tubo-ovarial abscess, and internal bowel fistula due to irradiation. Only 3 of 140 patients (2%) developed a hematoma, and there were no procedure-related deaths. Transrectal (GAZELLE et al. 1991; LOMAS et al. 1992) and paracoccygeal (LONGO et al. 1993) approaches have also been described as technically safe and effective in smaller studies.

### 37.2.6.3
### Chest

BARTON et al. (1992) retrospectively evaluated CT-guided drainage procedures performed in 39 patients with various intrathoracic fluid collections. Of the fluid collections, 61.5% were seen in the pleural space, 25.6% in the lungs, and 12.8% in the mediastinum. In 28 patients (71.8%), CT-guided percutaneous drainage was curative, whereas 9 patients (23.1%) were temporized until surgery was possible. Pneumothorax rate without further necessary treatment was 1/39 procedures (2.6%). The procedures were predominantly performed using the Seldinger technique (70%) and 8–12 French catheters.

### 37.2.7
### Complications

Complications are observed in approximately 10% of the patients undergoing percutaneous abscess and fluid drainage (Table 37.6). Because the abscess wall is highly vascularized, transient bacteremia is sometimes caused through the drainage catheter placement itself. Application of broad-spectrum antibiotics before the intervention will help prevent further consequences like septicemia. Hemorrhage is a complication relatively common for all interventional procedures, but the probability of relevant bleeding can be minimized through correction of any coagulation disorder prior to the drainage procedure. In well-vascularized organs like the spleen or liver, subcapsular or parenchymal bleeding can be avoided by using small catheters. The penetration of the capsule itself should be performed quickly in order to avoid laceration during the patient's respiratory excursions. Hemorrhage may stop spontaneously due to self-tamponade, or after insertion of drainage of a larger diameter. Otherwise, superselective transarterial embolization is an ultimate means of percutaneous, minimally invasive therapy. Unintended bowel perforation by a needle (Seldinger technique) or the drainage catheter itself (Trocar technique) represents a complication that requires a certain management: needle penetration of the bowels does usually not have further clinical consequences. If the drainage has successfully been placed within the abscess traversing the bowels, and one or more side-holes communicate with the bowel lumen, then the enteric fluid will drain through

**Table 37.6.** Specific major complications of percutaneous abscess and fluid drainage (compilation according to the Society of Interventional Radiology, based on published results (BAKAL et al. 2003))

| Complication | Rate (%) |
|---|---|
| Septic shock | 1–2 |
| Bacteremia requiring significant new intervention | 2–5 |
| Hemorrhage requiring transfusion | 1 |
| Superinfection (includes infection of sterile fluid collection) | 1 |
| Bowel transgression requiring intervention | 1 |
| Pleural transgression requiring intervention (abdominal procedures) | 1 |
| Pleural transgression requiring additional intervention (chest procedures) | 2–10 |

the drainage catheter. The drainage catheter is left in place for a period of 10 days until a fibrous channel has formed around the catheter. If the abscess has vanished, then the drainage is removed, and the fibrous channel will prevent leakage of enteric fluid into the peritoneal cavity and be closed within 1 day. In case the patient develops signs of peritonitis after drainage placement, immediate surgical intervention is necessary.

## 37.2.8
## Key Points

- Planning CT: additional arterial phase scan necessary in selected cases for differentiation of small arteries along access path (e.g., internal mammary artery, epigastric vessels)
- Planning CT: adequate bowel opacification necessary for clear differentiation of enteric abscesses and bowel loops
- Trocar technique for easy-to-access fluid collections
- Seldinger technique for more sophisticated, i.e., deep or small fluid collections adjacent to neurovascular structures or bowels
- Sump and non-sump catheters
- Diameter of suitable drainage catheter (8–28 French) depends on viscosity of fluid and size of fluid collection.

## References

Anderson JM et al. (2003) CT-guided lung biopsy: factors influencing diagnostic yield and complication rate. Clin Radiol 58:791–797

Arslan S et al. (2002) CT-guided transthoracic fine needle aspiration of pulmonary lesions: accuracy and complications in 294 patients. Med Sci Monit 8:CR493–497

Bakal CW et al. (2003) Quality improvement guidelines for adult percutaneous abscess and fluid drainage. J Vasc Interv Radiol 14:S223–S225

Barton P et al. (1992) [Percutaneous CT-guided catheter drainage of intrathoracic fluid accumulations.] (In German) Rofo 156:47–52

Bickels J et al. (1999) Biopsy of musculoskeletal tumors. Current concepts. Clin Orthop Relat Res 368:212–219

Brandt KR et al. (1993) CT- and US-guided biopsy of the pancreas. Radiology 187:99–104

Cantasdemir M et al. (2003) Computed tomography-guided percutaneous catheter drainage of primary and secondary iliopsoas abscesses. Clin Radiol 58:811–815

Cardella JF et al. (2003) Quality improvement guidelines for image-guided percutaneous biopsy in adults. J Vasc Interv Radiol 14:S227–S230

Carlson SK et al. (2001) Benefits and safety of CT fluoroscopy in interventional radiologic procedures. Radiology 219:515–520

Cox JE et al. (1999) Transthoracic needle aspiration biopsy: variables that affect risk of pneumothorax. Radiology 212:165–168

Daly B, Templeton PA (1999) Real-time CT fluoroscopy: evolution of an interventional tool. Radiology 211:309–3015

Elvin A et al. (1990) Biopsy of the pancreas with a biopsy gun. Radiology 176:677–679

Ferrucci JR Jr et al. (1980) Diagnosis of abdominal malignancy by radiologic fine-needle aspiration biopsy. AJR Am J Roentgenol 134:323–330

Fish GD et al. (1988) Postbiopsy pneumothorax: estimating the risk by chest radiography and pulmonary function tests. AJR Am J Roentgenol 150:71–74

Gazelle GS et al. (1991) Pelvic abscesses: CT-guided transrectal drainage. Radiology 181:49–51

Gouzi JL et al. (1999) [Percutaneous drainage of infected pancreatic necrosis: an alternative to surgery.] (In French) Chirurgie 124:31–37

Haage P et al. (1999) [CT-guided percutaneous biopsies for the classification of focal liver lesions: a comparison between 14 G and 18 G puncture biopsy needles.] (In German) Rofo 171:44–48

Harisinghani MG et al. (2003) Transgluteal approach for percutaneous drainage of deep pelvic abscesses: 154 cases. Radiology 228:701–705

Hashimoto L et al. (1995) Pyogenic hepatic abscess: results of current management. Am Surg 61:407–411

Hopper KD et al. (1993) Automated biopsy devices: a blinded evaluation. Radiology 187:653–660

Irie T et al. (2001) Biopsy of lung nodules with use of I-I device under intermittent CT fluoroscopic guidance: preliminary clinical study. J Vasc Interv Radiol 12:215–219

Jelinek JS et al. (2002) Diagnosis of primary bone tumors with image-guided percutaneous biopsy: experience with 110 tumors. Radiology 223:731–737

Kang M et al. (2007) Image guided percutaneous splenic interventions. Eur J Radiol 64:140–146

Kazerooni EA et al. (1996) Risk of pneumothorax in CT-guided transthoracic needle aspiration biopsy of the lung. Radiology 198:371–375

Klein JS et al. (1996) Transthoracic needle biopsy with a coaxially placed 20-G automated cutting needle: results in 122 patients. Radiology 198:715–720

Laurent F et al. (2000) CT-guided transthoracic needle biopsy of pulmonary nodules smaller than 20 mm: results with an automated 20-G coaxial cutting needle. Clin Radiol 55:281–287

Lechevallier E et al. (2000) Fine-needle percutaneous biopsy of renal masses with helical CT guidance. Radiology 216:506–510

Lee M (2004) Image-guided percutaneous biopsy In: Kaufman J, Lee M (eds) Vascular and interventional radiology: the requisites. Mosby, Philadelphia, pp 469–488

Li H et al. (1996) Diagnostic accuracy and safety of CT-guided percutaneous needle aspiration biopsy of the lung: comparison of small and large pulmonary nodules. AJR Am J Roentgenol 167:105–109

Llovet JM et al. (2001) Increased risk of tumor seeding after percutaneous radiofrequency ablation for single hepatocellular carcinoma. Hepatology 33:1124–1129

Lomas DJ et al. (1992) CT-guided drainage of pelvic abscesses: the peranal transrectal approach. Clin Radiol 45:246–249

Longo JM et al. (1993) CT-guided paracoccygeal drainage of pelvic abscesses. J Comput Assist Tomogr 17:909–914

Lucey BC et al. (2002) Percutaneous nonvascular splenic intervention: a 10-year review. AJR Am J Roentgenol 179:1591–1596

Lumachi F et al. (2001) Fine-needle aspiration cytology of adrenal masses in noncancer patients: clinicoradiologic and histologic correlations in functioning and nonfunctioning tumors. Cancer 93:323–329

Lumachi F et al. (2003) CT-scan, MRI and image-guided FNA cytology of incidental adrenal masses. Eur J Surg Oncol 29:689–692

Lüning M et al. (1984) [Analysis of the results of 96 CT-guided fine needle biopsies of liver masses.] (In German) Rofo 141:267–725

Lüning M et al. (1985) CT guided percutaneous fine-needle biopsy of the pancreas. Eur J Radiol 5:104–108

Memel DS et al. (1996) Efficacy of sonography as a guidance technique for biopsy of abdominal, pelvic, and retroperitoneal lymph nodes. AJR Am J Roentgenol 167:957–962

Mueller PR (1993) Pancreatic biopsy: striving for excellence. Radiology 187:15–16

Nahar Saikia U et al. (2002) Image-guided fine-needle aspiration cytology of deep-seated enlarged lymph nodes. Acta Radiol 43:230–234

Pagani JJ (1983) Biopsy of focal hepatic lesions. Comparison of 18 and 22 gauge needles. Radiology 147:673–675

Piccinino F et al. (1986) Complications following percutaneous liver biopsy. A multicentre retrospective study on 68,276 biopsies. J Hepatol 2:165–173

Poe RH et al. (1984) Predicting risk of pneumothorax in needle biopsy of the lung. Chest 85:232–235

Pramesh CS et al. (2001) Core needle biopsy for bone tumours. Eur J Surg Oncol 27:668–671

Quon D et al. (1988) Pulmonary function testing in predicting complications from percutaneous lung biopsy. Can Assoc Radiol J 39:267–269

Renfrew DL et al. (1991) CT-guided percutaneous transpedicular biopsy of the spine. Radiology 180:574–576

Salomonowitz (E 2001) MR imaging-guided biopsy and therapeutic intervention in a closed-configuration magnet: single-center series of 361 punctures. AJR Am J Roentgenol 177:159–163

Schweitzer ME et al. (1996) Percutaneous skeletal aspiration and core biopsy: complementary techniques. AJR Am J Roentgenol 166:415–418

Segal D et al. (2007) Acute necrotizing pancreatitis: role of CT-guided percutaneous catheter drainage. Abdom Imaging 32:351–361

Silverman SG et al. (1999) CT fluoroscopy-guided abdominal interventions: techniques, results, and radiation exposure. Radiology 212:673–681

Smith EH (1991) Complications of percutaneous abdominal fine-needle biopsy. Review. Radiology 178:253–258

Spivak H et al. (1998) Management of pancreatic pseudocysts. J Am Coll Surg 186:507–511

Swischuk JL et al. (1998) Percutaneous transthoracic needle biopsy of the lung: review of 612 lesions. J Vasc Interv Radiol 9:347–352

Takamori R et al. (2000) Needle-tract implantation from hepatocellular cancer: is needle biopsy of the liver always necessary? Liver Transpl 6:67–72

Thanos L et al. (2002) Percutaneous CT-guided drainage of splenic abscess. AJR Am J Roentgenol 179:629–632

Tomiyama N et al. (2000) CT-guided needle biopsy of small pulmonary nodules: value of respiratory gating. Radiology 217:907–910

Torzilli G et al. (1999) Accurate preoperative evaluation of liver mass lesions without fine-needle biopsy. Hepatology 30:889–893

Tsukada H et al. (2000) Diagnostic accuracy of CT-guided automated needle biopsy of lung nodules. AJR Am J Roentgenol 175:239–243

vanSonnenberg E, Casola G (1988) Interventional radiology 1988. Invest Radiol 23:75–92

vanSonnenberg E et al. (1988) Difficult thoracic lesions: CT-guided biopsy experience in 150 cases. Radiology 167:457–461

Welch TJ et al. (1989) CT-guided biopsy: prospective analysis of 1,000 procedures. Radiology 171:493–496

Wildberger JE et al. (2003) [Refinement of cytopathology of CT-guided fine needle aspiration biopsies with additional histologic examination of formalin-fixed blood-clots.] (In German) Rofo 175:1532–1538

Wutke R et al. (2001) [CT-guided percutaneous core biopsy: Effective accuracy, diagnostic utility and effective costs.] (In German) Rofo 173:1025–1033

Zangos S et al. (2003) [MR-guided biopsies of undetermined liver lesions: technique and results.] (In German) Rofo 175:688–894

Zwischenberger JB et al. (2002) Mediastinal transthoracic needle and core lymph node biopsy: should it replace mediastinoscopy? Chest 121:1165–1170

# Vertebroplasty

38

Tobias F. Jakobs

CONTENTS

## ABSTRACT

Percutaneous vertebroplasty (PV) is a safe and efficient therapeutic option for patients suffering from
otherwise untreatable pain and disability caused by
osteoporotic fracture or tumoral involvement of a
vertebra. Vertebroplasty provides nearly immediate pain relief and stabilization, leading to a high
rate of successful treatments with low morbidity,
no or only short hospitalization, and rare adverse
events. In addition, PV contributes to spinal stabilization and can be successfully combined with
chemotherapy, radiation therapy, tumor ablation,
and posterior laminectomy. Therefore, the number of procedures performed has continuously
increased over the last few years. However, indications and contraindications, technical aspects, and
possible complications of PV always have to be
taken into account by the interventional radiologist. The success rate strongly depends – besides
on the experience of the physician performing the
procedure – on the visualization equipment used,
such as CT fluoroscopy.

## 38.1
## Introduction

### 38.1.1
### Osteoporotic Vertebral Body Fracture

Vertebral body fracture is one of the main causes for severe debilitating back pain causing a reduction of life
quality, physical function, and survival (STALLMEYER et
al. 2003). A vast majority of the vertebral body fractures
is caused by an underlying osteoporosis. Vertebroplasty

T. F. JAKOBS, MD
Department of Clinical Radiology, Ludwigs-Maximilians-Uni-
versity of Munich, Munich University Hospitals, Marchioninistrasse 15, 81377 Munich, Germany

is a percutaneously performed minimally invasive treatment for painful vertebral body fracture using bone cement to strengthen a fractured vertebral body and for pain relief. The first percutaneous vertebroplasty (PV) was performed in 1984 by the interventional neuroradiologists Galibert and Deramond and reported first in the literature in 1987 for the treatment of a painful aggressive hemangioma of a vertebral body (Galibert and Deramond 1990). Since then, this technique has gained wide acceptance all over Europe and worldwide as a therapeutic option for patients suffering from otherwise intractable pain caused by osteoporotic fractures of the vertebral body (Diamond et al. 2006; Hoffmann et al. 2003).

## 38.1.2
## Tumoral Osteolysis

Metastatic spread to the vertebral column is the most common malignant disease of the skeletal system (Wong et al. 1990). Symptoms may be the consequence of a pathologic fracture secondary to vertebral destruction, with development of spinal instability and compression of adjacent neurological structures. In patients with spinal metastases, aggressive hemangiomas, or multiple myeloma, a pathologic vertebral compression fracture is a frequent cause of debilitating back pain resulting in deteriorated quality of life, physical function, and psychosocial performance (Stallmeyer et al. 2003). Even survival time for patients may be significantly reduced following fracture or spinal cord compression (Hill et al. 1993). Chemotherapy, hormonal therapy, and radiation therapy have proven to be effective in halting the tumorous process and reversing the neurological compromise; however, severe side effects, ineffectiveness, and delayed onset of the effect are major drawbacks of these aforementioned treatment options (Coleman 2005; Jacobs and Perrin 2001; Rades et al. 2006). Furthermore, these modalities cannot provide immediate stabilization to an unstable vertebral segment. Surgery enables restoration of spinal canal support and therefore facilitates nursing, improves neurological function, and supports pain control (Chataigner and Onimus 2000), but major surgery performed on severely ill patients carries a high risk of complications and therefore is usually not recommended in patients whose expected survival is limited (Pascal-Moussellard et al. 1998). PV is a minimally invasive, radiologically guided procedure in which bone cement [polymethylmethacrylate (PMMA)] is injected into structurally weakened vertebrae. PV has been pro-

gressively developed and adopted to treat spinal tumoral osteolysis, making it possible to provide biomechanical stability and pain relief (Ahn et al. 2006; Alvarez et al. 2003, 2006; Deramond et al. 1998; Gangi et al. 2003; Higgins et al. 2003).

## 38.2
## Patient Selection

### 38.2.1
### Osteoporotic Vertebral Body Fracture

The main indication for percutaneous vertebroplasty in osteoporotic fractures for selected patients is focal intractable or intense pain adjacent to the level of the fracture. The fracture must be proven by plain radiograph, CT, or MRI. Furthermore, MRI is able to evaluate the age of a fracture by visualizing the degree of a bone marrow edema (Do 2000). Suitable patients should have undergone conservative treatment for at least 3 to 4 weeks (Hide and Gangi 2004; Peh and Gilula 2005) without significant effect on the patient's situation or pain relief could only be obtained using high doses of analgesics causing severe side effects. Furthermore, another possibility is a combined treatment with a surgical dorsal stabilization using a fixateur interne and a further ventral stabilization by percutaneous vertebroplasty (Gangi et al. 2006) (Fig. 38.1a–d).

There are only few absolute contraindications for PV, which include non-correctable bleeding disorder, asymptomatic vertebral body fracture, an improvement of patients pain on medication, osteomyelitis, or any active systemic infection, allergy to bone cement, and prophylactic vertebroplasty.

Relative contraindications include radicular pain, inability to lie in a prone position for the duration of the treatment, a vertebral collapse of more than 70% of the original vertebral body height, retropulsion of a fragment into the spinal canal, lack of surgical or neurosurgical backup, and lack of patient monitoring facilities. Possible inability to lie in a prone position can be overcome using mild conscious sedation. Since there are continuous changes in indications and contraindications, it is highly recommended to review the guidelines of interventional societies such as CIRSE (Cardiovascular and Interventional Radiological Society of Europe) or SIR (Society of Interventional Radioloy) – for example, Gangi et al's (2006) recently published "Quality assurance guidelines for percutaneous vertebroplasty" for CIRSE.

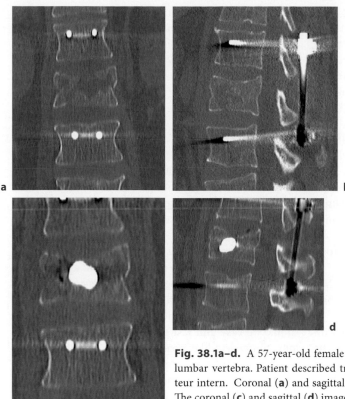

**Fig. 38.1a–d.** A 57-year-old female patient with a painful osteoporotic fracture of the 2nd lumbar vertebra. Patient described treatment-refractory pain after stabilization with a fixateur intern. Coronal (**a**) and sagittal (**b**) images show the osteoporotic fracture prior to PV. The coronal (**c**) and sagittal (**d**) images after PV demonstrate a nice cement deposition in the fractured area

## 38.2.2
## Tumoral Osteolysis

Treatment of tumoral osteolysis to the spine is complex and challenging, and requires systemic and local therapies. Because PV is only aimed at treating the pain and consolidating the weight-bearing bone, other specific tumor treatment is required for tumor management. Therefore, the decision to perform PV should be made by an interdisciplinary team consisting of interventional radiologists, radiation oncologists, spine surgeons, and oncologists to ensure appropriate adjuvant therapy and follow-up.

A detailed clinical history and examination, with specific emphasis on the neurological signs and symptoms, should be performed to confirm the underlying vertebral fracture as the cause of debilitating back pain and rule out other causes such as, e.g., degenerative spondylosis or radiculopathy. This should be correlated with the imaging studies, including magnetic resonance (MR) imaging, computed tomography (CT), and technetium 99m pertechnetate bone scintigraphy (PHILLIPS 2003; ZOARSKI et al. 2002). Whenever doubt persists, the lesion should be sampled for biopsy during the PV procedure. In metastatic disease, fractures might be present at multiple levels of the spine, not all of which require treatment with PV.

## 38.3
## Indications and Contraindications

### Indications

- Osteoporotic vertebral compression fracture with excruciating pain and/or adverse effects to opioid treatment or opioid tolerance developed in patients with formerly controlled pain. Failure of medical therapy is defined as minimal or no pain relief with the administration of analgesics for 3-4 weeks or achievement of adequate pain relief with only narcotic dosages that induce excessive intolerable adverse effects (constipation, urinary retention, and/or confusion).

- Painful vertebrae due to aggressive primary bone tumors such as hemangioma and giant cell tumor. In hemangiomas, treatment is aimed at pain relief, strengthening of bone, and devascularization. It can be used alone or in combination with sclerotherapy, especially in cases of epidural extension causing spinal cord compression.
- Painful vertebrae with extensive osteolysis with or without fracture of the affected vertebral body due to malignant infiltration by multiple myeloma, lymphoma, and metastasis. Because PV is only aimed at treating the pain and consolidating the weight-bearing bone, other specific tumor treatment should be given in conjunction for tumor management.
- Painful fracture associated with osteonecrosis (Kummel's disease).
- intended posterior surgical procedure for stabilization in which reinforcement of the affected vertebral body or pedicle is requested.
- Chronic traumatic fracture in normal bone with non-union of fracture fragments or internal cystic changes (HELMBERGER et al. 2003).

## Contraindications

### Absolute

- Patient improving well on appropriate analgesic medication
- Asymptomatic vertebral fracture and low risk for biomechanical instability and collapse
- Apparent systemic infection, osteomyelitis, discitis
- Local infection at the puncture site
- Uncorrectable coagulopathy
- Known allergy to any of the components used for PV
- Diffuse non-focal back pain.

### Relative

- Asymptomatic displacement of a fracture fragment producing spinal canal narrowing
- Radiculopathy
- Extension of the tumor into the spinal canal with or without cord compression
- Collapse of the posterior vertebral body wall (increased risk of PMMA leakage)
- Vertebra plana resulting in difficulties in needle placement

- Cardiorespiratory compromise such that safe sedation or anesthesia cannot be accomplished
- Lack of monitoring facilities and surgical back-up (HELMBERGER et al. 2003).

## Bone Cement

The bone cement used during augmentation of a fractured vertebral body/tumoral osteolysis or as an adjunct to surgical treatment requires specific mechanical and biological properties to support the spinal column. The bone cement is injected into the load-bearing part of the body; therefore, it has to withstand different strains. At the same time, due to the technique to approach the bone using a special type of needle, the cement has to have certain flow characteristic with an appropriate polymerization time. The ideal material for vertebroplasty should be easy and fast to prepare and should have a long toothpaste-like phase enabling the physician to perform the treatment without pressure of time. During the last years, polymethylmetacrylat (PMMA) has proven its properties as an inert, biomechanically adequate, and cost-effective substance, with a long history in surgical joint replacement. Up to now, other bone substitutes, such as ceramic bone cements and composite material, are still under development. However, there are some disadvantages of PMMA. Excessive inherent stiffness, high polymerization temperature, the lack of biologic potential to integrate into the bone, and possible monomer toxicity are the major drawbacks of this widely used bone cement. The key feature of the cement is its radio-opacity. The visibility of the material used has to be very good to make an early detection of a leak possible. The new intrinsically radio-opaque cements developed especially for vertebroplasty have solved problems caused by the addition of barium or tungsten to the older cements that interfered with the polymerization and changed its chemical properties.

## Preprocedural Evaluation

Patients' radiographs can be used to evaluate the degree of the compression after vertebral body fracture. Computed tomography is more exact in assessing the fractured vertebral body, its height loss on sagittal reconstruction, the presence or absence of any bone fragment within the spinal canal, the integrity of the posterior wall, and to rule out any unknown osteolytic process causing the vertebral body fracture. CT provides detailed information about the size and location of osteolytic tumors and is therefore an indispensable tool for the preprocedural workup. CT is furthermore able to give information about the size of the pedicles (and possible tumor involvement of the pedicles), the most suitable access path to the vertebral body, and which needle diameter should be used. However, it is impossible to differentiate chronic from acute compression fracture on plain film or CT examination without comparison films. If there are any doubts about the age of the fracture or which height should be treated in multilevel fractures and an additional adequate clinical examination is inconclusive, MRI helps to determine the site of acute fractures due to its sensitivity for bone marrow edema (especially STIR images) occurring in fresh fractures (Do 2000). Careful patient selection is mandatory and increases the likelihood of good treatment results (Do 2000; Mathis et al. 2001).

## 38.6
## Technique

During a preprocedural consultation with the patient, the procedure, intended benefits, and possible complications should be discussed and balanced. A patient informed consent is mandatory. Periprocedural application of antibiotics is mandatory in immunocompromised patients. Antibiotics are usually administered via a venous access 30 min ahead of the beginning of the procedure. However, there is no clear consensus in the literature (Alfonso et al. 2006; Soyuncu et al. 2006). During PV vital signs of the patient are monitored, and strict asepsis is maintained. Anatomic landmarks and structures differ according to the vertebral level to be treated.

In the cervical spine, a right anterolateral approach is used. The carotid-jugular complex has to be displaced gently downward and laterally and separated from the trachea and esophagus to expose an entry site for the needle.

Depending on the site of the neoplastic lesion/osteoporotic fracture in the thoracic and lumbar spine, three different approaches are feasible:

- The classic transpedicular route, which can be performed either by a unipedicular or bipedicular approach;
- the posterolateral approach, especially in the lumbar spine when a tumor lesion involves the pedicles;

- the intercostovertebral approach, especially used in the thoracic spine, which is more favorable when the pedicles are too small or destroyed by tumor. It has to be taken into account that this approach bears a higher risk of pneumothorax and paraspinal bleeding.

The PV can be performed either using biplane fluoroscopy guidance, dual guidance including CT and fluoroscopy, or CT-fluoroscopy alone.

### 38.6.1
### Biplane Fluoroscopy Guidance

The appropriate radiographic projection for the transpedicular approach is a straight anteroposterior (AP) view with 5°–10° angulation, in which the pedicle appears oval. Using AP and lateral views, the needle is forced through the upper and lateral aspect of the pedicle because of the reduced risk of harming the spinal cord and nerve roots. Using lateral fluoroscopy, the tip of the needle is positioned in the anterior third of the vertebral body or in the osteolytic lesion, with the shaft of the needle aligned parallel to the endplates of the affected vertebral body. Using this technique, the final endpoint of the needle tip is within the ipsilateral half of the vertebral body, therefore usually requiring a bipedicular approach for optimal filling of the vertebrae. The use of a beveled needle supports precise placement since rotating the beveled tip allows for distinct steering and therefore the tip can be positioned anteromedial in the vertebral body. Usually, this technique allows sufficient filling of the vertebral body making a bipedicular approach unnecessary.

### 38.6.2
### Dual Guidance

The advantage in combining CT and fluoroscopy is the precise needle placement, which is particularly important in the upper thoracic spine, tumor cases, and other difficult cases. This dual-guidance technique reduces complications and increases the comfort and the confidence of the interventional radiologist. It allows for visualization in three dimensions with exact differentiation of anatomic structures at risk. Fluoroscopy is provided by placing a mobile C-arm in front of the CT gantry. When the position of the needle tip is considered satisfactory, the imaging mode is switched to C-arm fluoroscopy for real-time visualization of cement application in an AP and lateral view.

### 38.6.3
### CT-Fluoroscopy Guidance

When the CT scanner is equipped with online CT fluoroscopy, it can be used for monitoring and guiding the whole procedure. A prerequisite is that the table can be moved by the interventional radiologist using a joystick from inside the room, maintaining strict asepsis. The entry point at the skin and advancing the needle through the vertebral body can be visualized at all times. Therefore, this technique allows for safe needle placement without harming critical structures (Fig. 38.2a–d). The cement application can be monitored online, and by moving the table back and forth the whole affected vertebral body can be covered easily. This allows for reliable detection of any cement leakage, especially into the spinal canal. Particularly in tumor cases, CT-fluoroscopy guidance facilitates the correct positioning of the needle in the osteolysis and permits to reliably assess potential bulging of the posterior vertebral wall when fractured (Fig. 38.3).

### 38.7
### Cement Application

After the needle (10–15 gauge) or in case of multiple affected vertebral bodies preferably up to three monolateral needles are carefully positioned, the cement is prepared. There are two options. To avoid contamination and the inclusion of air bubbles, the use of a closed mixing device is advocated. This system allows for homogenous mixing of the components and therefore increases its strength. If not available, the cement can also be mixed by hand in a sterile bowl. After 30–60 s of continuous mixing, the initially very fluid cement starts to get thick and pasty. Especially if only one vertebral body is supposed to get treated, it is advisable to wait an additional 60–90 s before injecting the cement into the vertebral body. If the cement is administered in this pasty polymerization phase, the risk of extravertebral leakage as well as venous intravasation is reduced.

For the administration of cement into the vertebral body, a dedicated screw-like injection set, provided by several manufactures, is usually employed. The advantage to using a dedicated set instead of a 2-cc Luer lock syringe is that the cement can be administered with continuous flow and minimal effort for the treating interventional radiologist. Furthermore, if a leak is noticed, the pressure can be stopped and reversed immediately.

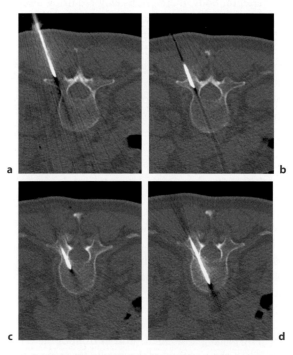

**Fig. 38.2a–d.** A 59-year-old female with an osteoporotic fracture of the 1st lumbar vertebra. Image series (**a–d**) demonstrates safe needle positioning in the anterior third of the altered vertebral body

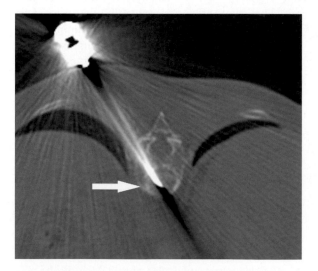

**Fig. 38.3.** A 64-year-old female patient with two painful osteolytic metastases affecting the 12th thoracic vertebra (*displayed*) and the 3rd lumbar vertebra. Needle placement using online CT-fluoroscopy guidance is demonstrated. The tip of the needle is positioned within the center of the osteolytic metastasis (*arrow*)

The injection of cement is observed under continuous lateral fluoroscopic or online CT-fluoroscopy control to allow for instant detection of leakage (Fig. 38.4). If a leakage is detected, it is very important to stop the procedure, reverse the pressure, and wait for up to 60 s. This time allows the cement to harden and probably seal the leak. If the leak then persists, the needle either has to be repositioned or the bevel direction should be modified. In cases in which these measures are not effective, the procedure should be abandoned. To complete the filling of the affected vertebral body, the contralateral approach could be used. In order the avoid cement leakage through the puncture canal, the initial needle should remain in place.

The procedure is completed when the osteolytic lesion within the vertebral body is completely or partially filled (Fig. 38.5a–f) or when the anterior two thirds of the fractured, osteoporotic vertebral body is filled and/or the cement is homogenously distributed between both endplates. It has to be taken into account that the cavity of the needle contains an additional 1–2 cc of cement. While the stylet of the needle is pushed forward, this cement is also injected into the vertebral body. This should be done under fluoroscopic control to avoid

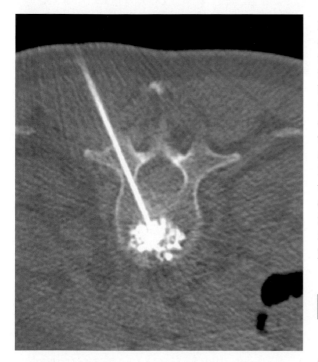

**Fig. 38.4.** Injection of cement observed by online CT-fluoroscopy, which allows instant detection of leakage. The whole vertebral body can be covered easily by stepwise movement of the table using a joystick mounted to the CT table

leakage. Especially in tumor vertebroplasty, the use of online CT-fluoroscopy is favorable, since not only cement leakage can be detected, but also bulging of soft tissue tumor components into the spinal canal can be depicted. The re-insertion of the stylet reduces the risk of a cement antenna in the paravertebral soft tissue. If the stylet is not completely repositioned, the interventional radiologist should wait until the cement is completely hardened. Then the cement antenna within the needle can be broken off and carefully removed together with the needle.

The time between mixing and hardening of the cement is approximately 8–10 min (room temperature, 20°C). Some manufacturers provide cement with longer setting times. Therefore, in case of multiple affected vertebral bodies, preferably up to three vertebral levels can be treated in a single session.

Concerning the cardiotoxicity of PMMA (especially when spilled into the venous circulation), no consistent data are published in the literature. The deteriorating baseline mean arterial blood pressure during PV is, according to the literature, most likely associated with the increase of pressure within the vertebral bodies rather than with the use of PMMA (AEBLI et al. 2003; KAUFMANN et al. 2002).

The pain relief in vertebral destructions due to malignant tumors is not directly proportional to the percentage of lesion filling (COTTEN et al. 1996). Therefore, the volume of cement as well as the number of injections performed to obtain complete lesion filling should be limited, especially when extensive cortical destruction is present. Consequently, it should decrease the risk of leaks of cement, particularly epidural, foraminal, and venous leaks. Discal and paravertebral leaks of PMMA seem to have no clinical importance for the patients. Depending on the size of the osteolytic lesion, smaller volumes (1.5–3 cc) are usually associated with good clinical results. In patients with osteoporotic vertebral fractures, usually 2.5–4 cc of cement provides good filling of the vertebra and achieves both consolidation and pain relief (Fig. 38.6a–d).

## 38.8
## Complications

Complications are classified into minor and major adverse events. Minor adverse reactions are defined as unexpected or undesirable clinical occurrences that require no immediate or delayed surgical intervention (MCGRAW et al. 2002). A major adverse event is defined as the occurrence of an unexpected or undesirable clini-

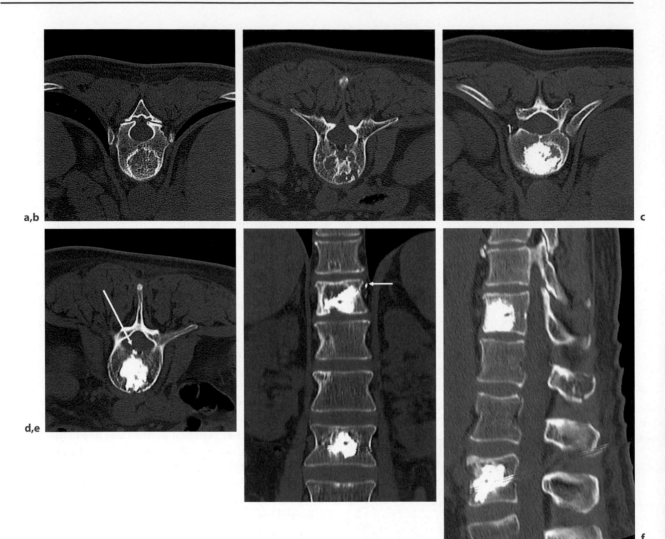

**Fig. 38.5a–f.** Same patient as in Fig. 38.3. Two osteolytic metastases involving the 12th thoracic vertebra (**a**) and the 3rd lumbar vertebra (**b**). The posterior wall of the 3rd lumbar vertebra is destroyed. The post-procedural CT scans [axial (**c**, **d**), coronal (**e**) and sagittal (**f**)] show partial filling of the lesion in the 12th thoracic vertebra and complete filling of the metastasis in the 3rd lumbar vertebral body. Initial leakage of cement in an epidural vein (**d**, *arrow*) with no significant narrowing of the spinal canal. In the coronal view a small cement leakage (**e**, *arrow*) in a paravertebral vein can be appreciated

cal event, which requires surgical intervention or results in death or significant disability. Published data have placed the complication rates in osteoporotic fractures treated with PV at <1%, while the rates in metastatic vertebrae with fractures may be as high as 10% (Dera-mond et al. 1998; McGraw et al. 2003).

Most complications, such as infection, fracture of ribs, posterior vertebral elements or pedicles, allergic reaction, as well as bleeding from the puncture site, have a reported incidence below 1% and are considered as minor complications (Diamond et al. 2003; Kallmes et al. 2002).

A recently published paper described six (5.1%) local and two (1.7%) systemic complications in 117 patients treated for vertebral metastases with PV (Barragan-Campos et al. 2006). Local complications consisted of hematoma at the puncture site (resolved uneventful with no further treatment required) and radicular pain

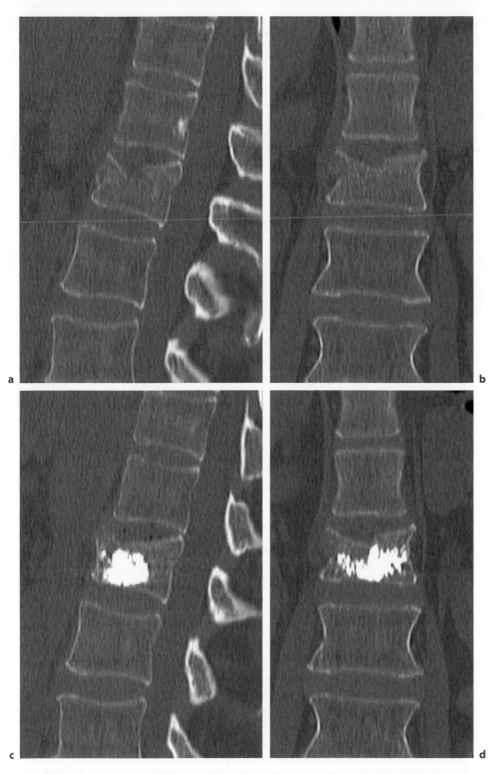

**Fig. 38.6a–d.** A 58-year-old female patient with a treatment-refractory painful osteoporotic fracture of the 1st lumbar vertebra. Sagittal (**a**) and coronal (**b**) images prior to PV illustrate the impression fracture of the cranial endplate and a height reduction in the center of the vertebral body of about 20%. After PV, sagittal (**c**) and coronal (**d**) images show sufficient cement filling of the vertebral body with a column between the endplates

due to ipsilateral foraminal venous cement leakage. The symptoms resolved under appropriate medication with non-steroidal anti-inflammatory drugs and a single bolus of prednisolon. None of the patients required surgical debulking of the cement. Interestingly, two patients developed pulmonary embolism (PE) detected on their post-procedural chest radiographs and CT scans. One patient did not develop any pulmonary or hemodynamic signs or symptoms of PE, while the other patient (adenocarcinoma of the lung) developed ventilatory and hemodynamic symptoms of PE and died despite treatment with anticoagulants 1 week after PV. In total, the per-procedure and per-patient morbidity rates were 5.0% (8 of 159 procedures) and 6.8% (8 of 117 patients), while the single death recorded meant that the procedural and patient mortality rates were 0.6% (1 of 159 procedures) and 0.9% (1 of 117 patients), respectively.

Although leakage of cement is well tolerated in most cases (NUSSBAUM et al. 2004), it is the main source of pulmonary and neurological complications. A transient neurological deficit is observed in 5% of patients with malignant etiology. Symptoms respond well to nerve-root blocks or oral medication; rarely do they require surgical decompression (COTTEN et al. 1996; WEILL et al. 1996). While leakages of cement into the spinal canal only infrequently lead to neurological complications or even paraplegia, intraforaminal leakage is more harmful. COTTEN et al. (1996) found that leakage into the spinal canal was well tolerated in all their 15 patients, while two of eight cases of foraminal leakage were associated with radiculopathy.

It has been reported that cement leakage is more common when PV is used for metastatic osteolytic tumors or myelomas of the spine than in osteoporotic fractures. However, VASCONCELOS et al. (2002) observed no major differences, although they noted venous leaks slightly more frequently in patients with metastatic lesions. When PV was performed in osteoporotic vertebral compression fractures, leakage into the disc space was more commonly observed. MOUSAVI et al. (2003) reviewed post-procedural CT scans in patients with osteoporotic vertebral compression fractures and metastatic lesions of the spine and concluded that in osteoporotic vertebrae leakage occurred mainly into the disc, whereas in metastatic lesions it was found in various different locations.

MCGRAW et al. (2002) found that intraosseous venography predicted the flow of PMMA during vertebroplasty in 83% of cases; however, this has not been confirmed by other authors, and the use of preprocedural venography has largely been abandoned except in hypervascular tumors (DO 2002; GAUGHEN et al. 2002). The viscosity of the cement has been shown to represent the most important factor for cement leakage. HEINI et al. (2002) described that the risk of cement intravasation is diminished if the flow of cement is directed in a medial direction within the vertebral body. Therefore, they suggested using a side-opening cannula.

## Postprocedural Care

After finishing the vertebroplasty and removing the needle, the patient should stay on the examination table until the cement is hardened, demonstrated by the rest of the cement in the mixing bowl. After moving the patient into the bed, the patient is at bed rest for at least 2 h, because the cement reaches 90% of its ultimate strength within the first hour. If there is an increase in pain or neurological deterioration, a CT examination has to be performed immediately to rule out any complications (bleeding) or an extravasation of the cement into the spinal canal or the neuroforamina. Anti-inflammatory drugs can be prescribed for 2 to 4 days to reduce the possible inflammatory reaction due to the heat caused by polymerization of PMMA (GANGI et al. 2006).

## Results

### 38.10.1
### Osteoporotic Vertebral Body Fractures

Published data available dealing with the analgesic effect of vertebroplasty are mainly observational studies. In these studies, some of the patients describe improvement of their complaints immediately after treatment; however, significant pain relief normally occurs within 24 h after treatment (COTTEN et al. 1998) and were demonstrated in up to 90% of patients suffering from osteoporotic fractures (DERAMOND et al. 1998; GANGI et al. 1998; HOCHMUTH et al. 2006; SINGH et al. 2006). However, sometimes it takes several days until the patient reports definite improvement of symptoms. The mechanism responsible for pain relief after PV indeed still remains unclear. Possible reasons are the mechanical stabilization of the fractured vertebral body, chemical toxicity, or thermal necrosis of surrounding tissues and nerve endings (LIEBERMAN et al. 2005). Interestingly, there are studies proving that the age of a fracture, from the onset of the symptoms, is not a predictor regarding success or failure of the treatment. Moreover, it has been shown that the age of the fracture was not independently associated with postprocedural pain (KAUFMANN et al. 2001). Furthermore, in the majority of cases, the procedure results not only in pain relief, but in the ability to significantly reduce the dosage of analgesics needed for pain palliation, an increase in physical mobility and therefore in a distinct improvement in quality of life (ZOARSKI et al. 2002; SINGH et al. 2006; EVANS et al. 2003). It was even shown that patients with severe osteoporotic fractures defined as a height loss of 60 to 70% of the fractured vertebral body do benefit from the treatment (O'BRIEN et al. 2000). Furthermore, studies dealing with the long-term effects of PV, with a follow-up of up to 48 months, were able to demonstrate that the benefits for these patients are persistent over a longer period of time (GRADOS et al. 2000; HODLER et al. 2003; PEREZ-HIGUERAS et al. 2002). However, a well designed controlled trial to demonstrate the effects of PV in comparison to open surgery or best supportive care is still needed.

## 38.10.2
## Tumoral Osteolysis

While in healthy vertebrae, burst fracture occurs only under high impact loading, patients with vertebral metastases may experience burst fractures under normal physiologic loading conditions (ROTH et al. 2004; WHYNE et al. 2003). Factors such as bone density and tumor volume as well as tumor location and shape have been shown to be important in assessing burst fracture risk (WHYNE et al. 2003; TSCHIRHART et al. 2004). The strengthening effect of the PMMA application is thought to provide stability and prevent fracture or further collapse of the affected vertebrae. Concerning pain relief, it is discussed that the vascular, chemical, and thermal forces associated with the inflammatory reaction to the heat of polymerization of PMMA probably have a more pronounced effect than the mechanical forces and may account for the clinical improvements of the patients (DERAMOND et al. 1999).

## 38.10.3
## Analgesic Effect

Clear improvement is usually defined as complete pain relief with no necessity for analgesic medication or enough of a decrease in pain that the dose of analgesic drugs can be reduced by at least 50%. Also the replacement from narcotic drugs to non-narcotic drugs

is considered to reflect clear clinical improvement. In vertebrae with metastases and debilitating pain, pain palliation can be achieved in 50–97% of the patients (ALVAREZ et al. 2003; COTTEN et al. 1996; BARR et al. 2000; FOURNEY et al. 2003; MARTIN et al. 1999; WINKING et al. 2004). These data are similar to those reported for surgical treatment (WEIGEL et al. 1999).

COTTEN et al. (1996) described partial or complete pain relief in 36 of 37 patients within 6–72 h of PMMA injection, independent from the percentage of cement fill in the vertebral body. Depending on the size of the osteolytic lesion, smaller volumes (1.5–3.5 cc) are usually sufficient to provide good results (LIEBSCHNER et al. 2001). In a retrospective analysis on 37 patients suffering from various primary tumors with metastatic spread to the spine, WEILL et al. (1996) described clear to moderate improvement in 35 patients. At the 1-month follow-up, there was no recurrence in pain in those patients who initially benefited from the procedure. At the 3-month follow-up, 9 of 14 patients presented with stable pain palliation. In those five patients with a variable degree of recurrence of pain, additional vertebrae involved by metastases adjacent to the formerly treated vertebral body were detected by MR imaging. This suggests that recurrence of pain is most likely due to the new lesions instead of failure of the initial procedure. This has been well described by HODLER et al. (2003).

ALVAREZ et al. (2003) demonstrated an immediate analgesic efficacy in 90% of 21 treated patients with a persistent pain relief in 67% of the patients over prolonged periods of time. Another important finding was that 69% of non-ambulatory patients became ambulatory after the PV procedure due to the substantial relief of pain.

## 38.10.4
## Biomechanical Stabilization

To date, the mechanical properties of the metastatic spine and the mechanisms of collapse have not been fully elucidated. Moreover, the correlation between vertebral body collapse and the location and extent of the metastatic tumor is not fully understood. TANEICHI et al. (1997) evaluated 100 thoracic and lumbar vertebrae (53 patients) with osteolytic lesions, determined risk factors for vertebral collapse, and estimated the probability of collapse under various states of metastatic vertebral involvement. The most important risk factor leading to vertebral collapse in the thoracic region was involvement of the costovertebral joint. Tumor size within the vertebral body was the second most important risk factor. Interestingly, destruction of the costovertebral joint more strongly induced vertebral body collapse than the size of metastatic tumor within the thoracic vertebral body. Under the condition that the metastatic lesion was confined to the vertebral body, impending collapse existed when the vertebral body involvement was 50-60% in the thoracic spine and 35-40% in the thoracolumbar and lumbar spine. This indicates that the thoracic vertebra has greater tolerance to collapse than the thoracolumbar and lumbar vertebrae as long as the costovertebral joint remains intact. The impact of metastatic pedicle involvement on vertebral collapse was much greater in the thoracolumbar and lumbar spine than in the thoracic spine. The involved vertebral body with pedicle destruction may be more vulnerable to axial overload than the vertebrae with intact pedicles. This might be attributed to the fact that posterior load-bearing structures (e.g., facet joints) can no longer support the involved vertebral body from the posterior aspect once disconnection between the vertebral body and the posterior elements occurs as a result of pedicle destruction

TSCHIRHART et al. (2005) published a study aimed to determine the effect of cement location and the volume of cement injected during percutaneous vertebroplasty on improving vertebral stability in a metastatically compromised spinal motion segment using a parametric poroelastic finite element model. Sixteen scenarios (different tumor locations within the vertebral body, different cement locations within the vertebrae) were investigated pre- and post-vertebroplasty using a serrated spherical representation of tumor tissue and various geometric representations of PMMA.

Vertebral bulge and vertebral axial displacement were used as a measure of stability. Vertebral bulge was defined as the maximum radial bulge of the vertebral body under load as a burst fracture predictor irrespective of endplate failure, and vertebral axial displacement represented the maximum axial displacement of the vertebral body under load as a predictor for burst fracture following endplate failure.

The results indicated that vertebral bulge and axial displacement decreased with the addition of cement in all scenarios, and therefore PV decreased the risk of burst fracture initiation. However, the magnitude of the increase in stability depended on the location and geometry of the cement injected. Burst fracture risk appeared to be minimized when cement was injected near the posterior wall of the vertebral body.

The cement volume required to restore vertebral stability to that of a baseline intact model was calculated. To significantly decrease vertebral bulge 16%–17% fill of the vertebral body was required for the posterolateral

and anterolateral PMMA deposition, whereas stabilization of the axial displacement required up to 32% fill of the metastatically involved vertebrae. This is especially noteworthy since other authors have indicated that cement leakage becomes imminent at approximately 20% cement volume of the involved vertebral body (HIGGINS et al. 2003). Therefore the authors concluded that it may not be necessary to exceed a volume of 20% of PMMA, especially since the vertebral bulge rather than the axial displacement has shown clinically to best predict burst fracture in the metastatic spine (ROTH et al. 2004). Further results of this study indicated that augmentation of metastatic vertebrae was beneficial for stabilization even when the PMMA was asymmetrically located and focused on areas of bone destruction.

These results are supported by AHN et al. (2006). They experimentally measured the load-induced spinal canal narrowing to determine the biomechanical stability of metastatically involved vertebrae following percutaneous vertebroplasty. Specimens with cement located in a posterior location showed reduced load-induced spinal canal narrowing of 39% following PV. Moreover, AHN et al. found that a reduction in load-induced spinal canal narrowing did not occur with PMMA located in the anterior portion of the vertebral body.

## 38.11
## Combination with Tumor Ablation

The location of cement injection relative to the tumor tissue is critical in attaining maximum vertebral stability following PV. Vertebrae with tumors located in the posterior region are at a higher risk for the occurrence of burst fractures due to their proximity to the posterior vertebral body wall (TSCHIRHART et al. 2004). TSCHIRHART et al. (2005) described that stabilization effects of PV on vertebrae with posterior tumors are not as positive as for tumors in other locations.

Using current methods for PMMA injection, there is a high risk of cement leakage into the spinal canal when the cement is injected in the posterior region of the vertebral body. However, the above-mentioned biomechanical studies indicate that cement injection in this region tends to provide improved biomechanical stability to the vertebral body (AHN et al. 2006). Cement leakage, particularly into the spinal canal, is still considered as the primary concern associated with PV. However, as the effects of cement location and volume become better understood, less cement injection may be required

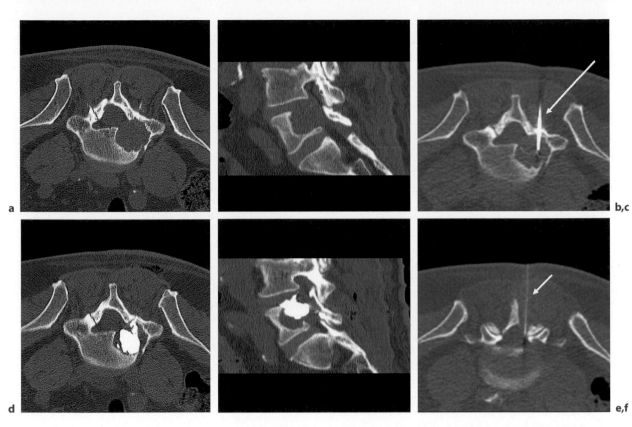

**Fig. 38.7a–f.** A 71-year-old male patient suffering from a painful and destabilizing osteolytic renal cell cancer metastasis of the 5th lumbar vertebra (**a, d**). In order to avoid radiculopathy as a result of cement contact with the adjacent nerve root and heating of the nerve tissue during tumor ablation (**c**, *long arrow* – RFA electrode within the metastasis) and the polymer- ization phase of the PMMA, a spinal needle was positioned in close proximity of the neuroforamina, and saline was injected slowly to cool the nerve root (**f**, *short arrow*). Post-procedural axial (**b**) and sagittal (**e**) scans show partial filling of the osteolytic metastasis. The patient developed no neurological symptoms, but significant pain relief

to provide adequate stability and at the same time reduces the risk of leakage. With online CT-fluoroscopy guidance and its excellent overview and spatial resolution, it is feasible to perform ablation on tumors located adjacent to the posterior wall of the vertebra, and it becomes feasible to inject the cement reliably into the region of the posterior vertebral body wall with minimal likelihood of leakage (Fig. 38.7a–f). Therefore, tumor ablation could decrease the tumor volume prior to PV, providing the space necessary for cement injection and allowing for a quasi-shell geometry of the cement to encapsulate the tumor with minimal risk for leakage. This is of special interest for stabilizing vertebrae with metastases in the posterior portion of the vertebral body. Recently published studies have shown improvement in vertebral stability and reduced PMMA leakage when tumor ablation was performed prior to PV (Buy et al. 2006; Masala et al. 2004; Schaefer et al. 2003).

## 38.12
## Conclusion

Percutaneous vertebroplasty is a safe and efficient therapeutic option for patients suffering from otherwise untreatable pain and disability caused by osteoporotic fracture or tumoral involvement of a vertebra. The vertebroplasty provides nearly immediate pain relief and stabilization, leading to a high rate of successful treatments with low morbidity, hospitalization, and adverse events. In addition, PV contributes to spinal stabilization and can be successfully combined with chemotherapy, radiation therapy, tumor ablation, and posterior laminectomy. Therefore, the number of procedures performed has continuously increased over the last few years. However, indications and contraindications, the technique, and possible complications of percutaneous vertebroplasty and its therapy always have to be taken into account by the experienced interventionalist, and the success rate strongly depends – beside on the experience of the interventionalist – on the visualization equipment used.

## References

Aebli N, Krebs J, Schwenke D, Davis G, Theis JC: Pressurization of vertebral bodies during vertebroplasty causes cardiovascular complications: an experimental study in sheep. Spine 2003;28:1513–9

Ahn H, Mousavi P, Roth S, Reidy D, Finkelstein J, Whyne C: Stability of the metastatic spine pre and post vertebroplasty. J Spinal Disord Tech 2006;19:178–82.

Alfonso Olmos M, Silva Gonzalez A, Duart Clemente J, Villas Tome C: Infected vertebroplasty due to uncommon bacteria solved surgically: a rare and threatening life complication of a common procedure: report of a case and a review of the literature. Spine 2006;31:770–3

Alvarez L, Perez-Higueras A, Quinones D, Calvo E, Rossi RE: Vertebroplasty in the treatment of vertebral tumors: postprocedural outcome and quality of life. Eur Spine J 2003;12:356–60

Alvarez L, Alcaraz M, Perez-Higueras A, Granizo JJ, de Miguel I, Rossi RE et al: Percutaneous vertebroplasty: functional improvement in patients with osteoporotic compression fractures. Spine 2006;31:1113–8.Chataigner H, Onimus M: Surgery in spinal metastasis without spinal cord compression: indications and strategy related to the risk of recurrence. Eur Spine J 2000;9:523–7

Barragan-Campos HM, Vallee JN, Lo D, Cormier E, Jean B, Rose M et al: Percutaneous vertebroplasty for spinal metastases: complications. Radiology 2006;238:354–62

Barr JD, Barr MS, Lemley TJ, McCann RM: Percutaneous vertebroplasty for pain relief and spinal stabilization. Spine 2000;25:923–8

Buy X, Basile A, Bierry G, Cupelli J, Gangi A: Saline-infused bipolar radiofrequency ablation of high-risk spinal and paraspinal neoplasms. AJR Am J Roentgenol 2006;186:322–6

Coleman RE: Bisphosphonates in breast cancer. Ann Oncol 2005;16:687–95

Cotten A, Dewatre F, Cortet B, Assaker R, Leblond D, Duquesnoy B et al: Percutaneous vertebroplasty for osteolytic metastases and myeloma: effects of the percentage of lesion filling and the leakage of methyl methacrylate at clinical follow-up. Radiology 1996;200:525–30

Cotten A, Boutry N, Cortet B, Assaker R, Demondion X, Leblond D et al: Percutaneous vertebroplasty: state of the art. Radiographics 1998;18:311–20

Deramond H, Depriester C, Galibert P, Le Gars D: Percutaneous vertebroplasty with polymethylmethacrylate. Technique, indications, and results. Radiol Clin North Am 1998;36:533–46

Deramond H, Wright NT, Belkoff SM: Temperature elevation caused by bone cement polymerization during vertebroplasty. Bone 1999;25:17S–21S.

Diamond TH, Bryant C, Browne L, Clark WA: Clinical outcomes after acute osteoporotic vertebral fractures: a 2-year non-randomised trial comparing percutaneous vertebroplasty with conservative therapy. Med J Aust 2006;184:113–7

Diamond TH, Champion B, Clark WA: Management of acute osteoporotic vertebral fractures: a nonrandomized trial comparing percutaneous vertebroplasty with conservative therapy. Am J Med 2003;114:257–65

Do HM: Magnetic resonance imaging in the evaluation of patients for percutaneous vertebroplasty. Top Magn Reson Imaging 2000;11:235–44.Galibert P, Deramond H: [Percutaneous acrylic vertebroplasty as a treatment of vertebral angioma as well as painful and debilitating diseases]. Chirurgie 1990;116:326–34

Do HM: Intraosseous venography during percutaneous vertebroplasty: is it needed? AJNR Am J Neuroradiol 2002;23:508–9

Evans AJ, Jensen ME, Kip KE, DeNardo AJ, Lawler GJ, Negin GA et al: Vertebral compression fractures: pain reduction and improvement in functional mobility after percutaneous polymethylmethacrylate vertebroplasty retrospective report of 245 cases. Radiology 2003;226:366–72

Fourney DR, Schomer DF, Nader R, Chlan-Fourney J, Suki D, Ahrar K et al: Percutaneous vertebroplasty and kyphoplasty for painful vertebral body fractures in cancer patients. J Neurosurg 2003;98:21–30

Gangi A, Guth S, Imbert JP, Marin H, Dietemann JL: Percutaneous vertebroplasty: indications, technique, and results. Radiographics 2003;23:e10

Gangi A, Sabharwal T, Irani FG, Buy X, Morales JP, Adam A: Quality assurance guidelines for percutaneous vertebroplasty. Cardiovasc Intervent Radiol 2006;29:173–8.

Gangi A, Dietemann JL, Mortazavi R, Pfleger D, Kauff C, Roy C: CT-guided interventional procedures for pain management in the lumbosacral spine. Radiographics 1998;18:621–33

Gaughen JR, Jr., Jensen ME, Schweickert PA, Kaufmann TJ, Marx WF, Kallmes DF: Relevance of antecedent venography in percutaneous vertebroplasty for the treatment of osteoporotic compression fractures. AJNR Am J Neuroradiol 2002;23:594–600

Grados F, Depriester C, Cayrolle G, Hardy N, Deramond H, Fardellone P: Long-term observations of vertebral osteoporotic fractures treated by percutaneous vertebroplasty. Rheumatology (Oxford) 2000;39:1410–4

Heini PF, Dain Allred C: The use of a side-opening injection cannula in vertebroplasty: a technical note. Spine 2002;27:105–9

Helmberger T, Bohndorf K, Hierholzer J, Noldge G, Vorwerk D: [Guidelines of the German Radiological Society for percutaneous vertebroplasty]. Radiologe 2003;43:703–8.

Hide IG, Gangi A: Percutaneous vertebroplasty: history, technique and current perspectives. Clin Radiol 2004;59:461–7

Higgins KB, Harten RD, Langrana NA, Reiter MF: Biomechanical effects of unipedicular vertebroplasty on intact vertebrae. Spine 2003;28:1540–7

Hill ME, Richards MA, Gregory WM, Smith P, Rubens RD: Spinal cord compression in breast cancer: a review of 70 cases. Br J Cancer 1993;68:969–73

Hochmuth K, Proschek D, Schwarz W, Mack M, Kurth AA, Vogl TJ: Percutaneous vertebroplasty in the therapy of osteoporotic vertebral compression fractures: a critical review. Eur Radiol 2006;16:998–1004

Hodler J, Peck D, Gilula LA: Midterm outcome after vertebroplasty: predictive value of technical and patient-related factors. Radiology 2003;227:662–8

Hoffmann RT, Jakobs TF, Ertl-Wagner BB, Wallnofer A, Reiser MF, Helmberger TK: [Vertebroplasty in osteoporotic vertebral compression]. Radiologe 2003;43:729–34

Jacobs WB, Perrin RG: Evaluation and treatment of spinal metastases: an overview. Neurosurg Focus 2001;11:e10.

Kallmes DF, Schweickert PA, Marx WF, Jensen ME: Vertebroplasty in the mid- and upper thoracic spine. AJNR Am J Neuroradiol 2002;23:1117–20

Kaufmann TJ, Jensen ME, Ford G, Gill LL, Marx WF, Kallmes DF: Cardiovascular effects of polymethylmethacrylate use in percutaneous vertebroplasty. AJNR Am J Neuroradiol 2002;23:601–4

Kaufmann TJ, Jensen ME, Schweickert PA, Marx WF, Kallmes DF: Age of fracture and clinical outcomes of percutaneous vertebroplasty. AJNR Am J Neuroradiol 2001;22:1860–3.

Lieberman IH, Togawa D, Kayanja MM: Vertebroplasty and kyphoplasty: filler materials. Spine J 2005;5:305S–16S

Liebschner MA, Rosenberg WS, Keaveny TM: Effects of bone cement volume and distribution on vertebral stiffness after vertebroplasty. Spine 2001;26:1547–54

Martin JB, Jean B, Sugiu K, San Millan Ruiz D, Piotin M, Murphy K et al: Vertebroplasty: clinical experience and follow-up results. Bone 1999;25:11S–5S

Masala S, Roselli M, Massari F, Fiori R, Ursone A, Fossile E et al: Radiofrequency Heat Ablation and Vertebroplasty in the treatment of neoplastic vertebral body fractures. Anticancer Res 2004;24:3129–33

Mathis JM, Barr JD, Belkoff SM, Barr MS, Jensen ME, Deramond H: Percutaneous vertebroplasty: a developing standard of care for vertebral compression fractures. AJNR Am J Neuroradiol 2001;22:373–81

McGraw JK, Heatwole EV, Strnad BT, Silber JS, Patzilk SB, Boorstein JM: Predictive value of intraosseous venography before percutaneous vertebroplasty. J Vasc Interv Radiol 2002;13:149–53

McGraw JK, Lippert JA, Minkus KD, Rami PM, Davis TM, Budzik RF: Prospective evaluation of pain relief in 100 patients undergoing percutaneous vertebroplasty: results and follow-up. J Vasc Interv Radiol 2002;13:883–6

McGraw JK, Cardella J, Barr JD, Mathis JM, Sanchez O, Schwartzberg MS et al: Society of Interventional Radiology quality improvement guidelines for percutaneous vertebroplasty. J Vasc Interv Radiol 2003;14:311–5

Mousavi P, Roth S, Finkelstein J, Cheung G, Whyne C: Volumetric quantification of cement leakage following percutaneous vertebroplasty in metastatic and osteoporotic vertebrae. J Neurosurg 2003;99:56–9

Nussbaum DA, Gailloud P, Murphy K: A review of complications associated with vertebroplasty and kyphoplasty as reported to the Food and Drug Administration medical device related web site. J Vasc Interv Radiol 2004;15:1185–92

O'Brien JP, Sims JT, Evans AJ: Vertebroplasty in patients with severe vertebral compression fractures: a technical report. AJNR Am J Neuroradiol 2000;21:1555–8

Perez-Higueras A, Alvarez L, Rossi RE, Quinones D, Al-Assir I: Percutaneous vertebroplasty: long-term clinical and radiological outcome. Neuroradiology 2002;44:950–4

Pascal-Moussellard H, Broc G, Pointillart V, Simeon F, Vital JM, Senegas J: Complications of vertebral metastasis surgery. Eur Spine J 1998;7:438–44

Peh WC, Gilula LA: Percutaneous vertebroplasty: an update. Semin Ultrasound CT MR 2005;26:52–64

Phillips FM: Minimally invasive treatments of osteoporotic vertebral compression fractures. Spine 2003;28:45–53.

Rades D, Fehlauer F, Schulte R, Veninga T, Stalpers LJ, Basic H et al: Prognostic factors for local control and survival after radiotherapy of metastatic spinal cord compression. J Clin Oncol 2006;24:3388–93

Roth SE, Mousavi P, Finkelstein J, Chow E, Kreder H, Whyne CM: Metastatic burst fracture risk prediction using biomechanically based equations. Clin Orthop Relat Res 2004;83–90.

Schaefer O, Lohrmann C, Markmiller M, Uhrmeister P, Langer M: Technical innovation. Combined treatment of a spinal metastasis with radiofrequency heat ablation and vertebroplasty. AJR Am J Roentgenol 2003;180:1075–7

Singh AK, Pilgram TK, Gilula LA: Osteoporotic compression fractures: outcomes after single- versus multiple-level percutaneous vertebroplasty. Radiology 2006;238:211–20.

Soyuncu Y, Ozdemir H, Soyuncu S, Bigat Z, Gur S: Posterior spinal epidural abscess: an unusual complication of vertebroplasty. Joint Bone Spine 2006

Stallmeyer MJ, Zoarski GH, Obuchowski AM: Optimizing patient selection in percutaneous vertebroplasty. J Vasc Interv Radiol 2003;14:683–96

Taneichi H, Kaneda K, Takeda N, Abumi K, Satoh S: Risk factors and probability of vertebral body collapse in metastases of the thoracic and lumbar spine. Spine 1997;22:239–45

Tschirhart CE, Roth SE, Whyne CM: Biomechanical assessment of stability in the metastatic spine following percutaneous vertebroplasty: effects of cement distribution patterns and volume. J Biomech 2005;38:1582–90

Tschirhart CE, Nagpurkar A, Whyne CM: Effects of tumor location, shape and surface serration on burst fracture risk in the metastatic spine. J Biomech 2004;37:653–60

Vasconcelos C, Gailloud P, Beauchamp NJ, Heck DV, Murphy KJ: Is percutaneous vertebroplasty without pretreatment venography safe? Evaluation of 205 consecutives procedures. AJNR Am J Neuroradiol 2002;23:913–7

Weigel B, Maghsudi M, Neumann C, Kretschmer R, Muller FJ, Nerlich M: Surgical management of symptomatic spinal metastases. Postoperative outcome and quality of life. Spine 1999;24:2240–6

Weill A, Chiras J, Simon JM, Rose M, Sola-Martinez T, Enkaoua E: Spinal metastases: indications for and results of percutaneous injection of acrylic surgical cement. Radiology 1996;199:241–7

Whyne CM, Hu SS, Lotz JC: Biomechanically derived guideline equations for burst fracture risk prediction in the metastatically involved spine. J Spinal Disord Tech 2003;16:180–5.

Winking M, Stahl JP, Oertel M, Schnettler R, Boker DK: Treatment of pain from osteoporotic vertebral collapse by percutaneous PMMA vertebroplasty. Acta Neurochir (Wien) 2004;146:469–76

Wong DA, Fornasier VL, MacNab I: Spinal metastases: the obvious, the occult, and the impostors. Spine 1990;15:1–4

Zoarski GH, Snow P, Olan WJ, Stallmeyer MJ, Dick BW, Hebel JR et al: Percutaneous vertebroplasty for osteoporotic compression fractures: quantitative prospective evaluation of long-term outcomes. J Vasc Interv Radiol 2002;13:139–48.

Zoarski GH, Stallmeyer MJ, Obuchowski A: Percutaneous vertebroplasty: A to Z. Tech Vasc Interv Radiol 2002;5:223–38

# CT-Guided Tumor Ablation

## 39

Ralf-Thorsten Hoffmann, Tobias F. Jakobs, Christoph Trumm
and Maximilian F. Reiser

CONTENTS

R.-T. Hoffmann, MD, PD
Department of Clinical Radiology, Ludwig-Maximilians-University, Munich University Hospitals, Marchioninistrasse 15, 81377 Munich, Germany

T. F. Jakobs, MD
Department of Clinical Radiology, Ludwig-Maximilians-University, Munich University Hospitals, Marchioninistrasse 15, 81377 Munich, Germany

C. Trumm, MD
Department of Clinical Radiology, Ludwig-Maximilians-University, Munich University Hospitals, Marchioninistrasse 15, 81377 Munich, Germany

M. F. Reiser MD
Department of Clinical Radiology, Ludwig-Maximilians-University, Munich University Hospitals, Marchioninistrasse 15, 81377 Munich, Germany

**ABSTRACT**

Percutaneous thermal ablation therapies have been receiving increasing attention as potential primary treatments for focal HCC and liver metastases. Possible advantages of ablative therapies as compared to surgical resection include a lower morbidity and mortality rate, lower costs, the suitability for real time imaging guidance, the option to perform ablative procedures on outpatients, and the potential application to a wider spectrum of patients, including those who are unsuitable as surgical candidates. Therefore, the major advantage of RFA is its ability to create a well-controlled focal thermal injury in the liver resulting in high success rates in treating HCC nodules and metastases smaller than 3 cm in diameter with long-term outcome results comparable to surgery. Besides the accepted application of thermal ablation in patients suffering from liver tumors, RFA has a rapidly growing role in tumors beyond the liver. Especially in renal and lung cancer, RF ablation shows very promising results; however, larger studies are still missing proving its effectiveness regarding the long-term follow-up.

## 39.1
### Introduction

CT-guided tumor ablation is one of the most challenging developments in the field of interventional radiology. The radiologist performing tumor ablation needs profound knowledge both in modern diagnostic and interventional radiology and in clinical and oncological patient care. These premises have to be fulfilled to be an accepted partner, especially for the surgeons—who often think that they are in competition for patients qualifying for minimally invasive therapies with interventional radiologists—as well as for the referring oncologists.

Thermal ablative techniques using heat (laser, radiofrequency, and microwave) or cold (cryotherapy) have shown rapid progress during the last 10 years, with its efficacy being confirmed by multiple large series and clinical follow-up since then. Especially in patients suffering from HCC in underlying liver cirrhosis, there is proof that radiofrequency ablation is superior to open surgery due to its less invasive character (HELMBERGER et al. 2007). However, even patients suffering from metastases within their liver—who are not surgical candidates because of inoperability—show significant benefit regarding survival compared to those patients undergoing chemotherapy only. Due to the rapidly growing acceptance of minimally invasive thermal therapy for liver malignancies, ablative therapies (especially radiofrequency ablation) are being increasingly used for the treatment of extrahepatic tumors, especially within the lung, kidney, and bone with both curative (osteoid osteoma) and palliative (osteolyses) intentions.

The aim of this chapter therefore is to describe technical details and the major applications. Furthermore, it will give a short summary of the latest literature–with an emphasis on RFA and especially RFA of the liver due to the widespread use of this technique and the clinically accepted indication for RF ablation of liver tumors.

## 39.2
## Technique

In principle, there are different types of energy sources causing either heat (RFA, laser, and microwave) or cold (cryoablation) and therapies such as ionizing radiation (stereotactic irradiation) or radiosurgery (cyber knife). While RFA is well known and used by many physicians, laser and especially cryotherapy are used only by a few centers due to several drawbacks. All heating techniques have to raise tissue temperatures to 60 to 100° C to cause sufficient coagulation necrosis, while cryotherapy freezes cells to death using tissue temperatures below –20° C.

## 39.2.1
## Radiofrequency Ablation

The first experiments in thermal ablation of living tissue were described by d'Arsonval as early as 1868, while the use of thermal ablation for treatment of malignant hepatic lesions was first suggested by MCGAHAN et al. and ROSSI et al. in 1990 (MCGAHAN et al. 1990). Radiofrequency ablation involves the delivery of high-frequency electrical current (375–480 kHz) into tissue, causing cell death. There are two different types of RFA. In monopolar systems, grounding electrodes have to be placed on the patient's thighs or back to allow current conduction, while in bipolar or multipolar systems, grounding pads are redundant as the electrical circuit is completed by either two electrodes, or both are mounted on a single needle (MCGAHAN et al. 1996). This high-frequency electrical current causes a rapid movement of ions within the tissue surrounding the electrode, leading to frictional heat (MCGAHAN et al. 1990). Reliable cell death only occurs if the temperature exceeds 60°C. However, temperatures of more than 105° are not as effective due to possible carbonization and vaporization around the RF probe. The maximal achievable necrosis within tissue is not only dependent on tumor type and surrounding vessels, but also on the shape of the electrode. Using needle-shaped electrodes, only tissue within a maximum diameter of 1.6 cm around the electrode can be destroyed. However, treatment of larger tumor volumes is possible with the development of different types of electrodes, including mounting of additional needles in a cluster-arrangement or umbrella-shaped electrodes with a diameter of up to 7 cm (GOLDBERG and GAZELLE 2001). Apart from tumor size and needle shape, the effect of radiofrequency ablation and its completeness is also dependent on vascularization of the tumor and the surrounding tissue. Large vessels can cause the so-called "heat-sink effect," describing the loss of temperature by cooling mediated by blood flow. This effect is well known, especially in liver tumors, and is most often caused by blood flow within branches of the portal vein, liver veins, or vena cava.

## 39.2.2
## Laser

Actually, there are two types of laser commercially available for image-guided laser ablation. Both types of laser (NdYAG with a wavelength of 1,064 nm and solid-state laser with a wave length of 805 nm) use photon absorption and heat conduction to create tissue heating and therefore a coagulation necrosis comparable to the effect of radiofrequency ablation. The laser energy is delivered via flexible laser fibers with diameters between 400 and 600 μm. While the point source at the tip of the bare laser fiber creates a more roundish necrosis, the fibers with the diffuser technique create a more elliptic lesion. A possible advantage of laser ablation is a more predictable size and shape of the achievable necrosis. However, compared to RF ablation, drawbacks of this technique are higher costs and the more invasive approach, especially in larger tumors due to the necessity for multiple fibers and therefore multiple introducer sheaths.

### 39.2.3
### Cryoablation

Cryotherapy uses liquid nitrogen and argon gas via cryoprobes as coolants to produce temperatures below –20°C. By repetitive freezing and thawing of the targeted tissue around the cryoprobe, a predictable thermal necrosis is achieved. The major disadvantage of the formerly used probes was the large size, and therefore the need for a laparoscopic approach has been overcome by the newly developed smaller probes; however, cryotherapy is said to cause more complications because of the missing coagulation of vessels and therefore the higher risk of bleeding compared to RF. The possibility to monitor the development of the ice ball using ultrasound or MRI with an accuracy of 1 to 5 mm could be an advantage with respect to a higher rate of complete tumor ablation.

## 39.3
## Clinical Applications

### 39.3.1
### Primary and Secondary Liver Tumors

In most patients with a history of cancer, liver metastases occur—depending on the tumor—in up to 70%. These metastases have the highest impact on a patient's long-term survival and are responsible for the largest part of cancer-related deaths worldwide (Tranberg 2004). In Europe and the USA, metastases of colorectal cancer and breast cancer are the most common indication for liver resection. Successful resection has a significant impact on the 3-, 5-, and 10-year survival rate, which is published to be as high as 45, 30 and 20%, respectively

(Scheele et al. 1995). Therefore, surgical resection is still considered to be the gold standard in liver metastases, while chemotherapy and radiation therapy are seen as palliative treatment options. However, due to risk factors only 10 to 25% of all patients suffering from liver metastases are suitable candidates for liver surgery. This has a major impact on the demand for minimally invasive treatments achieving an effective and reproducible percutaneous tumor ablation while simultaneously lowering both morbidity and costs.

### 39.3.1.1
### Indications and Contraindications

The indications for local ablative treatment are comparable to those established for resection—however, with some modifications (Table 39.1, Fig. 39.1). RFA is indicated for patients suffering from unresectable metastases due to tumor spread in both liver lobes or due to contraindications to surgical treatment. The combination of RFA with surgical resection as an adjuvant therapy or as a neoadjuvant therapy for bilobar tumors is an accepted indication. Most investigators have limited ablative treatment to patients with four or fewer hepatic tumors with a diameter of 4 to 5 cm or smaller because of a significantly higher local recurrence rate in tumors larger than 3 cm (Curley et al. 1999, 2000). Ideally, tumors are smaller than 3.5 cm in diameter and completely surrounded by hepatic parenchyma, with a distance of at least 1 cm to the liver capsule and of more than 2 cm to the large hepatic or portal veins. Contraindications include extrahepatic spread of the tumor, a tumor volume of more than 30% of the total liver volume, sepsis, and uncorrectable coagulopathies (Curley 2003). Additionally, tumor location next to the large portal triads is a relative contraindication due to the risk of harming the bile duct. Subcapsular liver tumors can be treated with RFA; however, the treatment is usually associated with greater procedural and post-procedural pain and is often associated with a higher complication rate (Lencioni et al. 2005b). Furthermore, tumors larger than 3–4 cm can be treated using newer RF generators, multiple needle positions, or angiographically assisted RFA. Tumors adjacent to large blood vessels are more difficult to treat because perfusion-mediated tissue cooling reduces the extent of coagulation necrosis produced by thermal ablation. The blood flow-mediated heat sink effect protects the vascular endothelium from thermal injury, allowing the placement of the electrodes as close as necessary to the vessels.

**Table 39.1.** Indications for local ablative treatment

| Indications | Contraindications |
| --- | --- |
| Single tumor less than 5 cm in diameter | Life expectancy <6 months |
| Maximum three lesions less than 3 cm in diameter | Current infection |
| Non-resectable | Treatment refractory coagulopathy |
| Recurrence after surgical resection | Treatment refractory ascites |
| Patient declined surgery | Portal hypertension |
| Combination with resection | Tumor size >5 cm$^{\lozenge}$ |
| | >4 lesions |
| | Extrahepatic spread * |
| | Tumor adjacent to structures at risk (main bile ducts, pericardium, stomach, or bowel)† |

$^{\lozenge}$In individual cases, depending on the location within the liver parenchyma, an ablation might be possible. †Only if a dissection of structures at risk by injection of air or glucose is not possible. *In selected patients, RFA is possible even if extrahepatic tumor (e.g., stable bone metastases, slow-growing lymph nodes) is present

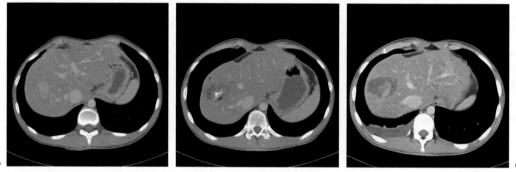

a,b                                                                                                                      c

**Fig. 39.1a-c.** A 25-year-old male patient with a history of a neuroendocrine tumor of the pancreas has developed a solitary liver metastasis. The patient was treated according to the local tumor board. **a** Shows the hypervascularized lesion located in segment 7 of the liver. Control scan (**b**) immediately after the ablation with the needle still in place showing a successful ablation confirmed in the scan 24 h after treatment (**c**)

### 39.3.1.2
### Results in Liver Metastases

Unfortunately, few studies exist with good long-term follow-up evaluating local recurrence, disease-free survival, and overall survival after ablation. However, proof exists that the completeness of tumor ablation is directly related to survival (BILCHIK et al. 2001), comparable to a free resection margin after surgery (OHLSSON et al. 1998; SCHEELE et al. 1995). Moreover, the local recurrence rate significantly depends on the size of the treated metastases (CURLEY 2003; SOLBIATI et al. 2001; WOOD et al. 2000). In the study by CURLEY (2003), a local relapse in only about 7% of the patients was shown after RFA of colorectal metastases—however, 80% of the local recurrences developed in the periphery of tumors larger than 5 cm in diameter.

DE BAERE and colleagues (2000) analyzed 68 patients with 121 hepatic metastases who underwent 76 sessions of RFA with or without additional surgery.

Forty-seven patients with 88 metastases ranging from 1 to 4.2 cm in diameter were treated with RFA alone, while the remaining 21 patients underwent a combination of surgery and intraoperative RFA for remaining small tumors. In 33 patients with 67 metastases who underwent percutaneous RFA, a follow-up of at least 4 months was available, showing a local relapse in only 10% of the lesions (21% of the patients). A mean follow-up of 13.7 months was available for all patients showing 79% of the patients treated with percutaneous RFA were alive, 42% had no evidence of new or recurrent malignant hepatic disease, but only 27% were completely tumor free (DE BAERE et al. 2000). A study recently published by GILLAMS et al. (2004) referred to a cohort of 167 patients with colorectal liver metastases treated with percutaneous RFA. The authors were able to show a median survival period of 38 months, with a 5-year survival rate of 30% after the diagnosis of liver metastases. Furthermore, a survival period of 31 months with a 5-year survival rate of 25% after the first ablation was reported. The authors concluded from their results that RFA increases the therapeutic options for patients with colorectal metastases.

### 39.3.1.3
### Results in HCC

Treatment success varies in HCC with the size of the lesion to be treated comparable to that of metastases as described above. The reported experience of BUSCARINI et al. (BUSCARINI and BUSCARINI 2001, BUSCARINI et al. 2001) in 88 patients showed that complete tumor necrosis is only achievable in tumors smaller than 3.5 cm in maximum diameter. Similar results were shown in a review by POON (2002) in which a complete tumor necrosis was achieved in 80%–90% of tumors smaller than 3–5 cm in size after a single treatment session.

A recently published prospective clinical trail performed on 187 patients showed promising results concerning long-term survival in HCC patients after RFA (LENCIONI et al. 2005a). Overall survival rates were 97% at the 1-year, 89% at the 2-year, 71% at the 3-year, 57% at the 4-year, and 48% at the 5-year follow-up. The survival rates of patients with a Child-Pugh class A cirrhosis ($n = 144$; 76% at 3 years and 51% at 5 years) were significantly higher than those of patients with a Child-Pugh class B cirrhosis ($n = 43$; 46% at 3 years and 31% at 5 years). The data published by TATEISHI et al. (2005) concerning percutaneous RF ablation of HCC in 664 patients are also very encouraging. The authors assessed the cumulative survival in patients who received RFA as the primary treatment ($n = 319$, naïve patients)

as well as in patients who received RFA for recurrent tumor ($n = 345$, non-naïve patients) after previous treatment including surgical resection, microwave coagulation therapy, PEI, and TACE. The cumulative survival rates at 1, 2, 3, 4, and 5 years were 94.7%, 86.1%, 77.7%, 67.4%, and 54.3% for naive patients, whereas the cumulative survival rates were 91.8%, 75.6%, 62.4%, 53.7%, and 38.2% for non-naive patients, respectively.

### 39.3.1.4
### Complications and Side Effects

The largest study regarding complications after radiofrequency ablation was published by LIVRAGHI et al. (2003) and reported the complication rates after treating 2,320 patients with a total number of 3,554 lesions. Six deaths (0.3%) were noted, including two fatalities caused by multiorgan failure following intestinal perforation. Furthermore, only 2.2 % of all patients suffered from major complications, with the most frequently observed complications being peritoneal hemorrhage, intrahepatic abscess formation, and intestinal perforation, while tumor seeding along the needle tract has been a rare complication as a track ablation was performed after every thermal ablation (LIVRAGHI and MELONI 2001). Risk factors for peritoneal hemorrhage were superficial metastases, whereas intrahepatic abscesses were mostly observed in diabetic patients without periprocedural antibiosis. Furthermore, thermal damage to adjacent organs (colon, stomach) has rarely been described (LIVRAGHI et al. 2003). Minor complications, including post ablation syndromes such as post- or periprocedural pain, fever, and asymptomatic pleural effusion, were observed in less than 5% of patients. Pleural effusion can be detected regularly, especially after using an intercostal approach. Furthermore, the authors (LIVRAGHI et al. 2003) reported the rate of complications to be directly related to the number of required RF sessions. In accordance with the experience of other authors, these results confirmed RFA to be a relatively low-risk procedure for the treatment of focal liver tumors (CURLEY et al. 2004; LIU et al. 2002; MULIER et al. 2002; PEREIRA et al. 2003).

### 39.3.2
### Renal Cell Carcinoma

CT-guided radiofrequency ablation as a minimally invasive therapy also shows promising results in the treatment of small renal masses. However, there are still insufficient data regarding long-term outcome after RFA (Fig. 39.2).

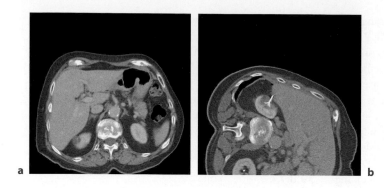

a                                                           b

**Fig. 39.2a,b.** An 85-year-old male patient suffering from a small RCC (**a**). Due to several risk factors, the patient was not regarded as suitable for surgery. Therefore, RFA was successfully performed under conscious sedation (**b**)

Therefore, partial nephrectomy and nephron-sparing surgery are considered to be the gold standard for the treatment of renal cell carcinoma. However, even in very experienced centers, the complication rate is described to be up to 30% (HABER and GILL 2006; UZZO and NOVICK 2001) after laparoscopic surgery with a notable amount (up to 2%) of renal insufficiencies. In comparison, the complication rate is very low in patients treated with RFA, and major complications are described to be 2.2% as a maximum (JOHNSON et al. 2004). Other authors who published their data on 82 RF cases were not able to show a significant impact on renal function measured by the mean serum creatinine level. Furthermore, partial nephrectomy or nephron-sparing surgery has to be performed under general anesthesia, while RFA can be performed under conscious sedation in most of the cases—enabling even patients with severe co-morbidities to undergo this type of treatment. In tumors larger than 5 cm, however, results are quite poor.

Due to the higher probability to develop a second tumor in the contralateral kidney after having suffered a RCC, these particular patients have to undergo regular follow-up examinations. If tumors are detected in the follow-up, they are usually small. Especially in tumors smaller than 3 cm, the success rate of RFA is nearly 100%. RFA requires less time and recovery, a shorter hospitalization, reduced pain, morbidity, and mortality in comparison to more invasive surgical methods (ALLAF et al. 2005; HACKER et al. 2005; MOURAVIEV et al. 2007) and is even less expensive compared to traditional methods (LOTAN and CADEDDU 2005).

### 39.3.3
### Lung Tumors

Radiofrequency ablation can also be used for the treatment of small primary and secondary tumors located in the lung (Fig. 39.3). Several hundred procedures have been performed and published worldwide, showing very good results at reasonable low complication rates. The overall pneumothorax rate is similar to that of CT-guided percutaneous lung biopsies, ranging between 20 and 40% with less than 20% requiring a drainage in-

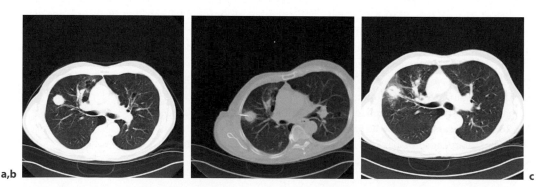

a,b                                                           c

**Fig.39.3a–c.** A 55-year-old male patient with a solitary pulmonary metastasis due to colorectal cancer. The patient did not want to undergo open surgery; therefore, RF ablation was performed using CT fluoroscopic guidance (**b**). Control scan (**c**) 24-h after treatment showed no complication and the lesion completely covered as indicated by the ground-glass opacities surrounding the metastasis

sertion (Hoffmann et al. 2006; Kelekis et al. 2006). Ideal tumors for RF treatment are smaller than 3 cm in diameter, located in the periphery, and should have a distance of at least 1 cm to large pulmonary vessels or bronchi. Furthermore, the number of tumors within each lung should not exceed three, and patients should not qualify for open surgery. For probe positioning, the use of CT together with CT fluoroscopy is recommended. However, there is no recommendation about whether the therapy should be done under general anesthesia or conscious sedation, but there is proof that there is no difference in using either of them (Hoffmann et al. 2006). A successful ablated tumor shows no further contrast enhancement and a ground-glass shadowing completely surrounding the tumor. Furthermore, ablated lung tumors seem to increase in size after 3 months due to necrosis of healthy surrounding tissue, but normally show significant shrinkage after 6 and 12 months due to progressive scarring.

Unfortunately, until now, the results published in the literature regarding technical feasibility, therapeutic response, and short-term survival (Kelekis et al. 2006) seem to be encouraging, but there is still no proof so far for a clinical benefit in the long-term follow-up.

## 39.3.4
## Bone and Soft Tissue Tumors

Radiofrequency ablation in the treatment of benign osteoid osteoma causing severe pain is a well known and clinically accepted indication and has replaced open surgery due to its less invasive character and higher success rate regarding clinical symptoms (Woertler et al. 2001).

Especially in palliative situations, radiofrequency ablation has successfully been applied to osteolytic metastases and soft tissue tumors involving the bone to relieve pain (Goetz et al. 2004) or as an adjunct to vertebro- or osteoplasty. Furthermore, RFA has also been used for tumor debulking if the tumor causes pressure symptoms such as dysphagia or dyspnea.

## 39.4
## Conclusion

Percutaneous thermal ablation therapies have been receiving increasing attention as a potential primary treatment for focal HCC and liver metastases. Possible advantages of ablative therapies as compared to surgical resection include a lower morbidity and mortality rate, lower costs, the suitability for real-time imaging guidance, the option to perform ablative procedures on outpatients, and the potential application to a wider spectrum of patients, including those who are unsuitable as surgical candidates. Therefore, the major advantage of RFA is its ability to create a well-controlled focal thermal injury in the liver resulting in high success rates in treating HCC nodules and metastases smaller than 3 cm in diameter with long-term results comparable to surgery. Besides the accepted application of thermal ablation in patients suffering from liver tumors, RFA has a rapidly growing role in tumors beyond the liver. Especially in renal and lung cancer, RF ablation shows very promising results; however, larger studies still have not been able to prove its effectiveness regarding the long-term follow-up.

## References

Allaf ME, Varkarakis IM, Bhayani SB et al. (2005) Pain control requirements for percutaneous ablation of renal tumors: cryoablation versus radiofrequency ablation—initial observations. Radiology 237:366–370

Bilchik AJ, Wood TF, Allegra DP (2001) Radiofrequency ablation of unresectable hepatic malignancies: lessons learned. Oncologist 6: 24–33

Buscarini L, Buscarini E (2001) Therapy of HCC radiofrequency ablation. Hepatogastroenterology 48:15–19

Buscarini L, Buscarini E, Di Stasi M et al. (2001) Percutaneous radiofrequency ablation of small hepatocellular carcinoma: long-term results. Eur Radiol 11:914–921

Curley SA, Izzo F, Delrio P et al. (1999) Radiofrequency ablation of unresectable primary and metastatic hepatic malignancies: results in 123 patients. Ann Surg 230:1–8

Curley SA, Izzo F, Ellis LM et al. (2000) Radiofrequency ablation of hepatocellular cancer in 110 patients with cirrhosis. Ann Surg 232:381–391

Curley SA (2003) Radiofrequency ablation of malignant liver tumors. Ann Surg Oncol 10:338–347

Curley SA, Marra P, Beaty K et al. (2004) Early and late complications after radiofrequency ablation of malignant liver tumors in 608 patients. Ann Surg 239:450–458

de Baere T, Elias D, Dromain C et al. (2000) Radiofrequency ablation of 100 hepatic metastases with a mean follow-up of more than 1 year. AJR Am J Roentgenol 175:1619–1625

Gillams AR, Lees WR (2004) Radio-frequency ablation of colorectal liver metastases in 167 patients. Eur Radiol 14:2261–2267

Goetz MP, Callstrom MR, Charboneau JW et al. (2004) Percutaneous image-guided radiofrequency ablation of painful metastases involving bone: a multicenter study. J Clin Oncol 22:300–306

Goldberg SN and Gazelle GS (2001) Radiofrequency tissue ablation: physical principles and techniques for increasing coagulation necrosis. Hepatogastroenterology 48:359–367

Haber GP, Gill IS (2006) Laparoscopic partial nephrectomy: contemporary technique and outcomes. Eur Urol 49:660–665

Hacker A, Vallo S, Weiss C et al. (2005) Minimally invasive treatment of renal cell carcinoma: comparison of four different monopolar radiofrequency devices. Eur Urol 48:584–592

Helmberger T, Dogan S, Straub G et al. (2007) Liver resection or combined chemoembolization and radiofrequency ablation improve survival in patients with hepatocellular carcinoma. Digestion 75:104–112

Hoffmann RT, Jakobs TF, Lubienski A et al. (2006) Percutaneous radiofrequency ablation of pulmonary tumors—is there a difference between treatment under general anaesthesia and under conscious sedation? Eur J Radiol 59:168–174

Johnson DB, Solomon SB, Su LM et al. (2004) Defining the complications of cryoablation and radio frequency ablation of small renal tumors: a multi-institutional review. J Urol 172:874–877

Kelekis AD, Thanos L, Mylona S et al. (2006) Percutaneous radiofrequency ablation of lung tumors with expandable needle electrodes: current status. Eur Radiol 16:2471–2482

Lencioni R, Cioni D, Crocetti L et al. (2005a) Early-stage hepatocellular carcinoma in patients with cirrhosis: long-term results of percutaneous image-guided radiofrequency ablation. Radiology 234:961–967

Lencioni R, Della Pina C, Bartolozzi C (2005b) Percutaneous image-guided radiofrequency ablation in the therapeutic management of hepatocellular carcinoma. Abdom Imaging 30:401–408

Liu LX, Jiang HC, Piao DX (2002) Radiofrequence ablation of liver cancers. World J Gastroenterol 8:393–399

Livraghi T, Meloni F (2001) Removal of liver tumours using radiofrequency waves. Ann Chir Gynaecol 90:239–245

Livraghi T, Solbiati L, Meloni MF et al. (2003) Treatment of focal liver tumors with percutaneous radio-frequency ablation: complications encountered in a multicenter study. Radiology 226:441–451

Lotan Y, Cadeddu JA (2005) A cost comparison of nephron-sparing surgical techniques for renal tumour. BJU Int 95:1039–1042

McGahan JP, Browning PD, Brock JM et al. (1990) Hepatic ablation using radiofrequency electrocautery. Invest Radiol 25:267–270

McGahan JP, Gu WZ, Brock JM et al. (1996) Hepatic ablation using bipolar radiofrequency electrocautery. Acad Radiol 3:418–422

Mouraviev V, Joniau S, Van Poppel H et al. (2007) Current status of minimally invasive ablative techniques in the treatment of small renal tumours. Eur Urol 51:328–336

Mulier S, Mulier P, Ni Y et al. (2002) Complications of radiofrequency coagulation of liver tumours. Br J Surg 89:1206–1222

Ohlsson B, Stenram U, Tranberg KG (1998) Resection of colorectal liver metastases: 25-year experience. World J Surg 22:268–276; discussion 276–267

Pereira PL, Trubenbach J, Schmidt D (2003) [Radiofrequency ablation: basic principles, techniques and challenges]. Rofo Fortschr Geb Rontgenstr Neuen Bildgeb Verfahr 175:20–27

Poon RT, Fan ST, Tsang FH et al. (2002) Locoregional therapies for hepatocellular carcinoma: a critical review from the surgeon's perspective. Ann Surg 235:466–486

Scheele J, Stang R, Altendorf-Hofmann A et al. (1995) Resection of colorectal liver metastases. World J Surg 19:59–71

Solbiati L, Ierace T, Tonolini M et al. (2001) Radiofrequency thermal ablation of hepatic metastases. Eur J Ultrasound 13:149–158

Tateishi R, Shiina S, Teratani T et al. (2005) Percutaneous radiofrequency ablation for hepatocellular carcinoma. An analysis of 1,000 cases. Cancer 103:1201–1209

Tranberg KG (2004) Percutaneous ablation of liver tumours. Best Pract Res Clin Gastroenterol 18:125–145

Uzzo RG, Novick AC (2001) Nephron sparing surgery for renal tumors: indications, techniques and outcomes. J Urol 166:6–18

Woertler K, Vestring T, Boettner F et al. (2001) Osteoid osteoma: CT-guided percutaneous radiofrequency ablation and follow-up in 47 patients. J Vasc Interv Radiol 12:717–722

Wood TF, Rose DM, Chung M et al. (2000) Radiofrequency ablation of 231 unresectable hepatic tumors: indications, limitations, and complications. Ann Surg Oncol 7:593–600

## 40

# Rotational C-Arm-Based CT in Diagnostic and Interventional Neuroradiology

ARND DOERFLER, GREGOR RICHTER and WILLI KALENDER

## CONTENTS

## ABSTRACT

C-arm-mounted flat detectors capable of volume scanning allow for CT-like imaging (FD-CT) in the angiography suite or in the operating room, respectively. The acquisition of 3D angiographies was introduced in the era of image intensifier C-arms. Several advancements in research and development concerning flat detectors have allowed imaging that provides real soft tissue resolution using rotating C-arms for the first time. This CT option of flat detector-equipped C-arms offers a large number of potential applications. The high spatial resolution of 3D angiography allows precise visualization of vascular pathologies, such as cerebral aneurysms and arteriovenous malformations. In addition, the soft tissue imaging option of FD-CT enables the neurointerventionalist to detect space-occupying intracranial lesions, in the first instance acute hemorrhage in patients suffering from vascular diseases. This allows to prove or to exclude bleeding or rebleeding in patients undergoing endovascular interventions without patient transfer to conventional CT. The high spatial resolution of FD-CT enables high quality imaging of small intracranial devices, such as microstents or cochlear implants. An additional, three-dimensional, multiplanar FD-CT of the spine may be helpful in vertebroplasties or kyphoplasties and for mylography. In the future, FD-CT data may possibly become important for procedures performed with 3D navigation.

A. DOERFLER, MD
Department of Neuroradiology, University of Erlangen-Nuremberg, Schwabachanlage 6, 91054 Erlangen, Germany

G. RICHTER, MD
Department of Neuroradiology, University of Erlangen-Nuremberg, Schwabachanlage 6, 91054 Erlangen, Germany

W. KALENDER, PhD
Department of Medical Physics, University of Erlangen-Nuremberg, Henkestrasse 91, 91052 Erlangen

## Introduction

Flat-panel detectors or, synonymic, flat detectors (FD) have been developed for use in radiography and fluoroscopy with the defined goal to replace standard X-ray film, film-screen combinations and image intensifiers by an advanced sensor system. FD technology in comparison to X-ray film and image intensifiers offers higher dynamic range, dose reduction, fast digital readout, and the possibility for dynamic acquisitions of image series, yet keeping to a compact design. Within a remarkably short time span, flat-panel detectors CT (FD-CT) using C-arm systems have gained recognition and acceptance as a dedicated application-specific CT implementation. Interventional and intraoperative imaging is most important at present, but quite a number of further FD-CT applications are on the horizon. As angiographic CT, FD-CT provides an efficient method of combining 2D radiographic, fluoroscopic, digital subtraction angiographic and 3D CT imaging. This chapter briefly reviews the technical principles of FD technology and then mainly focuses on its possible applications in diagnostic and interventional neuroradiology.

## Technical Principles

Flat-detector technology was initially developed for radiography and later for angiography in order to overcome insufficiencies of X-ray film and image intensifiers. The intent was to provide fast and repeated direct digital readout and a higher dynamic range. The basic design principle nevertheless still relies on the conversion of X-rays to light: a fluorescence scintillator screen, mostly a cesium iodide substrate, is used as X-ray converter. The light emitted is recorded by a regular array of photodiodes placed in immediate contact with the fluorescent screen. The selection of the entrance screen material and thickness, i.e., the X-ray sensor characteristics, is governed by the same criteria as in screen-film radiography. Greater thicknesses mean higher absorption efficiency; however, at the same time, spatial resolution is degraded since the light photons are emitted in all directions and propagate diffusely. Special efforts were directed at developing and manufacturing structured needle-type phosphors, which guide the light along these structures. These efforts have brought substantial improvements. Nevertheless, light is not guided perfectly along the needles, and there is still a degrada-

tion of spatial resolution. In any case, spatial resolution today is ultimately limited by the fluorescence screen even if very small pixel sizes defined through larger photodiode matrices become available. In consequence, efforts have been directed at so-called direct converters, which allow converting X-ray photons directly to electron charge, which then travels along the direction of an applied electric field and is collected without a significant loss of resolution.

Temporal response was no major concern in the design and development of flat detectors. Frame rates of five to ten images per second are typically available today for full matrix readout, which appears adequate for most fluoroscopic applications. Combining of pixels, the so-called binning process, allows for higher readout rates, e.g., up to 60 images per second with 4×4 binning, but at the expense of spatial resolution.

### 40.2.1
### Rotational
### C-Arm-Based Flat Detector CT (FD-CT)

Three-dimensional image reconstruction using rotational X-ray tubes generates a 3D data set from 2D X-ray input projections; the in vivo use of the technique (indeed with a modified CT gantry) for 3D angiography was described first in 1994 (SAINT-FELIX et al. 1994). FAHRIG et al. (1997) reported of the use of a C-arm system to generate true 3D computed rotational angiograms. Already in the era of conventional image intensifiers, the arithmetic operations necessary for this technique were improved several times, e.g., in 2000 (WIESENT et al. 2000). Another step in the technical development was ultra-high-resolution flat panel detector CT (GUPTA et al. 2006). Preliminary clinical application of C-arm-based flat-detector-equipped angiography prototypes started in the new millennium, first for 2D angiography imaging, later on resulting in the development of techniques for 3D imaging. The 3D angiography for high contrast imaging was introduced at first. ZELLERHOFF et al. (2005) published technical data concerning low-contrast 3D reconstruction from C-arm data. The in vivo use of C-arm-mounted, angiographic flat-panel detectors to generate both volume CT and 3D angiographic imaging was described first in 2005 (AKPEK et al. 2005).

C-arm systems are characterized by flexibility in their use, in particular by the possibility of choosing arbitrary angulations. The most important additional demand imposed by CT scanning is to allow for a circular scan over at least 180°. For high image quality a minimum angular range of 180° plus fan angle is required.

An additional requirement is related to mechanical stability: for good CT image quality exactly the same object section has to be viewed for all projections. This means that the desired perfect planar trajectory of focus and detector has to be realized with very high precision.

As angiographic computed tomography (ACT, synonymic FD-CT), this flat-panel detector application might offer high spatial resolution volumetric imaging. This technology is commercially available, offered by Philips Medical Systems (Allura Xpert FD20) and Siemens Medical Solutions (Axiom Artis Zee Biplane System).

For all cases presented in this contribution, data acquisition was performed on an Axiom Artis dBA Biplane System (Siemens Medical Solutions, Forchheim, Germany) using the 30×40-cm detector. Acquisition protocols requiring up to 20 s result in up to 538 projections over a partial rotation of at least 200°, with an increment of 0.4° per image. The standard system dose is 0.36×10$^{-6}$ Gy per image. For optimal detector performance, this system relies on a dose control system where the detector entrance dose is held constant by adjusting the X-ray tube current time product and regulating the tube voltage only if needed.

The 2D X-ray projections are subsequently sent to a workstation for 3D tomographic image reconstruction (Leonardo; Siemens Medical Solutions, Forchheim, Germany). The algorithm used accounts for irregular but stable scan trajectories. To achieve 3D soft tissue image quality, a sequence of correction algorithms is applied. They involve scatter correction, beam-hardening correction, truncation correction, and ring artifact correction. The enhanced 3D reconstruction algorithm is commercially marketed by Siemens Medical Solutions as DynaCT. DynaCT data sets can be secondarily reconstructed like CT volume data sets using volume-rendering (VRT), multiplanar reconstructions (MPR), and other visualization techniques. As opposed to high-contrast 3D imaging, e.g., 3D DSA with preferentially used maximum intensity projection (MIP) or VRT reconstructions, in low-contrast examinations for soft tissue visualization it may be preferentially MPR reconstructions that the physician has to examine. Especially thick MPRs (with a slice thickness of 5 to 10 mm) help quite a bit in detecting soft tissue objects.

DynaCT provides so-called HU (formerly called bone) and EE (vessel) kernels for 3D reconstruction. HU (bone) kernels are essential for correct tomographic gray level reconstruction (HU values). EE (vessel) kernels, on the other hand, involve edge-enhancement as indicated by their name. They can enhance the visual appearance of 3D vascular objects, but they should not be used for quantitative measurements. Three-dimen-

sional voxel data sets obtained with a 512×512 matrix and a 'full' volume of interest (VOI) usually have a voxel size of about 0.1 mm. Neighboring voxels may be averaged to reduce noise. This can be accomplished by selecting a 'thick MPR' viewing mode. These MPR and MIP reconstructions are especially helpful for visualization of inserted implants.

Rotational, three-dimensional angiography with automatic contrast agent injection (from 1.5 up to 2.5 ml s$^{-1}$, dependent on catheter position and vascular territory) is performed using a program with a single rotation time of 5 s (total contrast agent injection time 6.5 s, 1.5 s delay) after a 5-s native mask acquisition run.

Compared with conventional multislice CT scanners (MSCT), high isotropic spatial resolution is an outstanding advantage of current rotational C-arm systems. Similar to clinical CT, spatial resolution depends on focal spot size, detector element size, the geometry, and the reconstruction parameters (KALENDER 2003, KALENDER and KYRIAKOU 2007). The parameter modified most easily is the detector element size: it is enlarged effectively by binning. The n×n binning means that n×n pixels are combined and read out as one. Binning reduces noise and the amount of data and thereby can increase frame rates, but it also reduces spatial resolution as shown by modulation transfer function (MTF) and bar pattern measurements. The 10% MTF values amounted to 3.0 lp mm$^{-1}$ with no binning and 1.5 lp mm$^{-1}$ with 2×2 binning, respectively, visual evaluation of a bar pattern phantom confirms these results (KACHELRIESS et al. 2000). In any case, this exceeds the spatial resolution of MSCT, which typically provides up to 1.2–1.4 lp mm$^{-1}$ for high-resolution modes.

High contrast resolution is the ability to image small objects with a low contrast difference that is embedded into a large object. It depends very much on the size of the small object, on the size of the surrounding large object, on the contrast difference, and on dose. Right now in DynaCT we claim to see 10 HU for an object of a diameter of 10 mm in a 16-cm phantom at a CTDI dose of 20 mGy. Contrast detectability of small diameter objects seems to depend on tube voltage. Concerning the contrast detectability of small objects at a fixed dose, compared with higher tube voltages, lower tube voltages gave improved low contrast detectability (FAHRIG et al. 2006).

The standard 3D system dose today is 0.36 uGy. This dose is a factor of 10 less than a digital subtraction angiography (DSA) dose and a factor of 10 more than a fluoroscopy dose. Optionally, a second dose setting for 3D with 1.2 uGy is offered. The higher dose setting is provided for customers who want to achieve optimal signal to noise ratio for DynaCT applications.

In interventional angiography, the dose to the patient is usually quantified in entrance dose and in entrance dose-area product. The main problem in neuroradiological interventions is the accumulation of dose to the identical part of the body because of some ideal angulations that are not changed during the procedure ("hot spots"). FD-CT in this respect is different, and dose is equally spread over a partial rotation. Nevertheless, if it is requested to quantify a 3D dose in entrance dose, the comparison can be done as follows: The dose per frame is a factor of 10 less than for a DSA image. Two hundred fifty to 500 projections of a 3D run then are something like 25 to 50 DSA images, which is a number that may be typically reached with two DSA scenes.

## 40.2.2
## FD-CT Versus Regular CT

As of today, these are the main differences to a regular CT scanner:

1. The trajectory of the focal spot with respect to the patient is approximately planar, whereas it is a spiral on a CT scanner. The trajectory does not cover a full rotation in FD-CT.
2. The detector is really two-dimensional (with up to 1,920 rows and 2,480 columns), while on today's standard CT scanners it has 64 rows only (and 700 to 800 columns). The broad X-ray cone leads to a better usage of X-ray quanta, but, at the same time, to a higher degree of scattered radiation.
3. From a mathematical point of view, 1 and 2 enforce approximate reconstruction techniques. The standard approach for this type of cone-beam tomography is the so-called Feldkamp algorithm.
4. In radial direction the field of view (FoV) is more limited than on a CT scanner. The FoV has a diameter of 25 cm (zoom 0 of the angio FD), whereas on CT scanners, it has 50 cm. With the exception of the head, anatomy usually does not fit into a FoV of 25 cm, and projections are truncated.
5. One partial rotation is sufficient to scan a volume of an axial extent of about 20 cm. A CT scanner needs many rotations, which are acquired in shorter times (see next item), but can cover any axial length as the patient is moved.
6. Timing is very different. Mechanically, a partial scan with a C-arm takes a minimum 5 s (and up to date 8 s to 20 s for the scans with the potential of soft tissue imaging), but on a CT scanner it takes 1 to 0.33 s only for a 360° scan. The frame rates on a C-arm system are 30 to 60 frames s[-1], whereas the readout frequency of a CT detector is much higher (several

1000 s[-1]). The number of projections for a C-arm system today is up to about 500, and it is more than 1,000 on a CT scanner.
7. Today's two-dimensional X-ray detectors are optimized for the acquisition of 2D projection images (fluoro and acquisition), but do not necessarily fulfill all requirements of CT imaging.
8. The geometry of a C-arm system is not as well defined as the geometry for a CT gantry. Therefore, calibration of a rotational C-arm is a technical challenge.

## 40.3
## Applications of FD-CT in Diagnostic and Interventional Neuroradiology

The availability of FD technology in fluoroscopy and as rotational C-arm-based CT imaging (FD-CT) has stimulated a surprising number of novel developments for clinical imaging. Especially diagnostic and interventional neuroangiography profits from these innovative developments (HERAN et al. 2006).

### 40.3.1
### Imaging of Intracranial Hemorrhage

For diagnosis of acute subarachnoidal hemorrhage (SAH) due to its availability in emergency settings and high sensitivity, conventional CT is the modality of choice. CT offers rapid and reliable acquisition of the extent of SAH and width of ventricles. However, in the angiography suite conventional CT is not available. Transportation of the patient from angiography to CT is delaying the critical decision making. Ideally, a CT option would be available within the angiography room without the need of patient transportation, respectively, repositioning.

FD-CT might overcome this issue by providing morphological, CT-like images sufficient to visualize or exclude intracranial hemorrhage within the angio suite. Few data are available regarding visualization of SAH or ventricle width using FD-CT. According to our preliminary, not yet published data comparing FD-CT to conventional CT in the visualization of subarachnoidal hemorrhage in patients with acute SAH, FD-CT was inferior to CT, although FD-CT could sufficiently depict all relevant, space-occupying intracerebral hemorrhages (Fig. 40.1). The width of ventricles could be reliably visualized by FD-CT, respectively. Our results can be explained with the lower contrast resolution,

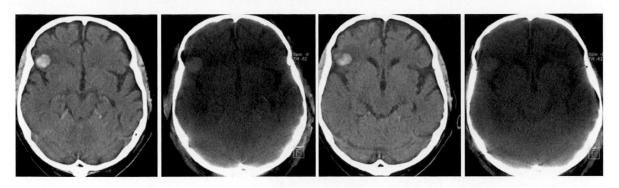

**Fig. 40.1.** Comparison of multislice-CT (*first* and *third image*) and FD-CT (*second* and *fourth*) in intracerebral hemorrhage

which is around 10 HU for FD-CT and 1 HU in helical CT. Regarding distinction of low contrast targets such as blood, ventricle, or brain parenchyma, the focus rests upon contrast resolution for soft tissue imaging. Subtle SAH can be depicted in high contrast in cranial CT while identification of subtle SAH in FD-CT may be problematic. Effective dose measurement of FD-CT has shown values below conventional CT (CTDI ~22 mGy). Recently, optional high-dose FD-CT protocols were implemented (CTDI ~66 mGy) with promising improvement of image quality, respectively.

In our institution, FD-CT is performed without contrast application and serves as postinterventional control after endovascular procedures such as aneurysm coiling, embolization of arteriovenous malformation (AVM), or intracranial angioplasty. In our experience this enables excluding space-occupying intracranial hemorrhage; thus, subsequent CT is no longer necessary. In our opinion, this time-saving approach improves the clinical work flow, since the patients arrive in the intensive or immediate care unit for further monitoring without time lag. Further data are necessary in imaging of low contrast targets such as SAH and intracerebral hemorrhage (Fig. 40.2; 40.3).

## 40.3.2
## Neurovascular Imaging and Interventions

Neurovascular interventions are still growing in importance. Angiographic FD-CT is particularly helpful during neurointerventional procedures, i.e., intracranial stenting for cerebrovascular stenoses, stent-assisted coil-embolization of wide-necked cerebral aneurysms, and embolizations of AVM of the brain. By providing morphologic CT-like images of the brain within the angio suite, FD-CT is able to work up periprocedural

hemorrhage in the rare cases of intraprocedural aneurysm or AVM rupture and may thus significantly improve immediate complication management without the need to transfer the patient to the CT scanner.

### 40.3.2.1
### Intracranial Aneurysms

Owing to its excellent spatial resolution, conventional DSA is still the gold standard in the diagnostic workup of cerebral aneurysms. Thus, cerebral angiography is performed as soon as possible in patients suffering from SAH. Cerebral angiography can localize the lesion, reveal the aneurysm shape and geometry, determine the presence of multiple aneurysms, define the vascular anatomy and collateral situation, and assess the presence and degree of vasospasm.

Precise visualizations of the aneurysm neck, the shape and the size of the aneurysm, and its relationship to parent vessels are important factors for deciding on therapeutic strategy. The endovascular therapy of ruptured subarachnoid aneurysms is associated with a more favorable clinical outcome compared to neurosurgical aneurysm clipping (MOLYNEUX et al. 2005). Rotational, 3D angiography represents a valuable supplement to standard biplane DSA. Using rotational angiography multiple oblique views are obtained as source for 3D reconstruction. Rotational angiography helps to define the aneurysm neck, to find the appropriate working position, and to perform accurate measurements. With the use of multiplanar cross-sectional images, high-resolution FD-CT hereby might improve planning of surgical and interventional procedures, especially in complex aneurysms (Fig. 40.4).

For patients undergoing aneurysm embolization, early recognition and management of complications

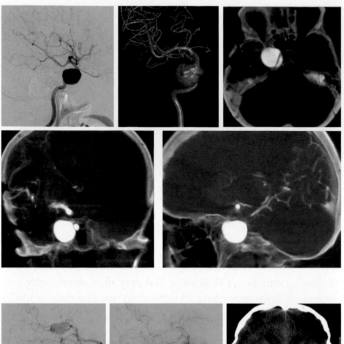

**Fig. 40.2** Fusiform acutely ruptured posterior cerebral artery aneurysm before and after parent artery coil occlusion (DSA). Postprocessing of FD-dataset with overlay of 3D-DSA vessel anatomy (displayed in *red colo*r) and soft tissue imaging of FD-CT

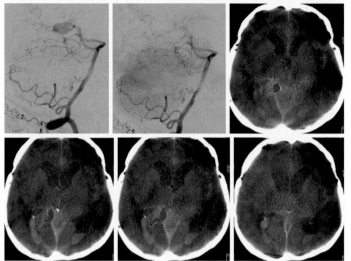

**Fig. 40.3** Primarily ruptured basilar tip aneurysm with re-rupture during the insertion of the first coil, comparison between conventional CT and FD-CT. 3D-DSA, conventional DSA with subarachnoidal rebleeding and extent of re-bleeding

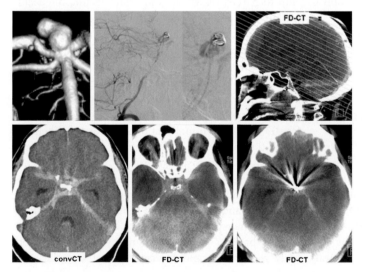

**Fig. 40.4.** FD-3D angiography provides high-resolution, precise visualization of the exact anatomy of the neck and relationship of tiny adjacent vessels to the aneurysm neck. DSA, surface-shaded VRT 3D DSA, tri-planar thin MIP-reconstructions

such as re-bleeding may significantly improve clinical outcomes (LEVY ET AL. 2001). Despite technical improvements in guide wires, catheters and coils, rupture of an aneurysm during endovascular treatment is one of the most feared complications of endovascular aneurysm therapy (DOERFLER et al. 2001). When a complication occurs during an endovascular procedure, the patient is usually transported emergently from the angiography suite to CT scanner to determine a diagnosis. The new combination of angiography with rotational CT suite overcomes this temporal delay for the transfer of the patient to the conventional CT. Although FD-CT images are not of the same quality as conventional CT, current FD-CT image quality seems to be sufficient to assess the extent of intracranial hemorrhage when a complication is suspected. Based on our preliminary experience we presume that especially periprocedural aneurysm rupture as a potential, serious complication seems to be detectable with FD-CT. Thus, this technique may improve procedural safety of aneurysm coiling, and it may enhance our understanding of aneurysm rupture during endovascular treatment by immediate visualization of the extent of subarachnoid hemorrhage (Fig. 40.2).

The illustrated case (Fig. 40.3) demonstrates that FD-CT may overcome the problem of delay in critical decision making, which would have resulted in the transport of the patient to the conventional CT scanner. As FD-CT showed no significant increase in subarachnoid hemorrhage, the patient did not have to rapidly undergo neurosurgical intervention due to a space-occupying bleeding. After immediate coil embolization to stop bleeding, the procedure could be finished without

pressure of time, an important presumption for a dense coil packing result.

In addition, FD-CT might demonstrate rebleeding before coil embolization, which otherwise would remain undetected until a post-procedural CT is performed, suggesting this bleeding to be related to endovascular treatment. In this respect, FD-CT may also have forensic impact on endovascular therapy.

Stent-assisted coil embolization using a scaffold to bridge the aneurysm neck with subsequent coiling through the stent interstices is a well-established therapy for broad-based cerebral aneurysms (WANKE ET AL. 2005). The current available, highly flexible self-expanding microstents enable treatment of patients with intracranial, even distally located, wide-necked aneurysms. However, fluoroscopic visibility of the stent is still poor, probably limited by the low profile of these highly flexible stents. Especially the stent struts are hardly visible in fluoroscopy, nonsubtracted angiographic and conventional X-ray, with only the proximal and distal radiopaque stent markers visible with these techniques.

FD-CT imaging in the angiography suite may enable adequate visualization of stent position and especially the stent struts with a high spatial resolution (RICHTER et al. 2007). The acknowledged advance offered by FD-CT with respect to image quality is the improved spatial resolution (Fig. 40.5).

The illustrated case shows a broad-based internal carotid giant aneurysm (Fig. 40.6). Multiplanar reconstructions (MPR) in axial and sagittal orientation to the stent and maximum intensity reconstructions (MIP) of the stent obtain excellent visualization after stent de-

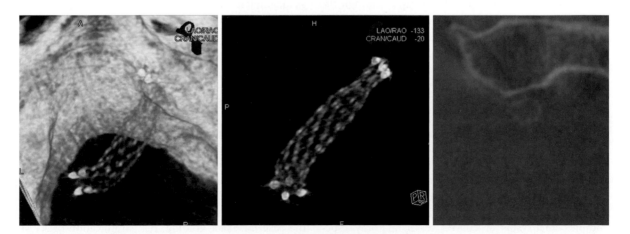

**Fig. 40.5.** FD-CT MPR and MIP images derived from one FD-CT run after application of a Neuroform stent in the basilar artery

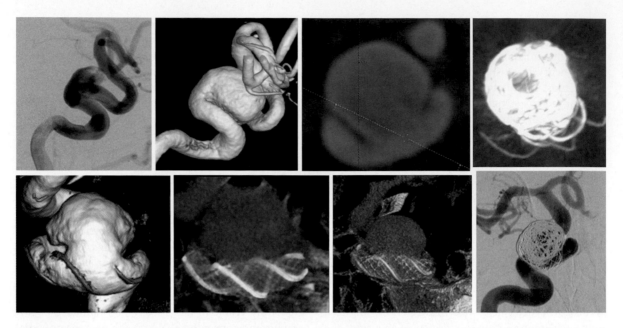

**Fig. 40.6.** Broad-based extradural, ophthalmoplegic giant internal carotid artery aneurysm. DSA, 3D DSA with VRT reconstruction, transversal MPR showing broad aneurysm neck and native DYNA-CT MIP after stent insertion and coil emboliza- tion (*upper row*). Dual-volume 3D-DSA (fusion of native mask run and 3D-DSA) and MIP reconstruction. Conventional DSA after coil embolization (*lower row*)

ployment and prior to the coiling procedure. According to the experience within our patient series, excellent or at least favorable overview of the stent with the adjacent coil package could be achieved in the cases with coil package diameter up to 10 mm. Due to beam-hardening artifacts, FD-CT stent visibility is poor in coiled aneurysms exceeding a diameter of 10 mm. ACT reconstructions (MIP and MPR) performed in our cases with aneurysm (coil package) size smaller than 10 mm allowed exclusion of coil prolapse through the stent struts, even when beam-hardening artifacts were distinctive (Fig. 40.7). This may be helpful, especially in cases with fusiform aneurysm geometry or at least a semi-circle coil package around the stent, when concise fluoroscopy projection is impossible.

The proximal and distal radiopaque markers are visible in fluoroscopy and provide gross overview of the stent position in situ. However, exact position of stent wall, adaptation of the stent to the vessel wall, and especially deployment of the stent struts at the aneurysm neck remain unclear. Even incomplete stent deployment or deficient fitting of the stent to the vessel wall may remain unnoticed. This deficit may play a role in complex aneurysms or curved vessel anatomy, especially, for instance, in cases with significant changing of parent vessel diameter and bifurcations. Additionally,

there are some reports available on fractures and kinkings of these dedicated aneurysm stents when placed in curved vessel segments (BENNDORF et al. 2006)–potentially leading to serious clinical complications. These single-center observations are confirmed by our own clinical experience.

For patients undergoing stent-assisted coil embolization of broad-based aneurysms, early recognition of procedure-related complications may be essential, such as incomplete stent deployment, stent migration during the coiling, or intracranial hemorrhage due to perforation of the aneurysm or the parent artery.

### 40.3.2.2
### Arteriovenous Malformations

DSA is still the gold standard in the diagnostic workup of cerebral AVM, the display of hemodynamic features of the AVM is possible with cerebral angiography only, and the exact anatomy of these lesions, accompanying pathologies, i.e., flow-related aneurysms or venous stenoses, have to be assessed angiographically. DSA is the base for exact grading, risk stratification of AVM, and planning of therapy as well.

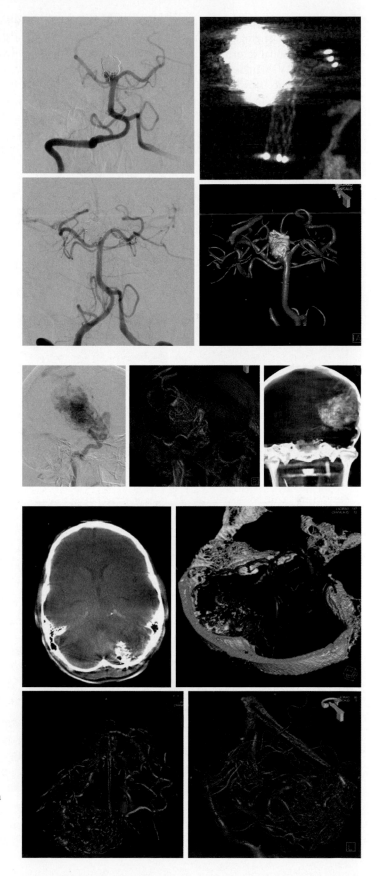

**Fig. 40.7.** DSA and FD-CT of a broad-based basilar tip aneurysm, initially treated with stent implantation and subsequent coiling. The displayed follow-up revealed some aneurysm reperfusion in the aneurysm neck (*upper row*). DSA and dual-volume fusion of native 3D-DSA mask run and subtracted dataset after re-coiling procedure (*lower row*)

**Fig. 40.8.** Large left hemispheric, high-flow AVM. DSA, 3D-DSA and MPR of the FD-CT dataset showing the anatomical extent of the AVM

**Fig. 40.9.** Left cerebellar AVM after partial glue embolization. Native transversal FD-CT single slice (*upper row, left side*). Dual-volume 3D fusion of native FD-CT dataset and 3D-DSA (*upper row, right side*). The glue is displayed in blue color in dual-volume fusion images (*lower row*) after the bone was removed manually

Rotational 3D angiography performed with flat-detector-equipped angiography provides high-resolution and cross-sectional information of AVMs. Exact delineation of the AVM nidus is possible with this technique; in our experience this is especially helpful for smaller AVM. In addition to high-contrast 3D-DSA, the acquisition of high-resolution FD-CT datasets with selective intra-arterial contrast-dye injection provides accurate topographic-anatomical information about AVM (Fig. 40.8). In our institution, planning of radiation therapy in the meanwhile is additionally based on these datasets. Furthermore, after endovascular AVM embolization, it is possible to display the anatomical distribution of the radiopaque glue material (Fig. 40.9).

The fundamental principles in the endovascular management of AVMs have not changed, with the primary objective to eliminate the arteriovenous shunt or to reduce the size of the nidus before surgery or radiation therapy. Exclusive endovascular embolization is curative only when complete AVM occlusion is achievable. This is possible in a small percentage of AVMs only, but endovascular glue embolization is recommended as part of a multimodal approach to reduce the size of a large AVM; the lesions then become more amenable to surgery or radiosurgery.

### 40.3.2.3
### Dural Arteriovenous Fistulae

Cranial dural arteriovenous fistulae may present with a wide spectrum of clinical findings from pulsatile tin-

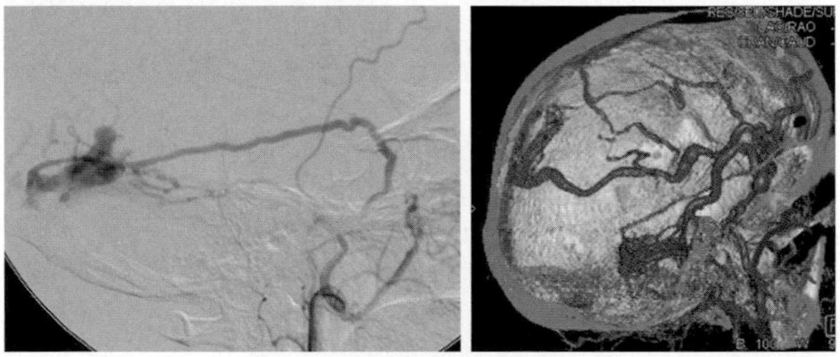

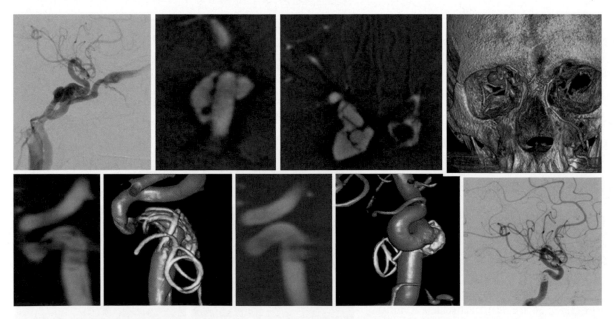

**Fig. 40.10.** Dural arteriovenous malformation. DSA shows arterial supply via the middle meningeal artery. Postprocessed dual-volume 3D image with the arteries and veins fused on the skull

**Fig. 40.11.** Traumatic direct carotid cavernous fistula in DSA. Cross-sectional imaging of 3D FD-CT data accurately depicts the fistulous arterio-venous vessel wall defect. The 3D fusion image demonstrates the contralateral superficial venous drainage. FD-CT during and after coil embolization displayed partial coil protrusion into the carotid artery, which was not visible in 2D DSA

nitus alone to intracranial hemorrhage. Selective angiography is essential for accurate assessment and prognostic classification. Endovascular treatment of dural arteriovenous fistulae can be performed using a transvenous, transarterial, or a combined approach, whereas the transvenous approach usually results in higher cure rates and demonstrated more stable therapeutic results (Fig. 40.10).

In the transvenous approach for treatment of direct carotid-cavernous sinus fistulae, unintentional coil prolapse in the supplying artery is a feared complication, which may result in embolic stroke. Due to dramatically reduced reconstruction times down to less than 1 min, FD-CT can be quickly performed and thus might be very helpful in the assessment of coil protrusions in the parent artery, otherwise not visible in 2D projections (Fig. 40.11).

### 40.3.2.4
### Intracranial Angioplasty and Stenting

Despite its frequency, the prognosis for patients with symptomatic intracranial stenosis is not well defined. A retrospective study with symptomatic intracranial vertebrobasilar stenosis found that 14% of the patients had another stroke over the 15-month follow-up interval. There has been increasing enthusiasm for endovascular treatment of intracranial artery stenosis (Fig. 40.12).

Intracranial angioplasty and stenting remain a high-risk procedure, which in our opinion is indicated only for highly selected patients symptomatic despite maximal anticoagulation therapy and judged to be at high risk for recurrent events. FD-CT provides imaging that allows accurate, 3D measurement of stenosis and may be helpful for stent imaging as well (BENNDORF et al. 2005).

### 40.3.2.5
### Intravenous FD-CT Angiography

Intracranial angioplasty and stenting may be associated with a high rate of restenosis; thus, consistent (ideally non-invasive) follow-up is mandatory. To avoid frequent invasive intra-arterial angiography, FD-CT with intravenously administered contrast agent may emerge as an alternative.

ACT for vascular imaging works with intravenously administered contrast agent as well: The automatic contrast injection is comparable to conventional CT angiography; we use 80 ml Imeron 400, flow rate 4 ml s$^{-1}$, injection time 20 s, and X-ray delay 20 s. The FD-CT does not provide a possibility to perform bolus-tracking up to now. The scan time for Dyna-CT is 20 s; thus, the intracranial veins show bouncing enhancement. Recently, there has been no possibility to perform subtraction of bony structures, but even small cerebral artery

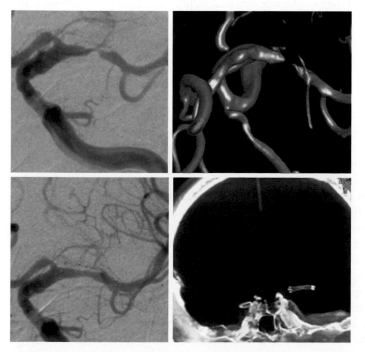

**Fig. 40.12.** Symptomatic high-grade stenosis of the middle cerebral artery. Stent angioplasty, DSA, 3D-DSA, and FD-3D-DSA. Result of angioplasty, native FD-CT showing the stent

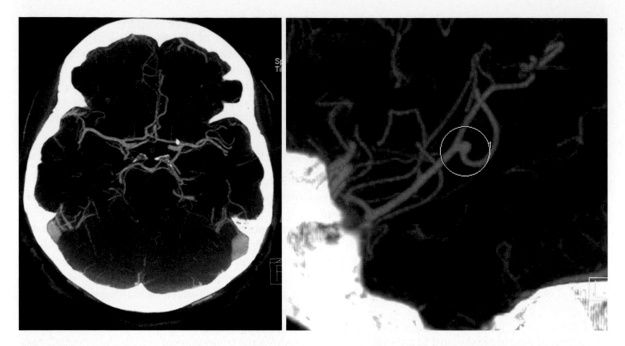

**Fig. 40.13.** Contrast-enhanced FD-CT with imeron administered intravenously. Transversal MIP, oblique MIP shows a right-sided small M2/M3 middle cerebral artery aneurysm, 1.5 mm in diameter (*circle*)

aneurysms seem be visible in high spatial resolution (Fig. 40.13).

Indications may be 3D imaging of contrast-enhancing intracranial tumors such as mengingiomas, non-invasive follow-up, e.g., for patients who obtained stent-assisted intracranial angioplasty, or for cerebrovascular imaging when arterial access is problematic. Our preliminary data are promising, and further research is required.

### 40.3.3
### FD-CT for Dedicated Maxillo-Facial Scanning

Imaging of the maxillo-facial skull has received growing attention in the past years as the number of image-guided procedures in dental and maxillo-facial surgery, in particular dental implants, is increasing. The introduction of FD technology has improved the diagnostic workup and intraoperative imaging in this field as well. CT is an essential imaging modality in evaluating the human skull base and the maxillofacial region. In addition to disease and trauma evaluation, CT now plays a growing role in treatment planning and intraoperative navigation. Despite recent developments in multislice CT, some structures are still beyond the resolu-

tion limits of MSCT and are, in addition, affected by relevant partial volume effects. Higher resolution CT imaging could therefore be beneficial. Thin bony structures would be less affected by the partial volume effect. Among others, reliability of diagnosis of lesions of the orbital wall or superior semicircular canal would increase with higher spatial resolution. Additionally, treatment planning and intraoperative navigation could be improved with the use of very high resolution datasets. Therefore, FD-CT may provide results superior to state-of-the-art MSCT.

Percutaneous sclerotherapy usually is performed under general anesthesia and with fluoroscopic monitoring, using pure (96%) ethanol, Ethibloc, and water-iodinated contrast material. FD-CT provides valuable cross-sectional visualization of deep compartments of facial venous malformations for better control and safety during embolization (Fig. 40.14).

### 40.3.4
### Temporal Bone

CT is an important diagnostic tool in temporal bone imaging. Despite all of these advances, numerous small and important anatomic structures in the temporal bone

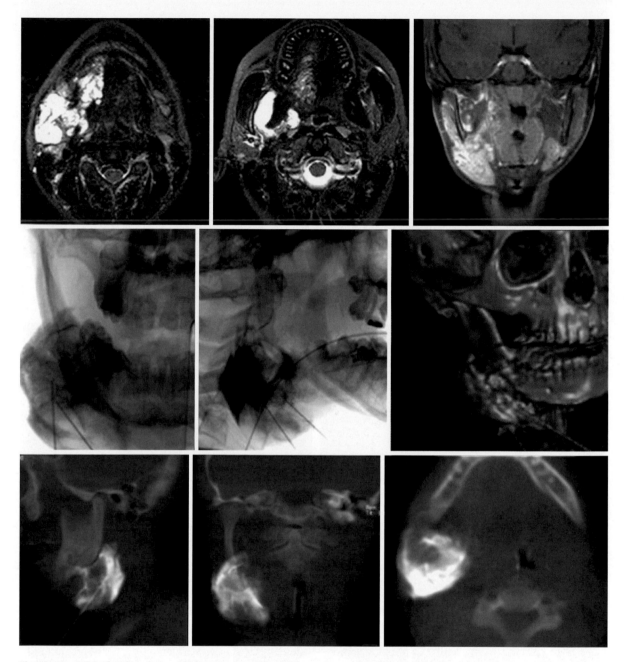

**Fig.40.14.** MRI of right submandibular arteriovenous malformation with progredient local pain and swelling (upper row). AP and lateral phlebogram, preceding sclerotherapy, 3D FD-CT (*middle row*). MPR reconstructions (*lower row*)

are still below this resolution limit; these structures are either blurred owing to partial volume effect or not seen at all. For example, assessment of otosclerosis, luxation of ossicles, the integrity of the round and oval window niche, malformations of the middle and inner ear, and many other diseases is often not possible by imaging alone. In addition, accurate post-surgical assessment

of middle- and inner-ear implants is limited because of metal artifacts. For treatment and surgical planning, accurate and repeatable visualization of these structures and the associated disease would be beneficial.

When compared with MSCT, FD-CT offers much smaller detector element size by fabricating them on an amorphous silicon wafer by using photolithographic

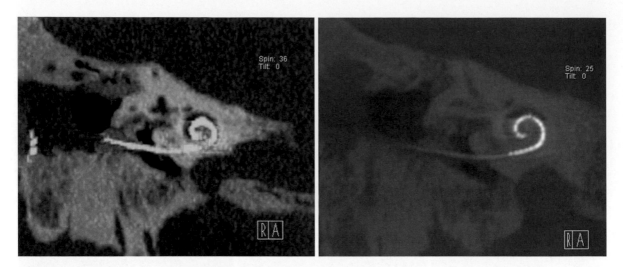

**Fig. 40.15.** Cochlear implant visualized by multislice CT (*left side*) and FD-CT

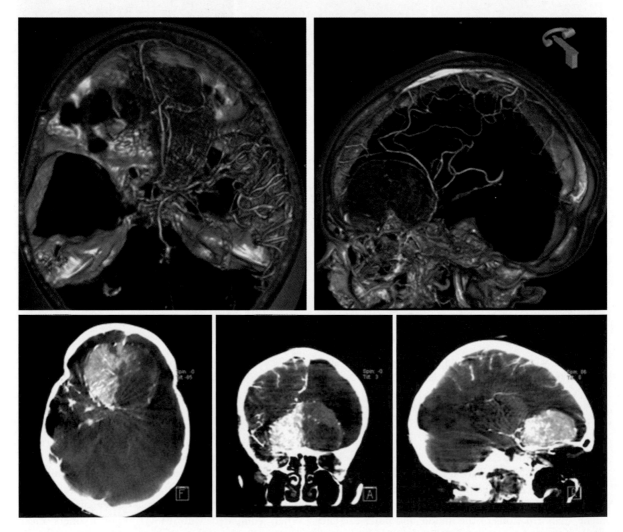

**Fig. 40.16.** Olfactorial meningioma. FD-CT reconstructions (*clip plane*), transversal and sagittal (*upper row*). Multiplanar MPR. The dataset was acquired during injection of 1.5 ml/s imeron with the catheter positioned in the right internal carotid artery

techniques. This results in higher spatial resolution. Because temporal bone imaging is often critically dependent on spatial resolution rather than soft tissue contrast, we hypothesized that such a scanner design could produce images of these structures superior to those rendered by the current state-of-the-art technique (Fig. 40.15).

## 40.3.5
## Intracranial Tumors

Besides the high spatial resolution of flat-panel detector technology for angiography, FD-CT provides good visualization of intracranial/extraaxial mass lesions and their topographic relation to cerebral arteries, allowing for improved preoperative or preinterventional planning. In the illustrated case the anterior cerebral arteries are displaced upwards and the middle cerebral arteries backwards, respectively (Fig. 40.16).

## 40.3.6
## Spinal Imaging and Interventions

Spinal examinations, such as myelography, or interventions, such as kyphoplasty or vertebroplasty, benefit from FD-CT, because on the one hand they have to be performed under fluoroscopy and on the other hand cross-sectional and three-dimensional imaging is helpful or sometimes even necessary.

## 40.3.6.1
## Myelography

As myelography and postmyelographic CT usually have to be performed using two separate imaging systems, these examinations can be carried out with flat panel volumetric computed tomography FD-CT in one step without the need of transportation of the patient. Using an angiographic system for myelography, postprocessing is done at the same workstation, hereby explicitly facilitating the workflow, which is an advantage of FD-CT. Additional applications, such as using the angiography suite for myelographic imaging, are possible: choosing the ideal projections from a three-dimensional MIP im-

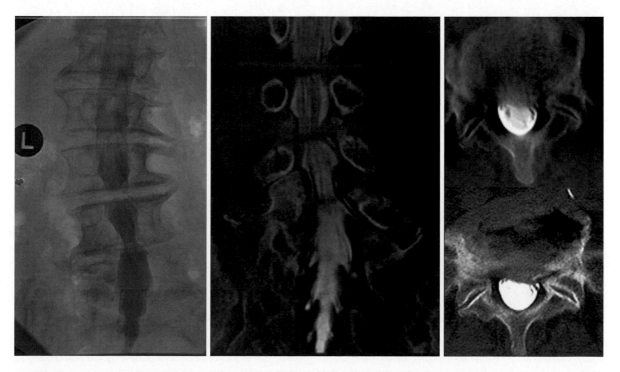

**Fig. 40.17.** Conventional lumbar myelography showing high grade, degenerative spinal stenosis, coronary and transversal MPR of FD-CT

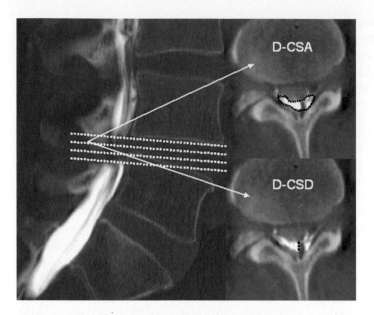

**Fig. 40.18.** Lateral FD-dataset derived MPR of massive lumbar intervertebal disc herniation, transversal MPR parallel to the lower vertebral endplate. Minimal D-CSA and D-CSD levels were measured

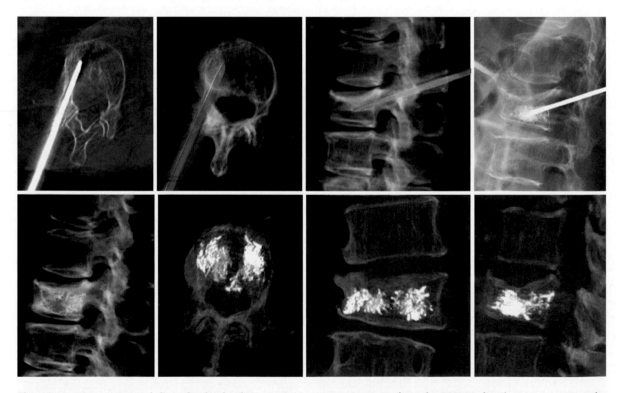

**Fig. 40.19.** Mono-segmental, bi-pedicular lumbar vertebroplasty, visualized by FD-CT. 3D imaging allows exact assessment of needle position. Procedure was started with the right pedicle. Exact survey of PMMA distribution is possible. MIP reconstructions show the PMMA distribution, respecting the dorsal border of vertebral body. Conventional radiography in the *upper row* on the *right side*

age derived from FD-CT performed right after intrathecal installation of contrast media could save fluoroscopy time to look for best projections and might be helpful for spinal interventions. Performing two examinations in a single session without the need of transportation of the patient also saves time and, in addition, by omitting conventional CT, the radiation dose could be further decreased. Moreover, the spatial resolution available with FD-CT enables the precise identification of small structures, and accurate assessment of the extent of disc herniations and spinal stenoses is possible (ENGELHORN et al. 2007) (Figs. 40.17, 40.18). In our experience, FD-CT demonstrated equal to multislice CT in analysis of lumbar spinal stenosis and degenerative disc disease and, at the same time, can decrease examination time and radiation dose.

## 40.3.6.2
## Vertebroplasty and Kyphoplasty

Vertebroplasty and kyphoplasty using polymethylmethacrylate (PMMA) have become a common procedure for treatment of vertebral compression fractures (LAYTON et al. 2007). Usually, the procedure is performed under fluoroscopy. Up to now, control CT was necessary to confirm correct distribution of PMMA after the procedure. FD-CT renders this control CT unnecessary; it provides all the information needed. A considerable advantage is the possibility to perform FD-CT in the angiography suite without moving the patient. This allows confirmation of correct needle position prior to PMMA injection as well (Fig. 40.19). Furthermore, in primarily intended mono-pedicular procedures, this allows accurate, three-dimensional assessment of PMMA distribution. This may be helpful for the decision whether an additional needle placement into the contralateral side is required.

## 40.4
## Novel Implementations and Potential Future Developments

Intraoperative imaging has shown an impressive upward trend just the same over the past few years. It is focused on orthopedic and trauma surgery such as joint replacements and spine surgery. Similar to the situation in the neurointerventional suite, FD-CT allows immediate and conclusive control of the surgical intervention, as, for example, the correct placement of screws without impairment of joint function (DALY et al. 2006). Navi-

gated biopsies or drug deliveries may be fields of application as well.

To combine the advantages of FD-CT with applications in radiation therapy, attaching a standard X-ray tube and an FD to a rotating linear accelerator may be trend-setting and would allow CT imaging of the patient on the therapy couch. It is the same rationale as in C-arm CT: the practical advantages of real-time control of patient positioning and tumor control and the option of real-time therapy planning outweigh potential disadvantages in image quality, which are to be acknowledged. The demanding diagnostic workup has usually been completed earlier by clinical CT or another modality; FD-CT image quality is adequate to accomplish the task at hand.

Last but not least, FD technology has also been integrated in standard CT designs. Respective efforts were labeled experimental and aimed at exploring so-called "volume CT" options. At present, they aim at pre-clinical imaging applications. It remains open if such designs will become acceptable for clinical CT; this will above all demand the development of FD designs improved with respect to dose efficiency and speed. In any case, such scanners are associated with high cost and the demand for a dedicated CT room, which is a disadvantage for most pre-clinical research laboratories.

Computer-assisted interventions and operations will increase in frequency and in importance as they provide higher precision and higher result quality. It is not only the difficult cases in interventions or operations that profit from the support by 3D image-guided planning and guidance by navigation systems.

Robotics will play an increasing role both for imaging and for therapy. Figure 40.20 (zeego, Siemens, Forchheim, Germany) shows a respective scenario of an interventional suite in the future, which may appear totally fictitious, but, in our opinion, is likely to appear. A large robot, either floor- or ceiling-mounted, moves the C-arm system at a speed and with mechanical precision higher than it is available today; fast and versatile imaging concepts are the motivation here. A second floor-mounted robot holds the patient bed and allows positioning the patient with higher versatility, e.g., adapting table height, swivel, and inclination with higher flexibility than available at present; the respective technology is already under evaluation for high-precision radiation and particle therapy. An additional small robot mounted to the patient bed on demand will support the interventional radiologist and the surgeon in positioning devices or implants; the respective technology is already under evaluation in the field of computer-assisted surgery (KALENDER and KYRIAKOU 2007) (Fig. 40.20).

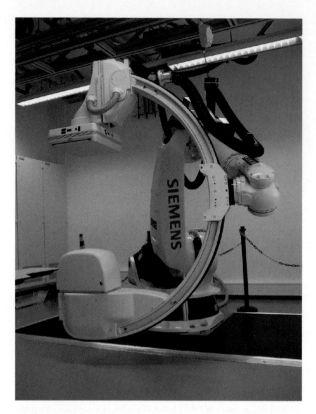

**Fig. 40.20.** Robotic C-arm, equipped with FD-technology (zeego, Siemens, Forchheim, Germany)

## Abbreviations

| | |
|---|---|
| ACT | Angiographic computed tomography |
| AVM | Arteriovenous malformation |
| CCT | Cerebral computed tomography |
| CTDI | Computed Tomography Dose Index |
| DSA | Digital subtraction angiography |
| FD | Flat detector |
| FD-CT | Flat detector computed tomography |
| FoV | Field of view |
| HU | Hounsfield unit |
| lp | Line pair |
| MIP | Maximum intensity projection |
| MPR | Multiplanar reconstruction |
| MSCT | Multislice computed tomography |
| MTF | Modulation transfer function |
| SAH | Subarachnoidal hemorrhage |
| VOI | Volume of interest |
| VRT | Volume-rendering technique |

## References

Akpek S, Brunner T, Benndorf G et al. (2005) Three-dimensional imaging and cone beam volume CT in C-arm angiography with flat panel detector. Diagn Interv Radiol 11:10–13

Benndorf G, Strother CM, Claus B et al. (2005) Angiographic CT in cerebrovascular stenting. Am J Neuroradiol 26:1813–1818

Benndorf G, Claus B, Strother CM et al. (2006) Increased cell opening and prolapse of struts of a neuroform stent in curved vasculature: value of angiographic computed tomography: technical case report. Neurosurgery 58 (Suppl 2):4

Daly MJ, Siewerdsen JH, Moseley D et al. (2006) Intraoperative cone-beam CT for guidance of head and neck surgery: Assessment of dose and image quality using a C-arm prototype. Med Phys 33:3767–3780

Doerfler A, Wanke I, Egelhof T et al. (2001) Aneurysmal rupture during embolization with Guglielmi detachable coils: Causes, management, and outcome. Am J Neuroradiol 22:1825–1832

Engelhorn T, Rennert J, Richter G et al. (2007) Myelography using flat panel volumetric computed tomography: a comparative study in patients with lumbar spinal stenosis. Spine 15;32:E523–527

Fahrig R, Fox S, Lownie S, Holdsworth DW (1997) Use of a C-arm system to generate true 3-D computed rotational angiograms: Preliminary in vitro and in vivo results. Am J Neuroradiol 18:1507–1514

Fahrig R, Dixon RL, Payne T et al. (2006) Dose and image quality for a cone-beam C-arm CT system. Med Phys 33:4541–4550

Gupta R, Grasruck M, Suess C et al. (2006) Ultra-high resolution flat-panel volume CT: fundamental principles, design architecture, and system characterization. Eur Radiol 16:1191–1205

Heran NS, Song JK, Namba K et al. (2006) The utility of DynaCT in neuroendovascular procedures. Am J Neuroradiol 27:330–332

Kachelrieß M, Schaller S, Kalender WA (2000) Advanced single-slice rebinning in cone-beam spiral CT. Med Phys 27:754–772

Kalender WA (2003) The use of flat-panel detectors for CT imaging. Der Einsatz von Flachbilddetektoren für die CT-Bildgebung. Der Radiologe 43:379–387

Kalender WA, Kyriakou Y (2007) Flat-detector computed tomography (FD-CT). Eur Radiol 17:2767–2779

Layton KF, Thielen KR, Koch CA et al. (2007) Vertebroplasty, first 1,000 levels of a single center: evaluation of the outcomes and complications. Am J Neuroradiol 28:683–689

Levy E, Koebbe CJ, Horowitz MB et al. (2001) Rupture of intracranial aneurysms during endovascular coiling: management and outcomes. Neurosurgery 49:807–811

Molyneux A J. Kerr R S, Yu L M et al. (2005) International subarachnoid aneurysm trial (ISAT) of neurosurgical clipping versus endovascular coiling in 2,143 patients with ruptured intracranial aneurysms: a randomised comparison of effects on survival, dependency, seizures, rebleeding, subgroups, and aneurysm occlusion. Lancet 3–9;366:809–917

Richter G, Engelhorn T, Struffert T et al. (2007) Flat panel detector angiographic CT for stent-assisted coil embolization of broad-based cerebral aneurysms. Am J Neuroradiol 28:1902–1908

Saint-Félix D, Trousset Y, Picard C et al. (1994) In vivo evaluation of a new system for 3D computerized angiography. Phys Med Biol 39:583–595

Wanke I, Doerfler A, Schoch B et al. (2003) Treatment of wide-necked intracranial aneurysms with a self-expanding stent system: initial clinical experience. Am J Neuroradiol 24:1192–1199

Wiesent K, Barth K, Durlak P et al. (2000) Enhanced 3-D reconstruction algorithm for C-arm systems suitable for interventional procedures. IEEE Trans Med Imaging 19:391–403

Zellerhoff M, Scholz B, Ruehrnschopf EP (2005) Low contrast 3D reconstruction from C-arm data. Proc SPIE 5745:646–655

# Abdominal Intervention with C-Arm CT

Christoph R. Becker

## ABSTRACT

Rotating C-arm CT is an emerging new option for digital angiography allowing display of contrast distribution in parenchymal organs while the catheter is placed in a certain position. The information from C-arm CT allows for a safer tumor targeting and prevention of any side structures outside the desired treatment volume. We have experienced the benefit of C-arm CT in particular for patients with liver metastases that were scheduled for radio-embolization. Prior to therapy, these patients undergo technetium angiography in order to determine the feasibility of the procedure. Metastases in the liver typically appear with a rim enhancement and a non-enhancing center. The hyperdense rim in C-arm CT corresponds to the area of hypermetabolism in PET with uptake of FDG. C-arm CT in these patients is well suited to determine a safe position of the catheter before treatment with radioactive microspheres. Another indication for C-arm CT may be intervention of the vasculature. For instance, in case of aortic dissection, C-arm CT is particularly useful to guide intervention by displaying the location of the catheter relative to the dissection membrane. Furthermore, this technique may also be used for planning embolization of uterine fibroids.

## 41.1

## Technical Background of C-Arm CT

Flat detector technology has gained in acceptance over the conventional X-ray film because of its higher absorption efficiency and wider dynamic range. Furthermore, flat detectors are capable of direct, several frames

C. R. Becker, MD
Department of Clinical Radiology, Munich University Hospitals, Ludwig-Maximilians-University, Marchioninistrasse 15, 81377 Munich, Germany

per second digital read out. For all these reasons, flat detectors are meanwhile more and more used in angiographic and interventional units. Since recently, in analogy to computed tomography, flat panel detectors mounted on a C-arm have been capable of providing a rotation around the patient in a rapid fashion. By taking projections from an angular range of 180° and more, these kinds of systems are able to reconstruct for CT image from these projections (KALENDER et al. 2007).

In theory, because of the wide dynamic range of flat detectors, soft tissue structures would be able to be delineated by C-arm CT as well as by conventional CT. However, the contrast resolution in C-arm CT images directly depends on the number of projections acquired and thereby on the rotation time of the C-arm. Short rotation times of just 5 s are only capable of imaging highly dense structures, such as the spine or contrast-filled vessels. Eight-second rotation protocols with a correspondingly higher number of projections already allow discrimination between different soft tissue structures, such as liver, fat and muscle. Long-lasting C-arm rotations of 20 s are capable of displaying even smaller contrast differences, such as bleedings or contrast extravasations.

Because of its properties, C-arm CT first was accepted into neuro-radiology because the head is a comparably small object and could easily be scanned in a patient even with long rotation times with only minor risks of motion artifacts. Detailed description about the application of C-arm CT in neuro-radiology is provided elsewhere in this book. Imaging of the abdomen with C-arm CT systems then requires a compromise between soft tissue resolution and acquisition times in order to avoid respiratory motion artifacts. Generally, we acquire C-arm CT images of the abdomen by an 8-s acquisition. During this period of time, it is easy to sustain the breath for most of the patients, even in expiration. Beside the drawback of limited soft tissue resolution, a 30 by 40-cm² flat panel detector in landscape format is able to acquire a field of view of 23 cm for a range of 8 cm. Acquisition of the entire liver with this technique requires either very careful patient positioning or rescanning the patients in different positions.

Recently, a new kind of system has been introduced to the market, where the C-arm is mounted on a robot, allowing for faster, more precise and more flexible data acquisition. Because of these new features, this system is capable of performing a complex movement around the patients. After having completed the first rotation, the system shifts the C-arm to a more lateral position and rotates then immediately back again. If the flat panel detector is brought into portrait mode, this option for data acquisition allows covering a 47-cm field

of view and a 13-cm range. In practice, we have realized that it is easy to scan the entire liver with this technique even in large patients. This acquisition mode is also less susceptible to different respiratory levels that could otherwise cause partial movement of the liver outside the scan range.

The drawback of the large-volume CT acquisition mode is the significantly longer acquisition time. Most of the patients may not be able to hold their breath in expiration for the duration of 24 s that is necessary for this double rotation of the C-arm. Instead of that, the acquisition may be performed in inspiration, which is well tolerated by most of the patients, even for that rather long period of time. The disadvantage of longer acquisition time is also the necessity to inject the contrast media for a longer period of time in order to achieve a constantly sufficient enhancement of the liver parenchyma.

C-arm CT images may not only suffer from motion artifacts, but also from streak artifacts caused by any dense objects, such as the catheter or high concentrations of contrast media. Ideally, the system is set up as in conventional CT with an automated two-syringe contrast injector that injects either diluted contrast media or at slow flow rates at a predefined time point ahead of the acquisition followed by a saline chaser bolus. This delay time between the contrast injection and the acquisition is essentially necessary to order to enhance the liver parenchyma and flush the arteries with saline.

The other concern about this new technique is related to radiation exposure. From our own measurements, we learned that the radiation exposure of a single-rotation C-arm CT of the liver is approximately the same as for a conventional mono-phase multi-slice CT of the same region (approximately 4 mSv effective dose). Also of concern is the scatter radiation for the investigator. In order to avoid unnecessary scatter radiation exposure, it is mandatory for the investigator to step back as far away as possible or ideally to leave the scan room and to start the whole procedure, including contrast injection and C-arm rotation, from the control room.

## 41.2
## Clinical Experiences

C-arm CT imaging for the brain became available in 2005 and for the abdomen in 2006. Therefore, only very little has been published about this technique being applied in the abdomen so far. VIRMANI et al. (2007) were the first to describe the application of this technique for intervention in the abdomen. Between March 2006 and September 2006, they gathered the experience they gained from 18 patients with unresectable liver tumors (15 patients with hepatocellular carcinoma and 3 patients with neuroendocrine tumors) that were treated by transarterial chemoembolization. Apart from the fact that C-arm CT imaging improved the diagnostic confidence of the selected catheter position in 14 of the 18 patients, they found that it also led to an altered catheter positioning anticipated by the attending interventional radiologist in 7 patients.

Wallace et al. applied this technique from May 2005 to March 2006 in 86 out of 240 different liver interventions (infusion, radioembolization, embolization and chemoembolization). They reported that C-arm CT added important information without impact on the procedure in 19% of the cases. In another 41%, C-arm CT, however, added information that had clear impact and might have even changed the carrying out of the procedure. Apart from all the other procedures, the highest benefit was seen for chemoembolization. The additional time needed to perform the procedure was 18 min at average (WALLACE et al. 2007).

Finally, KAKEDA et al. (2007) applied C-arm CT in 49 patients with hepatocellular carcinoma undergoing chemoembolization. They found that C-arm CT added further information in 81% of the cases. By their detailed analysis they reported that C-arm CT was particularly useful if the quality of the conventional DSA was graded as less than adequate in regard to tumor staining.

We were trying to apply this technique in a variety of different settings. We realized the advantage of C-arm CT in case of aortic dissection in order to follow the course of the catheter through the false and true lumen (Fig. 41.1). Also, in case of both sided hip endoprotheses where beam-hardening artifacts between the two metal pieces hinders conventional CT visualization of the structures in the small pelvis, C-arm CT was able to demonstrate the proximity of the internal iliac

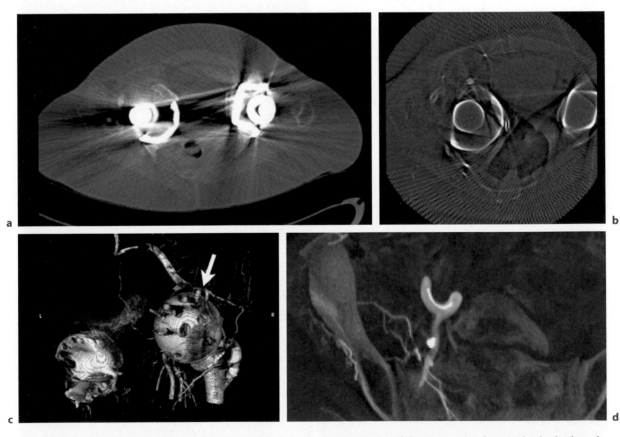

**Fig. 41.1a–d.** Beam-hardening causes severe artifact in the region of the small pelvis in conventional multi-slice CT (**a**). Because C-arm CT is based on projections, these artifacts are less likely to occur (**b**). Three-dimensional volume-rendering reconstruction of the C-arm CT dataset clearly displays the proximity of the screws (*arrow*) to the internal iliac artery. Three-dimensional (**c**) reconstruction and maximum intensity projection (**d**) of the C-arm CT dataset clearly.

artery relative to the screws of a protruded prothesis (Fig. 41.2).

We also applied this technique for different kinds of interventions of the liver and realized a particularly high potential for radio-embolization. For this kind of therapy, Yttrium-loaded microspheres are injected into the hepatic arteries. From the Yttrium emitted beta X-rays seem to be effective for the radiation treatment of a variety of different liver metastasis. Injecting Yttrium microspheres is far more critical than injecting any Gel-foam or Lipidol for chemoembolization. As any extra-hepatic application of the Yttrium microspheres may cause significant side effects and complications, including radionecrosis of the stomach or the gall bladder, it is absolutely mandatory to confirm a safe positioning of the catheter prior to administration (SALEM et al. 2004). For this reason, a planning and test procedure is performed where, instead of Yttrium microspheres, Technetium is injected via a catheter into the right and

left hepatic artery in order to detect any uptake, particularly in the lung, but also anywhere else outside the liver. Thereby, shunting into the lung is picked up easily by Technetium. However, it is often quite hard to understand the localization of extra-hepatic tracer uptake (SALEM et al. 2007).

In these circumstances, C-arm CT seems to be ideally suited to demonstrate that the tumor may safely be reached with the selected catheter position. However, C-arm CT may also confirm contrast reaching the stomach or the gall bladder. In this situation C-arm CT adds important information requiring either repositioning of the catheter or preventive occlusion of side branches by coiling.

We also had to understand that the image impression from C-arm CT is significantly different from conventional multi-slice CT. Contrast media injected into the superior mesenteric artery and scan acquisition about 60 s after the administration may result in images

**Fig. 41.2a–c.** Portal venous phase CT in a patient with cholangiocellular carcinoma (**a**). The corresponding FDG PET/CT (**b**) demonstrates vital tumor tissue at the rim. Corresponding C-arm CT with the catheter in the right hepatic artery (**c**) displays that the tumor must be supplied not only from the right, but also from the left hepatic artery. Furthermore, the area of high contrast enhancement in C-arm CT corresponds well to the location of the FDG uptake

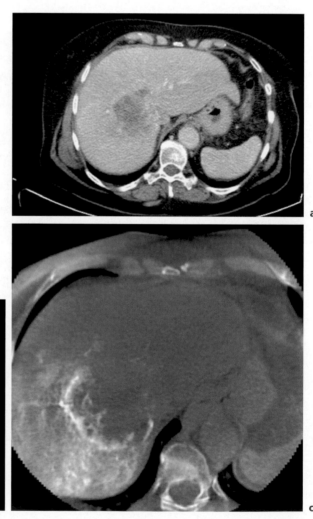

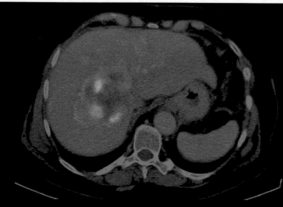

quite comparable to multi-slice CT images obtained in the portal venous phase. However, contrast media administered into the hepatic artery may lead to a typical ring enhancement in metastases that had exceeded a certain size. In comparison to PET/CT, it turned out that this ring enhancement in C-arm CT images commonly corresponds to the area of high metabolic activity within the tumor (Fig. 41.3).

We learned from C-arm CT in preparation for the radio-embolization that in 31.9% of patients we could confirm correct positioning of the catheter reaching the metastases. In another 25.5% of patients, C-arm CT had an impact on the interventional procedure either by the detection of contrast media outside the liver or by demonstrating the inability to reach the tumor from the any catheter position. One patient was even discharged from therapy because C-arm CT demonstrated an early portal-venous shunting that was not suspected from any other imaging modality.

## 41.3
## Other Applications and Future Outlook

C-arm CT may also be worth considereding not only for liver interventions, but also to aid in intervention for uterine fibroids. Here again, it might be difficult to confirm the appropriate catheter positioning from the DSA images only, whereas C-arm CT helps to see that the fibroids can be reached in the current position and other structures, such as the ovaries and the bladder, are not in danger of being embolized as well (Fig. 41.4).

The future set up of C-arm CT is very similar to conventional multi-slice CT. Once the patient has been prepared for scanning, the catheter will be connected to an automated contrast injector. C-arm CT may then be initiated from outside the scan room with automated contrast injection, patient breathing instruction and start of the scan after a predefined delay time. C-arm

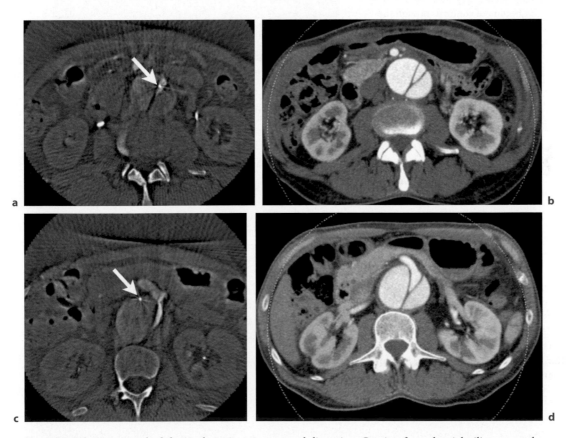

**Fig. 41.3a–d.** Patient with abdominal aortic aneurysm and dissection. Coming from the right iliac artery, the catheter passed through the true lumen (*arrow*) below the renal arteries (**a**) and through the false lumen (*arrow*) at the level of superior mesenteric artery (**c**). The C-arm CT is a 5-s acquisition primarily aimed at demonstrating high-contrast structures. The images on the right are the corresponding CT images from a dual source CT (**b** and **c**)

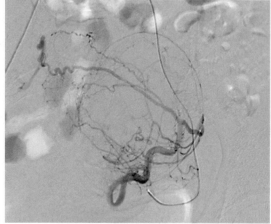

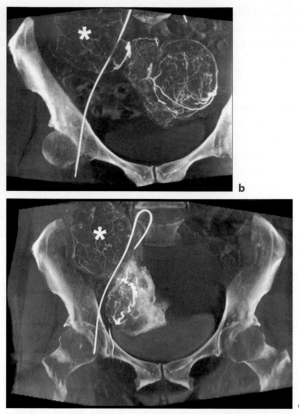

**Fig. 41.4a–c.** A 48-year-old female with uterine fibroid. The conventional DSA shows the extent of the fibroid as seen when contrast has been injected through the left internal iliac artery (**a**). C-arm CT clearly demonstrates that the same artery supplied multiple fibroids (**b**). With injection of contrast through the right internal iliac artery (**c**), one of the major fibroids seems to receive blood from both internal iliac arteries (*asterisk*)

CT images will firmly be integrated into the current intervention workflow. One of the other challenges is to integrate the data from C-arm CT into a navigation system that allows the support of particularly difficult procedures. Currently, neither navigation nor respiratory gating systems are available for the C-arm CT systems.

## References

Kakeda S, Korogi Y, Miyaguni Y et al. (2007) A cone-beam volume CT using a 3D angiography system with a flat panel detector of direct conversion type: usefulness for super-selective intra-arterial chemotherapy for head and neck tumors. AJNR 28:1783–1788

Kakeda S, Korogi Y, Ohnari N et al. (2007) Usefulness of cone-beam volume CT with flat panel detectors in conjunction with catheter angiography for transcatheter arterial embolization. J Vasc Interv Radiol 18:1508–1516

Kalender WA, Kyriakou Y (2007) Flat-detector computed tomography (FD-CT). Eur Radiol 17:2767–2779

Salem R, Lewandowski R, Roberts C et al. (2004) Use of Yttrium-90 glass microspheres (TheraSphere) for the treatment of unresectable hepatocellular carcinoma in patients with portal vein thrombosis. J Vasc Interv Radiol 15:335–345

Salem R, Lewandowski R, Sato K et al. (2007) Technical aspects of radioembolization with 90Y microspheres. Tech Vasc Intervent Radiol 10:12–29

Virmani S, Ryu RK, Sato KT et al. (2007) Effect of C-arm angiographic CT on transcatheter arterial chemoembolization of liver tumors. J Vasc Interv Radiol 8:1305–1309

Wallace MJ, Murthy R, Kamat PP et al. (2007) Impact of C-arm CT on hepatic arterial interventions for hepatic malignancies. J Vasc Interv Radiol 18:1500–1507

# Trauma Imaging / Acute Care

# CT Management of Multisystem Trauma

Markus Körner and Ulrich Linsenmaier

**ABSTRACT**

This chapter emphasizes on the use of MDCT in patients with multisystem trauma. These patients are usually seriously injured and require urgent operations or other therapeutic procedures. Consequently, CT examinations of this population differ significantly from dedicated examinations of defined body regions. Scanning protocols have to be adapted to the demand that imaging must be performed quickly, but remain accurate enough to safely rule out life-threatening injuries. Even if CT is well established in the diagnostic workflow of trauma patients, there is still discussion about how and when exactly to image patients sustaining multisystem trauma. Mass casualty incidents produce a large number of patients over a short period of time. Imaging during such an event is challenging and has to be prepared and exercised. This chapter also discusses how to handle a mass casualty incident from the radiologist's point of view.

## 42.1
## Introduction

Trauma remains the leading cause of death in people of age 45 and younger (Mutschler and Kanz 2002). Multisystem trauma (major trauma, polytrauma) is defined as injuries to more than one body region such as head, chest, abdomen, and extremities, one or the combination of which is potentially fatal to the patient (Trentz 2000). Trauma scores to define and characterize extend, severity, and prognosis of multisystem trauma were introduced nearly 30 years ago. Some of

M. Körner, MD
Department of Clinical Radiology, Ludwig-Maximilians-University of Munich, Munich University Hospitals, Nussbaumstrasse 20, 80336 Munich, Germany

U. Linsenmaier, MD
Department of Clinical Radiology, Ludwig-Maximilians-University of Munich, Munich University Hospitals, Nussbaumstrasse 20, 80336 Munich, Germany

them are widely accepted and in use all over the world. The Injury Severity Score (ISS) was introduced by S.P. Baker and allows objective characterization of injury severity according to an anatomical scale representing the three most involved organ regions. A score of 16 points and more (maximum of 75) is defined as multi-system trauma (Baker et al. 1974).

Management of multisystem trauma is an interdisciplinary challenge. Diagnostic workflow and urgent interventions to stabilize the patient such as fluid resuscitation or chest decompression have to be carried out immediately, because any delay in diagnostics or treatment will result in a deteriorated patient outcome and higher mortality (Cowley 1976; Clarke et al. 2002). Comprehensive diagnostic imaging is a key factor to help the clinicians to quickly establish the exact extent of injuries and to categorize the patient fast and accurate to enable priority-oriented treatment (Kanz et al. 2004).

The main tasks for the interdisciplinary cooperation of trauma surgeons, anesthesiologists, and radiologists in caring for patients with major trauma are to diagnose severe and life-threatening injuries and to initiate targeted and adequate treatment immediately. The priorities in the trauma room are as follows:

1. Immediate treatment of potentially fatal injuries and conditions.
2. Control of severe bleeding.
3. Treatment of elevated intracranial pressure if intracranial bleeding if present.
4. Stabilization for urgent operative, diagnostic and interventional procedures .
5. Completion of diagnostic procedures after the acute phase.

Diagnostic and therapeutic workflows should be organized, guided, and linked together by time-oriented algorithms. For therapeutic decisions, it is essential to recognize the exact pattern of injuries and categorize the resulting priorities for treatment, which is the main role of imaging in the acute phase of trauma care. Diagnostic imaging should therefore be carried out in a structured and problem-oriented workflow (Kanz et al. 1994, 2004; Hauser and Bohndorf 1998; Linsenmaier et al. 2002a; Mutschler and Kanz 2002; Boehm et al. 2004).

Before helical CT scanners were available, CT in multisystem trauma was limited to dedicated examinations of body parts such as head, chest, or abdomen because of the long scanning time and limited body volume coverage. With the introduction of helical CT, faster scanning times made scanning larger volumes

and combination of different protocols in different phases of contrast enhancement possible. Consequently, combined scans of more than one body region in patients sustaining multisystem trauma was introduced in trauma centers, even though the use of those quasi-whole-body protocols was heavily discussed (Low et al. 1997; Leidner et al. 1998; Linsenmaier and Pfeifer 1998, 1999; Novelline et al. 1999; Linsenmaier et al. 2000). The protocols used by that time usually consisted of a nonenhanced sequential head CT, which was followed by arterial-phase chest and portovenous-phase abdomen scans. However, the images were acquired at quite thick slices of usually 5 to 10 mm, and secondary reformations for evaluation of the spine and bones were of limited diagnostic value and not routinely computed.

The introduction of MDCT led to further advantages in imaging of trauma. Scan time was substantially reduced, and motion artifacts that were commonly seen with the slower scanners could be eliminated. Thinner primary slice collimation was introduced, allowing for high-quality secondary reformations in differently oriented planes whenever necessary (Dawson and Lees 2001; Kloppel et al. 2002; Linsenmaier et al. 2002a; Philipp et al. 2003a). Further techniques like volume rendering for 3D visualization of the dataset were also implemented.

## 42.2
## General Considerations about the Use of CT in Multisystem Trauma

Following the concept of the "golden hour" in trauma, time matters substantially in CT examinations of severely injured patients (Cowley 1976; Clarke et al. 2002). Not only the minimum achievable scanning speed, but also other factors have influence on total examination time.

Trauma algorithms are used to standardize trauma resuscitation and to coordinate the workflow of the different disciplines involved (Linsenmaier et al. 2001b). Algorithms should also help to avoid incomplete diagnostic imaging, resulting in missed relevant diagnoses. It is essential that algorithms are present for each single department and, of course, established and incorporated into daily routine by the staff. With regard to the algorithm of the radiology department involved in trauma room care, imaging modalities as well as their temporal order have to be defined precisely.

Acute trauma care consists of three different phases

(Table 42.1) (Kanz et al. 2004). During the first 5 min after admission (the primary phase) the patient is physically examined; life-threatening conditions have to be recognized and treated immediately. Imaging is limited to diagnostic means that are directly available in the resuscitation room, like mobile US machines and integrated X-ray units. Usually, the patient's status at that time does not allow transportation to other facilities such as CT at all.

The next phase is the secondary survey (5–30 min after admission). After initial patient stabilization, more sophisticated imaging should be done to rule out serious injuries that require treatment and that were not obvious after physical examination. If stabilization for transport cannot be achieved, then interventions or transfer to the operation theatre should follow without any further imaging.

The third phase, beginning 30 min after admission, initiates the definitive patient treatment and care after the entire diagnostic workflow has been completed. During this phase, further imaging such as additional CT scans or MRI can be performed, although this yet implies prior clearance of all life-threatening injuries.

Logistic concepts play a major role in handling patients with multisystem trauma. Patient preparation and transport time to our own data and experience contributes substantially to total examination time (Kanz et al. 2004). If the patient has to be transported from the resuscitation suite to the CT scanner over a long distance, then time can be lost resulting in possible life-threatening situations for the patient. In general, a well-organized floor plan with proximity of the trauma room and the CT scanner is essential; however, there are different solutions available to bring both units together (Krötz et al. 2002).

Dedicated trauma departments should have their own CT scanner available for their patients. This usually requires the department to be especially designed as an emergency department and constructed according to experiences being available from existing level I trauma centers. If possible, direct proximity and access of the trauma room and the CT scanner suite should be established. The most preferable way would be to equip the admitting area and trauma room unit with a dedicated CT scanner, which is the most effective but also most cost intensive way to integrate the scanner into the trauma room (Fig. 42.1).

Other concepts include the so-called sliding gantry, which allows the CT gantry to be moved instead of the patient being transferred by stretchers on different tables (Krötz et al. 2002; Wurmb et al. 2005). This model enables either parking the gantry far from the patient table within the scanner room, making the patient more accessible, or to use the gantry in two separate CT scanning rooms connected with a mobile wall. The latter solution enables to use the CT scanner in routine diagnosis while the trauma room is still busy but CT is no more needed.

If a logistic concept integrating the scanner into the resuscitation area cannot be achieved, then transportation has to be optimized. The patient can be placed on an X-ray permissive carbon spine board, which will not produce significant artifacts in CT images (Linsenmaier et al. 2001c). Using these flexible and modular boards, the patient can be moved easily from one table to a stretcher, another table, or a dedicated transportation trolley. Some vendors also offer transportation trolleys that can be used as CT scanner tables by connecting them to the scanner. However, every patient transfer from one table to another is time-consuming and must be limited by adequate radiology floor planning to the absolute necessary.

**Table 42.1.** Phases in handling multisystem trauma patients according to ATLS

| Phase | Time(min) | Radiologic modalities | Clinical treatment (ATLS) |
|---|---|---|---|
| I | 1–5 | US (FAST)<br>Chest radiograph (intubated patients) | Primary survey (ABCDE)<br>Resuscitation |
| II | 5–30 | MDCT scan and reading<br>MPR calculation | Secondary survey (from head to toe) |
| III | > 30 | Extremity radiographs<br>Additional CT scans | Definitive care |

*ABCDE* *a*irway, *b*reathing, *c*irculation, *d*isability, and *e*xposure

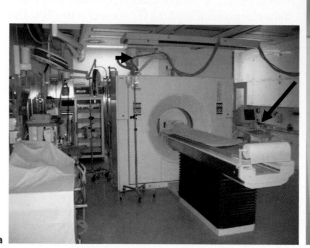

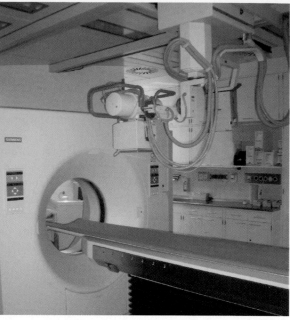

a

b

**Fig. 42.1.  a** Integration of a four-detector-row CT scanner in the trauma resuscitation room (Department of Trauma and Orthopedic Surgery, University Hospital Munich, Munich, Germany) After admission, the patient is positioned on the CT table. US can be performed prior to the CT scan (*long arrow*) The US machine is always available in this room. The digital radiography device is located behind the gantry in parking position (*short arrow*). **b** If chest radiography is needed prior to CT, the radiography device can be moved to the front of the gantry, and the image can be obtained

## 42.3
### Scanning Protocols

Standard scanning protocols for multisystem trauma should be defined and routinely be implemented on the CT scanner. Those protocols should be strictly used because remodeling protocols in emergencies is time-consuming and will significantly delay diagnostic and therapeutic procedures and result in variable unpredictable imaging results. Depending on the scanner type, adequate scanning protocols are needed for the technical capabilities of the equipment in use. Therefore, protocols vary somehow from generation to generation of CT scanner (Table 42.2).

The patient is positioned on the CT table in a supine position if possible. For the cranial CT scan, the arms should be placed next to the patient's body. For all other scans, it is useful to place the patient with both arms elevated in order to reduce artifacts. When arm elevation is not possible due to fractures or suggested injuries in non-addressable or endotracheally intubated patients, placing the arms crossed on the front of the chest or abdomen is preferable because the artifacts are reduced in contrast to having the arms placed parallel to each side

of the body (LINSENMAIER et al. 2002b; HOPPE et al. 2006). Repositioning the patient during the CT examination will take some time and should only be considered if the patient is stable and the need for immediate interventions is not obvious.

Whole-body CT (WB-CT) protocols in multisystem trauma usually consist of a non-contrast enhanced head CT, which is followed by a contrast-enhanced chest and abdominal CT. For evaluation of the spine, reformations from the chest and abdomen are of diagnostic image quality if the primary collimation was 2.5 mm or less, and dedicated scans of the spine are not obligatory (MANN et al. 2003). The cervical spine can be scanned separately with thin collimations after the head scan, or can be included in the chest scan. The latter option has the advantage that the cervical vessels are contrast-enhanced, and vascular injuries can be ruled out from the same dataset, sparing one additional scan.

In older scanner generations such as single- to four-detector-row scanners, the primary collimation usually has to be thicker than with scanners utilizing more than four detector rows. For cranial CT, collimation is 1 mm, while for chest and abdomen the collimation is 2.5 mm or larger. There are some reasons for the thicker collimation in these scanner generations: the time needed

**Table 42.2.** Typical scanning protocols for 4-, 16-, and 64-slice scanners

|  | Head | Chest | Abdomen | Spine (MPR) |
|---|---|---|---|---|
| kVp | 120 | 120 | 120 | |
| mAs | 210 | 140 (dose modulation) | 200 (dose modulation) | |
| Collimation (mm) | 1/0.75/0.6 | 2.5/1.5/0.6 | | |
| Slice thickness (mm) | 2 (base)<br>4 (brain)<br>2 (bone) | 5/3/3 (soft tissue)<br>3/2/2 (bone) | | 3/2/2<br>Sagittal/coronal |
| Table movement (mm) | 4/12/22 | 12.5/24/46 | 12.5/24/46 | |
| Kernel | Brain<br>Bone | Soft tissue<br>Lung/bone | Soft tissue<br>Bone | Bone<br>Soft tissue[a] |
| Intravenous contrast (ml) | ∅ | 140 (1.5–2 ml/kg/BW)[b] | | |
| Scan delay (s) | ∅ | 25[c] | 80[c] | |

*BW* body weight

[a]Additional soft tissue coronary and sagittal MPR of the chest and the abdomen can be useful

[b]With 16- and 64-slice scanners, the amount of contrast media can be reduced to 100 ml, followed by a 40-ml NaCl bolus

[c]Delays represent arterial-phase chest and portovenous abdomen

for scanning large volumes is longer the less scanning rows are installed, resulting in an increase of motion and breathing artifacts. Additionally, inhomogeneous contrast material distribution has to be considered with possible obscuring of lesions. Another important issue is that the tubes of those scanners are not as powerful as they are in newer generation scanners, resulting in tube overheating and the need for tube cooling, which also delays the workflow reasonably (KÖRNER et al. 2006).

With 16 and more detector rows, the WB-CT scan can be performed with collimations of 1 mm and less. From the primary data, secondary reformations can be obtained with high diagnostic quality, which can often replace repeat examinations of some body regions needed because of limited image quality in the first scan (Fig. 42.2). In addition, standard MPR of the abdomen and chest can be obtained if there are unclear findings.

Intravenous contrast material is needed by default for the chest and abdomen scan. Nonenhanced scans will not allow sufficient detection of vascular or solid organ injuries and should only be performed in patients with known reduced renal clearance, or if catheterization of a vein is impossible. In any case, the benefit of

a contrast-enhanced scan is often significantly higher than the risk of acute renal failure. The contrast medium can be any standard CT contrast agent. If used with an iodine concentration of 300 mg/ml, the amount should be 120–150 ml (1.5–2.0 ml per kilogram body weight) at a flow rate of 2.5–3.5 ml/s. For CTA, the flow rate can be increased to 5.0 ml/s if the intravenous access is capable of such high flows. A post-contrast saline flush of 40 ml can be helpful to reduce the amount of contrast material needed.

While intravenous contrast material is undisputedly needed in any multisystem trauma patient, the application of oral contrast material is not uniformly recommended. In patients with penetrating trauma to the chest, abdomen, or pelvis, oral and rectal contrast media application increases sensitivity for the detection of hollow organ injury (SHANMUGANATHAN et al. 2004; SAMPSON et al. 2006). However, installation of contrast fluids takes some time, and patients that are unable to swallow need a gastric tube before contrast material can be given. In blunt abdominal trauma, oral contrast application is not imperatively necessary to rule out bowel injuries because CT without oral contrast leads

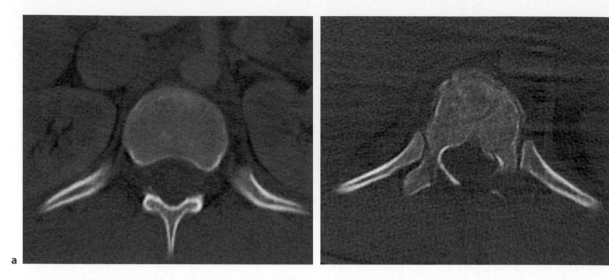

**Fig. 42.2. a** Image of a 43-year-old male who sustained a motorcycle crash. The image is a bone kernel reconstruction with a 3-mm slice thickness from a 2.5-mm collimation whole-body dataset obtained with a four-slice scanner. On this image, T12 does not show obvious signs of fractures. **b** After 3 days, the patient complained of persistent back pain, and a dedicated spine CT with the same scanner was obtained with a smaller FOV and a primary collimation of 1 mm. The compression fracture of T12 delineates quite clearly. Even with secondary reading of the first images, the fracture was not visible on the whole body CT scan with the thicker collimation

to similar results compared with CT with oral contrast (ALLEN et al. 2004; HOLMES et al. 2004; STUHLFAUT et al. 2004).

With faster scanners, multiphase imaging is possible. Usually, WB-CT protocols for trauma comprised an arterial phase scan of the chest and neck, and a portovenous phase scan of the abdomen (LINSENMAIER et al. 2002b; KANZ et al. 2004; WURMB et al. 2005). In cases of suspected pelvic fractures, arterial-phase imaging of the pelvis can be helpful to detect vascular injuries with active bleeding requiring intervention. If injuries of the abdominal aorta are suspected scanning the abdomen during arterial phase should be considered.

In trauma of the kidney, excretory-phase imaging after 3 to 10 min can provide valuable information about the extent of the injury into the renal collection system (Fig. 42.3) (PARK et al. 2006). When injuries to the spleen and liver are present, late-phase images help to plan interventions because they allow differentiating pseudoaneurysms from lacerations and active contrast material extravasations (MARMERY and SHANMUGANATHAN 2006).

Although more phases provide additional diagnostic information on injuries, the radiation dose applied to the patient will proportionally increase considerably with the covered scan volume and number of scans performed. In order to keep radiation as reasonably low as possible in major trauma patients, additional phases must be indicated individually on clinical suspicion or findings in the standard dataset rather than by default.

It is important to keep the number of images acquired at a straightforward quantity. Using standard reformations in three planes (axial, sagittal, and coronal) and in different kernels will result in up to several thousands of images. Reading those images will not only take a long time, but also the digital transfer to the picture archiving and communication systems (PACS) is a significant bottleneck, depending on the network speed and active network load (KÖRNER et al. 2006). A possible solution in an emergent situation is viewing the images directly on the CT operating workstation; consequently, the time for the transfer to the digital archive can be disregarded. If an additional workstation is available connected by a direct link to the CT operating computer, then image viewing and reformatting on this console should be strongly considered because images can easily be reformatted in different planes and slice thicknesses during the reading process.

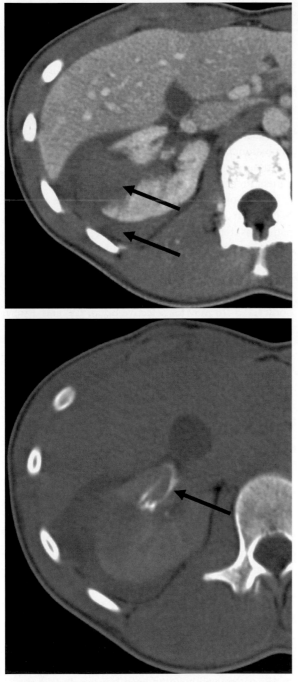

a

b

**Fig. 42.3 a** Axial CT portovenous phase images of the right kidney in a 16-year-old male soccer player who was struck by another player. There is a large hematoma in the renal parenchyma, expanding through the capsule of the kidney and pararenal free fluid (*arrows*). Due to possible expansion of the injury into the collecting system, late-phase images were obtained. **b** Delayed-phase CT image, obtained 10 min after infusion of intravenous contrast material, shows extravasation (*arrow*), a finding indicative of a rupture of the collecting system (Grade IV lesion).

42.4

## Controversies about CT in the Early Phase of Trauma Resuscitation

There is some discussion about whether plain radiography and US examinations are needed prior to the CT scan and in which extent they should be carried out. In the 1990s, there was general agreement in the Western world to use plain films of the head, spine, chest, and pelvis as well as a focused abdominal US (FAST) prior to CT (FRESHMAN et al. 1993; NAST-KOLB et al. 1994; HAUSER and BOHNDORF 1998; HAUSER 1999). This kind of basic radiological evaluation of injuries was needed to indicate CT of injured body regions, because standardized whole-body imaging was not possible at that time due to the slow scanners available. Even with faster scanners, the Advanced Trauma Life Support (ATLS) guidelines and surgical guidelines in many countries still insist on radiographs of the cervical spine, chest, and pelvis before taking the patient to the CT scanner (KANZ et al. 2004).

Radiography has certain limitations in patients with multisystem trauma. Patient positioning is not always possible in the required way, thus standard projections frequently cannot be achieved. Artifacts from clothing and technical equipment are often present and can obscure pathologic findings. Both factors contribute to poor image quality and reduced sensitivity in injury detection. Consequently, clearing the cervical spine with a single, lateral view is often not safely possible, which leads to recommendations to replace the lateral view by CT (KANZ et al. 2004; PLATZER et al. 2006). Furthermore, recent reports have shown the superiority of MDCT in detection of fractures compared with plain radiography. RESNICK et al. (1992) reported that about 80% of acetabular fractures are not shown on plain radiographs. Other authors who compared CT with conventional pelvic radiographs showed the superiority of CT for depiction and classification of pelvic fractures (WEDEGÄRTNER et al. 2003). Further examples of the superiority of CT are in the diagnosis of skeletal trauma in general (GEIJER and EL-KHOURY 2006), spinal fractures (BUCKWALTER et al. 2001; MANN et al. 2003; PHILIPP et al. 2003b; SCHRÖDER et al. 2003), and of blunt abdominal and thoracic trauma (FRESHMAN et al. 1993; LOW et al. 1997; LINSENMAIER et al. 2001a; POLETTI et al. 2002; RIEGER et al. 2002; MAHONEY et al. 2003; MATTHES et al. 2003).

The use of US in trauma patients as only imaging method for the abdomen is reported to be not sufficient to safely rule out injuries (POLETTI et al. 2004; KÖRNER et al. 2008). However, it can be useful in deciding whether the patient can be taken to the CT or needs immediate laparotomy (LINDNER et al. 2004; BAKKER et al. 2005). In some cases, US can help to exclude patients from unnecessary CT scans and radiation (MA et al. 2005).

Consequently, the method of choice in imaging critical patients with major trauma undisputedly is MDCT. The use of CT even during the first minutes of trauma resuscitation is highly preferable over all other imaging modalities, because it provides superior, volumetric image quality and reliably helps to identify injuries of all relevant body regions in short time. In contrast to single-detector CT, MDCT is significantly superior in terms of scanning spatial and temporal resolution, speed, and maximum volume coverage.

There is no general agreement so far about whether patients with unstable circulation can undergo CT examinations (KANZ et al. 2004). Although patient monitoring is possible throughout the whole stay in the scanning room, and fluid resuscitation can be achieved even during active scanning, some working groups do not agree with scanning semistable patients. LEIDNER et al. (1998) insisted on a complete examination that conformed to the ATLS rules, including radiographs of the chest, pelvis, and cervical spine, before CT. They also required a stable circulation. WILLMANN et al. (2002) requested MDCT in injured patients only if hemodynamic stability was achieved with a 2,000-ml infusion or less; otherwise, the patient's status was regarded as unstable, and CT was contraindicated. Hemodynamic instability was not regarded as a contraindication to CT in another study in patients (KLÖPPEL et al. 2002). In patients undergoing cardiopulmonary resuscitation (CPR), CT imaging should not be carried out because it might have a negative impact on the outcome when CPR is stopped during the scan.

All of the studies dealing with finding the best time for CT imaging in multisystem trauma were conducted using single- or four-detector-row CT scanners. To the authors' knowledge, there are no studies to this point that have investigated the outcome of unstable patients that were scanned with newer generation scanners. As trauma rooms with in-room CT scanners become more widespread, further investigation is needed to validate the given recommendations.

Despite unstable patients, the general recommendation for multisystem trauma patients is to image them as soon as possible with CT after admission. After excluding the need for immediate operation with US, CT should be performed without further delay. The goal is to have the first images available 30 min after admission. It is obvious that this time frame cannot be achieved in every patient. However, our working group was able to prove that in about 75% of all multisystem trauma patients WB-CT can be carried out within the first thirty minutes after hospital admission (KANZ et al. 2004). In the other 25% of patients, this time could not be achieved because of clinical problems that needed immediate therapies (i.e., chest drains, endotracheal intubation, CPR). This study also showed that most of the time during trauma resuscitation was needed for patient preparation and transportation.

Radiation dose is another important issue with WB-CT in trauma patients. As the average trauma patient is reported to be about 45 years old, dose reduction and radiation protection is needed where possible in order to reduce excess cancer risk in those patients. The effective radiation dose of trauma examinations is reported to be about 10–30 mSv for whole-body CT, 5–16 mSv for selective organ CT, and 2 mSv for a conventional radiography series (chest, vertebral column, pelvis), respectively (RUCHHOLTZ et al. 2002; PTAK et al. 2003; BRENNER and ELLISTON 2004; WEDEGÄRTNER et al. 2004; HEYER et al. 2005). However, specific organ doses can be significantly higher, above all when special protocols for gated cardiac and chest examinations are used, and an increase in excess cancer risk has to be considered (HURWITZ et al. 2007; TIEN et al. 2007). When comparing different WB-CT protocols, single-pass acquisition protocols demonstrated lower radiation exposure compared to segmented, partially overlapping examinations (PTAK et al. 2003; FANUCCI et al. 2007).

WB-CT is associated with an increased radiation exposure compared to selective-organ CT, but increase of diagnostic safety should result in better patient outcome and survival, consequently justifying the higher radiation dose and consequent use of those protocols. SALIM et al. (2006) demonstrated that the use of WB-CT resulted in a change of treatment in 19% of 1,000 patients without obvious signs of injuries. Another study was able to show a benefit of whole-body imaging in 457 patients with closed head injuries. In that study, unexpected findings were present in 38%; therapeutic changes were made in 26% of the patients (SELF et al. 2003).

The patients for WB-CT imaging have to be carefully selected and separated from those not needing a full-body scan. Table 42.3 shows parameters that are indicating suspicion of multisystem trauma. If any of these parameters is present, then WB-CT should be considered, even in younger subjects.

**Table 42.3.** Parameters indicating multisystem trauma

| Mechanism |
|---|
| Traffic accident: |
| • Bicyclist/pedestrian struck by vehicle with subsequent loss of consciousness |
| • High-speed collision (≥50 km/h / 30 mph) |
| • Rollover in vehicle |
| • Ejection of passenger from vehicle |
| • Airbag released |
| • Accompanying passengers killed |
| Fall from height: |
| • 5 m and higher |
| • Height not clear |
| • Fall from stairway, escalator, scaffold, or ladder, or of unknown cause |
| Other mechanisms: |
| • Buried under ground |
| • Trapped in crashed vehicle, etc. |
| • Explosion |
| • Exact mechanism unclear, severe trauma likely |

| Injury patterns |
|---|
| • Penetrating injury |
| • Gunshot wound to the trunk |
| • Stab wound to the trunk |
| • Open chest injury/unstable chest |
| • Unstable pelvic fracture |
| • Fractures of two or more extremity long bones |
| • Proximal amputation of limb |
| • Serial rib fractures in addition to other injuries |
| • Comminuted fractures |

| Vital parameters |
|---|
| • GCS <10 |
| • Systolic blood pressure <80 mmHg |
| • Respiratory frequency <10 or >29 per min |
| • Arterial oxygen saturation <90% |

## 42.5

## CT as a Triage Tool in Mass Casualty Incidents

Mass casualty incidents (MCI) are defined as situations with a larger number of casualties produced in a relatively short period of time, usually as the result of a single incident such as accidents, natural disasters, or acts of terrorism. These events are also expected to exceed normal capacities of health care systems in terms of logistics, personnel, and maximum achievable individual care (Levi et al. 2002; Arnold et al. 2003).

In order to provide appropriate individual treatment, it is essential to identify critically injured patients with potentially fatal injury patterns early and transport them to a trauma center, without any further delay. After these patients have arrived at the trauma center, secondary diagnostic tests have to be performed to further assess the injuries of the patients in order to set up a priority-based therapeutic regime.

In patients with multisystem trauma, CT has proven to be an adequate diagnostic tool for evaluating all critical organic traumas with a WB-CT scan, as stated above. Consequently, MSCT could be also very helpful in correctly triaging patients that have been wrongly

**Table 42.4** Modified scanning protocol for mass casualty incidents for a four-detector-row scanner, adapted from (Körner et al. 2006) The collimation for the head CT was increased to 2.5 mm, the chest and abdomen scan were fused, and the current–time product for the chest and abdomen had to be lowered because of tube cooling issues. There are no standard MPR or additional reformations in different kernels. After the acute setting has cleared, those reformations can be calculated

|  | Cardiac CT | Thoracic and abdominal CT |
|---|---|---|
| Tube voltage (kV) | 120 | 120 |
| Current–time (mA) | 210 | 120 |
| Collimation (mm) | 4 × 2.5 | 4 × 2.5 |
| Slice thickness (mm) | 5 | 5 |
| Table movement (mm) | 4 | 15 |
| Kernel | Brain | Soft tissue |
| Contrast media (ml) | ∅ | 140 (2 ml/kg/BW) |
| Delay after CM (s) | ∅ | 45 |

categorized into a lower (undertriage) or higher (overtriage) triage group. In multiple casualties, this is essential to avoid blocking of limited health care resources like operating room and intensive care unit capacities with patients suffering from noncritical injuries.

When it comes to larger number of patients in case of a multiple casualty incident, the CT scanner capacity will come to its limit and thus represents a significant bottleneck in the initial diagnostic phase. For such events, the scanning protocol and other CT workflow algorithms have to be adapted concentrating on the main issues and limiting the initial number of images to be handled.

Our workgroup developed a modified MCI CT scanning protocol that helped to improve the patient throughput from 2.3 to 6.7 per hour (Körner et al. 2006). In order to provide appropriate service during patient arrival after a mass casualty incident occurred, the scan parameters have to be adapted to such a situation (Table 42.4). For the first image reading, axial images should be sufficient to rule out life-threatening injuries. Secondary reformations can be obtained after the acute situation has been cleared, and the patients' treatment is initiated.

## Key Points

- Multisystem trauma is injury to more than one body region, one or the combination of these injuries being potentially fatal.

- MDCT, the diagnostic test of choice in multisystem trauma, produces fast, accurate high-quality images. Whole-body CT in multisystem trauma generally comprises a noncontrast-enhanced head scan, which is followed by a contrast-enhanced chest and abdominal scan.
- Newer scanners allow for multiphase imaging and help to prioritize therapeutic interventions.
- Some of the limitations of CT scanning in multisystem trauma are difficulty in patient positioning, and artifacts produced by clothing and equipment can obscure findings.

## References

Allen TL, Mueller MT, Bonk RT et al. (2004) Computed tomographic scanning without oral contrast solution for blunt bowel and mesenteric injuries in abdominal trauma. J Trauma 56:314–322

Arnold JL, Tsai MC, Halpern P et al. (2003) Mass-casualty, terrorist bombings: epidemiological outcomes, resource utilization, and time course of emergency needs (part I) Prehospital Disaster Med 18:220–334

Baker SP, O'Neill B, Haddon W Jr et al. (1974) The injury severity score: a method for describing patients with multiple injuries and evaluating emergency care. J Trauma 14:187–96

Bakker J, Genders R, Mali W et al. (2005) Sonography as the primary screening method in evaluating blunt abdominal trauma. J Clin Ultrasound 33:155–163

Boehm T, Alkadhi H, Schertler T et al. (2004) (Application of multislice spiral CT (MSCT) in multiple injured patients and its effect on diagnostic and therapeutic algorithms) Rofo 176:1734–1742

Brenner DJ, Elliston CD (2004) Estimated radiation risks potentially associated with full-body CT screening. Radiology 232:735–738

Buckwalter KA, Rydberg J, Kopecky KK et al. (2001) Musculoskeletal imaging with multislice CT. AJR Am J Roentgenol 176:979–986

Clarke JR, Trooskin SZ, Doshi PJ et al. (2002) Time to laparotomy for intra-abdominal bleeding from trauma does affect survival for delays up to 90 min. J Trauma 52:420–425

Cowley RA (1976) The resuscitation and stabilization of major multiple trauma patients in a trauma centre environment. Clin Med 83:14–19

Dawson P, Lees WR (2001) Multi-slice technology in computed tomography. Clin Radiol 56:302–309

Fanucci E, Fiaschetti V, Rotili A et al. (2007) Whole body 16-row multislice CT in emergency room: effects of different protocols on scanning time, image quality and radiation exposure. Emerg Radiol 13:251–257

Freshman SP, Wisner DH, Battistella FD et al. (1993) Secondary survey following blunt trauma: a new role for abdominal CT scan. J Trauma 34:337–340; discussion 340–341

Geijer M, El-Khoury GY (2006) MDCT in the evaluation of skeletal trauma: principles, protocols, and clinical applications. Emerg Radiol 13:7–18

Hauser H, Bohndorf K (1998) [Radiologic emergency management in multiple trauma cases.] (In German) Radiologe 38:637–644

Hauser HB (1999) Radiological emergency management of multiple trauma patients. Emerg Radiol 6:61–69

Heyer CM, Rduch G, Kagel T et al. (2005) [Prospective randomized trial of a modified standard multislice CT protocol for the evaluation of multiple trauma patients.] Rofo 177:242–249

Holmes JF, Offerman SR, Chang CH et al. (2004) Performance of helical computed tomography without oral contrast for the detection of gastrointestinal injuries. Ann Emerg Med 43:120–128

Hoppe H, Vock P, Bonel HM et al. (2006) A novel multiple-trauma CT-scanning protocol using patient repositioning. Emerg Radiol 13:123–128

Hurwitz LM, Reiman RE, Yoshizumi TT et al. (2007) Radiation dose from contemporary cardiothoracic multidetector CT protocols with an anthropomorphic female phantom: implications for cancer induction. Radiology 245:742–750

Kanz KG, Eitel F, Waldner H et al. (1994) [Development of clinical algorithms for quality assurance in management of multiple trauma.] (In German) Unfallchirurg 97:303–307

Kanz KG, Körner M, Linsenmaier U et al. (2004) [Priority-oriented shock trauma room management with the integration of multiple-view spiral computed tomography.] (In German) Unfallchirurg 107:937–944

Klöppel R, Schreiter D, Dietrich J et al. (2002) [Early clinical management after polytrauma with 1 and 4 slice spiral CT.] (In German) Radiologe 42:541–546

Körner M, Krötz M, Kanz KG et al. (2006) Development of an accelerated MSCT protocol (Triage MSCT) for mass casualty incidents: comparison to MSCT for single-trauma patients. Emerg Radiol 12:203–209

Körner M, Krötz M, Degenhart C et al. (2008) Current role of emergency ultrasound in patients with major trauma. RadioGraphics 28:246–252

Krötz M, Bode PJ, Hauser H et al. (2002) [Interdisciplinary shock room management: personnel, equipment and spatial logistics in 3 trauma centers in Europe.] (In German) Radiologe 42:522–532

Leidner B, Adiels M, Aspelin P et al. (1998) Standardized CT examination of the multitraumatized patient. Eur Radiol 8:1630–1638

Levi L, Michaelson M, Admi H et al. (2002) National strategy for mass casualty situations and its effects on the hospital. Prehospital Disaster Med 17:12–16

Lindner T, Bail HJ, Manegold S et al. (2004) [Shock trauma room diagnosis: initial diagnosis after blunt abdominal trauma. A review of the literature.] (In German) Unfallchirurg 107:892–902

Linsenmaier U, Pfeifer KJ (1998) Umstrittenes Konzept beim Polytrauma: Ganzkörper-CT als Nativuntersuchung. RoFo 168:306

Linsenmaier U, Pfeifer KJ (1999) Imaging of trauma patients in Germany. Emergency Radiology 6:74–76

Linsenmaier U, Rieger J, Brandl T et al. (2000) New method for fast spiral CT of trauma patients—RUSH CT. Emergency Radiology 7:135–141

Linsenmaier U, Kanz KG, Mutschler W et al. (2001a) [Radiological diagnosis in polytrauma: interdisciplinary management.] (In German) Rofo 173:485–943

Linsenmaier U, Kanz KG, Mutschler W et al. (2001b) Radiologische Diagnostik beim Polytrauma: Interdisziplinäres Management. RöFo Fortschr Geb Rontgenstr Neuen Bildgeb Verfahr 173:1–9

Linsenmaier U, Krötz M, Kanz KG et al. (2001c) Evaluation von Wirbelsäulenbrettern für die Röntgendiagnostik. RoFo 173:1041–1047

Linsenmaier U, Kanz KG, Rieger J et al. (2002a) [Structured radiologic diagnosis in polytrauma.] (In German) Radiologe 42:533–540

Linsenmaier U, Krötz M, Häuser H et al. (2002b) Whole-body computed tomography in polytrauma: techniques and management. Eur Radiol 12:1728–1740

Low R, Duber C, Schweden F et al. (1997) [Whole body spiral CT in primary diagnosis of patients with multiple trauma in emergency situations.] (In German) Rofo 166:382–288

Ma OJ, Gaddis G, Steele MT et al. (2005) Prospective analysis of the effect of physician experience with the FAST examination in reducing the use of CT scans. Emerg Med Australas 17:24–30

Mahoney EJ, Biffl WL, Harrington DT et al. (2003) Isolated brain injury as a cause of hypotension in the blunt trauma patient. J Trauma 55:1065–1069

Mann FA, Cohen WA, Linnau KF et al. (2003) Evidence-based approach to using CT in spinal trauma. Eur J Radiol 48:39–48

Marmery H and Shanmuganathan K (2006) Multidetector-row computed tomography imaging of splenic trauma. Semin UA CT MR 27:404–419

Matthes G, Stengel D, Seifert J et al. (2003) Blunt liver injuries in polytrauma: results from a cohort study with the regular use of whole-body helical computed tomography. World J Surg 27:1124–1130

Mutschler W and Kanz KG (2002) [Interdisciplinary shock room management: responsibilities of the radiologist from the trauma surgery viewpoint]. (In German) Radiologe 42:506–514

Nast-Kolb D, Waydhas C, Kanz KG et al. (1994) [An algorithm for management of shock in polytrauma.] (In German) Unfallchirurg 97:292–302

Novelline RA, Rhea JT, Rao PM et al. (1999) Helical CT in emergency radiology. Radiology 213:321–339

Park SJ, Kim JK, Kim KW et al. (2006) MDCT Findings of renal trauma. AJR Am J Roentgenol 187:541–547

Philipp MO, Kubin K, Hormann M et al. (2003a) Radiological emergency room management with emphasis on multidetector-row CT. Eur J Radiol 48:2–4

Philipp MO, Kubin K, Mang T et al. (2003b) Three-dimensional volume rendering of multidetector-row CT data: applicable for emergency radiology. Eur J Radiol 48:33–38

Platzer P, Jaindl M, Thalhammer G et al. (2006) Clearing the cervical spine in critically injured patients: a comprehensive C-spine protocol to avoid unnecessary delays in diagnosis. Eur Spine J 15:1801–1810

Poletti PA, Wintermark M, Schnyder P et al. (2002) Traumatic injuries: role of imaging in the management of the polytrauma victim (conservative expectation) Eur Radiol 12:969–978

Poletti PA, Mirvis SE, Shanmuganathan K et al. (2004) Blunt abdominal trauma patients: can organ injury be excluded without performing computed tomography? J Trauma 57:1072–1081

Ptak T, Rhea JT, Novelline RA (2003) Radiation dose is reduced with a single-pass whole-body multi-detector row CT trauma protocol compared with a conventional segmented method: initial experience. Radiology 229:902–905

Resnik CS, Stackhouse DJ, Shanmuganathan K et al. (1992) Diagnosis of pelvic fractures in patients with acute pelvic trauma: efficacy of plain radiographs. AJR Am J Roentgenol 158:109–112

Rieger M, Sparr H, Esterhammer R et al. (2002) [Modern CT diagnosis of acute thoracic and abdominal trauma.] (In German) Anaesthesist 51:835–842

Ruchholtz S, Waydhas C, Schroeder T et al. (2002) [The value of computed tomography in the early treatment of seriously injured patients.] (In German) Chirurg 73:1005–1012

Salim A, Sangthong B, Martin M et al. (2006) Whole body imaging in blunt multisystem trauma patients without obvious signs of injury: results of a prospective study. Arch Surg 141:468–473; discussion 473–475

Sampson MA, Colquhoun KB and Hennessy NL (2006) Computed tomography whole body imaging in multi-trauma: 7 years experience. Clin Radiol 61:365–369

Schroder RJ, Albus M, Kandziora F et al. (2003) [Diagnostic value of three-dimensional reconstruction in CT of traumatic spinal fractures.] (In German) Rofo 175:1500–1507

Self ML, Blake AM, Whitley M et al. (2003) The benefit of routine thoracic, abdominal, and pelvic computed tomography to evaluate trauma patients with closed head injuries. Am J Surg 186:609–613; discussion 613–614

Shanmuganathan K, Mirvis SE, Chiu WC et al. (2004) Penetrating torso trauma: triple-contrast helical CT in peritoneal violation and organ injury—a prospective study in 200 patients. Radiology 231:775–784

Stuhlfaut JW, Soto JA, Lucey BC et al. (2004) Blunt abdominal trauma: performance of CT without oral contrast material. Radiology 233:689–694

Tien HC, Tremblay LN, Rizoli SB et al. (2007) Radiation exposure from diagnostic imaging in severely injured trauma patients. J Trauma 62:151–156

Trentz O (2000) Polytrauma: pathophysiology, priorities and management. In: Rüedi T, Murphy WM (eds) AO principles of fracture management. Thieme, Stuttgart, pp 661–673

Wedegärtner U, Gatzka C, Rueger JM et al. (2003) [Multislice CT (MSCT) in the detection and classification of pelvic and acetabular fractures.] (In German) Rofo 175:105–111

Wedegärtner U, Lorenzen M, Nagel HD et al. (2004) [Diagnostic imaging in polytrauma: comparison of radiation exposure from whole-body MSCT and conventional radiography with organ-specific CT.] Rofo 176:1039–1044

Willmann JK, Roos JE, Platz A et al. (2002) Multidetector CT: detection of active hemorrhage in patients with blunt abdominal trauma. AJR Am J Roentgenol 179:437–444

Wurmb T, Fruhwald P, Brederlau J et al. (2005) [The Würzburg polytrauma algorithm. Concept and first results of a sliding-gantry-based computer tomography diagnostic system.] (In German) Anaesthesist 54:763–768; 770–772

# Subject Index

# List of Contributors

Hatem Alkadhi, MD
Associate Professor,
Section Head – Body Computed Tomography
Institute of Diagnostic Radiology
University Hospital Zurich
Raemisstrasse 100
8091 Zurich
Switzerland

Email: hatem.alkadhi@usz.ch


Gerald Antoch, MD
Department of Diagnostic and Interventional Radiology
and Neuroradiology
University Hospital Essen
Hufelandstrasse 55
45127 Essen
Germany

Email: gerald.antoch@uni-due.de


Ahmed Ba-Ssalamah, MD
Universitätsklinik für Radiodiagnostik
Medizinische Universität Wien
Währinger Gürtel 18–20
1090 Wien
Austria


Andrea Baur-Melnyk, MD, PD
Department of Clinical Radiology
University of Munich Hospitals
Ludwig-Maximilians-University
Marchioninistrasse 15
81377 Munich
Germany

Email: andrea.baur@med.uni-muenchen.de


Christoph R. Becker, MD
Department of Clinical Radiology
University of Munich Hospitals
Ludwig-Maximilians-University
Marchioninistrasse 15
81377 Munich
Germany

Email: christoph.becker@med.uni-muenchen.de


C. Behrmann, MD
Department of Diagnostic Radiology
University of Halle
Ernst-Grube-Str. 40
06097 Halle
Germany


Thorsten A. Bley, MD
Abteilung Röntgendiagnostik
Radiologische Universitätsklinik Freiburg
Hugstetter Str. 55
79106 Freiburg
Germany

Email: thorsten.bley@uniklinik-freiburg.de

presently:
Department of Radiology
University of Wisconsin
600 Highland Ave
Madison, WI, 53792
USA


Dittmar Böckler, MD
Department of Vascular and Endovascular Surgery
Ruprecht-Karls University Heidelberg
Im Neuenheimer Feld 110
69120 Heidelberg
Germany

Email: dittmar.boeckler@med.uni-heidelberg.de


Jan Boese, PhD
Siemens AG
Healthcare Sector
MED AX
Siemensstrasse 1
91301 Forchheim
Germany

Email: jan.boese@siemens.com

Gunnar Brix, PhD
Federal Office for Radiation Protection, Germany
Department of Radiation Protection and Health
Ingolstaedter Landstrasse 1
85764 Neuherberg
Germany

*Email: gbrix@bfx.de*


Thomas Brunner, PhD
Siemens AG
Healthcare Sector
MED AX
Siemensstrasse 1
91301 Forchheim
Germany

*Email: thomas.brunner@siemens.com*


Albert Dirisamer, MD
Department of Diagnostic and Pediatric Radiology
Medical University of Vienna
Waehringer Guertel 18–20
1190 Vienna
Austria

*Email: albert.dirisamer@meduniwien.ac.at*


Arnd Dörfler, MD
Professor, Department of Neuroradiology
University of Erlangen-Nuremberg
Schwabachanlage 6
91054 Erlangen
Germany

*Email: arnd.doerfler@uk-erlangen.de*


Birgit Ertl-Wagner, MD, PD
Department of Clinical Radiology
Ludwig-Maximilians-University of Munich
Munich University Hospitals
Marchioninistrasse 15
81377 Munich
Germany

*Email: birgit.ertl-wagner@med.uni-muenchen.de*

Dominik Fleischmann, MD
Associate Professor of Radiology
Department of Radiology
Stanford University Medical Center
300 Pasteur Drive, Room S-072
Stanford CA, 94305-5105
USA

*Email: d.fleischmann@stanford.edu*


Thomas Flohr, PhD
Siemens AG
Healthcare Sector
Business Unit Computed Tomography
Siemensstr. 1
91301 Forchheim
Germany

*Email: thomas.flohr@siemens.com*


Gary Glazer, MD, Professor
Departmentof Radiology
Stanford University, School of Medicine
Room P-263
1201 Welch Road
Palo Alto, CA 94304
USA

*Email: glazer@stanford.edu*


Anno Graser, MD
Department of Clinical Radiology
Ludwig-Maximilians-University of Munich
University of Munich Hospitals
Marchioninistrasse 15
81377 Munich
Germany

*Email: anno.graser@med.uni-muenchen.de*


Jürgen Griebel, MD
Federal Office for Radiation Protection, Germany
Department "Radiation Protection and Health"
Ingolstaedter Landstrasse 1
85764 Oberschleißheim
Germany

*Email: jgriebel@BfS.de*

Marcus Hacker, MD
Department of Nuclear Medicine
Munich University Hospitals
Ludwig-Maximilians-University of Munich
Marchioninistrasse 15
81377 Munich
Germany

Email: marcus.hacker@med.uni-muenchen.de


Peter Hallscheidt, MD
Professor and Section Chief, Department of Diagnostic
Radiology
University Hospital Heidelberg
Im Neuenheimer Feld 110
69120 Heidelberg
Germany

Email: peter.hallscheidt@med.uni-heidelberg.de


Cesare Hassan, MD
Gastroenterology and Digestive Endoscopy Unit
"Nuovo Regina Margherita" Hospital
Via Emilio Morosini 30
00153 Rome
Italy


Benno Heigl, PhD
Siemens AG
Healthcare Sector
MED AX
Siemensstrasse 1
91301 Forchheim
Germany

Email: benno.heigl@siemens.com


Christian J. Herold, MD
Professor, Department of Diagnostic and Pediatric
Radiology
Medical University of Vienna
Waehringer Guertel 18–20
1190 Vienna
Austria

Email: christian.herold@meduniwien.ac.at

Claus Peter Heussel, MD, PD
Department of Radiology
Chest-Clinic at University Hospital Heidelberg
Amalienstrasse 5
69126 Heidelberg
Germany

Email: heussel@uni-heidelberg.de


Christoph Hoeschen, PhD
Helmholtz Zentrum München
German Research Center for Environmental Health
Institute of Radiation Protection
Ingolstädter Landstraße 1
85764 Neuherberg
Germany

Email: christoph.hoeschen@gsf.de


Martin H.K. Hoffmann, MD
Klinik für Diagnostische und Interventionelle Radiologie
Unikliniken Ulm
Steinhoevelstrasse 9
89075 Ulm
Germany

Email: martin.hoffmann@uniklinik-ulm.de


Ralf-Thorsten Hoffmann, MD
Department of Clinical Radiology
Ludwig-Maximilians-University of Munich
University of Munich Hospitals
Marchioninistrasse 15
81377 Munich
Germany

Email: ralf-thorsten.hoffmann@med.uni-muenchen.de


Martin Hoheisel, PhD
Siemens AG
Healthcare Sector
MED AX
Siemensstrasse 1
91301 Forchheim
Germany

Email: martin.hoheisel@siemens.com

Franco Iafrate, MD
Department of Radiological Sciences
"Sapienza" - University of Rome, Polo Pontino
I.C.O.T. Hospital
Viale Franco Fagiana 43
04100 Latina
Italy


Lorenz Jäger, MD, PD
Diagnostisches Zentrum Garmisch Partenkirchen
Partnaachstrasse 65
82467 Garmisch Partenkirchen
Germany

Email: jaeger@radiologie-online.net


Tobias F. Jakobs, MD
Department of Clinical Radiology
Ludwig-Maximilians-University of Munich
Munich University Hospitals
Marchioninistrasse 15
81377 Munich
Germany

Email: tobias.jakobs@med.uni-muenchen.de


Thorsten R.C. Johnson, MD
Department of Clinical Radiology
Ludwig-Maximilians-University of Munich
Munich University Hospitals
Marchioninistrasse 15
81377 Munich
Germany

Email: thorsten.johnson@med.uni-muenchen.de


Willi A. Kalender, PhD
Professor, Department of Medical Physics
University of Erlangen-Nuremberg
Henkestrasse 91
91052 Erlangen
Germany

Email: willi.kalender@imp.uni-erlangen.de


Hans-Ulrich Kauczor, MD
Professor, Ärztlicher Direktor
Abt. Diagnostische und Interventionelle Radiologie
Universitätsklinikum Heidelberg
Im Neuenheimer Feld 110
69120 Heidelberg
Germany

Email: hu.kauczor@med.uni-heidelberg.de


Klaus Klingenbeck-Regn, PhD
Siemens AG
Healthcare Sector
MED AX
Siemensstrasse 1
91301 Forchheim
Germany

Email: klaus.klingenbeck-regn@siemens.com


Claus Kölblinger, MD
Universitätsklinik für Radiodiagnostik
Medizinische Universität Wien
Währinger Gürtel 18–20
1090 Wien
Austria


Markus Körner, MD
Department of Clinical Radiology
Ludwig-Maximilians-University of Munich
University of Munich Hospitals
Nussbaumstrasse 20
80336 Munich
Germany

Email: markus.koerner@med.uni-muenchen.de


Sabrina Kösling, MD
Professor, Department of Diagnostic Radiology
University of Halle
Ernst-Grube-Str. 40
06097 Halle
Germany

Email: sabrina.koesling@medizin.uni-halle.de


Andrea Laghi, MD
Department of Radiological Sciences
"Sapienza" - University of Rome, Polo Pontino
I.C.O.T. Hospital
Viale Franco Fagiana 43
04100 Latina
Italy

Email: andrea.laghi@uniroma1.it; andlaghi@gmail.com

GÜNTER LAURITSCH, PhD
Siemens AG
Healthcare Sector
MED AX
Siemensstrasse 1
91301 Forchheim
Germany

Email: guenter.lauritsch@siemens.com


ALEXANDER LEMBCKE, MD
Department of Radiology
Charité – University Medicine Berlin
Chariteplatz 1
10117 Berlin
Germany

Email: alexander.Lembcke@gmx.de


JULIA LEY-ZAPOROZHAN, MD
Pädiatrische Radiologie
Universitätsklinikum Heidelberg
Im Neuenheimer Feld 153
69120 Heidelberg
Germany

Email: julia.leyzaporozhan@gmail.com


ULRICH LINSENMAIER, MD
Department of Clinical Radiology
Ludwig-Maximilians-University of Munich
University of Munich Hospitals
Nussbaumstrasse 20
80336 Munich
Germany


JÜRGEN LUTZ, MD
Resident, Department of Radiology
Ludwig-Maximilians-University of Munich
Munich University Hospitals
Ziemssenstrasse 1
80336 Munich
Germany

Email: juergen.lutz@med.uni-muenchen.de


MICHAEL MACARI, MD
Department of Radiology
New York University Medical Center
560 1st Avenue
New York, NY 10016
USA


DAVID MAINTZ, MD
Associate Professor, Department of Clinical Radiology
University of Muenster
Albert-Schweitzer-Strasse 33
48149 Muenster
Germany

Email: maintz@uni-muenster.de


OLIVER MEISSNER, MD
Siemens AG
Healthcare Sector
MED AX
Siemensstrasse 1
91301 Forchheim
Germany

Email: oliver.meissner@siemens.com


DOMINIK MORHARD, MD
Department of Clinical Radiology
Ludwig-Maximilians-University of Munich
Munich University Hospitals
Marchioninistrasse 15
81377 Munich
Germany

Email: dominik.morhard@med.uni-muenchen.de


ULLRICH G. MUELLER-LISSE, MD, MBA
Attending Radiologist, Associate Professor of Radiology
Health Care Management
Department of Clinical Radiology
Ludwig-Maximilians-University of Munich
Munich University Hospitals
Ziemssenstrasse 1
80336 Munich
Germany

Email: ullrich.mueller-lisse@med.uni-muenchen.de


CHRISTINA MUELLER-MANG, MD
Department of Diagnostic and Pediatric Radiology
Medical University of Vienna
Waehringer Guertel 18–20
1190 Vienna
Austria

Email: christina.mueller-mang@meduniwien.ac.at

Markus Nagel, PhD
CAS innovations
Heusteg 47
91056 Erlangen
Germany

Email: markus.nagel@cas-innovations.de


Elke A. Nekolla, PhD
Federal Office for Radiation Protection, Germany
Department "Radiation Protection and Health"
Ingolstaedter Landstrasse 1
85764 Oberschleißheim
Germany

Email: enekolla@bfs.de


Kerstin Neumann, MD, PD
Department of Otorhinolaryngology
University of Halle
Ernst-Grube-Str. 40
06097 Halle
Germany


Konstantin Nikolaou, MD
Department of Clinical Radiology
Ludwig-Maximilians-University of Munich
University of Munich Hospitals
Marchioninistrasse 15
81377 Munich
Germany

Email: konstantin.nikolaou@med.uni-muenchen.de


Michael Owsijewitsch, MD
Department of Radiology
German Cancer Research Center (DKFZ)
Im Neuenheimer Feld 280
69120 Heidelberg
Germany

Email: m.owsijewitsch@dkfz.de


Marcus Pfister, PhD
Siemens AG
Healthcare Sector
MED AX
Siemensstrasse 1
91301 Forchheim
Germany

Email: marcus.pfister@siemens.com


Christina Plank, MD
Department of Diagnostic and Pediatric Radiology
Medical University of Vienna
Waehringer Guertel 18–20
1190 Vienna
Austria

Email: christina.plank@meduniwien.ac.at


Gabriele Pöpperl, MD, PD
Department of Nuclear Medicine
Ludwig-Maximilians-University of Munich
University of Munich Hospitals
Marchioninistraße 15
81377 Munich
Germany

Email: gabriele.poepperl@med.uni-muenchen.de


Dieter Regulla, PhD
Helmholtz Zentrum München
German Research Center for Environmental Health
Institute of Radiation Protection
Ingolstädter Landstraße 1
85764 Neuherberg
Germany


Maximilian F. Reiser, MD, Professor
Department of Clinical Radiology
Ludwig-Maximilians-University of Munich
Munich University Hospitals
Marchioninistrasse 15
81377 Munich
Germany

Email: mreiser@med.uni-muenchen.de


Gregor Richter, MD
Department of Neuroradiology
University of Erlangen-Nuremberg
Schwabachanlage 6
91054 Erlangen
Germany

Email: gregor.richter@UK-Erlangen.de


Helmut Ringl, MD
Department of Diagnostic and Pediatric Radiology
Medical University of Vienna
Waehringer Guertel 18–20
1190 Vienna
Austria

Email: helmut.ringl@meduniwien.ac.at

PATRIK ROGALLA, MD
AssociateProfessor, Department of Radiology
Charité Hospital
Humboldt-University Berlin
Schumannstrasse 20/21
10098 Berlin
Germany

*Email: patrik.rogalla@charite.de*


ERNST-PETER RÜHRNSCHOPF
Siemens AG
Healthcare Sector
MED AX
Siemensstrasse 1
91301 Forchheim
Germany

*Email: esruewald@aol.com*


ULRICH SAUERESSIG, MD
Abteilung Röntgendiagnostik
Radiologische Universitätsklinik Freiburg
Hugstetter Str. 55
79106 Freiburg
Germany

*Email: ulrich.saueressig@uniklinik-freiburg.de*


WOLFGANG SCHIMA, MD, MSc, Professor
Abteilung für Radiologie und bildgebende Diagnostik
KH Göttlicher Heiland
Dornbacher Strasse 20–28
1170 Vienna
Austria

*Email: wolfgang.schima@meduniwien.ac.at*


HELMUT SCHLATTL, PhD
Helmholtz Zentrum München
German Research Center for Environmental Health
Institute of Radiation Protection
Ingolstädter Landstraße 1
85764 Neuherberg
Germany

BERNHARD SCHOLZ, PhD
Siemens AG
Healthcare Sector
MED AX
Siemensstrasse 1
91301 Forchheim
Germany

*Email: bernhard.scholz@siemens.com*


BERND SCHREIBER, PhD
Siemens AG
Healthcare Sector
MED AX
Siemensstrasse 1
91301 Forchheim
Germany

*Email: bernd.bs.schreiber@siemens.com*


HARALD SEIFARTH, MD
Department of Clinical Radiology
University of Muenster
Albert-Schweitzer-Strasse 33
48149 Muenster
Germany


BERNHARD SOMMER, MD
Center of Diagnostic Radiology Munich Pasing
Pippinger Strasse 25
81245 Munich
Germany

*Email: sommer@rzm.de*


WIELAND H. SOMMER, MD
Department of Clinical Radiology
Ludwig-Maximilians-University of Munich
Munich University Hospitals
Marchioninistrasse 15
81377 Munich
Germany

*Email: wieland.sommer@med.uni-muenchen.de*


MARTIN SPAHN, PhD
Siemens AG
Healthcare Sector
MED AX
Siemensstrasse 1
91301 Forchheim
Germany

*Email: martin.spahn@siemens.com*

PAUL STOLZMANN, MD
Institute of Diagnostic Radiology
University Hospital Zurich
Raemisstrasse 100
8091 Zurich
Switzerland


NORBERT STROBEL, PhD
Siemens AG
Healthcare Sector
MED AX
Siemensstrasse 1
91301 Forchheim
Germany

Email: norbert.strobel@siemens.com


HENDRIK VON TENGG-KOBLIGK, MD
Department of Radiology
German Cancer Research Center (DKFZ)
Im Neuenheimer Feld 280
69120 Heidelberg
Germany

Email: h.vontengg@dkfz.de


DANIEL THEISEN, MD
Department of Clinical Radiology
Ludwig-Maximilians-University of Munich
Munich University Hospitals
Marchioninistrasse 15
81377 Munich
Germany

Email: daniel.theisen@med.uni-muenchen.de


CHRISTOPH G. TRUMM, MD
Department of Clinical Radiology
Ludwig-Maximilians-University of Munich
University of Munich Hospitals
Marchioninistrasse 15
81377 Munich
Germany

Email: christoph.trumm@med.uni-muenchen.de


STEFAN ULZHEIMER, PhD
Siemens Medical Solutions USA, Inc.
Computed Tomography Division
51 Valley Stream Parkway
Malvern, PA 19355
USA

Email: stefan.ulzheimer@siemens.com


TIM F. WEBER, MD
Department of Radiology
German Cancer Research Center
Im Neuenheimer Feld 280
69120 Heidelberg
Germany

Email: t.weber@dkfz.de


JOACHIM-ERNST WILDBERGER, MD, Professor
Department of Radiology
University Hospital Maastricht
P.O. Box 5800
6202 AZ Maastricht
The Netherlands

Email j.wildberger@mumc.nl


MAX WINTERMARK, MD
Department of Radiology
Neuroradiology Section
University of California
505 Parnassus Avenue, Box 0628
San Francisco, 94143-0628, CA
USA

Email: max.wintermark@radiology.ucsf.edu


BERND J. WINTERSPERGER, MD
Associate Professor, Department of Clinical Radiology
Ludwig-Maximilians-University of Munich
Munich University Hospitals
Marchioninistrasse 15
81377 Munich
Germany

Email: bernd.wintersperger@med.uni-muenchen.de


MARIA ZANKL, PhD
Helmholtz Zentrum München
German Research Center for Environmental Health
Institute of Radiation Protection
Ingolstädter Landstraße 1
85764 Neuherberg
Germany

CHRISTOPH J. ZECH, MD
Department of Clinical Radiology
Ludwig-Maximilians-University of Munich
Munich University Hospitals
Marchioninistrasse 15
81377 Munich
Germany

*Email: christoph.zech@med.uni-muenchen.de*

MICHAEL ZELLERHOFF, PhD
Siemens AG
Healthcare Sector
MED AX
Siemensstrasse 1
91301 Forchheim
Germany

*Email: michael.zellerhoff@siemens.com*

## DIAGNOSTIC IMAGING

**Innovations in Diagnostic Imaging**
Edited by J.H. Anderson

**Radiology of the Upper Urinary Tract**
Edited by E.K. Lang

**The Thymus - Diagnostic Imaging, Functions, and Pathologic Anatomy**
Edited by E. Walter, E. Willich, and W.R. Webb

**Interventional Neuroradiology**
Edited by A. Valavanis

**Radiology of the Pancreas**
Edited by A.L. Baert, co-edited by G. Delorme

**Radiology of the Lower Urinary Tract**
Edited by E.K. Lang

**Magnetic Resonance Angiography**
Edited by I.P. Arlart, G.M. Bongartz, and G. Marchal

**Contrast-Enhanced MRI of the Breast**
S. Heywang-Köbrunner and R. Beck

**Spiral CT of the Chest**
Edited by M. Rémy-Jardin and J. Rémy

**Radiological Diagnosis of Breast Diseases**
Edited by M. Friedrich and E.A. Sickles

**Radiology of the Trauma**
Edited by M. Heller and A. Fink

**Biliary Tract Radiology**
Edited by P. Rossi

**Radiological Imaging of Sports Injuries**
Edited by C. Masciocchi

**Modern Imaging of the Alimentary Tube**
Edited by A.R. Margulis

**Diagnosis and Therapy of Spinal Tumors**
Edited by P.R. Algra, J. Valk, and J.J. Heimans

**Interventional Magnetic Resonance Imaging**
Edited by J.F. Debatin and G. Adam

**Abdominal and Pelvic MRI**
Edited by A. Heuck and M. Reiser

**Orthopedic Imaging. Techniques and Applications**
Edited by A.M. Davies and H. Pettersson

**Radiology of the Female Pelvic Organs**
Edited by E.K. Lang

**Clinical Applications of Magnetic Resonance in Cardiovascular Disease**
Edited by J. Bogaert, A.J. Duerinckx, and F.E. Rademakers

**Modern Head and Neck Imaging**
Edited by S. Mukherji and J.A. Castelijns

**Radiological Imaging of Endocrine Diseases**
Edited by J.N. Bruneton - in collaboration with B. Padovani and M.-Y. Mourou

**Trends in Contrast Media**
Edited by H.S. Thomsen, R.N. Muller, and R.F. Mattrey

**Functional MRI**
Edited by C.T.W. Moonen and P.A. Bandettini

**Radiology of the Pancreas 2nd revised edition**
Edited by A.L. Baert, Co-edited by G. Delorme and L. Van Hoe

**Emergency Pediatric Radiology**
Edited by H. Carty

**Spiral CT of the Abdomen**
Edited by F. Terrier, M. Grossholz, and C. Becker

**Radiology of Peripheral Vascular Diseases**
Edited by E. Zeitler

**Liver Malignancies**
*Diagnostic and Interventional Radiology*
Edited by C. Bartolozzi and R. Lencioni

**Medical Imaging of the Spleen**
Edited by A.M. De Schepper and F. Vanhoenacker

**Diagnostic Nuclear Medicine**
Edited by C. Schiepers

**Radiology of Blunt Trauma of the Chest**
(Authors) P. Schnyder and M. Wintermark

**Portal Hypertension**
Edited by P. Rossi, P. Ricci, and L. Broglia

**Recent Advances in Diagnostic Neuroradiology**
Edited by Ph. Demaerel

**Virtual Endoscopy and Related 3D Techniques**
Edited by P. Rogalla, J. Terwisscha van Scheltinga, and B. Hamm

**Transfontanellar Doppler Imaging in Neonates**
(Authors) A. Couture and C. Veyrac

**Multislice CT**
Edited by M.F. Reiser, M. Takahashi, M. Modic, and R. Bruening

**Diagnostic and Interventional Radiology in Liver Transplantation**
Edited by E. Bücheler, V. Nicolas, C.E. Broelsch, and X. Rogiers

**Pediatric Uroradiology**
Edited by R. Fotter

**Radiology of AIDS.**
*A Practical Approach*
Edited by J.W.A.J. Reeders and P.C. Goodman

**Pediatric Chest Imaging**
*Chest Imaging in Infants and Children*
Edited by J. Lucaya and J.L. Strife

**Radiological Imaging of the Small Intestine**
Edited by N. Gourtsoyiannis

**Magnetic Resonance Angiography.**
**2nd Revised Edition**
Edited by I.P. Arlart, G.M. Bongartz, and G. Marchal

**CT of the Peritoneum**
(Authors) A. Rossi and G. Rossi

**Pediatric ENT Radiology**
Edited by S.J. King and A.E. Boothroyd

**Applications of Sonography in Head and Neck Pathology**
Edited by J.N. Bruneton. In Collaboration with C. Raffaelli and O. Dassonville

**Radiological Imaging of the Ureter**
Edited by F. Joffre and Ph. Otal

**Imaging of the Knee.**
*Techniques and Applications*
Edited by A.M. Davies and V.N. Cassar-Pullicino

**Radiology of Osteoporosis**
Edited by S. Grampp

**Gastrointestinal Tract Sonography in Fetuses and Children**
Edited by A. Couture

**Imaging of Orbital and Visual Pathway Pathology**
Edited by W.S. Müller-Forell

**Imaging of the Larynx**
Edited by R. Hermans

**3D Image Processing.**
*Techniques and Clinical Applications*
Edited by D. Caramella and C. Bartolozzi

**Imaging and Intervention in Abdominal Trauma**
Edited by R.F. Dondelinger

**Perinatal Imaging. From Ultrasound to MR Imaging**
Edited by F. Avni

**Interventional Radiology in Cancer**
Edited by A. Adam, R.F. Dondelinger, and P.R. Mueller

**Radiological Imaging of the Neonatal Chest**
Edited by V. Donoghue

**Imaging of the Foot & Ankle.**
*Techniques and Applications*
Edited by A.M. Davies, R.W. Whitehouse, and J.P.R. Jenkins

**Pelvic Floor Disorders**
Edited by C.I Bartram and J.O.L. DeLancey
Associate Editors: S. Halligan, F.M. Kelvin, J. Stoker

**Imaging of the Pancreas.**
*Cystic and Rare Tumors*
Edited by C. Procacci and A. J. Megibow

**High-Resolution Sonography of the Peripheral Nervous System**
Edited by S. Peer and G. Bodner

**Radiology of the Petrous Bone**
Edited by M. Lemmerling, K. Marsot-Dupuch, and S.S. Kollias

**Imaging of the Shoulder.**
*Techniques and Applications*
Edited by A.M. Davis and J. Hodler

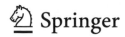

## RADIATION ONCOLOGY

**Lung Cancer**
Edited by C.W. Scarantino

**Innovations in Radiation Oncology**
Edited by H.R. Withers and L.J. Peters

**Radiation Therapy of Head and Neck Cancer**
Edited by G.E. Laramore

**Gastrointestinal Cancer - Radiation Therapy**
Edited by R.R. Dobelbower, Jr.

**Radiation Exposure and Occupational Risks**
Edited by E. Scherer, C. Streffer,
and K.-R. Trott

**Radiation Therapy
of Benign Diseases - A Clinical Guide**
S.E. Order and S.S. Donaldson

**Interventional Radiation
Therapy Techniques - Brachytherapy**
Edited by R. Sauer

**Radiopathology of Organs and Tissues**
Edited by E. Scherer, C. Streffer,
and K.-R. Trott

**Concomitant Continuous Infusion
Chemotherapy and Radiation**
Edited by M. Rotman and C.J. Rosenthal

**Intraoperative Radiotherapy - Clinical
Experiences and Results**
Edited by F.A. Calvo, M. Santos,
and L.W. Brady

**Radiotherapy of Intraocular
and Orbital Tumors**
Edited by W.E. Alberti
and R.H. Sagerman

**Interstitial
and Intracavitary Thermoradiotherapy**
Edited by M.H. Seegenschmiedt
and R. Sauer

**Non-Disseminated Breast Cancer**
*Controversial Issues in Management*
Edited by G.H. Fletcher and S.H. Levitt

**Current Topics
in Clinical Radiobiology of Tumors**
Edited by H.-P. Beck-Bornholdt

**Practical Approaches
to Cancer Invasion and Metastases**
*A Compendium of Radiation Oncologists'
Responses to 40 Histories*
Edited by A.R. Kagan with the Assistance
of R.J. Steckel

**Radiation Therapy in Pediatric Oncology**
Edited by J.R. Cassady

**Radiation Therapy Physics**
Edited by A.R. Smith

**Late Sequelae in Oncology**
Edited by J. Dunst and R. Sauer

**Mediastinal Tumors. Update 1995**
Edited by D.E. Wood and C.R. Thomas, Jr.

**Thermoradiotherapy and
Thermochemotherapy**
*Volume 1: Biology, Physiology, and Physics
Volume 2: Clinical Applications*
Edited by M.H. Seegenschmiedt,
P. Fessenden, and C.C. Vernon

**Carcinoma of the Prostate**
*Innovations in Management*
Edited by Z. Petrovich, L. Baert,
and L.W. Brady

**Radiation Oncology of Gynecological Cancers**
Edited by H.W. Vahrson

**Carcinoma of the Bladder**
*Innovations in Management*
Edited by Z. Petrovich, L. Baert,
and L.W. Brady

**Blood Perfusion
and Microenvironment of Human Tumors**
*Implications for Clinical Radiooncology*
Edited by M. Molls and P. Vaupel

**Radiation Therapy of Benign Diseases.**
*A Clinical Guide*
2nd revised edition
(Authors) S.E. Order and S.S. Donaldson

**Progress and Perspectives
in the Treatment of Lung Cancer**
Edited by P. Van Houtte, J. Klastersky,
and P. Rocmans

**Combined Modality Therapy
of Central Nervous System Tumors**
Edited by Z. Petrovich, L.W. Brady,
M.L. Apuzzo, and M. Bamberg

**Age-Related Macular Degeneration.**
*Current Treatment Concepts*
Edited by W.E. Alberti, G. Richard,
and R.H. Sagerman

**Radiotherapy
of Intraocular and Orbital Tumors**
2nd revised edition
Edited by W.E. Alberti
and R.H. Sagerman

**Clinical Target Volumes in Conformal
and Intensity Modulated Radiation Therapy**
*A Clinical Guide to Cancer Treatment*
Edited by V. Grégoire, P. Scalliet,
and K.K. Ang

**Palliative Radiation Oncology**
(Authors) R.G. Parker, N.A. Janjan,
and M.T. Selch

**Modification of Radiation Response**
Edited by C. Nieder, L. Milas,
and K.K. Ang

**Advances in Radiation Oncology in Lung
Cancer**
Edited by B. Jeremic

**Technical Basis of Radiation Therapy**
*Practical Clinical Applications*
**4th Revised Edition**
Edited by S.H. Levitt, J.A. Purdy,
C.A. Perez, and S. Vijayakumar

**New Technologies in Radiation Oncology**
Edited by W. Schlegel, T. Bortfeld,
and A.-L. Grosu

**Medical Radiology volume on Multimodal
Concepts for Integration of Cytotoxic Drugs
and Radiation Therapy**
Edited by J.M. Brown, M.P. Mehta,
and C. Nieder

**Clinical Practice
of Radiation Therapy for Benign Diseases**
*Contemporary Concepts and Clinical Results*
Edited by M. H. Seegenschmiedt,
H.-B. Makoski, K.-R. Trott,
and L.W. Brady

**CURED I – LENT - Late Effects of Cancer
Treatment on Normal Tissues**
Edited by P. Rubin, L.S. Constine,
L.B. Marks, and P. Okunieff

**CURED II LENT - Cancer Survivorship
Research and Education**
*Late Effects of Cancer Treatment on Normal
Tissues*
Edited by P. Rubin, L.S. Constine,
L.B. Marks, and P. Okunieff

**Radiation Oncology**
*An Evidence-Based Approach*
Edited by J.J. Lu and L.W. Brady

**Primary Optic Nerve Sheath Meningioma**
Edited by B. Jeremić and S. Pitz

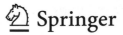